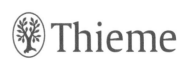

Synopsis of Orthopaedic Trauma Management

Brian H. Mullis, MD
Professor and Program Director
Department of Orthopaedic Surgery
Indiana University School of Medicine
Indianapolis, Indiana, USA

Greg E. Gaski, MD
Orthopaedic Trauma Surgeon
Department of Orthopaedic Surgery
Inova Fairfax Medical Campus
Falls Church, Virginia, USA

565 illustrations

Thieme
New York • Stuttgart • Delhi • Rio de Janeiro

Library of Congress Cataloging-in-Publication Data is available with the publisher.

Important note: Medicine is an ever-changing science undergoing continual development. Research and clinical experience are continually expanding our knowledge, in particular our knowledge of proper treatment and drug therapy. Insofar as this book mentions any dosage or application, readers may rest assured that the authors, editors, and publishers have made every effort to ensure that such references are in accordance with **the state of knowledge at the time of production of the book.**

Nevertheless, this does not involve, imply, or express any guarantee or responsibility on the part of the publishers in respect to any dosage instructions and forms of applications stated in the book. **Every user is requested to examine carefully** the manufacturers' leaflets accompanying each drug and to check, if necessary in consultation with a physician or specialist, whether the dosage schedules mentioned therein or the contraindications stated by the manufacturers differ from the statements made in the present book. Such examination is particularly important with drugs that are either rarely used or have been newly released on the market. Every dosage schedule or every form of application used is entirely at the user's own risk and responsibility. The authors and publishers request every user to report to the publishers any discrepancies or inaccuracies noticed. If errors in this work are found after publication, errata will be posted at www.thieme.com on the product description page.

Some of the product names, patents, and registered designs referred to in this book are in fact registered trademarks or proprietary names even though specific reference to this fact is not always made in the text. Therefore, the appearance of a name without designation as proprietary is not to be construed as a representation by the publisher that it is in the public domain.

Thieme Medical Publishers New York
333 Seventh Avenue
New York, New York 10001 USA
+1 800 782 3488, customerservice@thieme.com

Georg Thieme Verlag KG
Rüdigerstrasse 14, 70469 Stuttgart, Germany
+49 [0]711 8931 421, customerservice@thieme.de

Thieme Publishers Delhi
A-12, Second Floor, Sector-2, Noida-201301
Uttar Pradesh, India
+91 120 45 566 00, customerservice@thieme.in

Thieme Publishers Rio de Janeiro,
Thieme Publicações Ltda.
Edifício Rodolpho de Paoli, 25° andar
Av. Nilo Peçanha, 50 – Sala 2508,
Rio de Janeiro 20020-906 Brasil
+55 21 3172-2297

Cover design: Thieme Publishing Group
Typesetting by DiTech Process Solutions, India

Printed in USA by King Printing Company, Inc.   5 4 3 2 1

ISBN 978-1-62623-918-0

Also available as an e-book:
eISBN 978-1-62623-919-7

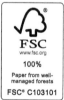

FSC
www.fsc.org
100%
Paper from well-
managed forests
FSC® C103101

To the many mentors and partners over the years who have inspired me to be a better surgeon,
and to my loving wife, Lani, and kids, Hunter, Colton, and Taylor,
who have inspired me to be a better man.

-Brian H. Mullis

To my loving wife Tricia for her unwavering support, my kids, Griffin and Scarlett
who make every day better than the last, my mom and dad for making everything possible,
my mentors that pushed me to always strive for excellence,
and to the residents and fellows I've had the privilege to train.

-Greg E. Gaski

Contents

Contents

Contents

Preface

There are a number of reference materials available to orthopaedic surgeons which give extensive detail to the expert for specific musculoskeletal conditions; however, there are few easily accessible resources available for treatment of musculoskeletal trauma patients. This text has been written by leading experts in the field as a resource for the initial provider which might include but is not limited to a nurse, an emergency department physician, a general surgeon, an orthopaedic surgeon, a resident, a medical student, or an advanced provider. The book was written to serve as a quick reference to initiate immediate treatment and to help serve as a primer for definitive treatment and rehabilitation. A major emphasis has been placed on the inclusion of up-to-date clinically relevant information with intentional omission of traditional dogma.

The bullet format was designed to be quickly and easily navigated. Original illustrations and radiographic examples efficiently supplement the written content. The e-book gives additional resources including a video library. Written chapters and videos have been performed by nationally recognized experts in the field. Content experts present the most pertinent information in a concise fashion through an outline format enhanced by figures to help the non-expert gain confidence in the initial treatment and management of specific musculoskeletal conditions. The book will also provide an improved comprehension of definitive treatment principles and rehabilitation of patients following injury. In addition to specific chapters discussing injuries, there is a general section to help with the understanding of the basic science and other treatment principles for musculoskeletal trauma.

Brian H. Mullis, MD
Greg E. Gaski, MD

Contributors

Timothy S. Achor, MD
Associate Professor
Department of Orthopaedic Surgery
University of Texas Health Science Center
  at Houston
Houston, Texas, USA

Kevin C. Anderson, MD
Associate Professor
Department of Orthopaedic Surgery
Beacon Bone and Joint Specialists;
Indiana University School of Medicine;
Michigan State University College of
  Human Medicine;
South Bend, Indiana, USA

Michael T. Archdeacon, MD, MSE
Peter J. Stern Professor and Chairman
Department of Orthopaedic Surgery
University of Cincinnati College of Medicine
Cincinnati, Ohio, USA

Frank R. Avilucea, MD
Director of Orthopaedic Research
Department of Orthopaedics
Orlando Health Orthopaedic Institute
Orlando, Florida, USA

Michael G. Baraga, MD
Associate Professor
Sports Medicine Institute
University of Miami Miller School of Medicine
Coral Gables, Florida, USA

Eric A. Barcak, DO
Assistant Professor
Department of Orthopaedic Trauma Surgery
John Peter Smith Hospital Orthopaedic Surgery
  Residency Program
Acclaim Bone and Joint Institute
Fort Worth, Texas, USA

Scott R. Bassuener, MD
Orthopaedic Trauma and Adult Reconstruction
Department of Orthopaedic Surgery
Gundersen Health System
La Crosse, Wisconsin, USA

Carlo Bellabarba, MD
Professor and Vice Chair
Department of Orthopaedics and Sports Medicine
University of Washington School of Medicine;
Chief of Orthopaedics
Harborview Medical Center
Seattle, Washington, USA

Richard J. Bransford, MD
Professor
Department of Orthopaedics and Sports Medicine
Harborview Medical Center
University of Washington School of Medicine
Seattle, Washington, USA

Brian Buck, DO
Associate Professor
Department of Orthopaedic Surgery
University of Arizona College of Medicine
Phoenix, Arizona, USA

Camden Burns, MD
Assistant Professor of Orthopaedic Surgery
Department of Orthopaedic Surgery
Indiana University School of Medicine
Indianapolis, Indiana, USA

John J. Callaci, PhD
Associate Professor
Department of Orthopaedic Surgery
Loyola University Chicago
Maywood, Illinois, USA

David H. Campbell, MD
Resident
Department of Orthopaedic Surgery
University of Arizona College of
  Medicine – Phoenix
Phoenix, Arizona, USA

Lisa K. Cannada, MD
Orthopaedic Trauma Surgeon
Department of Orthopaedics
Hughston Clinic
Jacksonville, Florida, USA

Jue Cao, MD
Upper Extremity and Pediatric
    Orthopaedic Surgeon
Department of Orthopaedic Surgery
Kaiser Permanente
Denver, Colorado, USA

Eben A. Carroll, MD
Director of Orthopaedic Trauma Service and
    Associate Professor
Department of Orthopaedic Surgery
Wake Forest University School of Medicine
Winston-Salem, North Carolina, USA

Brett D. Crist, MD
Associate Professor
Department of Orthopaedic Surgery
University of Missouri
Columbia, Missouri, USA

Nicholas E. Crosby, MD
Clinical Instructor
Department of Hand, Upper Extremity, and
    Microsurgery
Indiana Hand to Shoulder Center
Indianapolis, Indiana, USA

Jean-Claude G. D'Alleyrand, MD, MSE
Chief of Orthopaedic Traumatology
Department of Orthopaedic Surgery
Walter Reed National Military Medical Center
Bethesda, Maryland, USA

Hannah L. Dailey, PhD
Assistant Professor
Department of Mechanical Engineering and
    Mechanics
Lehigh University
Bethlehem, Pennsylvania, USA

Elizabeth P. Davis, MD
Resident
Department of Orthopaedic Surgery
McGovern Medical School at UTHealth Houston
Houston, Texas, USA

Gregory J. Della Rocca, MD, PhD, FACS
Associate Professor
Department of Orthopaedics
University of Missouri
Columbia, Missouri, USA

David Donohue, MD, MBA
Assistant Professor
Department of Orthopaedics
University of South Florida;
Staff Traumatologist
Florida Orthopaedic Institute
Tampa, Florida, USA

Christopher Doro, MD
Assistant Professor
Department of Orthopaedics
University of Wisconsin
Madison, Wisconsin, USA

Hayley E. Ennis, MD
Resident
Sports Medicine Institute
University of Miami Miller School of Medicine
Coral Gables, Florida, USA

Reza Firoozabadi, MD, MA
Associate Professor
Department of Orthopaedics and Sports Medicine
University of Washington
Seattle, Washington, USA

Mark J. Gage, MD
Assistant Professor
Department of Orthopaedic Surgery
Duke University
Durham, North Carolina, USA

George Gantsoudes, MD
Assistant Clinical Professor
Department of Orthopaedics
Georgetown University
Washington, D.C., USA;
Orthopaedic Surgeon
Pediatric Specialist of Virginia
Merrifield, Virginia, USA

Joshua L. Gary, MD
Associate Professor
Department of Orthopaedic Surgery
McGovern Medical School at UTHealth Houston
Houston, Texas, USA

Greg E. Gaski, MD
Orthopaedic Trauma Surgeon
Department of Orthopaedic Surgery
Inova Fairfax Medical Campus
Falls Church, Virginia, USA

Alexander Ghasem, MD
Fellow
Department of Orthopaedics
University of Miami Health System
Miller School of Medicine
Miami, Florida, USA

Joseph P. Gjolaj, MD
Associate Professor of Clinical Orthopaedics
Department of Orthopaedics
University of Miami
Miller School of Medicine
Miami, Florida, USA

Vaida Glatt, PhD
Assistant Professor and Director of Basic
    Science Research
Department of Orthopaedic Surgery
University of Texas Health Science Center
San Antonio, Texas, USA

Dylan N. Greif, BA
Medical Student
Sports Medicine Institute
University of Miami Miller School of Medicine
Coral Gables, Florida, USA

Michael M. Hadeed, MD
Resident
Department of Orthopaedic Surgery
University of Virginia
Charlottesville, Virginia, USA

Jonah Hebert-Davies, MD FRCS(c)
Assistant Professor
Department of Orthopaedics
University of Washington, Harborview
    Medical Center
Seattle, Washington, USA

Michael D. Hunter, MD
Resident
Department of Orthopaedic Surgery
Prisma Health–Upstate
Greenville, South Carolina, USA

D. Landry Jarvis, MD
Sports Medicine Surgery Fellow
Department of Orthopaedic Surgery
Duke University School of Medicine
Durham, North Carolina, USA

Kyle J. Jeray, MD
Department Chair
Department of Orthopaedic Surgery
Prisma Health–Upstate
Greenville, South Carolina, USA

Aaron Johnson, MD
Assistant Professor
Department of Orthopaedics
University of Maryland School of Medicine
Baltimore, Maryland, USA

Steven P. Kalandiak, MD
Assistant Professor
Department of Orthopaedics
University of Miami
Miller School of Medicine
Miami, Florida, USA

Meghan Kelly, MD
Resident
Department of Orthopaedics
University of Rochester
Strong Memorial Hospital
Rochester, New York, USA

Laurence B. Kempton, MD
Associate Professor of Orthopaedic Surgery
Department of Orthopaedic Surgery
Atrium Health Musculoskeletal Institute
Carolinas Medical Center
Charlotte, North Carolina, USA

John Ketz, MD
Associate Professor
Department of Orthopaedics
University of Rochester
Strong Memorial Hospital
Rochester, New York, USA

Jannat M. Khan, MD
Resident Physician
Department of Orthopaedic Surgery
William Beaumont Hospital
Royal Oak, Michigan, USA

Conor P. Kleweno, MD
Associate Professor
Orthopaedic Surgery and Sports Medicine
Harborview Medical Center/University
    of Washington
Seattle, Washington, USA

Shan Lansing, MS
Medical student
The Ohio State University College of Medicine
Columbus, Ohio, USA

Christopher Lee, MD
Assistant Professor
Department of Orthopaedic Surgery
University of California, Los Angeles
Los Angeles, California, USA

Nikola Lekic, MD
Fellow
Department of Orthopaedics
University of Miami Health System
Miller School of Medicine
Miami, Florida, USA

Frank A. Liporace, MD
Chairman and Vice President
Division of Orthopaedic Trauma and Complex
    Adult Reconstruction
Department of Orthopaedic Surgery
Jersey City Medical Center—Robert Wood Johnson
    Barnabas Health
Jersey City, New Jersey, USA

Jason A. Lowe, MD
Associate Professor
Department of Orthopaedic Surgery
The University of Arizona College of
    Medicine—Tucson
Tucson, Arizona, USA

Thuan V. Ly, MD, FAOA
Associate Professor and Director of
    Orthopaedic Trauma
Department of Orthopaedic Surgery
The Ohio State University
Columbus, Ohio, USA

Christiaan N. Mamczak, DO, FAOAO
Volunteer Assistant Professor
Department of Orthopaedic Surgery
Indiana University School of Medicine
South Bend, Indiana, USA

Alejandro Marquez-Lara, MD, PhD
Resident Physician
Department of Orthopaedic Surgery
Wake Forest University School of Medicine
Winston-Salem, North Carolina, USA

Michael D. McKee, MD, FRCSC
Professor and Chair
Department of Orthopaedic Surgery
University of Arizona College of
    Medicine—Phoenix
Phoenix, Arizona, USA

Hassan R. Mir, MD, MBA
Professor and Director of Orthopaedic
    Residency Program
Department of Orthopaedics
University of South Florida;
Director of Orthopaedic Trauma Research
Florida Orthopaedic Institute
Tampa, Florida, USA

Roman M. Natoli, MD, PhD
Assistant Professor
Department of Orthopaedic Surgery
Indiana University
Indianapolis, Indiana, USA

Aaron Nauth, MD, MSc
Assistant Professor
Department of Surgery
University of Toronto
St. Michael's Hospita
Toronto, Ontario, Canada

Robert V. O'Toole, MD
Hansjörg Wyss Medical Foundation Professor in
    Orthopaedic Trauma
Department of Orthopaedics
University of Maryland School of Medicine
Baltimore, Maryland, USA

William T. Obremskey, MD, MPH, MMHC
Professor and Vice Chair Orthopaedic Surgery;
Director
Division of Orthopaedic Trauma Research;
Executive Medical Director
Technology Assessment and Product Acquisition
    Center for Musculoskeletal Research
Vanderbilt University Medical Center
Nashville, Tennessee, USA

Ugochi Okoroafor, MD
Fellow
Department of Orthopaedics and Sports Medicine
University of Washington
Seattle, Washington, USA

Stephen Oleszkiewicz, MD
Orthopaedic Trauma Fellow
Department of Orthopaedic Surgery
University of Miami
Jackson Memorial Hospital
Miami, Florida, USA

Raymond Pensy, MD
Associate Professor
Department of Orthopaedics
University of Maryland Medical Center
Baltimore, Maryland, USA

Edward A. Perez, MD
Professor
Orthopaedic Trauma Surgery
Broward Health Medical Center
Ft Lauderdale, Florida, USA

Laura S. Phieffer, MD, FAOA
Associate Professor
Department of Orthopaedics
The Ohio State University
Columbus, Ohio, USA

Joel M. Post, DO
Staff Surgeon
Department of Orthopaedic Oncology and
    Traumatology
Memorial Hospital and Cancer Center
South Bend, Indiana, USA

Stephen Matthew Quinnan, MD
Associate Professor Orthopaedic Surgery
Department of Orthopaedic Surgery
University of Miami/Jackson Health System
Miami, Florida, USA

Robert Andrew Ravinsky, MDCM, MPH, FRCS(C)
Clinical Assistant Professor
Department of Orthopaedic Surgery
University of Arizona College of
    Medicine—Phoenix
Phoenix, Arizona, USA

David Ring, MD, PhD
Associate Dean for Comprehensive Care
Department of Surgery and Perioperative Care
Dell Medical School—The University of Texas
Austin, Texas, USA

Matthew I. Rudloff, MD
Assistant Professor
Department of Orthopaedic Surgery
University of Tennessee-Campbell Clinic
Memphis, Tennessee, USA

Thomas A. Russell, MD
Retired Professor
Campbell Clinic Department of
    Orthopaedic Surgery
University of Tennessee Center for Health Sciences
Memphis, Tennessee, USA

Claire B. Ryan, MD
Orthopaedic Surgery Resident
Department of Surgery and Perioperative Care
Dell Medical School—The University of Texas
Austin, Texas, USA

Adam P. Schumaier, MD
Resident
Department of Orthopaedic Surgery
University of Cincinnati College of Medicine
Cincinnati, Ohio, USA

Kyle M. Schweser, MD
Associate Professor
Department of Orthopaedics
University of Missouri
Columbia, Missouri, USA

Marcus F. Sciadini, MD
Professor
Department of Orthopaedics
University of Maryland School of Medicine
Baltimore, Maryland, USA

Brandon R. Scott, MD
Attending
Department of Orthopaedics
Kansas University School of Medicine—Wichita
Wichita, Kansas. USA

Jodi Siegel, MD
Assistant Professor
Department of Orthopaedics
UMass Memorial Medical Center
Worcester, Massachusetts, USA

Gerard P. Slobogean, MD, MPH, FRCSC
Associate Professor
Department of Orthopaedics
University of Maryland School of Medicine
R Adams Cowley Shock Trauma Center
Baltimore, Maryland, USA

Christopher B. Sugalski, MD
Orthopaedic Surgeon—Orthopaedic Trauma and
  Reconstructive Surgery
Department of Orthopaedic Surgery
Ochsner Medical Center
New Orleans, Louisiana, USA

Kevin Tetsworth, MD, FRACS
Senior Consultant Surgeon
Department of Orthopaedic Surgery
Royal Brisbane and Women's Hospital
Brisbane, Queensland, Australia

Rahul Vaidya, MD, FAOA, FRCSc
Chief of Orthopaedic Surgery
Detroit Receiving Hospital;
Professor of Orthopaedic Surgery
Fellowship Director Orthopaedic Trauma
Wayne State University
Detroit, Michigan, USA

Krishna Chandra Vemulapalli, MD
Orthopaedic Trauma Fellow
Department of Orthopaedic Surgery
UTHealth McGovern Medical School
Houston, Texas, USA

J. Tracy Watson, MD
Professor, Orthopaedic Surgery;
Chief, Orthopaedic Trauma Service
Department of Orthopaedic Surgery
Saint Louis University School of Medicine
Saint Louis University Health Sciences Center
Saint Louis, Missouri, USA

David B. Weiss, MD
Associate Professor and Division Head
  Orthopaedic Trauma
Department of Orthopaedic Surgery
University of Virginia
Charlottesville, Virginia, USA

Robert J. Wetzel, MD
Orthopaedic Trauma Surgeon and
  Assistant Professor
Department of Orthopaedic Surgery
University Hospitals Cleveland Medical Center
Case Western Reserve School of Medicine
Cleveland, Ohio, USA

Benjamin M. Wheatley, MD
Fellow
Department of Orthopaedic Surgery
Allegheny General Hospital
Pittsburgh, Pennsylvania, USA

Jason Wild, MD
Orthopaedic Surgeon
Department of Orthopaedics
Banner Thunderbird Medical Center;
Banner-University Medical Center South
Colorado Springs, Colorado, USA

Raymond D. Wright, Jr., MD
Associate Professor
Orthopaedic Surgery and Sports Medicine
University of Kentucky Chandler Medical Center
Lexington, Kentucky, USA

John Michael Yingling, DO
Chief Resident
Division of Orthopaedic Trauma and Adult
  Reconstruction
Jersey City Medical Center—Robert Wood Johnson
Barnabas Health
Jersey City, New Jersey, USA

Richard S. Yoon, MD
Director, Orthopaedic Research
Division of Orthopaedic Trauma and Adult
  Reconstruction
Jersey City Medical Center—Robert Wood Johnson
  Barnabas Health
Jersey City, New Jersey, USA

Haitao Zhou, MD
Acting Instructor
Department of Orthopaedics and Sports Medicine
Harborview Medical Center
University of Washington School of Medicine
Seattle, Washington, USA

Videos

Video 33.1 Femoral head fractures.
This video is provided courtesy of Robert P. Wessel III.

Video 37.1 The multiple ligament knee injury.
This video is provided courtesy of Roman M. Natoli and Patrick Siparsky.

Video 39.1 Quadriceps and patellar tendon injuries.
This video is provided courtesy of Abhi Seetharam, Brian H. Mullis, Robert P. Wessel III.

Video 40.1 An overview of tibial plateau fractures.
This video is provided courtesy of Camden Burns and Tyler Robert McCarroll.

Video 43.1 A basic guide for recognizing and reducing unstable ankle fractures.
This video is provided courtesy of Adam P. Schumaier and Michael T. Archdeacon.

Video 44.1 Mini-open repair of Achilles tendon rupture with longitudinal incision.
This video is provided courtesy of David Porter.

Video 47.1 ORIF of the Lisfanc.
This video is provided courtesy of David Porter.

Video 49.1 Gardner-Wells tong application.
This video is provided courtesy of Barrett Boody and Daniel Leas.

Video 50.1 Thoracolumbar Spine Trauma.
This video is provided courtesy of Joseph P. Gjolaj and Alexander Ghasem.

Section I

General Principles of Orthopaedic Trauma

I

1 Physiology of Fracture Healing

Roman M. Natoli and John J. Callaci

Introduction

Fracture fixation is an important part of orthopaedic trauma. Understanding the physiology of fracture healing will provide insight into the biologic and mechanical factors at play in bone healing. This chapter provides an overview of the components of fracture healing, how a fracture heals, and the clinical relevance of these topics (▶**Video 1.1**).

I. Fracture Healing Components

A. Bone blood supply and the effects of fracture and reaming

    1. Endosteal blood flow from high-pressure system nutrient arteries creates a centrifugal (inside to out) pattern of blood flow.

    2. Periosteal blood flow from low-pressure system supplies the outer ~one-third of bone cortex.

    3. Fracture disrupts blood flow causing acute hematoma to develop at the injury site.

    4. Reaming damages the endosteal blood supply and temporarily changes the blood flow pattern to centripetal (outside to in).

B. Cells

    1. Mesenchymal stem cells (MSCs)—precursors to blood vessels, muscle, fat, cartilage, and bone. Differentiate down different pathways depending on the mechanical and biologic signals received (▶**Fig. 1.1**). Can come from remote or local cell populations. In bone, local populations are periosteal, endosteal, muscle, blood vessels, and bone marrow.

    2. Chondrocytes—derived from MSCs and form cartilage intermediate during endochondral bone formation.

    3. Osteoblasts—derived from MSCs or via transdifferentiation of hypertrophic chondrocytes. Produce collagens and other proteins (e.g., osteocalcin, osteopontin) to form extracellular matrix (ECM) and also secrete regulatory proteins (e.g., osteoprotegerin [OPG], receptor activator of nuclear factor kappa-B [RANK] ligand, bone morphogenetic proteins [BMPs]) that affect fracture healing processes. They have parathyroid and vitamin D receptors and are responsible for matrix production during intramembranous and endochondral bone formation.

    4. Osteocytes—fully differentiated osteoblasts that exist in mature bone matrix. They respond to parathyroid hormone (PTH) or mechanical loading and secrete sclerostin to help regulate osteoblastic bone formation or osteoclastic bone resorption.

    5. Osteoclasts—derived from monocytes/macrophages, not from MSCs. These cells are responsible for bone resorption during intramembranous bone formation and remodeling. These attach to bone surfaces via integrin receptor signaling. Once attached, a ruffled border is created forming a local acidic environment to dissolve hydroxyapatite. Osteoclasts have the RANK receptor. PTH stimulates bone resorption by increasing osteoclast activity indirectly via osteoblast production of RANK ligand (RANKL).

C. Extracellular matrix (ECM)

    1. Organic component of ECM consists of different collagens and other stored proteins responsible for cell adhesion and signaling. The collagen expressed varies throughout the different stages of secondary fracture healing. The organic component of mature bone tissue is known as osteoid.

    2. Inorganic component is predominantly hydroxyapatite ($Ca_5(PO_4)_3OH$). Mineralization of osteoid results in mature bone tissue.

D. Cytokines (proteins that modulate immune response and cellular communication), growth factors (proteins that affect cell differentiation, proliferation, and function), and transcription factors

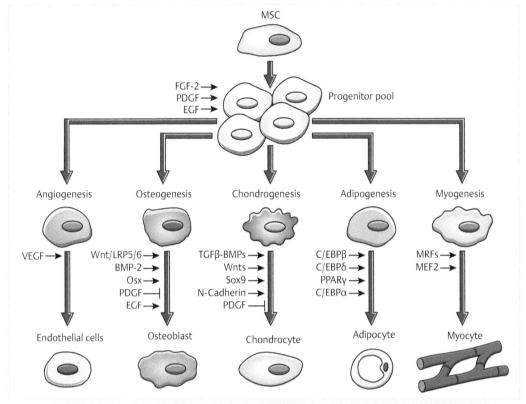

Fig. 1.1 Factors involved in differentiation of mesenchymal stem cells (MSCs). Depending on the signals received, MSCs can differentiate into blood vessels, bone, cartilage, muscle, or fat. Arrows are positive signals promoting differentiation into that cell type. ⊣'s are negative signals preventing differentiation into that cell type. BMP-2, bone morphogenetic protein 2; C/EBP, CCAAT-enhancer-binding proteins; EGF, epidermal growth factor; FGF-2, fibroblast growth factor 2; LRP5/6, low-density lipoprotein receptor-related protein 5/6; MEF2, myocyte enhancer factor-2; MRF, muscle regulatory factors; Osx, osterix; PDGF, platelet-derived growth factor; PPAR, peroxisome proliferator-activated receptor; TGF-β transforming growth factor beta; VEGF, vascular endothelial growth factor.

(intracellular DNA-binding proteins that modulate gene transcription): There is a myriad of these. Their function depends on location and time of expression during fracture healing.

1. Proinflammatory cytokines (e.g., tumor necrosis factor alpha [TNF-α], interleukin-1 [IL-1], IL-6)—recruit inflammatory cells, promote angiogenesis, modulate osteoblast/osteoclast differentiation, and affect cellular gene expression.

2. Transforming growth factor beta (TGF-β) superfamily, including BMPs—carry out MSC recruitment and differentiation into chondrocytes or osteoblasts and cellular proliferation. These proteins are stored in bone ECM in latent form.

3. Vascular endothelial growth factor (VEGF), angiopoietins—vascular ingrowth, neoangiogenesis, and revascularization of callus.

4. Wnt/β-catenin—canonical Wnt pathway regulates the amount of β-catenin transcription factor present intracellularly, guides differentiation of MSCs into osteoblasts, and regulates osteoblast activity during bone formation. Wnt signaling also inhibits osteoclastogenesis by increasing osteoblast synthesis of OPG.

5. Sclerostin—secreted by osteocytes and inhibits Wnt signaling.

6. OPG/RANKL—OPG is a decoy receptor for RANKL. RANKL produced by osteoblasts stimulates osteoclastogenesis. Their balance leads to resorption of mineralized cartilage and formation of woven bone.

E. Metabolic/endocrine components

1. Calcium.

2. Vitamin D—necessary for bone mineralization.

3. Vitamin C—necessary for collagen production.

4. PTH—important homeostatic regulator of serum calcium level and vitamin D metabolism by actions on bone, kidneys, and intestine. It also regulates endochondral bone formation. In recombinant form (Forteo®) it used to increase bone mass. It has also been used in treatment of nonunions, though clinical evidence of efficacy for this indication remains to be proven.

II. Types of Fracture Healing—Putting it All (and the Bone) Back Together

Bone is one of the few tissues that will heal without a scar (i.e., bone will absolutely become bone again). It is in contrast with healing in most of other tissues where there is some component of fibrous tissue (i.e., scar) at the repair/regeneration site. Bone is composed of cells and ECM. Woven bone is immature bone with randomly organized collagen fibers. Lamellar bone is composed of parallel layers of collagen fibers. The physiology of fracture healing remains incompletely understood. However, there are two well-described pathways of fracture healing: primary and secondary.

A. Primary (direct, intramembranous): This process of fracture healing occurs when a fracture is rigidly fixed (e.g., lag screw and neutralization plate, compression plate; ▶Fig. 1.2).

1. MSCs differentiate directly into osteoblasts. Based on Perren's strain theory, this is a low-strain environment (< 2%).

2. Cutting cones of osteoclasts followed by osteoblasts laying down osteoid which eventually mineralizes. This recreates Haversian canals/osteons directly across the fracture site.

B. Secondary (indirect, endochondral): This process of fracture healing occurs in mechanical environments with relative stability (e.g., cast, intramedullary nail [IMN], bridge plate, external fixation; ▶Fig. 1.3).

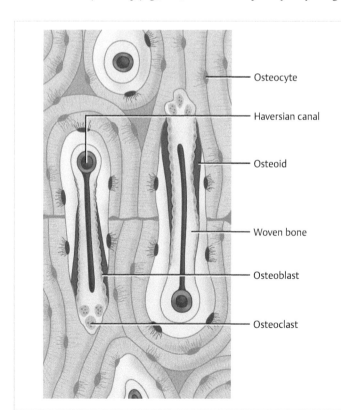

Osteocyte

Haversian canal

Osteoid

Woven bone

Osteoblast

Osteoclast

Fig. 1.2 Primary bone healing. Emanating from a Haversian canal a cutting cone is created. At the lead end of the cone are osteoclasts resorbing bone. They are followed by osteoblast that lay down osteoid. Osteoid eventually mineralizes to become new bone tissue.

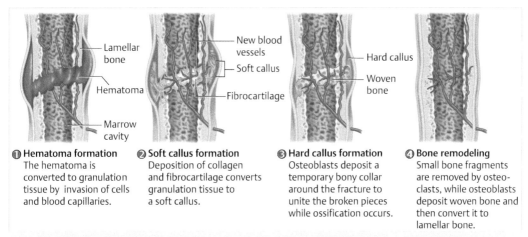

① Hematoma formation
The hematoma is converted to granulation tissue by invasion of cells and blood capillaries.

② Soft callus formation
Deposition of collagen and fibrocartilage converts granulation tissue to a soft callus.

③ Hard callus formation
Osteoblasts deposit a temporary bony collar around the fracture to unite the broken pieces while ossification occurs.

④ Bone remodeling
Small bone fragments are removed by osteoclasts, while osteoblasts deposit woven bone and then convert it to lamellar bone.

Fig. 1.3 Secondary bone healing. Following fracture, an acute inflammatory response occurs including the production and release of growth factors and cytokines, and the recruitment of mesenchymal cells to differentiate into chondrocytes. A cartilaginous intermediate is formed that then becomes vascularized. Osteoblasts and osteoclasts get recruited and the cartilage intermediate becomes mineralized and ultimately bone matrix is formed. Finally, this bone is remodeled to fully restore a normal bone structure.

1. Based on Perren's strain theory, this is a moderate-strain environment (~2–10%). The amount of strain present decreases over time as the stiffness of the tissues bridging the fracture changes.

2. Following fracture, an acute inflammatory response occurs including the production and release of growth factors and cytokines and the recruitment of mesenchymal cells to differentiate into chondrocytes. A cartilaginous intermediate is formed that then becomes vascularized. Osteoblasts and osteoclasts get recruited and the cartilage intermediate becomes mineralized and ultimately bone matrix is formed. Finally, this bone is remodeled to fully restore a normal bone structure. Classically, the process is divided into four stages:

    a. Inflammatory/hematoma—inflammatory cells (e.g., macrophages, neutrophils) and platelets debride the wound and release cytokines and cell recruitment factors. Early granulation tissue forms. This stage occurs immediately and up until ~2 weeks after injury.

    b. Soft callus (cartilaginous)—MSCs aggregate and differentiate into chondrocytes. An intermediate cartilage scaffold is formed bridging the fracture site. This stage occurs ~2 to 6 weeks after injury.

    c. Hard callus (endochondral bone formation)—chondrocytes hypertrophy (characterized by collagen X) and intermediate cartilage scaffold is degraded by matrix metalloproteinases and ultimately calcifies. Blood vessels invade and bring cells that differentiate into osteoblasts. Woven bone is laid down. This occurs ~6 weeks till injury site bridged.

    d. Remodeling—woven bone is slowly replaced by lamellar bone. Osteoblasts form new bone while osteoclasts resorb the woven bone. Restoration of bone marrow cavity starts. This occurs after hard callus has formed until bone is fully remodeled according to Wolff's law. It can take years to complete.

These are idealized stages of secondary fracture healing that in reality occur along a continuum overlapping in time.

III. Strategies to Manage Bone Defects or Augment and Accelerate Fracture Healing

Autograft, allograft, demineralized bone matrix, ceramics (e.g., tricalcium phosphate), growth factors (e.g., BMP-2 and BMP-7), platelet-rich plasma, bone marrow aspirate, electrical stimulation, and ultrasound are some strategies that have been used to either manage bone defects or augment and accelerate fracture healing. (see Chapter 8, Biologics, for more discussion on biologics in orthopaedic trauma).

IV. Clinical Rationale to Review Fracture Healing

Sections I and II surveyed "microscopic" physiology as it relates to fracture healing. We will now look in more detail at the macroscopic aspects.

A. Purpose of fracture management (four AO principles)

1. Reduce and fixate fractured bone/joint surface to restore anatomical relationships.

2. Provide absolute or relatively stable fixation based on the "personality" of the fracture, patient, or injury.

3. Preserve blood supply to soft tissue and bone by careful reduction techniques and tissue handling.

4. Safe and appropriately timed mobilization and rehabilitation of the injured extremity and entire patient.

B. At their core, principles 1 through 3 emphasize respect for fracture physiology. A theoretical reason to do a particular surgery is to alter the risk–benefit ratio of the natural history in a favorable way compared to a different procedure or nonoperative care.

1. Six typical outcomes for fractures in orthopaedic trauma patients are success, infection, malunion/nonunion, post-traumatic arthritis, joint stiffness/instability, and pain not otherwise specified (NOS).

2. Physiology of fracture healing is pertinent to the outcome of nonunion (see Chapter 7, Nonunion and Malunion, for further discussion on nonunions). Nonunions have a profound negative effect on patient's quality of life, far worse than many medical conditions (e.g., diabetes, acute myocardial infarction).

C. Multiple factors can contribute to impaired fracture healing (delayed union, nonunion).

1. Infection (see Chapter 6, Acute Infection Following Musculoskeletal Surgery, for more discussion on infection in orthopaedic trauma).

2. Biologic factors can be modifiable or nonmodifiable. Effort should be made, where appropriate, to optimize modifiable factors in favor of the physiology of fracture healing. See ▶ Table 1.1 for a list of purported biologic factors at play in the physiology of fracture healing. Aberrations in these higher-level physiologic systems manifest as alterations in the "microscopic" processes.

Table 1.1 List of purported biologic factors at play in the physiology of fracture healing. While some risk factors are modifiable, others are not

Biologic risk factors for non-union	
Nonmodifiable	Potentially modifiable
Polytrauma/multiple injury patient	Various medications (e.g., chemotherapy, steroids, anticonvulsants, anticoagulants)
Bone	NSAID use
Location within bone	Smoking
Fracture pattern	Malnutrition
Open fracture	Alcohol abuse
High-energy injury	Diabetes
Age	Vitamin D deficiency
Sex	Endocrine disorder (e.g., hyperthyroid/hyperparathyroid)
Prior irradiation	Time to weight bearing
Arthritis	Renal disease[b]
HIV	Liver disease[b]
Osteoporosis[a]	
Obesity[a]	

Abbreviations: HIV, human immunodeficiency virus; NSAID, nonsteroidal anti-inflammatory drugs.
[a]Not likely sufficiently alterable during the course of normal healing.
[b]May not be modifiable depending on specific diagnosis and stage of disease.

3. Mechanical factors: Improper surgical technique and mechanical stabilization can be detrimental to fracture healing physiology and increase nonunion rates. A multitude of chapters in this book are devoted to optimal nonoperative and operative procedures in fracture care. Two governing mechanical principles for fracture healing physiology are Perren's strain theory and Wolff's law.

   a. *Perren's strain theory* (▶ **Fig. 1.4**): The strain (change in length with load/initial length) seen at the fracture site determines the type of tissue that forms.

   b. *Wolff's law* (▶ **Fig. 1.5**): Bone will remodel in adaptation to the stress environment it experiences.

4. Orthopaedic fracture care interventions (nonoperative splints/casts/slings, percutaneous pinning, plating, intramedullary nailing, external fixation, arthroplasty, arthrodesis, and amputation) are limited in number. Understanding the physiology of fracture healing allows the surgeon to apply these methods to a given injury to promote a biologically favorable environment for bony union.

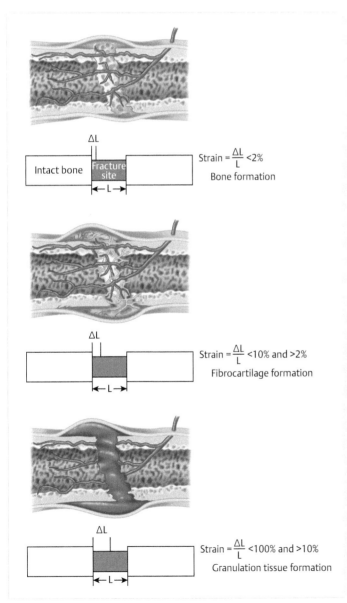

Fig. 1.4 Perren's strain theory. The strain experienced at the fracture site determines the type of tissue formed. Strain is the ratio of elongation to initial length. Bone forms in low-strain environments.

$$\text{Strain} = \frac{\Delta L}{L} < 2\%$$
Bone formation

$$\text{Strain} = \frac{\Delta L}{L} < 10\% \text{ and } > 2\%$$
Fibrocartilage formation

$$\text{Strain} = \frac{\Delta L}{L} < 100\% \text{ and } > 10\%$$
Granulation tissue formation

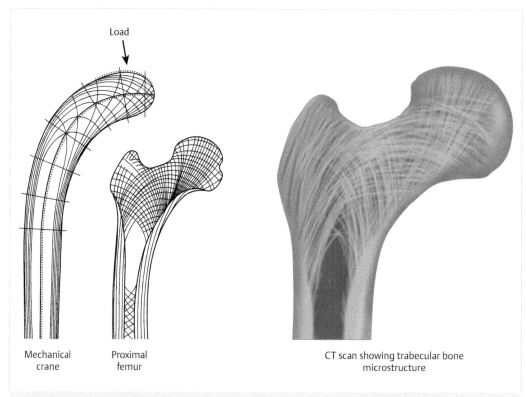

Mechanical crane

Proximal femur

CT scan showing trabecular bone microstructure

Fig. 1.5 Wolff's law. Bone models/remodels itself according to the mechanical environment it experiences. The image shows idealized stress distribution in the proximal femur subject to axial loading. The adjacent image is a computed tomography cut showing how trabecular bone is laid down in a strikingly similar pattern.

Summary

A. Physiology of fracture healing is an orchestrated set of events from the organ system level to the cellular level, down to and including complex intracellular processes.

B. Multiple organ systems are involved including bone, endocrine, vascular, gastrointestinal (e.g., overall nutrition and vitamin D), kidneys, immune, and respiratory systems.

C. At the local bone level there are two types of fracture healing, primary/intramembranous and secondary/endochondral.

D. Formation of new bone at a fracture site is the ultimate macroscopic outcome of cellular and intracellular events.

E. The goal of fracture surgery is to create a mechanical environment that optimizes the biology of fracture physiology to promote bony union.

Suggested Readings

Brinker MR, O'Connor DP, Monla YT, Earthman TP. Metabolic and endocrine abnormalities in patients with nonunions. J Orthop Trauma 2007;21(8):557–570

O'Keefe RJ, Jacobs JJ, Chu CR, Einhorn TA (2013). Orthopaedic Basic Science, Foundations of Clinical Practice, Fourth Edition. Rosemont, IL: American Academy of Orthopaedic Surgeons.

Schenker ML, Wigner NA, Lopas L, Hankenson KD, Ahn J (2014). Fracture Repair and Bone Grafting. In L.K. Cannada (Ed.), Orthopaedic Knowledge Update 11. Rosemont, IL: American Academy of Orthopaedic Surgeons.

Schottel PC, O'Connor DP, Brinker MR. Time trade-off as a measure of health-related quality of life: long bone nonunions have a devastating impact. J Bone Joint Surg Am 2015;97(17):1406–1410

Yang L, Tsang KY, Tang HC, Chan D, Cheah KS. Hypertrophic chondrocytes can become osteoblasts and osteocytes in endochondral bone formation. Proc Natl Acad Sci U S A 2014;111(33):12097–12102

Zura R, Mehta S, Della Rocca GJ, Steen RG. Biological risk factors for nonunion of bone fracture. JBJS Rev 2016;4(1): 01874474-201601000-00005

Zura R, Xiong Z, Einhorn T, et al. Epidemiology of fracture nonunion in 18 human bones. JAMA Surg 2016;151(11):e162775

2 Open Fractures and Principles of Soft Tissue Management

Mark J. Gage and Robert V. O'Toole

Introduction

Open fractures are fractures with an associated breach in the surrounding soft-tissue envelope. This results in a communication between the fracture and the outside environment, and increased risk of surgical site infection compared to closed injuries. These injuries typically represent a higher-energy injuries with more significant associated soft tissue and blood supply disruption. As a result, goals of treatment for this unique scenario are focused on reducing risk of infection and avoiding complications.

Keywords: open fracture, compound fracture, limb salvage, soft tissue injury, soft tissue reconstruction, wound infection, debridement

I. Mechanism of Injury

A. Blunt injuries

    1. These are the results of a direct blow leading to a focal area of injury (▶ **Fig. 2.1**).

    2. This is the most common mechanism for open fractures.

B. Ballistic injuries

    1. Determine between low- (i.e., handguns) and high- (i.e., military and hunting rifles) velocity injuries and high-mass injuries (close-range shotgun).

        a. Low-velocity ballistic fractures often can be treated as closed fractures. Weak evidence for antibiotic prophylaxis in these injuries.

        b. High-energy (high-velocity or high-mass) ballistic injuries are associated with significant soft tissue compromise and require surgical debridement.

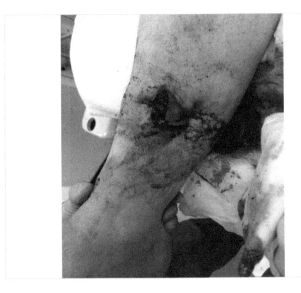

Fig. 2.1 An example of an open tibia fracture sustained after a blunt injury mechanism.

C. Blast injuries

1. These are divided into three different types of injuries:

   a. Primary: initial blast wave energy dissipated onto the body.

   b. Secondary: fragments emitted from the explosive device lodge into the body.

   c. Tertiary: resulting injury from victim being projected against ground or solid objects.

II. Classification

A. Gustilo–Anderson classification

1. Originally based on open tibial fractures and the size of associated soft-tissue wound but commonly applied to all open fractures. Classification is made in the operating room at time of the final debridement. Infection rates increase dramatically between lower types and IIIB and IIIC fractures.

   a. Type 1—skin laceration < 1 cm in length and low-energy fracture pattern.

   b. Type 2—1 to 10 cm wound length without extensive soft tissue damage or high-energy fracture pattern.

   c. Type 3A—open wound > 10 cm in length that can be closed primarily or with a skin graft. Smaller wounds are included if extensive stripping of periosteum, heavy contamination, or high-energy fractures (segmental or highly comminuted) are present.

   d. Type 3B—extensive soft tissue loss, typically a wound that requires rotational or free tissue transfer for closure when bone is at anatomic length. A fracture would be considered to be classified as a 3B type if shortening of the limb is required to allow for wound closure.

   e. Type 3C—arterial vascular injury in the affected extremity that requires vascular repair for limb viability. Repairs to vessels in limbs that have adequate perfusion are not 3C injuries.

B. Orthopaedic Trauma Association open fracture classification

1. Initially it was utilized in research setting to describe soft-tissue injuries in greater detail.

2. Numerical score from 1 (least severe) to 3 (most severe) for each of the following five categories of open fracture assessment: skin injury, muscle injury, arterial injury, degree of contamination, and bone loss.

III. Principles of Open Fracture Management in the Emergent Setting

A. Clinical assessment and initial management

1. Neurovascular evaluation:

   a. Vascular compromise is common.

   b. Abnormal pulse exam following fracture reduction necessitates further evaluation with ankle brachial indices (ABI) and/or computed tomography angiogram to diagnose vascular injury.

   c. Assess for neurologic deficit.

   d. Limbs with open fractures can still develop compartment syndrome.

2. Soft tissue assessment:

   a. Careful evaluation of all wounds and abrasions in fractured limbs is done for making the diagnosis of an open fracture. Be aware that the wound may be at some distance from the fracture location as the bone may have displaced during the injury.

   b. Evaluate degree of contamination, wound size, and potential need for soft tissue reconstruction (rotational flap, free tissue transfer). High level of contamination may warrant more urgent operative debridement.

    c. Entrapped tendons may prevent joint or fracture reduction.

    d. Completely devitalized bone should be removed, unless it contains articular cartilage.

    e. Sterile gauze should be applied to open wound either alone or with antiseptic solution. Consider packing wound with mild compression to control bleeding when clinically warranted.

B. Role of antibiotic treatment

    1. There is level 1 evidence to support that antibiotic treatment prior to the operation has a protective effect against early infection compared to no antibiotics or placebo.

    2. Antibiotics should be started as soon after injury as possible.

    3. Weak evidence to support the best type of antibiotic to be administered, but consensus opinion is an intravenous administration of first-generation cephalosporin for all open fractures. Local differences or protocols may exist at trauma centers.

    4. Gentamicin or equivalent is frequently supplemented for more contaminated injuries to give additional coverage against gram-negative bacteria.

        a. Aminoglycosides carry an increased risk of nephrotoxicity in trauma patients.

    5. Consider adding penicillin G or equivalent for gross contamination (fecal/soil/marine) for additional anaerobic bacterial coverage.

    6. Clindamycin is an alternative to cephalosporin treatment in penicillin-allergic patients.

    7. Piperacillin/tazobactam are acceptable alternative to cefazolin and gentamicin.

    8. No consensus on length of antibiotic treatment warranted for therapeutic benefit. Many centers recommend 24 to 48 hours of treatment after each debridement until definitive soft-tissue closure or coverage.

C. Radiographic evaluation

    1. X-rays should be performed primarily to assess the extent of osseous injury and guide the appropriate immobilization needed to stabilize the injury.

    2. Consider CT imaging if further bone detail is warranted prior to surgical intervention.

IV. Surgical Management of Open Fractures

A. Goals of debridement

    1. Open fractures are contaminated. Consider the level of contamination, severity of the wound, and the health of the patient when determining the risk of infection.

    2. Timing of surgical debridement:

        a. A recent meta-analysis found no difference between debridements performed before and after 12 hours from time of injury.

        b. Data from the LEAP study found no difference in timing of debridement; however, timing of arrival to the definitive treatment center was correlated with infection.

        c. It is recommended that open fractures should undergo surgical irrigation and debridement within the first 24 hours after injury when the patient is appropriately resuscitated and medically optimized for surgery, but this time point is based mostly on expert opinion. There may be open fractures where more urgent debridement is necessary such as associated vascular injuries or grossly contaminated wounds.

    3. Surgical approach:

        a. Removal of all devitalized and contaminated tissue to minimize infection.

        b. Excision of bone fragments devoid of soft tissue attachment except when that bone has significant portions of the joint attached to it.

    c.   There is wide variation among surgeons regarding the extent of osseous debridement necessary. For example, aggressive debridements may reduce the risk of infection, but large bone defects create challenges with initial limb stabilization and may be associated with more complex reconstructive paths to achieve healing.

B. Irrigation

    1. Types and application:

        a.   Purpose of irrigation is to help create a clean healing base by decreasing bacterial load, removing foreign bodies and detached necrotic tissue.

        b.   It should be performed after complete surgical debridement.

        c.   Normal saline is the most commonly used irrigant with poor support for other adjuvants to the solution.

        d.   Irrigant may be administered in a low-pressure manner by saline bags passing through cystoscopy tubing by gravity.

        e.   High-pressure irrigation is an alternative form with increased irrigant velocity thought to enhance debridement. Potential disadvantages outlined in basic science studies suggest an additional insult to bone and soft tissue, and concern for propulsion of bacteria deeper into tissues.

        f.   FLOW study: level 1 multicenter study comparing irrigation types in open fractures.

            i.   No clinical difference in reoperation rates between high-pressure, low-pressure, and gravity-rate irrigation.

           ii.   Higher reoperation rates in patients randomized to soap irrigation compared to saline.

C. Fracture stabilization

    1. External fixation:

        a.   It provides preliminary temporary skeletal stabilization in an expeditious manner or it can be used as definitive fixation. This is important not only to stabilize the bone but may also help in stabilizing the soft-tissue injury.

        b.   Soft-tissue injury can make pin placement difficult. Pins can be placed either at a distance from the wound or directly in the wound depending on size and morphology.

        c.   Consider for severe trauma/polytrauma, associated vascular injury, and highly contaminated open injuries that may require multiple surgical debridements.

        d.   External fixation is often advantageous in these situations as it is easy to obtain full access to the wound by displacing the bones which is more difficult to do once internal fixation is in place.

    2. Internal fixation:

        a.   Performed after debridement and irrigation is complete.

        b.   May be performed in the same surgical setting after debridement for open fractures that have a low likelihood for persistent contamination and infection.

        c.   Many surgeons prefer to limit the time between definitive fixation and flap coverage, and recent data supports that longer times (7 days or more) between fixation and flap coverage are associated with higher infection rates.

        d.   Temporary internal fixation, known as "damage-control plating," has recently been described as an effective means to stabilize open fractures prior to repeat surgical debridement with significantly lower costs (25%) incurred.

D. Infection prevention: local antibiotic delivery

    1. Antibiotic bead placement:

        a.   This serves as an easily retrievable method for high-dose local antibiotic delivery to prevent infection although there is little data looking at their use (▶ **Fig. 2.2**).

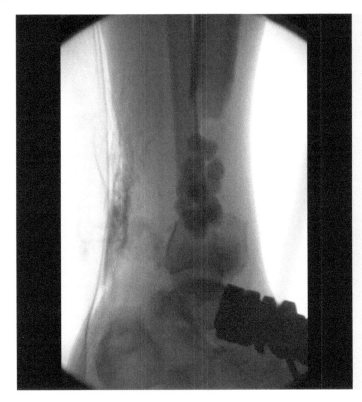

Fig. 2.2 An example of an open distal tibia fracture with bone loss and gross contamination being treated with antibiotic beads fabricated by polymethylmethacrylate combined with antibiotic powder.

    b. Antibiotic powder is combined with polymethylmethacrylate cement and shaped into beads.

    c. Vancomycin and tobramycin are commonly used although other heat-stable options exist.

    d. Capable of delivering very high local antibiotic concentrations and avoid the potential systemic antibiotic side effects.

    e. Beads are typically strung onto wire or suture to keep them localized in the wound and are often removed at the time of final wound closure.

  2. Antibiotic spacer placement:

    a. Composition similar to that of antibiotic beads.

    b. Administered in the form of a cement block.

    c. In addition to providing high concentrations of local antibiotic delivery, this technique, when placed into a bone void can provide additional skeletal stability.

  3. Antimicrobial implants:

    a. Antibiotic cement may be used to coat orthopaedic implants when infection risk is high. Some implants exist with antimicrobial coatings but their clinical impact is unknown.

E. Indications for serial debridement

  1. Intraoperative findings during the initial debridement dictate the need for subsequent debridement.

  2. High levels of contamination and tissue nonviability will necessitate repeat surgical debridements (▶ **Fig. 2.3**) as these wounds often evolve and more necrotic tissue will be observed at subsequent debridements.

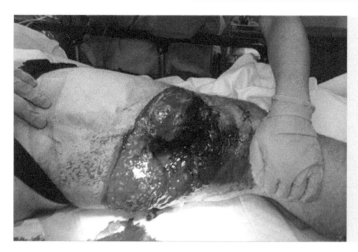

Fig. 2.3 Large open and grossly contaminated wounds typically require multiple surgical debridements.

V. Soft Tissue Management in Extremity Injuries

A. Negative pressure wound therapy

1. Negative pressure applied creates unique environment encouraging for wound healing (▶ **Fig. 2.4**).

2. Ideal for soft tissue defects that will heal through secondary intention or require skin grafting.

3. Helpful in the prevention of wound desiccation, reduction of microbial contamination that may occur with dressing changes, and aid in facilitation of wound drainage.

4. Effective way to downscale the complexity of soft tissue reconstruction by promoting granulation tissue.

5. Avoid direct contact with blood vessels, nerves, exposed bone, or tendon without paratenon as it may desiccate or damage these tissues.

6. It will not remove contaminated tissue by itself and basic science data shows it does not lower bacterial counts as much as antibiotic beads.

B. Primary wound closures and skin grafting

1. Open fractures are frequently associated with significant soft-tissue injury and subsequent edema making primary wound closure challenging.

2. Closure should be performed with techniques to preserve the soft tissue integrity and viability.

3. Relaxing incisions adjacent to the wound can be utilized to prevent excessive tension on wound edges when attempting primary closure.

4. Skin grafting is a coverage option for wounds that cannot be closed primarily and have a healthy underlying wound bed of muscle, paratenon, or subcutaneous tissue.

C. Soft tissue flap coverage

Flaps are dictated by the location and size of the soft tissue defect when primary closure is no longer possible. They are indicated for coverage of exposed vital structures including bone, artery, nerve, or tendon without paratenon.

1. Rotational flap coverage:

   a. Mobilization of local tissue with its vascular pedicle to an area in need of soft tissue coverage (▶ **Fig. 2.5**).

   b. This is a commonly needed option when addressing soft tissue loss in the leg. The local flap of choice is dictated by the defect location.

   c. Flap tissue cannot be from an already devitalized area involved in the initial zone of injury.

2. Free tissue transfer:

   a. The process of harvesting tissue with its blood supply and relocating it to a different anatomic location through a new vascular anastomosis.

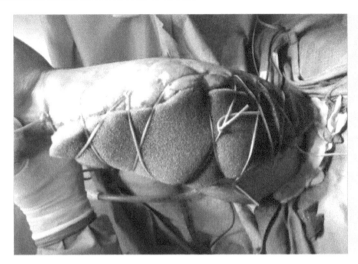

Fig. 2.4 Negative pressure wound therapy is helpful in soft tissue management by reducing microbial contamination between debridements and facilitation of wound drainage.

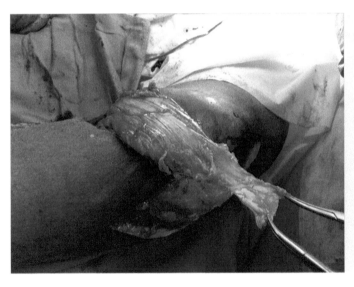

Fig. 2.5 The gastrocnemius rotational flap is an excellent treatment option for significant soft tissue defects of the proximal tibia.

    b. This provides vascularized tissue to the damaged area.

    c. Avoids further functional deficits to an already injured area potentially seen in rotational coverage.

3. Timing of soft tissue coverage:

    a. Controversy exists regarding the ideal timing of soft tissue coverage with wide variation in practice from center to center.

    b. Current recommendations are to attempt to achieve wound coverage within 7 days of the initial injury but the availability of a flap surgeon and need for multiple debridements may make this a very difficult goal to achieve in some situations.

Summary

Open fractures are associated with a breach in the surrounding soft-tissue envelope leading to direct communication between fractured bone and the outside world. These are often complex injuries commonly associated with significant soft tissue disruption, concomitant neurovascular injuries, and difficult-to-treat fractures that warrant careful assessment and important changes in treatment compared to a similar closed fracture. Thorough excisional debridement of devitalized tissue and contamination, early intravenous antibiotics, local wound antibiotic delivery, fracture stabilization, and timely soft tissue coverage are important components of open fracture management aimed at mitigating complications.

Suggested Readings

Bhandari M, Jeray KJ, Petrisor BA, et al; FLOW Investigators. A trial of wound irrigation in the initial management of open fracture wounds. N Engl J Med 2015;373(27):2629–2641

D'Alleyrand JC, Manson TT, Dancy L, et al. Is time to flap coverage of open tibial fractures an independent predictor of flap-related complications? J Orthop Trauma 2014;28(5):288–293

Gosselin RA, Roberts I, Gillespie WJ. Antibiotics for preventing infection in open limb fractures. Cochrane Database Syst Rev 2004(1):CD003764

Patzakis MJ, Bains RS, Lee J, et al. Prospective, randomized, double-blind study comparing single-agent antibiotic therapy, ciprofloxacin, to combination antibiotic therapy in open fracture wounds. J Orthop Trauma 2000;14(8):529–533

Patzakis MJ, Harvey JP Jr, Ivler D. The role of antibiotics in the management of open fractures. J Bone Joint Surg Am 1974;56(3):532–541

Pollak AN, Jones AL, Castillo RC, Bosse MJ, MacKenzie EJ, Group LS; LEAP Study Group. The relationship between time to surgical debridement and incidence of infection after open high-energy lower extremity trauma. J Bone Joint Surg Am 2010;92(1):7–15

Weber D, Dulai SK, Bergman J, Buckley R, Beaupre LA. Time to initial operative treatment following open fracture does not impact development of deep infection: a prospective cohort study of 736 subjects. J Orthop Trauma 2014;28(11):613–619

3 Closed Fracture Management/Casting

Rahul Vaidya

Introduction

Closed treatment has been the standard of care for all fractures until the 20th century. It remains the most widely used method of fracture management and in one recent review of 7,863 cases, 67% of all fractures were managed nonoperatively. This chapter will provide an overview of reduction techniques, indications for nonoperative fracture management, and outline principles of splint and cast application (▶Video 3.1–▶Video 3.3).

I. Specific Reduction Techniques and Principles of Casting and Splinting

A. Nondisplaced fractures

    1. Almost all nondisplaced fractures can be treated nonoperatively with the exception of the femur and some unusual conditions.

    2. The methods of immobilization include: slings, splints, casts, traction, or simply avoiding weight-bearing through the limb.

    3. Immobilization will allow secondary bone healing to take place and function to return by 6 weeks to 3 months depending on the bone.

B. Displaced fractures

    1. Trauma strong enough to cause a fracture will cause surrounding soft tissue injury including periosteal disruption.

    2. Bones are attached to muscles which contract, shorten, angulate, and rotate fracture fragments.

        a. The fracture will often heal in the displaced position but the deformities that result may leave the limb or patient compromised and potential loss of function.

        b. Most displaced fractures should be reduced to minimize deformity and soft tissue complications, including those that ultimately require operative fixation.

        c. Splints provide initial stabilization of displaced fractures. They should allow for swelling and all bony prominences should be adequately padded.

C. Indirect or closed reduction of fractures

    1. Adequate analgesia and muscle relaxation are critical for success.

        a. Hematoma block—aspirate hematoma and place 10 cm^3 of lidocaine at fracture site.

           i. May be less reliable than other methods.

           ii. Fast and easy.

        b. Intravenous sedation:

           i. Versed (0.5–1 mg q 3 minutes up to 5 mg).

           ii. Morphine (0.1 mg/kg).

           iii. Demerol (1–2 mg/kg up to 150 mg).

           iv. Beware of pulmonary complications with deep conscious sedation—consider anesthesia service assistance if there is concern.

           v. Physician should be credentialed for "conscious sedation."

           vi. Pulse oximeter and careful monitoring are recommended.

        c. Bier block—It results in superior pain relief, greater relaxation, and less premedication is needed.

           i. Double tourniquet is inflated on proximal arm and venous system is filled with local.

           ii. Lidocaine is preferred for fast onset.

           iii. Volume = 40 cm^3.

           iv. Adults: 2–3 mg/kg, children: 1.5 mg/kg.

      v. If tourniquet is deflated after < 40 minutes then deflate for 3 seconds and reinflate for 3 minutes—repeat twice.

      vi. Watch closely for cardiac and neurologic side effects, especially in the elderly patients.

2. Reduction is accomplished by some form of traction and force directed against the deformity to correct the length, alignment, and rotation of the bone and it may be specific for fracture location and pattern.

    a. Reduction may require reversal of mechanism of injury, especially in children with intact periosteum.

    b. When the bone breaks because of bending, the soft tissues disrupt on the convex side and remain intact on the concave side.

    c. Longitudinal traction may not allow the fragments to be disimpacted and brought out to length if there is an intact soft-tissue hinge (typically seen in children who have strong periosteum that is intact on one side).

    d. Reproduction of the mechanism of fracture to hook on the ends of the fracture angulation beyond 90 degree is usually required.

3. Immobilization:

    a. Fractures must be immobilized to include the joint above and below.

    b. Maintain the position of the bone fragments to the point of healing.

    c. Use splints initially to accommodate for potential swelling.

    d. Three-point contact (mold) is necessary to maintain closed reduction.

    e. Cast must be molded to resist deforming forces.

4. Cast padding:

    a. Roll the padding distal to proximal.

    b. Use 50% overlap.

    c. Four layers minimum.

    d. At bony prominences, use extra padding: fibular head, malleoli, patella, and olecranon.

5. Plaster versus fiberglass:

    a. Plaster is better for molding, use cold water to maximize molding time.

    b. Fiberglass is more difficult to mold but is more durable and 2 to 3 times stronger. It is also more resistant to breakdown.

    c. Width of roll: 6 inch for thigh; 3 to 4 inch for lower leg; 3 to 4 inch for upper arm; and 2 to 3 inch for forearm.

II. Nonoperative Treatment of Displaced Fractures of the Upper and Lower Extremity

A. Nonoperative treatment with immobilization or closed reduction is suitable for many displaced fractures such as clavicle, scapula, proximal humerus, humeral shaft, ulna, distal radius, vertebral fractures, pelvis, tibia, and ankle fractures.

B. Patients who are not amenable to operative treatment due to medical comorbidities are candidates for nonoperative treatment.

C. Clavicle fractures

1. Non or minimally displaced clavicle fractures:

    a. These fractures heal well with a sling, physical therapy, and range of motion (ROM) exercises.

    b. These return to normal function in 6 to 10 weeks or sooner in children and adolescents.

2. Midshaft clavicle fractures with > 100% displacement or shortened > 2 cm:

    a. Nonunion rate up to 15% with nonoperative treatment.

    b. These may heal with a symptomatic malunion.

D. Scapula fractures

1. Nonoperative management is indicated for the vast majority of extra-articular scapula fractures.

2. Treatment consists of sling immobilization with early motion as tolerated and physical therapy as needed.

3. Consideration for operative fixation should be made in cases involving glenohumeral instability, displaced glenoid fractures, and significant medial displacement of the lateral border.

E. Proximal humerus fractures

1. Nonoperative management is often recommended for minimally displaced fractures in all patients.

2. Some studies have reported little or no benefit of operative fixation for 3- and 4-part proximal humerus fractures in elderly low-demand patients.

3. Conservative treatment involves initial sling application with a progressive physical therapy regimen at 1 to 2 weeks post injury as pain subsides.

4. A thorough discussion of the indications for operative management of proximal humerus fractures can be found in Chapter 21, Proximal Humerus Fractures.

F. Humeral diaphysis

1. The treatment of displaced humeral shaft fractures has been traditionally nonoperative with low nonunion rates and good outcomes.

2. A modern trend of operative fixation has been generating substantial interest.

    a. Potential indications for surgical management are polytrauma, open fractures, vascular injury, inability to tolerate splinting, body habitus, and pathologic fractures.

3. Nonoperative management:

    a. Initial treatment with coaptation splint (laterally above shoulder, around elbow, and along the medial arm; pad armpit well).

    b. Conversion to functional bracing within 1 to 2 weeks.

    c. Immobilization with a brace should be employed for 6 to 12 weeks with confirmation of fracture healing radiographically.

    d. Elbow mobilization should begin shortly after the brace has been fitted.

    e. Humerus easily tolerates coronal and sagittal malalignment and 3 cm of shortening. Cosmetic deformities have been noted with 30 degrees of coronal angulation and 20 degrees of sagittal deformity.

    f. Dr. Sarmiento's series of 620 patients treated with functional bracing for humeral shaft fractures had the following results:

        i. Six percent nonunion in open fractures and < 2% nonunion in closed fractures.

        ii. Most patients healed with < 16 degrees of anterior and varus angulation and achieved good to excellent function.

G. Forearm

1. Isolated ulna fractures can be treated with immobilization if there is acceptable alignment (less than 50% translation and less than 15 degrees angulation).

    a. Some authors recommend initial immobilization of both the wrist and elbow, while others feel the elbow can be left free.

    b. Consider transition to ulna fracture bracing at 1 to 2 weeks post injury.

2. Most isolated radial shaft and both bone forearm fractures benefit from operative fixation in adults as it is difficult to maintain reduction with cast immobilization.

3. Nonoperative treatment in adults may lead to loss of pronation and supination.

4. Nonoperative treatment is the standard of care in children if alignment can be maintained in a cast (see Chapter 12, Principles of Pediatric Fracture Management, for specific guidelines).

H. Distal radius

1. Many displaced distal radius fractures can be treated with closed reduction and immobilization in a cast or splint.

2. Traction followed by reduction in flexion and ulnar deviation is usually required to reduce a Colles fracture (two-part extra-articular fracture; Chapter 28, Distal Radius and Galeazzi Fractures, ▸Fig. 28.4).

3. Immobilize in a splint with molding on the dorsum of the distal radius with slight flexion and ulnar deviation.

4. Assuming acceptable reduction is obtained, the injury should be closely monitored for maintenance of reduction.

5. Indications for surgical management of distal radius fractures are discussed in detail in Chapter 28, Distal Radius and Galeazzi Fractures.

6. Operative treatment, compared to nonoperative treatment, of displaced distal radius fractures in elderly patients has shown better radiographic results but no improvement in functional outcome.

I. Pelvis

1. The majority of minimally and nondisplaced pelvic fractures can be treated nonoperatively.

2. See Chapter 30, Pelvic Ring Injuries, for a detailed discussion of initial and definitive treatment.

J. Femoral shaft

1. Nonoperative treatment of femoral shaft fractures occurs in some third-world hospitals or in patients who are not amenable to operative treatment.

2. The results of Perkins' traction (skeletal traction which allows movement of the knee) is reported to have a nonunion/malunion rate up to 10%, pin infection incidence of 30%, and an average hospital stay of 8 weeks.

3. Intramedullary nailing of femur fractures has been one of the great success stories of 20th century and is the standard of care even in remote hospitals with union rates > 98%.

K. Tibial shaft

1. These fractures were commonly treated nonsurgically through the 1970s until intramedullary nailing became more popular.

2. Techniques such as long leg casting with wedging to correct angular deformity and transition to patellar tendon bearing casts and cast bracing were the standard of care.

   a. Patients were placed in above knee long leg casts and switched to functional braces after 3 to 5 weeks.

3. Sarmiento reported a 2.5% nonunion rate and < 10% malunion rate in a series of 780 tibial fractures (241 were open).

   a. Union occurred at an average of 17 weeks for closed fractures and 22 weeks for open fractures.

4. Generally acceptable parameters for closed treatment include < 5 to 10 degrees varus or valgus angulation, < 15 degrees in the sagittal plane, < 15 degrees internal rotation, < 20 degrees external rotation, and < 2 cm of shortening.

L. Ankle fractures

1. Most unimalleolar nondisplaced ankle fractures are treated closed.

2. Unstable displaced ankle fractures are typically treated surgically.

3. Displaced ankle fractures can be treated nonoperatively if tibiotalar joint congruity is obtained following reduction.

4. Indications for closed treatment of ankle fractures include:

   a. Isolated lateral malleolus fracture with < 4 mm medial clear space widening on external rotation or gravity stress views.

   b. Isolated medial malleolus fractures where reduction can be maintained in cast.

   c. Elderly low-demand patients or poorly controlled diabetics with high risk for surgical complications.

5. Displaced bimalleolar and trimalleolar ankle fractures should be promptly reduced even if surgical management is planned.

6. Typical reduction maneuver for a supination—external rotational injury with lateral talar displacement:

   a. The Quigley maneuver classically describes suspension of the great toe with the patient supine. This facilitates reduction by adduction, internal rotation, and supination of the foot.

   b. Treated with below knee casting for 4 weeks or longer depending on healing.

III. Casting Techniques

A. Short leg cast

   1. Support metatarsal heads.

   2. Flex the knee to relax the gastrocnemius muscle.

   3. Position the ankle in neutral dorsiflexion.

   4. Ensure freedom of the toes.

   5. Build up heel for walking casts—fiberglass much preferred for durability.

B. Long leg cast

   1. Apply the below knee portion first with a thin layer proximally.

   2. Flex the knee 5 to 20 degrees.

   3. Mold the supracondylar femur for improved rotational stability.

   4. Apply extra padding anterior to the patella.

C. Short arm cast

   1. Metacarpophalangeal joints free and thumb free to the base of the metacarpal.

   2. Distal extent of the cast ends at the proximal palmar crease.

   3. Opposition of the thumb to the small finger should be unobstructed.

D. Ulnar gutter: https://www.youtube.com/watch?v=kx2YBmq7oS0.

E. Volar/dorsal hand: https://www.youtube.com/watch?v=Iv-Nigb6aN8.

F. Thumb spica: https://www.youtube.com/watch?v=864h9gVgmKs.

IV. Traction Pin Placement

A. Create a sterile field with the limb exposed.

B. Administer local sedation +/– sedation.

C. Insert the pin from the known area of neurovascular structure.

D. Distal femoral traction

   1. It is the method of choice for acetabular and proximal femur fractures.

    2.   Indicated in the presence of a knee ligament injury for femoral shaft fractures instead of proximal tibial traction.

    3.   Insert the pin from medial to lateral at the adductor tubercle—slightly proximal to epicondyle.

E.   Proximal tibia traction

    1.   It is the method of choice for femoral shaft fractures.

    2.   Insert the pin 2 cm posterior and 1 cm distal to the tibial tubercle from lateral to medial.

    3.   Incise skin and avoid the anterior compartment by mobilizing the muscle posteriorly with the pin or hemostat.

F.   Calcaneus traction

    1.   Typically used when proximal tibia and distal femur traction pins are contraindicated.

    2.   Insert the pin medial to lateral 2 to 2.5 cm posterior and inferior to the medial malleolus.

G.   Place sterile dressing around pin site.

H.   Place protective caps over sharp pin ends.

I.   Hang weight from the traction bow.

    1.   Fifteen percent of the body weight for distal femur traction.

    2.   Ten percent of the body weight for proximal tibia and calcaneus traction.

V. Complications of Closed Treatment

A.   For select fractures treated nonoperatively, especially those requiring a cast, complication rates can be as high as seen with surgical intervention.

B.   If an unacceptable degree of malalignment develops, it usually occurs early. Correction can be achieved with surgery or cast wedging in select cases.

C.   Cast wedging can be used to improve alignment early in the treatment period.

    1.   Measuring the deformity with orthogonal films in the coronal and sagittal planes.

    2.   The cast is cut circumferentially leaving a hinge on the convexity of the deformity.

    3.   The cast is then distracted on the concave side and a spacer (cork, balsa wood, plastic) is inserted.

    4.   The size of the spacer can be approximated by the angle of deformity requiring correction (10 degree correction generally achieved with a 10-mm spacer).

    5.   The cast is overwrapped with plaster or cast material.

D.   Casts and splints carry the risk of causing a pressure sore.

    1.   Typically occurs over a bony prominence.

    2.   Be particularly vigilant if the patient has an impaired level of consciousness, decreased peripheral sensation (e.g., diabetic neuropathy), or has poor nutrition.

    3.   The risk of pressure sores can be reduced by appropriately padding all areas at risk.

    4.   Counterintuitively, total-contact casts are used in high-risk patients with less padding that allow less friction and a lower risk of wound development; however, this should only be applied by an experienced professional and not attempted by someone inexperienced.

Conclusion

Closed treatment can be applied to a wide variety of fractures with minimal risk to the patient. If a patient is not a good candidate for surgery, nonoperative methods can be attempted even in the most difficult cases. It is important for the surgeon to be aware of nonsurgical alternatives and methods of fracture treatment.

Suggested Readings

Court-Brown CM, Aitken S, Hamilton TW, Rennie L, Caesar B. Nonoperative fracture treatment in the modern era. J Trauma 2010;69(3):699–707

Egol KA, Walsh M, Romo-Cardoso S, Dorsky S, Paksima N. Distal radial fractures in the elderly: operative compared with nonoperative treatment. J Bone Joint Surg Am 2010;92(9):1851–1857

Gregson PA, Thomas PB. Tibial cast wedging: a simple and effective technique. J Bone Joint Surg Br 1994;76(3):496–497

Makwana NK, Bhowal B, Harper WM, Hui AW. Conservative versus operative treatment for displaced ankle fractures in patients over 55 years of age. A prospective, randomised study. J Bone Joint Surg Br 2001;83(4):525–529

McKee MD, Wild LM, Schemitsch EH. Midshaft malunions of the clavicle. J Bone Joint Surg Am 2003;85(5):790–797

Olerud P, Ahrengart L, Ponzer S, Saving J, Tidermark J. Internal fixation versus nonoperative treatment of displaced 3-part proximal humeral fractures in elderly patients: a randomized controlled trial. J Shoulder Elbow Surg 2011;20(5):747–755

Sarmiento A, Zagorski JB, Zych GA, Latta LL, Capps CA. Functional bracing for the treatment of fractures of the humeral diaphysis. J Bone Joint Surg Am 2000;82(4):478–486

Sarmiento A, Gersten LM, Sobol PA, Shankwiler JA, Vangsness CT. Tibial shaft fractures treated with functional braces. Experience with 780 fractures. J Bone Joint Surg Br 1989;71(4):602–609

4 Biomechanics of Internal Fracture Fixation

Jason A. Lowe, Hannah L. Dailey, and Jason Wild

Introduction

A proper discussion of biomechanics necessitates knowledge and understanding of key concepts. Since the definitions are complex, the concepts in this chapter will prove difficult without a command of the language of biomechanics.

Keywords: fracture biomechanics, bone healing, construct design, stress, strain, strength, implant, failure, elasticity, plasticity

I. Definitions

A. *Stress* is a force applied to an object distributed over the area that bears the load and is measured in Newtons per meter squared N/m² (pascal).

B. *Strain* describes a change in shape in response to an applied stress. In axial loading, strain is the change in length of an object over the original length. In fracture management, multiplanar motion at the fracture site gives rise to complex three-dimensional strains.

C. A *stress–strain curve* is the experimentally observed relationship between applied load (stress) and deformation (strain) for a given material (see ▶**Fig. 4.1**). This curve also defines other material properties.

D. *Young's modulus of elasticity* (*E*) describes the stiffness of a material and is defined by the slope of linear portion on a stress–strain curve. The modulus *E* is measured in megapascals (MPa) and is intrinsic to the material, so it does not depend on material geometry. The more stress it takes to deform an object, the steeper the curve (higher *E*).

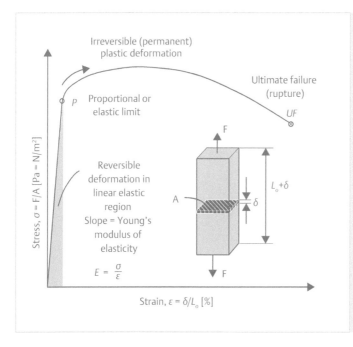

Fig. 4.1 Representative material stress–strain graph showing Young's modulus of elasticity (*E*), proportional limit (*P*), yield strength (σ_y), and ultimate strength (σ_u).

E. *Proportional limit* (*P*) of a material is the point on the stress–strain curve of a material after which any additional applied stress will cause nonelastic permanent deformation. For many materials, including implant-grade metals, the proportional limit is equal to the *elastic limit.*

F. *Elastic deformation* is the change in shape that is completely reversible when the applied stress is removed.

G. *Plastic deformation* or *permanent set* is deformation that does not completely resolve when stress is removed. When plastic deformation occurs, the object's shape is permanently altered because of damage to the material microstructure.

H. *Strength* is the ability of a material to withstand applied loading without failure (breakage) or plastic deformation.

I. *Yield strength* (σ_Y) is the stress at which a material starts to experience plastic deformation and it typically coincides with the proportional limit (*P*).

J. *Ultimate strength* (σ_U) is the stress in a material when catastrophic failure occurs following a one-time overloading event and corresponds to point *UF* of the stress–strain curve.

K. *Fatigue strength* (σ_N) is the maximum stress a material can withstand for *N* cycles of repeated loading. Trauma implant components are typically designed to withstand at least several hundred thousand cycles of weight bearing loading before *fatigue failure* (▶ Fig. 4.2).

L. *Endurance limit* (σ_E) is the stress at which a ferrous material, such as stainless steel, can experience infinite cyclic loading without failing. Nonferrous metals including implant-grade titanium alloys have a *fatigue limit*, which is the stress corresponding to failure at a defined limit such as 500 million loading cycles.

M. *Stiffness* describes the ability of a material or of a manufactured part to resist deformation in response to an applied load. The *material* stiffness, or Young's modulus *E*, does not depend on part geometry. The *part* stiffness is a function of the part geometry, the material's Young's modulus *E*, and the mode of loading (e.g., axial tension/compression, bending, or torsion). Choosing a larger part (e.g., thicker plate, larger-diameter nail or screw) always increases construct stiffness.

N. *Flexural rigidity* is a measure of the force required to bend an object and is the product of the material Young's modulus of elasticity (*E*) and a geometric factor. For a plate with rectangular cross section, the flexural rigidity is proportional to the plate thickness to the third power (h^3). For a

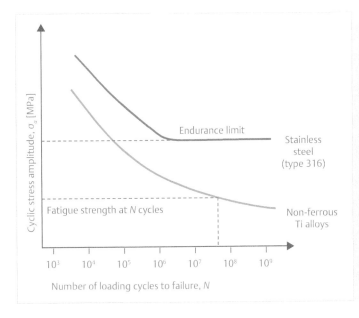

Fig. 4.2 Representative fatigue life curves for metals. Higher applied loads (higher cycle stress amplitude, σ_a) are associated with earlier fatigue failure.

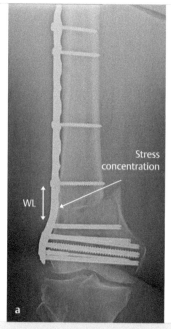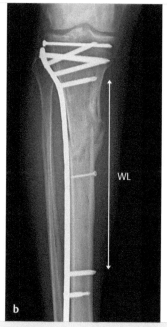

Fig. 4.3 (a) Six-month follow-up anteroposterior distal femur with plate osteosynthesis with a large fracture gap (malreduction). The working length (WL, distance between screws immediately adjacent to the fracture) is small creating a rigid implant. While the plate length (greater than 3 × WL) and screw density (< 50%) are appropriate, the screw very close to the fracture site limits the WL of the plate. The absence of callous at 6 months is due to the low-strain environment at the fracture site. The plate is experiencing high stress concentration right at the fracture site and may be subjected to failure. (b) Comminuted fracture fixed with a more flexible implant with longer WL. Callus formation is present at 3 months. Plate has stress spread across entire WL therefore minimizing strain and stress concentration. Interfragmentary screw may increase strain at main fracture site and may also cause formation of hypertrophic nonunion due to excessive strain at fracture site.

screw or pin with a circular cross section, the flexural rigidity is proportional to the radius to the fourth power (r^4).

O. *Stress concentration* or a **stress riser** describes the local high stresses that arise near a defect such as a notch or hole. Locally high stresses also occur around loading contact points, such as near bone screws or where a nail contacts the endosteal cortex.

P. *Fracture working length* is the length between fracture ends.

Q. *Implant working length* is the distance between the closest fixation points (▶Fig. 4.3).

II. Implant Construct Design and the Mechanobiology of Fracture Healing

These definitions are important to clinical practice because the mechanics of fracture fixation are an exercise in modulating strain (fracture motion) to promote the desired mode of fracture healing (primary vs. secondary).

A. Primary bone healing

1. Occurs in the presence of bony contact and the absence of fracture motion.

2. This is classically observed with simple fractures and is accomplished with interfragmentary compression.

3. Strain must be less than 2%, which is achieved with compression and the absence of a fracture gap.

B. Secondary bone healing

1. Any gap at the fracture line or flexibility in the fixation construct will allow some relative motion between the bone fragments and result in secondary healing.

2. Characterized by the formation, ossification, and later remodeling of a bridging cartilaginous callus.

3. Preferred for comminuted fractures as well as simple long bone fractures treated with intramedullary implants.

4. The magnitude and direction of the micromotion occurring at the fracture site are known to influence the speed and course of secondary healing. In general, moderate axial strains (approximately 2–10%) support callus formation maturation, whereas shear or torsional strains may disrupt callus and delay healing.

5. Excessive strain (motion) at the fracture gap may lead to nonunion.

C. Modulating strain

1. Given the absence of intraoperative "strain gauges," the surgeon must try to anticipate the postoperative demands on the construct as a result of the fracture's natural stability, patient body mass, and weight bearing restrictions.

2. Surgeons attempt to control interfragmentary strain by modulating construct stiffness. This concept bears clinical significance because a mismatch between desired healing mode and construct stiffness will lend itself to nonunion, and a fixation construct that is not strong enough or has a significant amount of strain concentrated over a small working length will fatigue prior to osseous union.

D. Example of excessive stiffness

1. Comminuted distal femur fracture with large original length where secondary bone healing is desired.

2. Application of an excessively stiff implant limits movement in a fracture that requires micromotion for callus formation.

3. In the presence of a large fracture gap or complex fracture, interfragmentary strains may be too low to allow secondary healing to occur. This can be observed clinically in locked plating constructs where no callus forms or asymmetrical callus forms only at the far cortex where some motion occurs as a result of plate bending.

4. In the absence of callus formation to support load sharing, the implant experiences high stresses during weight bearing and the construct may experience early fatigue failure.

5. To avoid this outcome, the surgeon would choose to apply implants that are less stiff/more flexible to allow some interfragmentary motion, and would design a construct that spreads the stress over a greater length.

E. Example of excessive strain

1. A simple fracture stabilized with a relatively flexible construct.

2. A very small gap such that even small relative motions between the bone ends can cause large strains because the original length across the gap is small (▶ Fig. 4.3a).

3. The excessive tissue strains may induce some resorption at the bone ends to effectively lengthen the gap and reduce the strain to more optimal levels for secondary healing.

4. However, if this does not occur, the fracture may go on to nonunion as the strain is too high for bone to bridge the gap.

5. To avoid this situation, the surgeon should be particularly wary of the simple fracture that has been compressed and stabilized with a plate that is too thin, too short, or has insufficient number of screws.

6. This situation may lead to motion at the fracture site resulting in secondary rather than primary bone healing and a greater likelihood of the construct failing before union.

F. Given the importance of interfragmentary strain for controlling the healing outcome, how then can construct stiffness be modulated to produce the desired response? The following sections provide a series of simple and intuitive guidelines to follow when considering the implant configuration and may serve as a guide to understanding and applying the biomechanical principles of fracture fixation.

III. Strategies for Modulating Stiffness, Strength, Stress, and Strain

A. Implant material

1. Titanium alloy (Ti-6Al-4V ELI or Ti-6Al-7Nb)—choose for applications requiring lower stiffness and higher strength: Young's modulus of elasticity, E = 105 to 120 GPa, tensile yield strength, $\sigma_y \geq 760$ MPa.

2. Stainless steel (AISI Type 316L)—choose for applications requiring higher stiffness and lower strength: Young's modulus of elasticity, E = 193 GPa, tensile yield strength, $\sigma_y \geq 490$ MPa.

B. Considerations for plate fixation

1. Working length:

a. Fracture working length is the distance between the closest points of fixation or the distance between screws immediately adjacent but on opposite ends of the fracture (▶ **Fig. 4.3**).

b. Working length is the most important factor affecting construct stiffness, strain at the fracture site, and stresses in the implant components.

c. Increasing the working length decreases construct stiffness and increases interfragmentary strain. Omitting screws immediately adjacent to the fracture reduces bending stresses on the plate near the fracture line and reduces the risk of premature fatigue failure. This also decreases axial and torsional stiffness thus allowing higher strains during weight bearing, so should be undertaken with caution in simple fractures if direct healing is intended.

2. Screw type:

a. Screws are often subjected to bending loads. Screw bending stiffness, or flexural rigidity, depends on the choice of material (titanium alloy or stainless steel) and screw diameter, with larger-diameter screws being exponentially stiffer than smaller-diameter screws.

b. Stability of nonlocking screws is dependent upon bone quality and friction between the bone ends (lag screw) or the plate–bone interface. Target compressive force for nonlocking screws is 3 N.

c. Locking screw stability is dependent upon the plate–screw locking mechanism.

d. Locking screw push-out strength is decreased if the screw is inserted off-axis.

e. Locking screws increase construct stiffness compared to nonlocking screws. Placing a locking screw at the end of a plate in osteoporotic bone creates a stress riser that can result in a peri-implant fracture.

f. Unicortical locking screws (screws placed into the near cortex only) are less stiff than bicortical locking screws.

g. Far cortical locking screws allow axial motion and decrease stiffness. By engaging only the far cortex while the near cortex is relatively overdrilled, these screws allow symmetric motion at the near and far cortex as the locking screw is able to bend. This theoretically leads to symmetric callus formation.

3. Screw number:

a. Increasing the screw number (plate screw density) increases construct stiffness and construct strength.

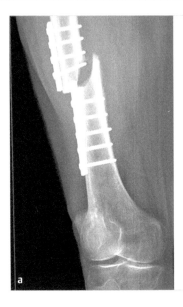 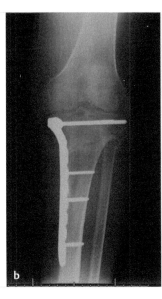

Fig. 4.4 (a) Anteroposterior radiograph of a simple femoral shaft fracture shows stress concentration over a single empty screw hole (high screw density) that may result in fatigue failure. **(b)** Anteroposterior radiograph of a tibia metaphyseal fracture stabilized with a compression plate. Distribution of screws through the plate decreases peak stress adjacent to the fracture line.

      i. Three screws on either side of a fracture maximize axial stiffness.

      ii. A fourth screw on either side of a fracture increases torsional stiffness compared to three screws.

   b. Increasing the screw number increases stress concentrations in the plate near the fracture site and can lead to fatigue failure with prolonged weight bearing in cases of delayed union or nonunion, especially when there is no bony contact for load sharing (▶ Fig. 4.4).

   c. Plate screw density is the ratio of the number of screws inserted to the number of holes in the plate.

      i. Ideal screw density for comminuted fractures is > 0.5.

      ii. Ideal screw density for simple fractures is < 0.3.

      iii. Screw density has a greater effect on stiffness in simple fractures than in comminuted fractures.

4. Plate length:

   a. Longer plates decrease the stress across the construct and increase bending flexibility (deflection) proportionally to the plate length.

   b. Longer plates decrease pullout load at each screw.

   c. Longer plates decrease peak stresses adjacent to the fracture line and therefore decrease risk of implant fatigue failure (more important for bridging constructs but also applicable to simple fractures; ▶ Fig. 4.4b).

   d. For bridging constructs, the plate length should approach three times the fracture working length.

      i. Longer plates afford lower screw density and balanced fixation which results in better distribution of stress across the construct rather than concentrating stress at empty screw holes over the fracture (▶ Fig. 4.4).

      ii. Shorter plates require increased screw density and concentrate stress at the fracture and any open screw holes.

      iii. Short plate constructs are reserved for simple fractures that are fixed with interfragmentary compression (▶ Fig. 4.5).

5. Plate thickness:

   a. Increasing plate thickness increases bending stiffness (flexural rigidity) to the third power.

   b. Thicker plates with increased prominence may cause soft tissue irritation.

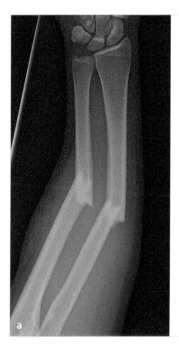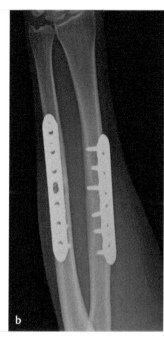

Fig. 4.5 (a, b) Simple transverse fractures fixed with interfragmentary compression and short constructs. Notice direct healing of fracture at 3 months with no callous formation. Direct bony contact protects the plate from stress during loading. The same construct with a residual fracture gap would create a high stress concentration at the plate near the fracture site due to the short construct and high screw density.

   c. Thicker plates may cause stress shielding of the underlying bone leading to resorption and a greater stress concentration at the terminal ends of the plate–bone interface. It may also cause symptomatic implants, peri-implant fracture, and greater refracture rate after implant removal.

C. Considerations for intramedullary nailing—reamed, locked intramedullary nails (IMN) are the standard of care for most diaphyseal adult fractures. Advances in nail design, interlocking screw configuration, and angularly stable interlocking screws have enhanced the biomechanical properties of IMN, and therefore extended their indications to metaphyseal and simple intra-articular fractures.

   1. Nail geometry:

      a. Slotted: A slotted nail increases friction between nail and endosteal bone through radial compression of the nail, but at the expense of torsional and bending rigidity. Historically, these nails were designed to obtain better stability within the bone before interlocking was developed.

      b. Terminal slotting: This clothespin-shaped relief slot may be found at the terminal end of a nail. This type of nail is designed to decrease rigidity and lessen the stress concentration at the terminus of the nail.

      c. Fluting: Fluting along the working length increases torsional interference between nail and bone, and decreases flexural rigidity which may be important especially in larger-diameter nails.

      d. Cannulation: Most modern nails utilize a cannulated design to facilitate nail insertion over a guide wire without compromising size of the outer nail diameter.

      e. Diameter: Nail diameter is chosen to suit patient anatomy and ensure good cortical contact after reaming (if done). A larger diameter increases bending stiffness (flexural rigidity) and torsional stiffness in proportion to $(r_{outer}^4 - r_{inner}^4)$ for cannulated nails. Larger nails typically accommodate larger screws and so have reduced risk of early construct fatigue failure.

      f. Length: Nail length is chosen to suit patient anatomy, except in short nails which produce stiffer constructs due to their shorter working length and which typically terminate in the isthmus.

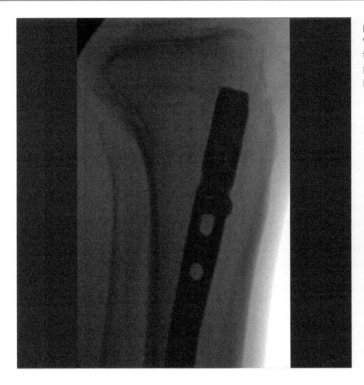

Fig. 4.6 Screw in the dynamic slot. When loading a length unstable fracture, the nail will migrate proximally around the screw in the proximal end of the slot.

g. Anterior bow of the femur: Mismatch between nail and femur anterior bow increases point contact and frictional fit. The point contact can result in malreduction, iatrogenic fracture, or anterior cortical perforation.

2. Reaming:

a. Allows a larger-diameter nail with benefits stated above (i.e., increased stiffness, larger screws, reduced risk of fatigue failure).

b. Increases the area of direct contact between endosteal bone and nail, which can help minimize undesirable interfragmentary shear and increase load sharing by the bone to decrease risk of fatigue failure.

3. Interlocking screws:

a. Static screws: Screws placed in tightly fitting holes allow very little relative movement and this provides axial and rotational stability for the construct.

b. Dynamic screw: A single screw placed in a short slot can allow axial shortening for use in intraoperative fracture compression or as postoperative intervention in cases of delayed union or nonunion (▶ Fig. 4.6). In length-stable fractures, this allows compression with weight bearing and may stimulate healing.

c. Screw diameter: Larger-diameter screws have increased bending stiffness (flexural rigidity) and reduced risk of fatigue failure. Choosing a large diameter increases bending strength of screw and reduces construct failure especially in length unstable fractures.

d. Angularly stable screws: Some implant systems have design features that enable mechanical coupling between one or more screws and the nail body to increase the rigidity of the construct, particularly in torsion. Examples include threaded or partially threaded screw holes, polymer bushings in the screw holes or sleeves added to the screw prior to insertion, and locking or compression endcaps.

e. Number of screws: Addition of a third screw increases stiffness in the proximal tibia metaphysis. This benefit is not observed in the distal tibia.

    f. Screw distance to fracture: Screws positioned closer to metaphyseal fractures afford greater rotational control, but do not increase axial stability.

    g. Screw orientation: Oblique interlocking screws increase stability of proximal one-third tibia constructs but not distal one-third tibia constructs.

Summary

Bone fracture healing is a complex mechanoresponsive process that is biologically regulated by the mechanical conditions at the fracture site over the course of healing. In fracture management, surgeons may stabilize broken bones with plates, intramedullary devices, external fixators, or external splints, casts, or braces. These constructs allow the surgeon to tailor the mechanical environment to suit the individual needs of the patient by selecting the implant length, implant thickness or diameter, screw number, screw type, and screw configuration. Each decision alters the fracture's biomechanical environment, which in turn determines if the fracture will attempt to heal with callus (relative stability leading to secondary healing) or without callus (absolute stability or interfragmentary compression leading to primary healing). A sound understanding of fracture fixation biomechanics is the foundation upon which a surgeon's treatment will succeed or fail. This chapter introduced basic definitions and principles of biomechanics as they apply to trauma implants and describe techniques for altering the implant construct mechanics to achieve the desired mode of healing and minimize the risk of premature construct failure.

Suggested Readings

Bottlang M, Doornink J, Lujan TJ, et al. Effects of construct stiffness on healing of fractures stabilized with locking plates. J Bone Joint Surg Am 2010;92(Suppl 2):12–22

Perren SM. Evolution of the internal fixation of long bone fractures. The scientific basis of biological internal fixation: choosing a new balance between stability and biology. J Bone Joint Surg Br 2002;84(8):1093–1110

Stoffel K, Dieter U, Stachowiak G, Gächter A, Kuster MS. Biomechanical testing of the LCP: how can stability in locked internal fixators be controlled? Injury 2003;34(Suppl 2):B11–B19

Törnkvist H, Hearn TC, Schatzker J. The strength of plate fixation in relation to the number and spacing of bone screws. J Orthop Trauma 1996;10(3):204–208

5 How to Analyze a Journal Article?

Gregory J. Della Rocca

Introduction

This original chapter breaks down the basic components of a journal article. Common statistical methods are introduced and different types of scientific studies are defined. Insight is provided on how to critically analyze scientific literature.

Keywords: journal article, levels of evidence, statistics, scientific studies

I. Components of a Standard Article

A. Introduction
   1. Sets the groundwork for the manuscript.
   2. Provides background information detailing why the research question is being asked:
      a. Typically acknowledges gaps in knowledge.
      b. Reinforces the clinical relevance of the topic.
   3. Clearly defines the research question(s).

B. Methods
   1. Should be sufficiently complete to allow the reader to duplicate the study, if desired.
   2. Description of the inclusion/exclusion criteria, intervention (i.e., study arms), how data was gathered and analyzed, and ethical approval (if applicable).

C. Results
   1. Succinct and clear presentation of study findings. A well-written results section is organized and follows a logical progression. When applicable, data presentation should mimic the order in which research questions are posed in the last paragraph of the introduction.
   2. Figures/tables should always be referenced in the text of the manuscript.
   3. Interpretation of study findings should not be included in this section.

D. Discussion
   1. Perhaps the least relevant part of the manuscript for the knowledgeable reader.
   2. Perhaps the most important part of the manuscript for the reader with minimal knowledge.
   3. Recognize that author opinions are often expressed in this section (these may be incorrect).
   4. Pay close attention to a description of study weaknesses.
      a. Study limitations should be appropriately identified.
      b. The impact of limitations and weaknesses should be explained.
   5. Allows study results to be placed into context of the recent literature.
   6. Directions of future investigations outlined.

E. Abstract
   1. Should provide concise summary of study.
   2. Often the only part of the article that is read by the public.
   3. If findings are interesting, care is required to verify if the abstract and the body of the manuscript are consistent with each other.
   4. Do the authors draw conclusions based upon their data? (Answer: not always).

F. Title

1. Should grab attention without being flashy.

2. Is the title an accurate portrayal of the study report? (Answer: not always).

II. Types of Studies

A. Experimental (▶ **Fig. 5.1**)

1. Prospective, randomized controlled trial:

    a. One or more interventions with a "control" group.

    b. Patient enters study at beginning of treatment via a randomization process and data is gathered moving forward.

    c. Defined end points.

        i. Primary outcome: Did the intervention change the rate of occurrence of this outcome? For example, did infection of an open fracture requiring surgical intervention occur more or less frequently with the intervention than in the control group? These are usually discrete (yes/no, defined time points, quantifiable).

        ii. Secondary outcomes: Did the intervention change rates of occurrence for one or more other outcomes? For example, did patients with open fractures in the intervention group report improved or poorer outcomes than in the control group? These should be as discrete as possible but could be qualitative.

2. Prospective cohort comparison study (nonrandomized controlled trial):

    a. Gathers data moving forward for similar patients provided two or more differing treatments determined by other factors besides randomization.

    b. Less controlled studies at risk of selection bias (e.g., surgeon preference, patient desires, etc.).

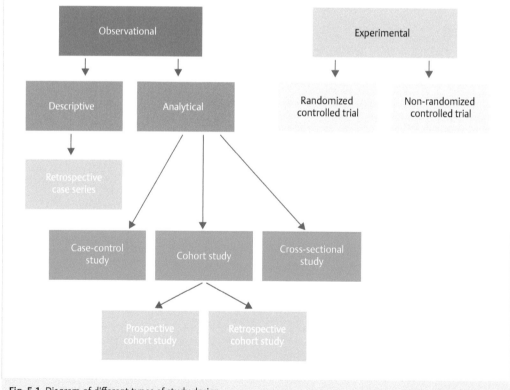

Fig. 5.1 Diagram of different types of study design.

B. Observational
 1. Descriptive:
  a. Retrospective case series:
   i. Report of a group of patients with a similar condition and/or treatment without any comparison group.
   ii. Often represents a report of a single individual's or institution's experience.
   iii. May be beneficial if reporting a group of patients with bad outcomes, in that it can help guide physicians away from dangerous interventions (e.g., Kirschner wire fixation of femur fractures results in 100% nonunion rates and 95% infection rates).
   iv. Limited value if reporting a group of patients with good outcomes, in that it does not provide evidence that the intervention is better or worse than other commonly accepted interventions.
 2. Analytical:
  a. Prospective cohort study:
   i. Gathers data moving forward on a novel treatment without a different intervention group.
   ii. Patients are identified based on exposure (e.g., femur fracture) and followed over time to determine who develops a particular outcome of interest (e.g., infection, nonunion).
   iii. Prospective cohort study with historical controls. Data collected are analyzed and compared to data already in existence at a given institution or to historical reports in the literature.
  b. Retrospective cohort comparison studies:
   i. Data is already in existence at the time of study development.
   ii. Normally entail medical record review (and radiographic review if applicable).
   iii. Two or more different treatments are then compared based upon data already in existence with respect to the development of an outcome(s) of interest.
   iv. Disadvantage—if data points do not exist, then a potentially important question may not be answered.
  c. Case-control study:
   i. Retrospective study that determines if an exposure is associated with an outcome.
   ii. Patients with a specific outcome or disease such as arthritis ("the cases") are compared to patients without arthritis ("the control") and the incidence of potential risk factor(s), such as obesity, are explored in both groups.
   iii. Better for rare outcomes as smaller numbers are necessary.
  d. Cross-sectional study.

III. Levels of Evidence

A. Types of studies
 1. Diagnostic—investigates a diagnostic test/protocol.
 2. Prognostic—investigates a characteristic of patients and its effect on disease outcomes.
 3. Therapeutic—most common in orthopaedics; investigates the results of a treatment.
 4. Economic—generally related to cost/value proportions.
B. Retrospective versus prospective
 1. A retrospective study has the study question formulated AFTER data acquisition.
 2. A prospective study has the study question formulated PRIOR to acquisition of any data.
C. Levels (for diagnostic, prognostic, and therapeutic studies)
 1. Level I—randomized controlled trials, inception cohort studies, testing of previously developed diagnostic tests.

2. Level II—prospective cohort (comparative) studies, development of diagnostic criteria (rigorous standards of references and blinding), dramatic effect observational studies.

3. Level III—case-control studies, retrospective cohort (comparative) study, diagnostic studies without consistently applied reference standards.

4. Level IV—case series, patient series with historical control group, poor reference standard diagnostic studies.

5. Level V—opinions (reasoning).

6. Systematic reviews/meta-analyses—level is determined based upon quality of evidence reviewed.

   a. These types of manuscripts represent studies of results from at least two previously published studies.

   b. Level I—review of randomized controlled studies (homogeneity of studies is necessary).

   c. Level II—review of cohort studies (or heterogeneous [inconsistent results noted between] randomized controlled studies).

   d. Level III—review of case-control studies.

IV. Basic Statistical Interpretation

A. Definitions

1. Null hypothesis:

   a. According to this, in a population, two interventions (or an intervention and a nonintervention) will result in no difference in outcomes.

   b. Often presented in the negative (i.e., an intervention being studied will NOT affect the outcome).

2. Alternative hypothesis:

   a. In a population, an intervention will result in a difference in outcome.

   b. Often presented in the positive (i.e., an intervention being studied WILL affect the outcome).

3. *P*-value:

   a. A probability that the null hypothesis will be accepted (and the alternative hypothesis will be rejected).

   b. Often set at < 0.05 for statistical significance (i.e., there is < 5% chance that the null hypothesis will be accepted).

4. Power:

   a. A trial should be big enough to detect a statistically significant effect, if it exists, and to be reasonably sure that no effect exists if none detected by the trial.

   b. Calculation based upon data in existence (such as previously published) or based upon assumptions.

   c. Authors need to determine a minimum clinically important difference (MCID) in order to perform this calculation.

   d. Underpowered studies may not be clinically relevant, even if the *p*-values indicate statistical significance (a larger sample size may cause a change in the results).

5. Fragile *p*-value:

   a. Beware when one group in a comparison study has zero events.

      i. Were there no events because there never will be events, or were there no events because the sample size was not big enough?

      ii. The *p*-value could change substantially if one event occurs.

    b. Beware when a small sample size results in outcomes that are marginally different between the two cohorts and yet result in a *p*-value that is significant (e.g., 10 coin flips give 4 heads and 6 tails; it is unlikely that tails are the more likely result, and instead 100 flips might demonstrate that the results are closer to 50:50).

6. Confidence interval (CI):

    a. Generally provided as 95% CI—there is a 95% chance that a repeat of a study will demonstrate differences or similarities within the range given. For example, medication A reduces systolic blood pressure by 12 points and medication B reduces systolic blood pressure by 20 points. The average reduction is 8 points, with a 95% CI of 3–12. So, 95% of trials that are duplicates of this study should yield a reduction in systolic blood pressure of 3 to 12 points.

    b. Larger trials result in smaller CIs.

7. Diagnostic parameters (▶ **Fig. 5.2**):

    a. Sensitivity—how good is the test at picking up a condition (true positives)?

    b. Specificity—how good is the test at excluding those without a condition (true negatives)?

    c. Positive predictive value—if a test reveals that a condition exists, how likely is it that the condition exists (probability)?

    d. Negative predictive value—if a test reveals that the condition does not exist, how likely is it that the condition does not exist (probability)?

B. Tests used routinely in orthopaedic trauma manuscripts

1. Chi-square (χ^2) test—tests the likelihood that two separate samples are different:

    a. Comparison of *categorical* variables (e.g., yes/no; infection present or absent).

    b. Fisher's exact test similarly compares categorical variables and is typically used when sample sizes are small; chi-square test is used when sample sizes are large.

		TRUTH	
		Disease present (tibia infection)	Disease absent (no tibia infection)	
TEST	Test positive for infection (new culture swab positive)	60 (true positive; TP)	30 (false positive; FP)	Positive predictive value = TP / (TP + FP) = 60/90 = 67%
	Test negative for infection (new culture swab negative)	20 (False negative; FN)	200 (True negative; TN)	Negative predictive value = TN / (FN + TN) = 200/220 = 91%
		Sensitivity = TP / (TP + FN) = 60/80 = 75%	Specificity = TN / (FP + TN) = 200/230 = 87%	

Fig. 5.2 Example of a sensitivity and specificity table evaluating a new test (culture swab) for diagnosis of a disease (tibia infection).

2. One-sample (paired) *t* test or Wilcoxon rank sum test—tests the likelihood that two different measurements in the same sample are different. Comparison of *continuous* variables.

3. Two-sample (unpaired) *t* test or Mann–Whitney U test—tests the likelihood that two separate samples from the same population are different.

4. Analysis of variance (ANOVA)—tests the likelihood that three or more sets of observations made on a single sample are different.

5. Pearson's or Spearman's test—if a straight-line association exists between two continuous variables, what is the strength of that association?

6. Linear regression—describes a numerical relationship between two variables.

7. Multiple regression—describes a numerical relationship between one dependent variable and multiple (at least two) other covariates.

V. Critical Analysis of a Journal Article

A. Review the abstract first.
   1. Does it catch your attention?
   2. Does the research question make sense? Does it matter?
   3. Are the authors' conclusions derived from the data presented?
   4. Is it clearly presented?

B. Review methods next.
   1. Careful review of inclusion/exclusion criteria and interventions (and control groups).
   2. Can the study be duplicated based upon the method presented (i.e., if the methods are followed by another group, can the study be performed by them?)?
   3. Was ethical approval obtained?
   4. Are there any sources of bias?
      a. Check conflicts of interest.
      b. Selection bias—occurs when the sample analyzed is not representative of the intended population. Problematic with retrospective trials as treatments provided may have been selected based upon surgeon preference, for example, unblinding of interventions in randomized trials.
      c. Interventions are applied by standardization of application (i.e., all patients with condition X received either treatment A or B in a randomized fashion).
      d. Outcomes are presented by standardized measurements (i.e., all patients who received a given treatment provided patient-centered outcomes scores, and objective clinical outcomes as measured clinically and radiographically were also consistently reported).
   5. Is there sufficient follow-up to determine efficacy in a therapeutic trial?

C. Review the results.
   1. Are the results presented in abstract consistent with results presented in body of manuscript?
   2. Often, more results are presented in manuscript body than in the abstract.
   3. Carefully pay attention to figures and tables (some journals require that all results be presented in table and figure form in addition to prose).

D. Introduction and discussion
   1. These sections are potentially more beneficial for the novice reader.
   2. Often set the context for the research question and can provide context for use of the results in the scheme of current practice.
   3. These sections often represent authors' opinions and are potentially least helpful to the intermediate/expert reader.

E. References
    1. Pay attention to references from reputable journals.
        a. A foreign journal is not disreputable.
        b. Some open-access journals are very respectable.
    2. If many references are from textbooks, be wary.
        a. Textbooks/review articles may quote literature incorrectly.
        b. A reference to a textbook or review article which misquotes the literature is misleading (perhaps unintentionally).
        c. Always go back to source literature (primary research articles), when possible.

Suggested Readings

Greenhalgh T. How to Read a Paper. 5th ed. Wiley Blackwell and BMJ Books, West Sussex, United Kingdom; 2014

JBJS Inc. Levels of Evidence, https://journals.lww.com/jbjsjournal/Pages/Journals-Level-of-Evidence.aspx. Accessed January 17, 2018

Kirkwood BR, Sterne JAC. Essential medical statistics, 2nd ed. Blackwell Science Ltd, Oxford, United Kingdom; 2003

6 Acute Infection Following Musculoskeletal Surgery

Frank R. Avilucea and William T. Obremskey

Introduction

Postoperative infection following internal fixation involves the soft tissues (skin, subcutaneous tissues, muscle fascia, and muscle), hardware, and potentially the bone. The infection is typically bacterial (▶**Video 6.1**).

I. Preoperative

A. History and physical exam
   1. Presentation:
      a. Purulent discharge from the surgical site and/or incision with or without associated erythema, tenderness, or fever.
      b. Symptoms (local or regional pain or joint stiffness) which may be less obvious signs of infection.
      c. Absence of radiologic evidence of bone healing after several months, with or without fixation failure, may also suggest infection.
      d. Intermittent fevers, chills, sweats (particularly, night sweats in the setting of chronic infections), and general malaise are common symptoms.
      e. An untreated infection may progress rapidly and threaten the limb, lead to septic shock, or even lead to death.
   2. Physical exam findings at the surgical site:
      a. Pain.
      b. Erythema or overlying cellulitis (▶**Fig. 6.1**).
      c. Drainage.
      d. External appearance may be benign with deep space infection.
   3. Host risk factors for developing infection:
      a. Diabetes mellitus.
         i.   Perioperative hyperglycemia.
         ii. Micro- and macrovascular disease.
         iii. Immunologic dysfunction.
      b. Peripheral vascular disease.
      c. Malnutrition.

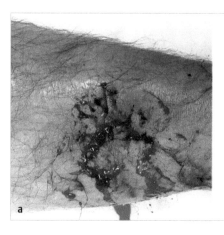
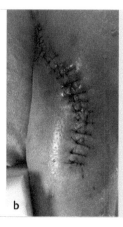

Fig. 6.1 Clinical photos demonstrating varied clinical presentation of deep infection (**a, b**). High suspicion is necessary for post-operative surgical sites with atypical findings or patient reporting increased pain.

    d. Obesity.

    e. Advanced age.

    f. Immunocompromised (HIV).

    g. Immunomodulating drugs:

        i. Steroid treatment.

        ii. Chemotherapy (cancer treatment).

        iii. Disease-modifying anti-rheumatic drugs (DMARDs) for autoimmune disorders.

    h. Polytrauma.

II. Anatomy of Infection

A. Superficial surgical site infection

    1. Early fracture site colonization and proliferation.

    2. Affects the incision but does not extend to the fracture site and remains superficial to the level of the fascia.

B. Deep surgical site infection

    1. Infection that penetrates deep to fascia and involves the fracture site.

    2. Surgical devices represent a substrate for microbial colonization and biofilm-associated infection.

      a. Variety of organisms have been associated with indwelling implants, some of the most common are:

        i. Staphylococcus (aureus, epidermidis).

        ii. Streptococcus pyogenes.

        iii. Klebsiella pneumoniae.

        iv. Pseudomonas aeruginosa.

        v. Acinetobacter baumannii.

        vi. Escherichia coli.

    3. Pathogenesis of biofilm includes following four stages (▶ Fig. 6.2):

      a. Planktonic—free-floating which represents the inoculation phase.

      b. Sessile phase: bacteria settle and form a mature biofilm.

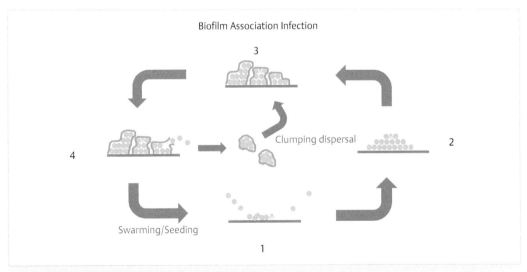

Fig. 6.2 Biofilm pathogenesis. 1. Planktonic bacteria attachment: reversible and bacteria susceptible to antibiotics and rinsing. 2. Micro-colonies develop: reversible and bacteria susceptible to antibiotics and rinsing. 3. Continued cell division: more adhesion sites, matrix formation, and biofilm maturation. 4. Detachment: liberate planktonic bacteria or small segments and plankontic bacterial may relocate and colonize other surfaces.

    c. Persister cells: dormant, multidrug tolerant cells that live within mature biofilm and have the ability to repopulate the biofilm.

    d. Quorum-sensing molecules: chemomodulators within a mature biofilm permitting intercellular communication to permit bacterial resistance.

III. Serologic Analysis

A. Subacute postoperative period

    1. Markers of inflammation, such as erythrocyte sedimentation rate (ESR) and C-reactive protein (CRP), are routinely elevated in response to traumatic and surgical events (low specificity for infection diagnosis).

    2. The magnitude of inflammatory marker elevation may be valuable.

    3. The change of CRP over time is helpful rather than the overall value.

B. Chronic infection

    1. ESR and CRP are sensitive markers of infection and relatively nonspecific.

    2. Twenty percent of patients undergoing nonunion repair with normal preoperative inflammatory markers may be culture-positive at the time of surgery.

IV. Imaging

A. Diagnostic imaging in the weeks immediately following operative care often fails to show changes that are commonly seen over the course of time.

B. Computed tomography or ultrasound may provide findings of an abscess or presence of air. Such findings may either guide percutaneous drainage with a needle or direct surgical debridement.

V. Classification

Infections are typically referred to as superficial or deep according to whether the infection has penetrated deep to the fascia.

VI. Treatment

A. Surgical debridement (▶ Fig. 6.3)

    1. Excision of all infected and nonviable tissue may require several operations.

    2. Retention versus removal of implants with staged internal fixation after temporary fixation (typically external fixation).

    3. Mechanical debridement of implant surfaces.

    4. Local antibiotic delivery.

    5. Soft tissue coverage as necessary.

B. Antibiotic therapy

    1. Six weeks of intravenous (IV) antibiotics is a commonly employed regimen.

    2. No conclusive evidence on the effectiveness of IV compared to PO regimens. Basic science and clinical series have not shown a clear benefit of IV antibiotics to date; although, both are routinely used in clinical practice.

C. Modifiable risk factors should be addressed to optimize treatment(s) as local host factors related to reduced host vascularity, neuropathy, trauma, and immunodeficiency increase the likelihood of infection.

D. Predictors of eradication of infection and limb salvage

    1. Short-term implant.

    2. Absence of a sinus tract.

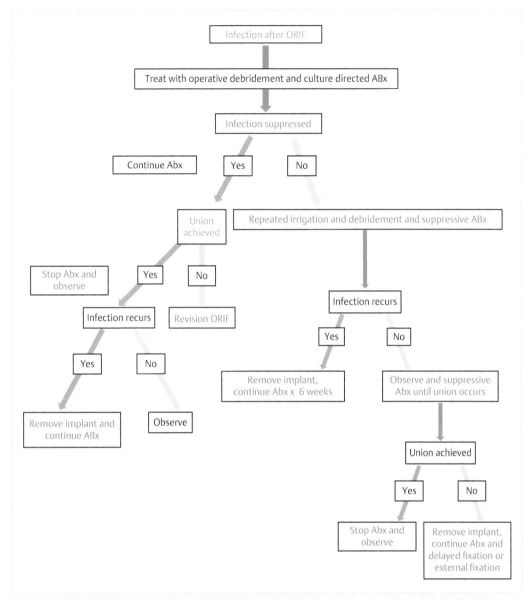

Fig. 6.3 Treatment algorithm for acute infection following internal fixation for trauma. ORIF, open reduction and internal fixation.

3. Known pathogen susceptible to antibiotics.

4. Stable implant.

E. Predictors of treatment failure include:

1. Intramedullary rod placement.

2. Smoking.

3. *Pseudomonas* infection.

F. Biopsy

1. Several deep tissue samples should be taken.

   a. These should be taken as far apart as possible to represent the entire wound.

   b. Superficial swabs may only identify local flora and are discouraged.

G. Factors that prompt implant removal
   1. Persistent infection.
   2. Loose hardware.
   3. Fracture displacement.
H. If implants are removed prior to fracture healing, ensure that fracture stabilization is achieved.
   1. Splinting.
   2. Revision internal fixation.
   3. External fixation.
I. If implants are removed and bone resection is necessary
   1. External fixation
      a. Place antibiotic spacer and proceed with Masquelet technique.
      b. Bone transport.

VII. Outcomes

A. Implant retention—success rates of curing early postoperative infection with maintenance of hardware range from 68 to 90% with surgical debridement and treatment with culture-specific antibiotics.
   1. Consider elective removal of hardware after bony union.
B. Implant removal—successful eradication of infection reaches 92% before bony union.
   1. Must outweigh the benefits of fracture stabilization.
   2. Consider an alternative method of fracture stabilization.
C. Factors increasing risk of treatment failure.
   1. Smoking.
   2. *Pseudomonas* infection.
   3. Intramedullary nail (IMN).
   4. Tibia.
   5. Need for two or more debridements.

VIII. Complications

A. Recurrence of infection following successful bony healing requires removal of hardware, debridement, and treatment with antibiotics.
B. Infected nonunion
   1. Removal of hardware, aggressive debridement.
   2. Culture-directed antibiotic treatment for 6 weeks.
   3. Repeat open reduction and internal fixation versus external fixation.
C. Septic arthritis.
D. Osteomyelitis.
E. Amputation.

IX. Special Considerations—Pediatric Population

A. Concern for septic arthritis due to bacterial seeding.
B. Inability to ambulate with a remote history of trauma may suggest infection.

Conclusion

Infection after internal fixation of fractures is one of the most common complications. Infections significantly increase the cost and the morbidity of an injury. By following standardized diagnosis and treatment regimens outcomes can be optimized. Surgeons need to assure diagnosis of infection, optimize the patient by improving host factors as much as possible and utilizing a multidisciplinary team. A thorough operative debridement of all necrotic and infected tissue is critical. The surgeon then needs to decide to retain or remove implants with a immediate or staged revision fixation. Antibiotics should be culture driven if possible and can be administered intravenous or by oral methods. Adequate soft tissue coverage may require a rotational or free flap. Without a standardized process and multidisciplinary team patients are at risk for persistent infection and/or amputation.

Suggested Readings

Berkes M, Obremskey WT, Scannell B, Ellington JK, Hymes RA, Bosse M; Southeast Fracture Consortium. Maintenance of hardware after early postoperative infection following fracture internal fixation. J Bone Joint Surg Am 2010;92(4):823–828

Darouiche RO. Treatment of infections associated with surgical implants. N Engl J Med 2004;350(14):1422–1429

Lawrenz JM, Frangiamore SJ, Rane AA, Cantrell WA, Vallier HA. Treatment approach for infection of healed fractures after internal fixation. J Orthop Trauma 2017;31(11):e358–e363

Meehan AM, Osmon DR, Duffy MC, Hanssen AD, Keating MR. Outcome of penicillin-susceptible streptococcal prosthetic joint infection treated with debridement and retention of the prosthesis. Clin Infect Dis 2003;36(7):845–849

Rightmire E, Zurakowski D, Vrahas M. Acute infections after fracture repair: management with hardware in place. Clin Orthop Relat Res 2008;466(2):466–472

Stucken C, Olszewski DC, Creevy WR, Murakami AM, Tornetta P. Preoperative diagnosis of infection in patients with nonunions. J Bone Joint Surg Am 2013;95(15):1409–1412

Trebse R, Pisot V, Trampuz A. Treatment of infected retained implants. J Bone Joint Surg Br 2005;87(2):249–256

Zimmerli W, Widmer AF, Blatter M, Frei R, Ochsner PE; Foreign-Body Infection (FBI) Study Group. Role of rifampin for treatment of orthopedic implant-related staphylococcal infections: a randomized controlled trial. JAMA 1998;279(19):1537–1541

7 Nonunion and Malunion

David B. Weiss and Michael M. Hadeed

Introduction

The goal of orthopaedic fracture care is to treat fractures in a way that minimizes complications while maximizing functional outcomes. This includes both operative and nonoperative management.

Bone healing is typically robust and dependable; however, it can fail. When it does, it can result in a nonunion or a malunion. It is critical to understand both the natural history and effect of interventions on bone healing as operative indications are often based on the ability to decrease the chance of nonunion and malunion.

When a patient develops a nonunion or a malunion, the cost to the health care system and society is great, as it typically results in multiple surgical procedures and extended time away from normal activities. A tibial nonunion has been compared to having an effect on health and wellbeing similar to some cancer or other chronic illness diagnoses.

To understand malunions and nonunions, it is critical to have a basic understanding of bone healing and the biomechanics of fracture repair (discussed in depth in Chapter 1, Physiology of Fracture Healing, and Chapter 4, Biomechanics of Internal Fracture Fixation). When approaching these difficult cases, it is important to have a stepwise, reproducible approach, make the diagnosis using the history, physical exam, laboratory and radiographic data. Try to determine the causative factor. Based on patient-specific variables, develop a treatment plan with a reasonable chance of success (▶**Video 7.1**).

Keywords: nonunion, malunion, hypertrophic, atrophic, bone graft

I. Assessment of Nonunions

Factors leading to nonunion can generally be grouped into two categories: biologic and mechanical. The assessment is a gathering of data on known factors which may have contributed to a failure of the biologic and mechanical success of the fracture healing.

A. History

    1. Common presenting symptoms:

        a. Pain at the fracture site (increased with weightbearing).

        b. Subjective feelings of instability in the affected bone.

        c. Symptoms (or history of symptoms) associated with infection: erythema, swelling, drainage, fevers, chills.

    2. The data of patient-specific risk factors is obtained after completing a thorough history with each individual patient.

        a. Demographic/patient directed risk factors:

            i. Smoking has negative effects on many pathways necessary for bone healing.

            ii. Nicotine diminishes arterial blood flow.

            iii. Nonsteroidal anti-inflammatory drugs negatively affect the pathways responsible for bone healing.

            iv. In some studies, female patients and older patients had an increased rate of nonunion.

            v. Poor nutrition is associated with nonunion.

        b. Associated comorbidities:

            i. Metabolic and endocrine dysfunction can impair fracture healing.

            ii. Diseases that negatively affect vascularity, such as diabetes mellitus and other vascular disorders, can impair fracture healing.

3. Fracture-dependent risk factors are independent of the patient; each practitioner must have an adequate baseline knowledge of previous reported literature on fracture healing.

    a. Certain bone-specific anatomy is associated with nonunion, often due to poor vascularity in these areas. Examples include:

        i. Open tibia fractures.

        ii. Intracapsular hip fractures.

        iii. Talar neck fractures.

        iv. Proximal metadiaphyseal fifth metatarsal fractures.

    b. Open fractures and bone loss are associated with increased nonunion rates. The higher the open fracture type, the greater is the risk of nonunion (and infection).

4. Risk factors from previous care:
These can be investigated using previous operative reports and medical documentation from the original perioperative period.

    a. Soft tissue destruction impairs the vascularity at the fracture site.

        i. Traumatic or surgical disruption—this can be due to vascular damage or due to excessive soft tissue stripping either from the injury or from a surgical procedure which was not biologically friendly.

    b. Interposed soft tissue at the fracture site if the fracture was not opened and debrided.

    c. History of infection at the fracture site:

        i. Previously undiagnosed infection.

        ii. Important to determine if the patient had cellulitis, wound drainage, or other concerning symptoms after the original treatment.

    d. Improper fixation—too much or too little strain at the fracture site (refer to Chapter 4, Biomechanics of Internal Fracture Fixation, for additional details).

        i. Doctor needs to critically assess the method of fixation and correlate it to the desired mode of healing at the fracture site.

        ii. Too rigid fixation in a zone of comminution will lead to a lack of callus formation.

        iii. Too flexible or inadequate fixation may cause excess soft callus to form without eventual maturation to rigid callus.

    e. Improper fixation—residual fracture gap, especially if > 1 cm.

B. Physical exam

    1. Inspection:

        a. Deformity at the fracture site—look for alterations in length, alignment, and rotation. Note if deformity occurs with passive motion or only with active motion or weight bearing.

        b. Current soft tissue envelope is very important in developing a treatment plan.

            i. Ulceration.

            ii. Open wounds.

            iii. Exposed hardware.

            iv. Damaged tissue.

        c. Evidence of decreased vascularity to the region:

            i. Previous scars.

            ii. Thin or damaged skin.

            iii. Atrophic or damaged muscle.

        d. Evidence of vascular disease:

            i. Varicosities.

            ii. Cool limbs.

            iii. Poor hair/nail growth.

            iv. Chronic erythema of skin.

2. Palpation:
   a. Tenderness at the fracture site.
   b. Pathologic motion at the fracture site (should not have any detectable motion).
   c. Palpable distal pulses indicate reliable overall vascularity.
   d. Decreased sensation distal to the fracture site is a marker for neuropathy or nerve injury.
   e. Evaluate motion at the joints above and below the nonunion site and test them both actively and passively.

3. Gait evaluation:
   a. Observe for signs of muscle weakness:
      i. Antalgic gait.
      ii. Trendelenburg gait.

C. Imaging
   1. Radiographs:
   These are the mainstay of the assessment; it is important to obtain historical imaging if the patient has been treated at other facilities. Obtain full-length anteroposterior and lateral X-rays of the involved bone. Additional oblique or specialty views may be necessary depending on the location.
   a. Expected results:
   It is important to understand what to expect on an X-ray based on the previous method of fixation (refer to Chapter 1, Physiology of Fracture Healing, for additional information).
      i. Primary bone healing—no callus.
      ii. Secondary bone healing—callus formation.
   b. General signs of nonunion:
      i. Absence of bone bridging at the fracture site/persistent fracture line. Particularly the lack of progression on serial radiographs.
      ii. Sclerotic edges at the fracture site.
      iii. Implant loosening or breakage can be indicative of pathologic motion from a nonunion.
      iv. Change in fracture alignment.
      v. Typically painful for the patient.
   c. General classification of nonunions:
   It is important to have a good working knowledge of bone healing and the biomechanics of fracture repair.
      i. Primarily mechanical issues.
      ii. Primarily biologic issues.
      iii. Combination of mechanical and biologic factors.
      iv. Several classification schemes have been developed, however understanding the principles at play is the critical aspect as the treatment will be based on addressing the mechanical and biologic factors.
      v. Weber–Cech System (▶Fig. 7.1a–c) uses the most common general descriptive breakdown based on radiographs.
         • Hypertrophic: abundant callus often indicates reasonable fracture biology but improper mechanical properties.
         • Oligotrophic: no obvious (or only a small amount) callus changes at the fracture site from bone resorption.
         • Atrophic: minimal/no callus and bone edges typically become sclerotic- must address biology (see ▶Fig. 7.2 for clinical example).
   d. Common fracture healing scores—RUST score:
      i. "Radiographic union scale in tibial" fractures.
      ii. Callus is evaluated at each of the four cortices on standard anteroposterior and lateral radiographs.

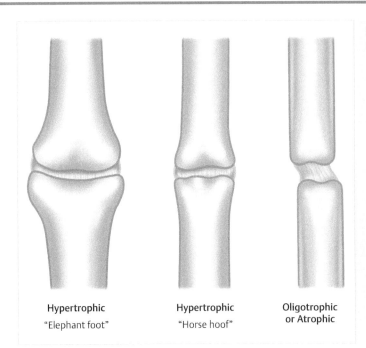

Fig. 7.1 Weber–Cech classification of nonunions.

Hypertrophic
"Elephant foot"

Hypertrophic
"Horse hoof"

Oligotrophic
or Atrophic

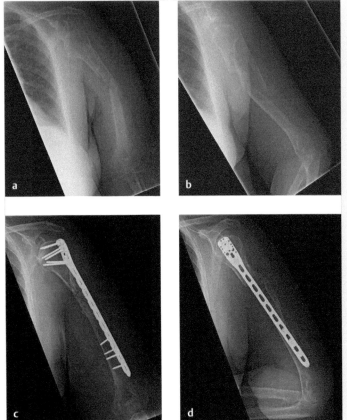

Fig. 7.2 (a, b) Anteroposterior and lateral humerus views of a 77-year-old female with an atrophic nonunion 8 months following the closed treatment with a fracture brace. Note that the bone edges appear thinned with no callus seen. The metabolic workup was negative. (c, d) Seven months after nonunion repair with rigid fixation and autogenous bone grafting demonstrating healing.

      iii. Each of the four cortices is scored between 1 and 3 and then added together for a total score of 4 to 12.
- 1 point = no callus.
- 2 points = visible fracture line with callus.
- 3 points = no fracture line with bridging callus.

      iv. A score of 9 or higher is considered a radiographically healed fracture (must match with clinical findings).
- Food and Drug Administration definition of nonunion: failure of fracture union by 9 months post injury. Clinicians will commonly use a time frame of 6 months assuming the fracture is reasonably well aligned and stable with no gaps > 1 cm. Absence of progressive signs of healing on successive radiographs can also be an indicator for nonunion.

2. Other imaging modalities:
    a. Computed tomography:
        i. One study demonstrated a significant false positive rate for nonunion.
        ii. Helpful to evaluate three-dimensional anatomy and look at the location and volume of callus, if present.
        iii. Gives an estimate of bone density and helps locate areas for future fixation if revision surgery is planned.
        iv. The image is somewhat affected by local hardware but this can be minimized with mono-energy techniques.
    b. Ultrasound:
        i. Has been shown to have very good sensitivity and specificity for tibia fracture healing.
        ii. User dependent.
        iii. Advantage of being able to adjust the beam to work around hardware but requires an experienced technician and radiologist to interpret the images.
        iv. Advantage of being a dynamic exam and so could potentially visualize motion at a nonunion site.
    c. Fluoroscopy:
        i. Beneficial when evaluating for pathologic motion.
        ii. Ability to adjust the limb in real time to obtain oblique or special images more accurately.
        iii. Images are not as crisp as standard X-rays.
    d. Bone scan:
        i. Aids in determining vascularity and ability of a fracture to heal.
        ii. Tagged white blood cell (or indium) scans are of limited value and may not be cost effective in evaluating for infection as a source of nonunion.
    e. Magnetic resonance imaging:
        i. Can be particularly helpful in cases of infection.
        ii. More susceptible to artifact from previous hardware (especially stainless steel).

D. Laboratory testing
1. Concern for infection:
    a. Infection is high on the list of differential diagnoses when searching for the etiology of a nonunion.
    b. Important to rule out infection prior to choosing a treatment plan.
    c. Lab testing can be helpful when determining whether an infection is present.
    d. Preoperatively, common laboratory values to evaluate are:
        i. Complete blood count (CBC)—often normal but may be elevated in acute osteomyelitis.
        ii. Erythrocyte sedimentation rate (ESR)—tends to rise and fall more slowly.
            - Elevation within days of insult (injury, inflammation, or infection).
            - Normalization may take up to several weeks after the insult is removed.

      iii. C-reactive protein (CRP)—tends to rise and fall quickly.
- Elevation can be observed within 4 to 6 hours of the insult.
- Reaches maximum value within 24 to 48 hours.
- Resolution within days after the insult is removed.

      iv. Both ESR and CRP may be normal or only mildly elevated in the setting of chronic osteomyelitis.

      v. ESR and CRP should be significantly elevated if acute osteomyelitis is present. The absolute values may be less important than the trend toward normal as treatment progresses appropriately.

  e. If there is a pseudoarthrosis or fluid collection adjacent to the fracture site, it is possible to aspirate the area and send it for cell count, differential, and culture with gram stain.

  f. Intraoperative tissue samples should also be sent for pathology and culture if infection is considered in the differential. If possible, have the patient discontinue any current antibiotics approximately 5 days prior to the surgery and wait on preoperative antibiotics until after cultures are obtained. This should increase the positive intraoperative culture yield.

2. Nutritional, metabolic, and endocrine:

  a. If there is clinical concern for nutritional deficiency, metabolic derangement, or endocrine abnormality which may be contributory, lab testing can often aid the diagnosis.

  b. Consultation and referral to general medicine or endocrinology is reasonable if clinical concern exists.

  c. Typical labs include infection (CBC, ESR, CRP), Vitamin D (most common associated endocrine abnormality), and nutrition (albumin, prealbumin, and total protein). Other labs to consider as more rare causes include the following: basic chemistry including calcium, magnesium, phosphorous, alkaline phosphatase, thyroid function tests, parathyroid hormone, iron studies, growth hormone, cortisol, and testosterone.

E. When to intervene operatively?

1. This is a difficult question to answer with a large subjective component; however, it is the most important decision on which all others are based.

2. Nonoperative treatment is always an option.

3. Ultimately, each case is unique and must be examined independently.

4. Several factors can help determine when to intervene:

  a. How much does the malunion/nonunion impact the patient's daily life?

  b. How much patient function can you improve with surgery?

  c. Is there a surgical option which can increase that function without exposing the patient to extreme risk?

  d. Does the surgeon have the skills and equipment necessary to complete the operation and deal with any potential intraoperative complications, or should it be referred to a specialist?

  e. Investigation of patient support system and motivation.

II. Treatment of Nonunions

A. The critical factor in finalizing a treatment plan is determining the cause of the nonunion and trying to counteract it.

1. Nonunion repair requires both the appropriate biology and the necessary mechanical stability for fracture healing.

2. The cause of nonunion can be multifactorial.

B. A comprehensive treatment is necessary to maximize chances of a successful outcome and minimize risks of complications.

C. If needed, it is imperative to consult with other specialists including infectious disease, general medicine, and endocrinology, among others.

D. Preoperative planning

1. Adequate imaging will be the foundation of the treatment plan.

2. From the imaging and previous records, it is critical to determine what, if any, implants are retained.

3. If the types of implants are unknown, the surgeon must be equipped to deal with any removal necessary to achieve the objectives of the operation.

4. With that in mind, it is important to minimize the destruction of the surrounding bone and soft tissue, if removing an implant is not critical to the success of the operation. Operative principles for most nonunions include:

   a. Exposure and debridement at the fracture site (may not be required if hypertrophic).

   b. Supplementation with biologic augments as needed. Autogenous bone graft, demineralized bone matrix, bone marrow aspirate.

   c. Rigid fixation—IM nails, plates and screws, or multiplanar external fixator.

   d. Preservation of soft tissues.

   e. Adequate treatment of known risk factors to provide an optimal chance at recovery.

   f. A frank understanding of the surgeon's limitations and abilities so that the patient is not subjected to undue risk.

   g. As a general rule:

      i. Hypertrophic nonunions require increased stability and rarely any biological augmentation.

      ii. Atrophic nonunions require biologic augmentation and typically some adjustment in mechanical stability such as compression at the fracture site to reduce gaps (▶Fig. 7.2).

5. Biologic augments:

   There are three basic properties:

   a. Osteoconductive—the graft acts as a structural frame for bone growth.

   b. Osteoinductive—stimulates bone growth by the induction of stem cells.

   c. Osteogenic—contain cells that promote bone healing.

Classes of Bone Graft (Refer to Chapter 8, Biologics, for additional information).

III. Malunion

Many of the principles discussed above in relation to nonunion also apply to malunion, particularly, the evaluation of when to intervene. For surgical correction to be considered, the malunion must be causing an unacceptable functional or cosmetic deformity.

A. Assessment

1. History:

   a. How much does the malunion affect the current activities of daily living, employment, and desired activities of the patient.

   b. What is the psychologic effect of the deformity on the patient is important to determine, yet treatment should be directed towards functional gain.

   c. Were there any issues during the previous injury or surgery which may have interfered with healing or which may have contributed to forming a malunion?

2. Physical exam—the evaluation of adjacent structures and functional impacts of malunion is critical. When evaluating and deciding whether to address a malunion with operative intervention, there are several characteristics to consider which are as follows:

   a. Limb length discrepancy (typically > 2 cm in lower extremity, 3 cm upper extremity).

   b. Clinically relevant malrotation (typically > 15–20 degrees).

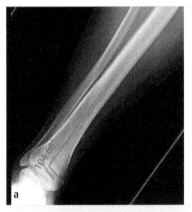 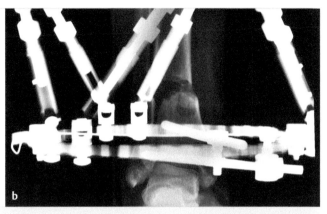

Fig. 7.3 **(a)** A 29-year-old male with a congenital 14-degree valgus deformity and 2 cm of shortening. **(b)** Osteotomy and application of circular ring fixator to gradually fix both length (via distraction osteogenesis) and alignment.

    c. Angular alignment of the deformed limb (> ~10 degrees for lower extremity and higher for upper extremity).

    d. Adjacent joint range of motion, particularly if there are contractures present.

  3. Imaging:

    a. For lower extremity deformity correction, full-length standing radiographs (anteroposterior and lateral) are extremely helpful in the evaluation and treatment planning stages.

    b. Computed tomography is particularly helpful in assessing rotation/torsion. It may be necessary to have both the affected and contralateral extremity in the scanner to provide comparison to the normal side.

B. Treatment

  1. Treatment protocols are site specific.

  2. Based on the location and extent of the deformity, it must be decided to address the issue with an acute or gradual correction.

  3. If considering a gradual correction, particularly with an external fixator, it is critical to assess the social environment of the patient to ensure that it will not place them at an unnecessarily high risk for infection or other complication.

  4. Surgical correction typically requires an osteotomy through or near the area of maximum deformity.

    a. This requires careful preoperative templating to assess the degree of correction required, and the location and position of the osteotomy.

    b. Planning will also have to account for changes in limb length and will likely determine which implant options are available and/or desirable.

    c. Typical options are plates and screws, IM nails, or external fixation.

    d. Internal fixation is typically better tolerated by patients, but the deformity must be amenable to an acute correction.

    e. For severe angular or rotational deformities or severe shortening, an external fixation-driven gradual correction is the best option (▶**Fig. 7.3**). However, there are new IM nails which can expand or contract by the daily application of external magnets and may provide an alternative to circular frames for lengthening procedures.

Conclusion

A. Nonunions and malunions are challenging problems as they are associated with high complication rates and high cost to the health care system and society.

B. Understanding the causative factor is critical to developing a successful treatment plan for nonunions. Correction of medical or other associated comorbidities (if present) is of paramount importance for a surgical procedure to be successful.

C. Understanding a patient's functional limitations due to malunion and understanding the different options available to correct them is important in developing deformity correction treatment plans.

D. Whether addressing malunion or nonunion, the decision when and on whom to intervene is of the utmost importance; nonoperative treatment is always possible.

E. A successful result is physician- and patient-dependent.

F. Understanding your own limitations will help maintain safety and minimize complications.

Suggested Readings

Brinker MR, O'Connor DP, Monla YT, Earthman TP. Metabolic and endocrine abnormalities in patients with nonunions. J Orthop Trauma 2007;21(8):557–570

Bishop JA, Palanca AA, Bellino MJ, Lowenberg DW. Assessment of compromised fracture healing. J Am Acad Orthop Surg 2012;20(5):273–282

Calori GM, Colombo M, Mazza EL, et al. Validation of the non-union scoring system in 300 long bone non-unions. Injury 2014; 45(Suppl 6):S93–S97

Cierny G III, Mader JT, Penninck JJ. A clinical staging system for adult osteomyelitis. Contemp Orthop 1985(10):17–37

Weber BG, Brunner C. The treatment of nonunions without electrical stimulation. Clin Orthop Relat Res 1981(161):24–32Nauth A, Lane J, Watson JT, Giannoudis P. Bone graft substitution and augmentation. J Orthop Trauma 2015;29(Suppl 12):S34–S38

8 Biologics

J. Tracy Watson

Introduction

This chapter reviews stages of fracture healing and the therapeutics that inhibits or augments fracture healing. Multiple adjuvants are clinically available for use. The biology of graft substitutes and mechanisms of action are discussed with each major category of adjuvant reviewed.

I. The Biology of Bone Grafts

The biology of bone grafts and their substitutes is appreciated from an understanding of the bone formation processes of osteogenesis, osteoinduction, and osteoconduction.

A. *Osteogenesis*: The ability of cellular elements within a donor graft, which survive transplantation, to synthesize new bone at the recipient site. Transplantation of marrow elements alone have demonstrated the ability to survive and form bone.

B. *Osteoconduction:* Substrate site for cellular attachment with the appropriate three-dimensional architecture to allow for these cells to proliferate. Material acts as a scaffolding through which to build bone. This three-dimensional process involves vascular proliferation and ingrowth of capillaries along the open spaces in the substrate. Therefore, the porosity of these materials is critical.

C. *Osteoinduction*: A process that supports the mitogenesis of undifferentiated mesenchymal cells leading to the formation of osteoprogenitor cells which have the capacity to form new bone. Thus, any material that induces this process could be considered to be osteoinductive material.

   1. All skeletal tissues evolve from undifferentiated mesenchymal stem cells and make a genetic commitment to a particular cellular lineage early in the developmental or repair process. The stimulus that causes these undifferentiated mesenchymal cells to differentiate along a chondro-osteogenic pathway is known as an inductive factor.

   2. These cells are influenced by multiple factors which cause them to migrate, attach, and multiply at the locale that provides a competent osteoconductive substrate as a site of cellular attachment.

   3. Osteoinductive new bone formation is realized through the active recruitment of host mesenchymal stem cells from the surrounding tissue which differentiate into bone-forming osteoblasts. This process is facilitated by the presence of "inductive" growth factors within the graft.

II. Influence of Growth Factors and Antagonists on the Phases of Fracture Healing

A. Inflammatory phase—most important for fracture healing to progress. It starts with injury and is complete within 2 to 3 weeks or earlier (▶Fig. 8.1).

   1. Hematoma invasion by macrophages, leukocytes, and lymphocytic cells.

      a. Platelets degranulate releasing signaling molecules.

         i. Transforming growth factor-beta (TGF-β) and platelet-derived growth factor (PDGF).
         ii. Promote chemotaxis, angiogenesis, and proliferation and differentiation of the cells that have migrated to the fracture.

      b. Characterized by neovascularization and ingrowth of proliferative blood vessels.

      c. Cellular attachment to extracellular matrix (ECM) and conductive substrate occurs. Integrins are membrane receptors that facilitate cell adhesion and attachment.

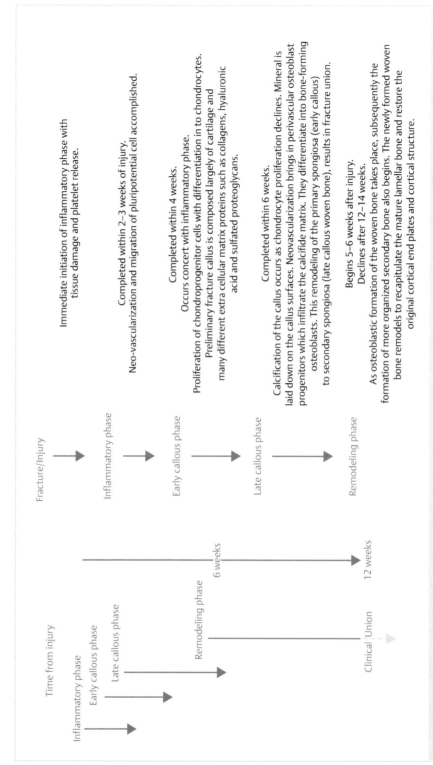

Fig. 8.1 Time table for the stages of fracture healing. This is a continuum, with all phases occurring in a sequential fashion with each phase overlapping.

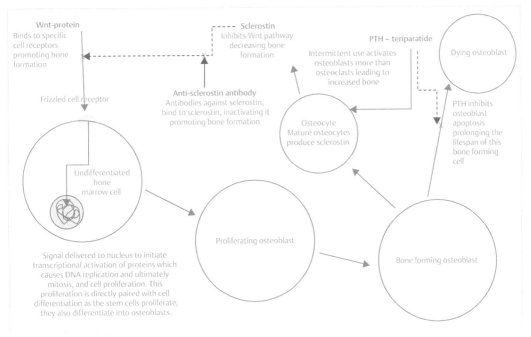

Fig. 8.2 Wnt signaling pathway, its antagonists and actions of parathyroid hormone (PTH).

2. Factors influencing the inflammatory phase—arachidonic acid metabolism.
   a. Enzymes cyclooxygenase (COX)-1 and -2 metabolize arachidonic acid to prostaglandin.
      i. COX inhibitors prevent the production of prostaglandin products. It inhibits *all* phases of the inflammatory process.
      ii. Important to refrain from these medications for the first 2 to 3 weeks post injury until inflammatory phase is complete.
   b. COX inhibitors are nonsteroidal anti-inflammatory drugs (NSAIDs). Largest effect on basic science models is either right before fracture or within the first few days following fracture.
   c. COX-2 inhibitors target COX-2 which is responsible for inflammation and pain.
   d. Targeting selectivity for COX-2 reduces peptic ulceration, but still has fracture healing side effects of NSAIDs and risk for fracture healing.
3. Wnt pathway (▶Fig. 8.2).
   a. Wnt are signal transduction pathways made of proteins that pass signals from outside a cell through cell surface receptors to the inside of the cell.
   b. Wnt regulates gene transcription conversion of undifferentiated mesenchymal stem cells into an osteoblastic lineage.
   c. Induction of the Wnt promotes bone formation; inactivation leads to osteopenia.
      i. Sclerostin produced by osteocytes inhibits the Wnt signaling pathway.
      ii. Wnt pathway inhibition leads to decreased bone formation.
4. Anti-sclerostin antibody (Romosozumab)—antibodies against sclerostin promote bone formation and increased callous size.

B. Callous phase of healing involves migration, proliferation, and differentiation of chondroprogenitor cells into chondrocytes. Cartilage callus provides immediate mechanical stability and promotes sites for cell attachment and new bone formation.

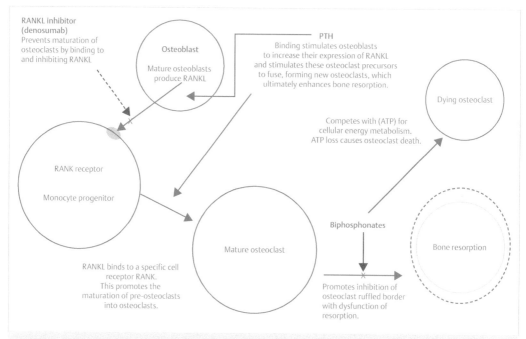

Fig. 8.3 Receptor activator of nuclear factor kappa-B ligand pathway and mechanism of action for bisphosphates.

1. Factors influencing callous phase of fracture healing (▶Fig. **8.1**).
   a. TGF-β activates fibroblasts to induce collagen formation, endothelial cells for angiogenesis, chondroprogenitor cells, and mesenchymal cells.
   b. PDGF stimulates cellular replication (mitogenesis), increasing cell populations of mesenchymal and osteoprogenitor cells.
   c. PDGF activates macrophages resulting in further debridement and triggers a second source of growth factors released from the host tissues by macrophages.
2. Mature callous phase involves mineralization of the cartilaginous callus matrix. Chondrocyte proliferation declines and hypertrophic chondrocytes predominate. Chondroclasts remove the calcified cartilage, and blood vessels develop with perivascular mesenchymal stem cells that differentiate into bone-forming osteoblasts.
3. Remodeling phase (▶Fig. **8.1**).
   a. Osteoclasts are responsible for fracture callus remodeling.
   b. Interaction between osteoblastic and osteoclastic function leads to successful remodeling.
4. Juvenile osteoblasts secrete factors that induce fully differentiated osteoblasts to express ligands that regulate the activity of osteoclasts.
5. Receptor activator of nuclear factor kappa-B ligand (RANKL), found on osteoblasts, activates osteoclasts (▶Fig. **8.3**).
   a. Osteoclastic activity is triggered by osteoblasts' surface-bound RANKL activating the osteoclasts' surface-bound RANK.
   b. Activation of RANK by RANKL promotes the maturation of preosteoclasts into osteoclasts.
6. RANKL inhibitor, denosumab prevents maturation of osteoclasts by binding to and inhibiting RANKL.

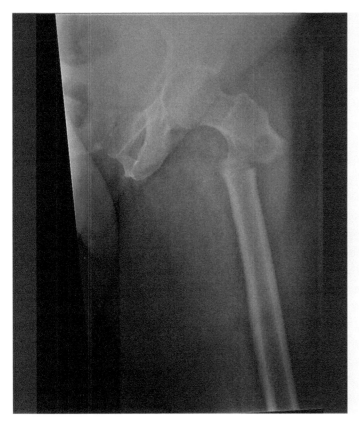

Fig. 8.4 Radiograph of a patient with a complete atypical femoral fracture. Note the substantially transverse orientation of the fracture line at the lateral cortex, the medial spike, and the generalized cortical thickening.

7. Estrogen inhibits the formation and activation of the bone-resorbing osteoclasts via suppression of RANKL signaling within the osteoclast.

8. Parathyroid hormone (PTH) binds to osteoblasts (osteoclasts *do not* have a receptor for PTH) stimulating them to increase expression of RANKL.

    a. PTH also inhibits osteoblast expression of osteoprotegerin (OPG).

    b. The binding of RANKL to RANK stimulates osteoclast precursors to fuse, forming new osteoclasts, which enhances bone resorption.

    c. Teriparatide (Forteo) is the recombinant form of PTH. Intermittent use activates osteoblasts more than osteoclasts and leads to an overall increase in bone.

    d. Teriparatide is used in the treatment of some forms of osteoporosis.

9. Bisphosphonates inhibit the digestion of bone by encouraging osteoclasts to undergo apoptosis which leads to slowing of bone loss (▶ Fig. 8.3).

    a. There are two classes of bisphosphonates: the *N*-containing and non-*N*-containing bisphosphonates.

        i.   Non-nitrogenous bisphosphonates (diphosphonates) are metabolized and replace terminal pyrophosphate moiety of adenosine triphosphate (ATP), forming a nonfunctional molecule. It competes with ATP for cellular energy metabolism. ATP loss causes osteoclast death, with decrease in the breakdown of bone.

        ii. Nitrogenous bisphosphonates promote inhibition of osteoclast ruffled border with dysfunction of resorption.

    b. Long-term bisphosphonate use can result in oversuppression of bone turnover (atypical femoral fractures; ▶ Fig. 8.4).

III. Categories of Available Biologic Adjuvants for Clinical Use

A. Autogenous cellular materials (osteogenic) (▶Table 8.1).

1. Autogenous iliac crest bone graft (AICBG, gold standard)—other sites include posterior iliac crest, proximal tibia, distal femur, calcaneus, and distal radius. Rapid revascularization occurs and performs best in well-vascularized beds.

   a. Approximately 30 mL of graft reliably harvested from an anterior iliac crest.

   b. Complications related to the harvest and limited availability.

2. Reamer Irrigator Aspirator (RIA; Synthes, Paoli, PA)—the medullary canal of the femur or tibia is reamed with a collection device and delivers 30 to 90 mL for grafting.

   a. Elevated osteoinductive growth factors, osteoprogenitor/endothelial progenitor cell types are used compared to AICBG.

   b. Cell viability and osteogenic potential is equal in both RIA and AICBG.

3. Bone marrow aspirate concentrate (BMAC; ▶Fig. 8.5).

   a. BMAC has a high concentration of viable connective tissue progenitors for grafting.

   b. Bone formation is dependent on the number of cells available in the graft.

      i. Technologies include methods for harvest and concentration of bone-forming cells.

      ii. Implanted BMAC combined with bioactive scaffold matrix allow differentiation into an osteoblastic cell lineage for bone repair.

      iii. Allogeneic human undifferentiated mesenchymal "stem cell grafts" from cadaver donors are clinically available. There is limited clinical data available for these, therefore use with caution.

4. Platelet concentrates (PC)—platelet activation following injury or surgical insult. Platelets release protein content (degranulation) of more than 30 bioactive proteins. Primary factors include PDGF and TGF-β.

   a. The PDGF

      i. Primary function of PDGF is to stimulate cellular replication (mitogenesis).

      ii. It increases cell populations of mesenchymal stem cells and osteoprogenitor cells.

      iii. It also activates macrophages resulting in debridement of the surgical or traumatic site.

   b. Transforming growth factor β (TGF-β)

      i. It stimulates proliferation of osteoblast precursor cells and collagen.

      ii. Increases osteoblast cell line, and the upregulation of osteoblasts.

Table 8.1 Available fracture healing adjuvants with their inherent properties

	Osteoconductive scaffold	Osteoinductive growth factors	Osteogenic living cells
Banked demineralized bone matrix	•	•	
Marrow concentrates			•
Platelet-rich concentrates		Osteopromotive indirect cellular effect No direct intracellular transcription Stimulates cells to amplify their current functions	
Autograft	•	•	•
Bone morphogenic proteins		Direct intracellular transcription of cells to bone forming lineage	
Synthetic Ca⁺ ceramics	•		
Allograft	•		

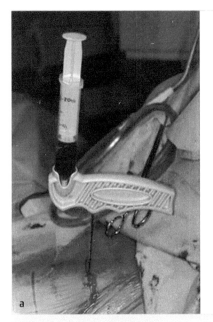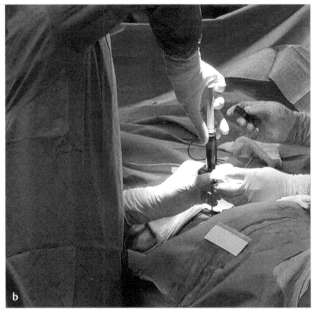

Fig. 8.5 (a, b) The aspiration technique is very specific in order to maximize the number of effective progenitor cells per unit. No more than 2 mL should be aspirated from any given area to avoid dilution with peripheral blood. The concentrate is then loaded onto a conductive substrate for implantation (composite grafting).

    c. PC stimulate the formation of blood vessels by invasion of pluripotential mesenchymal stem cells, monocytes, and macrophages. PC factors direct chemotactic and mitogenic effects on osteoblasts and osteoblast precursors.

    d. Level I evidence is lacking to indicate PC, alone or in combination, has a substantial effect on rates of bone healing.

      i. PC may have a positive effect as an adjunct to local bone graft.

      ii. Soft tissue effects: published series for clinical trials covering eight clinical conditions, such as rotator cuff, tennis elbow, with PC augmentation. Insufficient evidence to support PRP for musculoskeletal soft-tissue injuries.

    e. PC may have beneficial effects for knees with early degenerative changes.

  5. Recombinant PDGF (rh-PDGF) plus calcium phosphate matrix (rhPDGF/TCP) is an alternative to autogenous bone graft (Augment). Rh-PDGF is efficacious for diabetic fracture treatment and approved for defect management for foot and ankle indications.

B. Osteoconductive substrates with porous structures mimics cancellous architecture.

  1. Facilitate migration, attachment, and proliferation of mesenchymal stem cells.

  2. Calcium ceramics are the primary type of conductive materials.

    a. Calcium sulfate substitutes

      i. Calcium sulfate is minimally porous.

      ii. Rapid degradation by chemical process with loss of compressive strength.

      iii. Current best use is as carrier for adjuvant antibiotics. Material properties are advantageous for delivering high-dose antibiotics to infected defects.

    b. Calcium phosphate substitutes (▶ Fig. 8.6).

      i. Available in a variety of delivery forms such as solids, powders, and cements.

      ii. Slow degradation by biological process with maintained compressive strength.

      iii. Highly crystalline structures with variable porosity and rates of osteointegration based on crystalline structure and pore size.

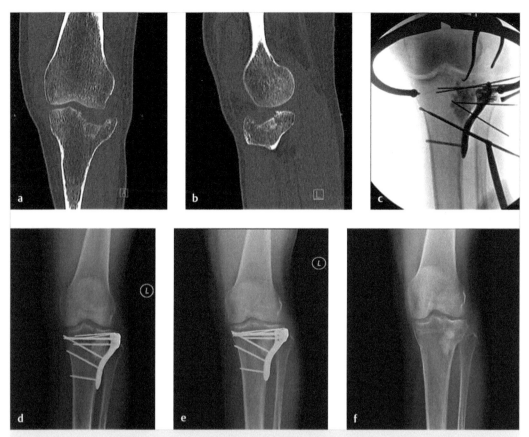

Fig. 8.6 (**a, b**) Computed tomography scan of plateau fracture demonstrating subchondral defect. (**c**) Elevated joint surface supported with particulate and injectable CaPO$_4$ conductive substrate. (**d**) 1-month post surgery with material present and maintenance of reduction. (**e**) 4-months post surgery with incorporation of graft substitute and articular surface maintained. (**f**) 10 months post surgery with nearly all material osteointegrated and articular surface well maintained.

c. Hydroxyapatite

    i. Crystalline structure dictates the rate of osteointegration. Materials integrate via a cell-mediated response and pore structure allows for cellular attachment.

    ii. Prolonged osteointegration because of the paucity of cellular interactions. High compressive strength.

    iii. Brittle mechanics and slow bone formation, hydroxyapatite alone is not commonly used as a conductive bone substitute nowadays.

d. Tricalcium phosphate (TCP)

    i. Less brittle and faster resorption due to increased porosity.

    ii. Also delivered in an injectable form. Timing of fracture fixation hardware is material dependent.

    iii. Level I studies document superiority to autograft for support of subchondral bone defects in tibial plateau fractures and other articular injuries.

    iv. Composite grafts available such as BMAC combined with scaffolding properties of TCP to stimulate cell proliferation and differentiation.

C. Demineralized bone matrix (DBM), allogenic bone:

    1. Formed by acid extraction of the mineralized ECM of allograft bone.

    2. Contains type-1 collagen, noncollagenous proteins, osteoinductive growth factors including bone morphogenetic proteins (BMPs) and other inductive factors.

    a. Effectiveness of autogenous BMPs in the DBM is in question.

        i. Differences in the growth factor concentrations between individual products.

        ii. Potencies of each available growth factor within each product is variable.

    b. DBM is available as freeze-dried powder, granules, gel, putty, strips, or in combination with allogeneic bone chips or calcium sulfate granules.

    c. Sterile processing and carrier molecules influence effectiveness of these materials.

3. DBM is highly osteoconductive due to its particulate/porous nature/increased surface area.

4. Preclinical data documents DBM forming de novo bone in lesser animal models.

5. Human data is limited to isolated case reports and uncontrolled retrospective reviews.

6. Effectiveness of DBM as a stand-alone graft is equivocal and not recommended.

7. Best evidence suggests comparable efficacy when combined with autograft compared to autograft alone. Use DBM as graft extender.

D. Bone morphogenic proteins (BMPs)—true "osteoinducers." Factors stimulate circulating undifferentiated mesenchymal cells changing them directly into osteoprogenitor cells.

    1. Mode of action

        a. BMPs bind at specific cell surface receptors TGF-β ligands.

        b. Protein complexes (intracellular messengers) form to trigger downstream molecular signals and transmit them to the nucleus. SMADs are intracellular proteins that transduce extracellular signals from surface ligands to the nucleus. Gene transcription is activated to modulate cell function.

        c. BMPs direct conversion of cells into a bone-forming lineage.

    2. Rh-BMP-2, Infuse, is approved for use for augmentation of an interbody fusion device during an anterior lumbar interbody fusion (ALIF) or oblique lateral interbody fusion (OLIF) procedures. Single level involvement. Rh-BMP-2 is approved for use within 10 days for open tibia fractures treated with an intramedullary (IM) nail. It is the graft substitute applied to defects at the time of delayed closure.

    3. Level 1 data demonstrating efficacy equal to that of autogenous bone graft.

        a. Complications of use in lumbar spine surgery include heterotopic ossification (HO), graft osteolysis, increased infection, arachnoiditis, increased neurological deficits, and retrograde ejaculation.

        b. Complications in cervical spine fusion include tracheal edema with air restriction.

        c. Heterotopic ossification is the most common complication for trauma-related conditions.

E. Extracellular matrices (ECM)

    1. Tissue-derived (bovine intestine, porcine bladder, etc.) scaffolds contain native collagens, glycosaminoglycans, and growth factors.

        a. ECM have an intact epithelial basement membrane layer, and are available as micronized powder and lyophilized sheets.

        b. This biologic scaffold presents a tremendous surface area for attachment of fibroblasts for the deposition and substitution with collagen.

        c. ECM degradation peptides are chemoattractive to appropriate progenitor cells, for constructive remodeling response and multilayer tissue regeneration.

        d. ECM have also been demonstrated to have antimicrobial activity in vitro, to augment clinical performance in infected wounds.

    2. Indications for use include the management of complex full-thickness wounds including exposed tendons, bone, and orthopaedic hardware.

        a. Especially useful in patients who were not deemed suitable candidates for routine surgical management with standard local or free flap techniques.

        b. Tissue regeneration covers defects, tendons, and hardware for skin graft coverage over durable tissue layers.

Suggested Readings

Blank A, Riesgo A, Gitelis S, Rapp T. Bone grafts, substitutes, and augments in benign orthopaedic conditions current concepts. Bull Hosp Jt Dis (2013) 2017;75(2):119–127

Hegde V, Jo JE, Andreopoulou P, Lane JM. Effect of osteoporosis medications on fracture healing. Osteoporos Int 2016;27(3):861–871

Kadam A, Millhouse PW, Kepler CK, et al. Bone substitutes and expanders in spine surgery: a review of their fusion efficacies. Int J Spine Surg 2016;10:33

Kim JH, Liu X, Wang J, et al. Wnt signaling in bone formation and its therapeutic potential for bone diseases. Ther Adv Musculoskelet Dis 2013;5(1):13–31

Marcucio RS, Nauth A, Giannoudis PV, et al. Stem cell therapies in orthopaedic trauma. J Orthop Trauma 2015;29(Suppl 12):S24–S27

Zhang D, Potty A, Vyas P, Lane J. The role of recombinant PTH in human fracture healing: a systematic review. J Orthop Trauma 2014;28(1):57–62

9 Polytrauma

Timothy S. Achor and Krishna Chandra Vemulapalli

Introduction

Orthopaedic surgeons face numerous challenges when treating multiply injured patients with orthopaedic injuries. The initial evaluation focuses on life and limb threatening conditions. Early identification and appropriate immobilization of pelvis and extremity injuries (open/closed fracture, vascular insult, compartment syndrome) may improve pain, aid in systemic resuscitation, and limit blood loss. This chapter will explore injury characteristics and factors of patient physiology that influence fracture treatment toward damage-control temporizing measures with external fixation versus initial definitive management. Finally, potential complications of poorly timed and executed fracture interventions in polytrauma patients are discussed.

Keywords: polytrauma, damage control orthopaedics, early appropriate care

I. Priorities and Goals of Treatment

A. Trauma is the leading cause of death in the United States for patients < 45 years of age and is a significant source of morbidity.
B. The emergent evaluation and management of the polytraumatized patient requires a coordinated effort between the emergency room physicians, trauma surgeons, and orthopaedic consultant.
C. Patients with multiple fractures frequently have associated injuries to the head, neck, chest, and/or abdomen.
D. Hemodynamic status and systemic physiology are intimately related to musculoskeletal injury.
   1. Life—immediately identify and emergently manage life-threatening injuries.
   2. Limb—identify and emergently manage limb-threatening injuries.
   3. Function—identify and treat injuries that can cause long-term disability.

II. Evaluation

A. Advanced Trauma Life Support (ATLS) and physical examination.
   1. Sixty percent of trauma patients have injuries to the musculoskeletal system.
B. Primary survey—it reveals obvious life- and limb-threatening injuries and begins the resuscitation process. Brief history from patient and/or EMS (age, mechanism, extrication time, fatalities at scene, obvious injuries and wounds) with simultaneous vital signs and airway, breathing, and circulation (ABC).
   1. Airway:
      a. Ability to protect airway.
      b. Intubate the patient if necessary.
   2. Breathing:
      a. Measure respiratory rate, oxygenation.
      b. Assess breath sounds and utilize needle decompression or chest tube as necessary.
   3. Circulation:
      a. Assess hemodynamic status and external sites of hemorrhage.
      b. Apply pressure and dressings to wounds.
      c. Utilize tourniquet for uncontrollable bleeding or mangled limbs.
      d. Obtain intravenous access and begin fluid resuscitation.

4. Disability:
   a. Perform a neurologic exam.
   b. Glasgow Coma Scale.
5. Environmental exposure:
   a. Remove all clothes and maintain patient body temperature.
   b. Warm the trauma bay.
   c. Use a fluid warmer and warm blankets.
6. Fractures:
   a. Identify obvious injuries.
   b. Apply splints/traction.
C. Secondary survey—it reveals less obvious injuries and requires vigilance and a head-to-toe exam.
D. History
   1. Past medical history: identify relevant medical conditions that may impact early decision-making and/or benefit from optimization (if obtainable).
   2. Past surgical history: relevant prior operations (if obtainable).
   3. Allergies.
E. Physical exam
   1. Complete visual inspection and examination.
   2. Take down all dressings, remove tourniquets, and clothing.
   3. Head-to-toe examination with palpation of all extremities including pelvis and spine.
   4. Range all joints and perform a ligamentous examination of suspected injuries.
   5. Vascular exam: palpate pulses in all extremities and utilize Doppler and ankle–brachial index (ABI) when indicated.
   6. A lower limb with an ABI < 0.90 warrants additional investigation with either computed tomography (CT) angiogram, formal angiogram, or vascular consultation.
   7. Motor and sensory examination with documentation.
   8. Compartment syndrome—increased intracompartmental pressure causing decreased limb perfusion.
      a. Identify injuries and patients at risk, and remain vigilant.
      b. High-energy injuries, tibia fractures, forearm fractures, segmental injuries, open fractures, and severe swelling all should raise concern.
      c. Diagnosis:
         i. Accuracy of the traditional "5 Ps" (pain with passive stretch, paresthesias, paralysis, pulselessness, and pallor) has been questioned. Refer to Chapter 13, Acute Compartment Syndrome, for a more in-depth discussion.
         ii. Typical exam findings include:
            • Pain out of proportion.
            • Pain with passive stretch of the muscle in the affected compartment.
            • Paresthesias.
            • Anesthesia or decreased sensation.
            • Muscle weakness or paralysis.
            • Tense compartment on palpation.
   9. Tertiary examination in 48 to 72 hours once distracting injuries have been stabilized.
F. Imaging
   1. Traditional—three radiographs are obtained urgently to aide in identifying life-threatening injuries: lateral cervical spine (c-spine), chest, anteroposterior pelvis.

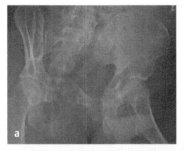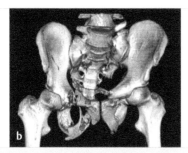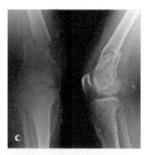

Fig. 9.1 (a–c) Index case: Initial imaging and three-dimesional reconstructions of a 33-year-old male status post-industrial crush injury with open volume-expanding pelvic ring disruption and ipsilateral distal femur and tibial plateau fractures with vascular compromise.

2. Many trauma centers no longer obtain c-spine X-ray, as CT scan imaging can be performed quickly and can accurately identify injuries.

   a. Less urgent imaging studies: X-rays of all injured or suspected injured skeletal structures above and below level of injury.

   b. Any tenderness, swelling, crepitus, or skin break warrants further evaluation.

   c. CT—2 mm fine cuts and three-dimensional reconstructions can improve diagnostic accuracy and assist in preoperative planning (▶ Fig. 9.1).

3. Shock:

   a. Hypovolemic—caused by hemorrhage and dehydration. Treatment includes control of hemorrhage and volume replacement.

   b. Cardiogenic—caused by inability of heart to sustain circulation due to causes such as cardiac tamponade, aortic dissection, myocardial infarction, or dysrhythmia. Treatment includes inotropes or extracorporeal membrane oxygenation (ECMO).

   c. Neurogenic—the loss of peripheral vascular tone secondary to spinal cord injury or traumatic brain injury. Treatment includes vasopressors and volume replacement.

   d. Anaphylactic—an antigen–antibody reaction which causes distributive loss of circulatory volume. Treatment includes epinephrine and volume replacement.

   e. Septic—the distributive loss of circulatory volume (peripheral vasodilation) secondary to infection and the resulting inflammatory response. Treatment includes antibiotics and volume replacement.

III. Treatment/Interventions

A. Initial management

   1. In the face of chaos, it is critical for the physician to obtain and maintain control.

   2. Traditional resuscitation efforts are changing. More trauma centers are replacing blood loss with blood products, including whole blood.

   3. Thromboelastography (TEG) is more commonly being used at trauma centers for guided resuscitation and treatment of coagulopathy.

   4. Persistent hemodynamic instability and evidence of intra-abdominal or intrathoracic injury: emergent exploratory laparotomy.

   5. Life-threatening head injuries and intracranial bleeding—emergent craniotomy.

   6. Mangled extremities—urgent surgery for:

      a. Hemorrhage control, wound debridement, and temporary skeletal stabilization for potentially salvageable injuries.

      b. Amputation, if the limb is nonsalvageable.

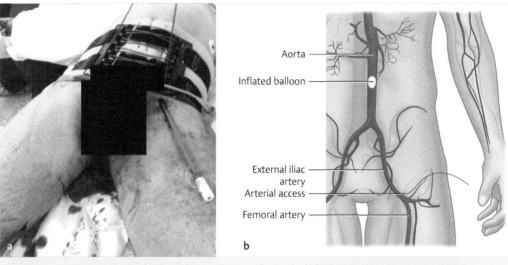

Fig. 9.2 (a) Application of pelvic binder and resuscitative endovascular balloon occlusion of the aorta (REBOA) catheter for open volume-expanding pelvic ring. (b) REBOA—a catheter is inserted via the femoral artery and introduced into aorta. A balloon is inflated to occlude the aorta and allow for distal control of hemorrhage.

7. Impending or active compartment syndrome—emergent fasciotomies.

8. Embolization in the interventional radiology suite may be appropriate for patients with solid organ injury or pelvic fractures with active extravasation noted on CT.

9. Occasionally, patients will benefit from both exploratory laparotomy as well as angioembolization.

10. Resuscitative endovascular balloon occlusion of the aorta (REBOA)—it is an emerging technology. Catheter is inserted via femoral artery and introduced into aorta. Balloon can be inflated to partially or completely occlude aorta and allow for distal control of hemorrhage. Functionally, an "internal tourniquet" (▶Fig. 9.2a, b).

11. Dislocations should be urgently reduced. Irreducible dislocations should go to the operating room for an open reduction to decrease likelihood of soft tissue or neurovascular compromise.

12. Open fractures can be provisionally treated in the emergency room (ER).

    a. Early appropriate antibiotic coverage is critical.

    b. Gross contamination can be removed in the ER.

    c. Irrigation with sterile saline can be performed, along with application of sterile dressings.

    d. Photographs, where institutionally and regionally appropriate, may improve communication between providers.

    e. Splint and/or traction can decrease additional soft tissue damage.

13. Skeletal traction may be appropriate for femur fractures, acetabular fractures, vertically unstable pelvic fractures, and hip dislocations.

    a. Distal femur versus proximal tibial traction pin is patient-, injury-, and practitioner-specific.

    b. The size of the traction pin (5-mm pin vs tensioned 2.0-mm wire) is debatable and institution-/practitioner-dependent.

    c. If proximal tibia is selected, care must be taken to ensure there are no knee ligamentous injuries.

    d. Skeletal traction may be indicated when patients with femur fractures cannot be definitely managed in an expeditious manner.

14. Application of a pelvic binder or sheet is appropriate for volume-expanding, unstable pelvic ring injuries.

a. A well-placed binder will decrease the pelvic volume, reduce anterior-posterior compression (APC)-type injuries, decrease pain, stabilize the blood clot, and potentially limit blood loss.

b. The binder can be left in place until the patient is stabilized for either internal or external fixation (▶ **Fig. 9.2a**).

c. Some surgeons advocate removing the binder within 24 hours to minimize the risk of soft-tissue necrosis. Consider removing the binder in surgery at the time of skeletal stabilization (external fixation and/or internal fixation).

IV. Orthopaedic Surgical Management

A. Early appropriate care (EAC)

1. Definitive skeletal stabilization of fractures within 24 to 48 hours.

2. May be appropriate for resuscitated, physiologically stable trauma patients.

3. Decision to proceed with EAC is based on many factors, including patient overall physiologic status, number and complexity of fractures, and the patient's tolerance of the ongoing operation.

   a. Labs such as a complete blood count, lactate, pH, base deficit, and TEG may all be useful markers to gauge the patient's physiologic state. For example, pH ≤ 7.25; BD ≥ −4; lactate ≥ 2 can all be markers that further resuscitation is required.

4. Benefits include decreased pulmonary complications and shorter intensive care unit (ICU) and hospital stay, improved mobilization.

5. Pitfalls include potential for exacerbation of lung injuries (in part from reaming of long bones) and inability to meet resuscitative demands.

B. Damage control orthopaedics (DCO)

1. Provisional stabilization of injured extremities.

2. Recognize life- and limb-threatening injuries and prioritize.

3. Terminology borrowed from US Navy—"damage control" is a way to keep vessels afloat and functional, even in the setting of severe structural damage.

4. Stabilization techniques include temporizing external fixation, provisional plate fixation, splinting, and traction application (▶ **Fig. 9.3a, b**).

5. Pitfalls include need for additional procedures/anesthesia, and risks associated with provisional external fixation including pin tract infection.

C. Decision-making (EAC vs. DCO)

1. First, 'Do no harm'—do not make a bad situation worse with prolonged anesthesia, surgical insult, and excessive blood loss.

2. Conversely, physiologically stable patients undergoing early definitive stabilization may benefit from improved short-term outcomes (fewer ICU days, hospital days, earlier mobilization).

3. Management of polytraumatized patients requires a multidisciplinary approach, including input from all relevant teams (ER, trauma, orthopaedic, anesthesia, critical care, neurosurgery, urology, vascular, plastics, etc.).

4. Patients with pulmonary issues including severe pulmonary contusions and high ventilator settings with difficulty maintaining oxygen saturation are candidates for DCO.

5. Patients with increased intracranial pressures secondary to intracranial hemorrhage and patients with renal failure should not be subjected to surgeries with a potential for large volume shifts and blood loss.

6. Patients with multiple extremity injuries and long bone injuries may be candidates for DCO, if they do not respond well to resuscitative efforts.

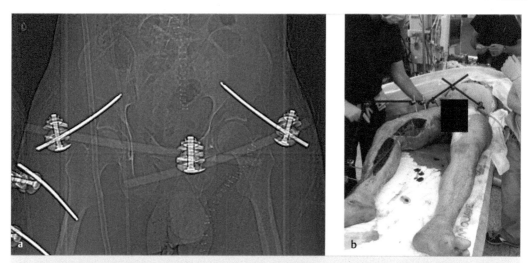

Fig. 9.3 (a, b) Index patient after emergent initial irrigation and debridement, fasciotomies, temporizing external fixation application and revascularization.

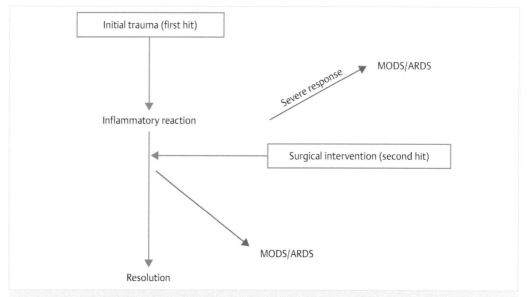

Fig. 9.4 The first hit is the inciting traumatic event, and the second hit is the definitive surgical intervention, usually femoral nailing. ARDS, adult respiratory distress syndrome; MODS, multiple organ dysfunction syndrome.

D. Sequelae and complications

   1. Second hit phenomenon (▶ **Fig. 9.4**):

      a. Concept that an ill-timed secondary intervention (surgery, excessive blood loss) may induce an additional inflammatory insult which may lead to multiple organ dysfunction or acute respiratory distress syndrome.

      b. It must be mitigated and accounted for in order to appropriately time and sequence surgical intervention to optimize outcome of the severely traumatized patient.

      c. Multiple laboratory markers, such as hematocrit, pH, base excess, and lactate, can been used to monitor the physiologic state of the patient through this time period in order to determine appropriate clearance for definitive surgical management.

      d. Immunologic markers, such as interleukin-6, have been demonstrated to be elevated in nonsurvivors.

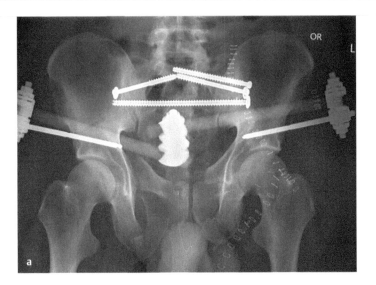

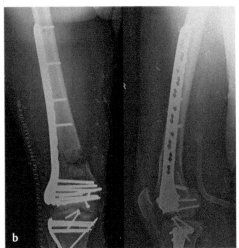

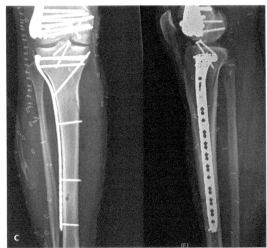

Fig. 9.5 (a–c) Index patient after definitive fixation with percutaneous iliosacral screw fixation of his posterior pelvic ring and open reduction and internal fixation of his distal femur and tibial plateau.

2. Etiology of decompensation:

   a. 50%–60% of deaths happen at the scene of trauma.

   b. Roughly 30% of deaths occur within the first 24 hours after arrival to a trauma center and are generally the result of hemorrhage or neurologic injury.

   c. The remaining 20% of deaths occur after the first 24 hours of hospitalization as a result of infection, multiple organ dysfunction syndrome (MODS), neurologic injury, or ongoing hemorrhage. As 24-hour survival rates have improved over the last decade, the incidence of multiple organ failure has risen.

   d. There is a complex interplay between the initial systemic inflammatory response to trauma and the body's counter anti-inflammatory response, and a balance must be struck to optimize clinical resolution.

   e. The role of the orthopaedic surgeon is vital to the initial stabilization effort and the decision between DCO and EAC can easily swing the pendulum between survival and morbidity and mortality. Thoughtful consideration of the patient's overall status is paramount when planning surgical intervention (▶ Fig. 9.5).

3. Nosocomial infection:
   a. Occur in up to 30% of multiple-injury patients.
   b. Include pneumonia, urinary tract infection, bloodstream infection, wound infection, and *Clostridium difficile* infection.
   c. Multiple organ failure is leading cause of death in multiple-injury patients that survive the initial insult.

Summary

Polytrauma patients present unique challenges to the orthopaedic surgeon. Patients can have life- and limb-threatening injuries, and timely evaluation, diagnosis, and management are essential. A coordinated effort between emergency room physicians, trauma surgeons, orthopaedic surgeons, and anesthesiologists is critical. A thorough history and physical exam are key to initial evaluation. The primary survey reveals obvious, life-threatening injuries, and the secondary survey requires diligence and a complete head-to-toe examination. "Damage control orthopaedics" can be utilized for severely injured patients who may not be physiologically optimized for lengthy, definitive operations. Provisional skeletal stabilization including splints, traction, and external fixation can decrease pain, blood loss, and local tissue damage while facilitating patient mobilization. "Early appropriate care" may be undertaken for patients who are physiologically and hemodynamically stable. Trends in vital signs and serum lab values can aide in decision-making for timing as well as type of operative intervention.

Suggested Readings

Bone LB, Giannoudis P. Femoral shaft fracture fixation and chest injury after polytrauma. J Bone Joint Surg Am 2011;93(3):311–317

Childs BR, Nahm NJ, Moore TA, Vallier HA. Multiple procedures in the initial surgical setting: when do the benefits outweigh the risks in patients with multiple system trauma? J Orthop Trauma 2016;30(8):420–425

Giannoudis PV, Giannoudi M, Stavlas P. Damage control orthopaedics: lessons learned. Injury 2009;40(Suppl 4):S47–S52

Nicola R, Total E, Etc C. Early total care versus damage control: current concepts in the orthopedic care of polytrauma patients. ISRN Orthop 2013;2013:329–452

Pape HC, Giannoudis P, Krettek C. The timing of fracture treatment in polytrauma patients: relevance of damage control orthopedic surgery. Am J Surg 2002;183(6):622–629

Roberts CS, Pape HC, Jones AL, Malkani AL, Rodriguez JL, Giannoudis PV. Damage control orthopaedics: evolving concepts in the treatment of patients who have sustained orthopaedic trauma. Instr Course Lect 2005;54(2):447–462

Vallier HA, Wang X, Moore TA, Wilber JH, Como JJ. Timing of orthopaedic surgery in multiple trauma patients: development of a protocol for early appropriate care. J Orthop Trauma 2013;27(10):543–551

10 Osteoporosis

David Donohue and Hassan R. Mir

Introduction

Osteoporosis is defined as decrease in bone mass and microarchitecture deterioration ultimately leading to a **decrease in bone strength** and **increased risk of fragility fracture.** In the United States, 44 million women and men over 50 years of age are either osteoporotic or osteopenic. Throughout the world, 200 million people are osteoporotic. Fragility fractures of the hip, spine, wrist, and pelvis are associated with significant morbidity and mortality, including 20% mortality following hip fracture. There are high costs associated with treatment and recovery from fragility fractures, with an estimated 19 billion dollars in the United States alone.

Keywords: osteoporosis, fragility fractures, dual energy X-ray absorptiometry (DEXA), bisphosphonates, calcium, vitamin D

I. Bone Health

A. Peak bone mass is achieved in early adulthood (early 20s).

1. Most important risk factor for osteoporosis is **low peak bone mass.**

2. Determined by genetics, physical activity, nutrition, and hormonal balance.

3. Bone mass begins to decrease in the fourth decade of life due to shift of balance to favor bone resorption.

II. Bone Physiology

The skeletal system serves two primary functions: mechanical support to the body and mineral homeostasis. Bone formation is coupled with bone resorption to allow reorganization of bony architecture along lines of stress (Wolff's law; Chapter 1, Physiology of Fracture Healing, ▶ **Fig. 1.5**) thus providing maximal structural support, and to allow liberation and sequestration of the body's calcium stores.

A. The remodeling process depends on the function of three cell types.

1. Osteoblasts—form bone

   a. Secrete type I collagen in addition to noncollagenous proteins that compose **osteoid.** Type I collagen forms a triple helix (two $\alpha 1$ chains and one $\alpha 2$ chain) arranged in parallel array with gaps between the ends of the molecule (hole zones) and in the parallel spaces (pores). Mineralization of bone (inorganic phase composed of calcium hydroxyapatite) begins in the hole zones.

   b. Maturation is induced by transcription factors $Runx_2$ and Osterix.

   c. Secrete receptor activator of nuclear factor-$\kappa\beta$ ligand (RANKL) and macrophage colony-stimulating factor (M-CSF) which stimulate osteoclast differentiation.

2. Osteoclasts—break down bone

   a. Monocyte lineage, differentiate after expression of transcription factor PU.1 which leads to expression of M-CSF receptor and RANK.

   b. RANKL, a cytokine secreted by osteoblasts and member of the TNFα family, is the most critical and terminal factor necessary for the differentiation of the osteoclast from the monocytic precursor cells.

   c. Form ruffled border (increased surface area) and bind to $\alpha_v\beta_3$ integrin to create a sealed pocket into which carbonic acid (breaks down mineralized bone) and cathepsin K (breaks down organic matrix of bone) are pumped.

d. Balanced by secretion of osteoprotegerin (OPG) by the osteoblast. This is a "decoy receptor" for RANKL. Denosumab (antiresorptive medication) is a synthetic version OPG.

e. Amount of bone resorbed depends on the number of mature osteoclasts, their lifespan, and activity level. While the former is governed by the ratio of RANKL/OPG, the latter two are increased in the presence of inflammatory cytokines (IL-1, IL-6, M-CSF, TNFα).

f. Secrete bone morphogenetic protein (BMP) to stimulate differentiation of osteoblasts.

3. Osteocytes—derived from osteoblasts that become encapsulated in the bone matrix they secreted.

a. Most abundant cells in bone (95%).

b. Cytoplasmic processes extend to adjacent cells through canaliculi and serve as the "neural network" of the bone.

i. Facilitate mechanical signal transduction via the piezoelectric effect, and mediate the remodeling process such that more bone is deposited in areas where greater force is detected (again, Wolff's law).

B. Imbalance in the remodeling process in favor of bone resorption leads to decrease in bone mineral density and trabecular microarchitecture. This results in weakening of the material and structural properties of bone, and thus increase in the risk of fracture.

III. Types of Osteoporosis

A. Primary

1. **Type 1:** Postmenopausal—decrease in net bone formation.

a. Due to low estrogen levels (low 17β estradiol results in increased levels of circulating pro-inflammatory cytokines).

b. Bone loss is rapid immediately following menopause and tapers as time goes on (less trabecular architecture to resorb).

2. **Type II:** Senile—age-related decline in osteoblast function.

a. Usually seen in patients over the age of 70 years.

b. Affects both trabecular and cortical bone.

B. Secondary (**Type III**)—results from medical illness, medication or lifestyle derangement (see risk factors below):

1. The list is quite inclusive, and the mechanisms by which each condition causes osteoporosis are often multifactorial and overlapping.

2. These diseases and their sequelae either result in an impediment to achievement of peak bone mass during youth or increase the rate of bone loss during the remodeling process.

IV. Nonmodifiable Risk Factors for Osteoporosis

A. Female gender

1. Women have lower peak bone mass and postmenopausal decrease in estrogen.

2. Lower risk in elderly men due to peripheral aromatization of testosterone to estrogen. In general, men have greater bone mineral density, larger bone cross-sectional area, and cortical thickness.

B. Increased age

1. 90% of fragility fractures occur in patients > 50 years old.

C. Small/thin body size

1. Increased body weight and body mass index (BMI) are associated with decreased rates of osteoporosis, most likely due to increased mechanical load and peripheral conversion of androgens to estrogen in adipose tissue.

2. BMI < 20 (thin frame) is associated with increased risk of fracture.

D. Ethnicity: Caucasian and Asian women are at the highest risk due to lower peak bone mass.

E. Family history of fragility fracture.

V. Modifiable Risk Factors for Osteoporosis

A. Estrogen deficiency—postmenopausal, hypogonadism, low caloric intake, excessive exercise.

B. Medical conditions

1. Genetic: Ehlers–Danlos syndrome, Marfan's syndrome, Gaucher's disease, hemochromatosis, homocystinuria, hypophosphatasia, cystic fibrosis.

2. Inflammatory—rheumatoid arthritis.

3. Endocrine: Cushing's syndrome, hyperthyroidism, hypothyroidism, hyperparathyroidism, hypogonadism, androgen insensitivity, anorexia nervosa, hyperprolactinemia, premature menopause, Turner's syndrome, athletic amenorrhea, Klinefelter's syndrome.

4. Gastrointestinal—celiac disease, chronic liver disease, malabsorption, vitamin D deficiency.

5. Renal—chronic kidney disease.

6. Neurologic—epilepsy.

7. Malignancy—multiple myeloma, leukemia, lymphoma.

C. Medications—heparin, antiepileptics, immunosuppressive medication (cyclosporine, tacrolimus), chemotherapy, glucocorticoids, lithium, methotrexate, thyroxine, total parenteral nutrition.

D. Sedentary lifestyle and prolonged recumbence.

1. Mechanical loading of bone by muscle pull is more anabolic to bone than weight born due to obesity.

E. Diet—deficiency in calcium, vitamin D, or magnesium.

F. Excessive alcohol use

1. Has a direct inhibitory effect on new bone formation and slows remodeling.

2. Leads to poor nutrition.

3. The direct effects of alcohol are quickly reversible (2–3 weeks).

G. Smoking

1. Mechanism is unclear, however some evidence suggests that nicotine impairs new bone formation.

2. May also be due to lower body weight and BMI among smokers, or promotion of a pro-inflammatory state which tips the remodeling balance in favor of bone resorption.

VI. Diagnosis

A. Dual-energy X-ray absorptiometry (standard of care)

1. Two X-ray beams of different energy are passed through tissue.

2. The two energy peaks correspond to soft tissue and bone, thus the absorption of bone in the absence of soft tissue can be calculated.

3. Measured in the lumbar spine (composite score from L2–L4), hip, radius, calcaneus, and whole body.

4. Generates three data points:

   a. Bone mineral density (BMD)—expressed as volumetric BMD in g/cm^3 or areal BMD in g/cm^2.

   b. T-score—comparison of measured BMD to normal, young (age 30), same sex controls (US uses same ethnicity; WHO uses white female reference).

   i. Used in postmenopausal females and males aged > 50 years.
   ii. Score reported as an integer representing the number of standard deviations from the young, normal, control value.
   c. Z-score—comparison of measured BMD to patients of similar age.
      i. Used in premenopausal females and males aged < 50 years.
5. Weaknesses:
   a. No normalized data for races other than Caucasian.
   b. Not weight adjusted.
   c. Bone architecture not considered.
   d. Bone turnover not measured.
   e. Can be influenced by osteoarthritic changes in the spine and hip, which are common in the elderly population.
   f. Error rate up to 20%.

B. Quantitative computed tomography (QCT)
   1. Special type of CT scan using routine phantom calibration. It allows volumetric assessment of BMD (g/cm^3) which can be converted to areal BMD (g/cm^2) and separation of cortical from trabecular bone. The g/cm^2 values generated with this modality have been shown to be predictive of fragility fracture and have been incorporated into the FRAX calculator.
   2. Disadvantages of this modality include limited availability of the software and variations of measurement from machines of different manufacturers.

C. Diagnostic CT (i.e., routine CT scans)
   1. Automated exposure control adjusts the tube current based on the attenuation of the signal after passage through the body. Results in uniform measurements of signal attenuation without the use of phantom calibration.
   2. Expressed in Hounsfield Units (HU), which is a coefficient of attenuation measured on a scale in which air is measured as 1000 HU and water as 0 HU.
   3. Currently under investigation as an opportunistic screening tool in the diagnosis of osteoporosis as over 80 million CT scans are performed annually in the United States for reasons unrelated to osteoporosis.

D. World health organization (WHO) criteria for diagnosis of osteoporosis
   1. Normal: T-score over −1.0.
   2. Osteopenia (low bone mass): T-score between −1.0 and −2.5.
   3. Osteoporosis: T-score below −2.5.
   4. Severe osteoporosis: T-score below −2.5 with a history of a fragility fracture.
   5. Additional criteria for diagnosis of osteoporosis
      a. Radiographs—routinely ordered to investigate suspected fragility fracture. At least 30% BMD must be lost before osteopenia is evident on radiographs.
      b. MRI scan indicated to evaluate for nondisplaced femoral neck fractures and sacral insufficiency fractures.
      c. Routine laboratory analysis:
         i. Low 25 hydroxycholecalciferol D level.
         ii. Normal or low serum calcium level:
      d. Additional markers of bone resorption include:
         i. Collagen telopeptide (collagen degradation).
         ii. Tartrate-resistant acid phosphatase (osteoclast numbers).

e. Markers of bone formation include:
   i. Alkaline phosphatase (osteoblast numbers).
   ii. Osteocalcin (osteoblast numbers).
   iii. Collagen propeptides (type 1 collagen synthesis).

VII. Treatment and Indications for Pharmacotherapy

A. Postmenopausal women and men over 50 years of age with history of hip fracture or vertebral fracture.

B. Severe osteoporosis: T-score below −2.5 with a history of a fragility fracture.

C. T-score < −2.5—diagnostic for osteoporosis.

D. T-score between −1.0 and −2.5 at the femoral neck or spine, and 10-year risk of hip fracture over 3% or 10-year risk of major osteoporotic fracture over 20% (calculated by FRAX).

   1. Lifestyle modifications—healthy, balanced diet, smoking cessation, limit alcohol intake, regular exercise (improved coordination reduces fall risk, slows bone resorption, improves mental well-being).

   2. Dietary supplementation: 1000 mg calcium/day for premenopausal women and men over 50 years; 1,200–1,500 mg calcium/day for postmenopausal women; 800–1000 international units (IU) vitamin D/day over 50 years.

   3. Treatment of secondary causes (treating or stabilizing medical conditions and adjusting medications).

E. Pharmacologic agents

   1. Antiresorptive medications:

      a. Bisphosphonates (first line):
         i. High affinity for calcium and binds to exposed calcium in areas of high bone turnover.
         ii. Osteoclast activity liberates the medication from bone, but it remains in bone for a long time (half-life ~ 10 years), thus rebound bone resorption does not occur.
         iii. Two mechanisms of action:
            • Nitrogen containing bisphosphonates **inhibit farnesyl pyrophosphate synthase** (pamidronate, alendronate, risedronate, zoledronate, ibandronate).
            • Non-nitrogen containing bisphosphonates **disrupt the ATP metabolic pathway by generating synthetic ATP analogue leading to osteoclast apoptosis** (etidronate, cloduronate, tiludronate).
         iv. Adverse events:
            • Gastrointestinal upset, esophagitis, esophageal ulcers. Contraindicated in patients who are unable to swallow or sit upright for 30 minutes following administration.
            • Osteonecrosis of the jaw—rare, more common in patients with dental problems.
            • **Atypical femur fractures**—subtrochanteric/proximal femoral shaft; associated with minimal or no trauma; radiographic features include transverse or short oblique, minimal comminution, medial spike, lateral cortical thickening. Risk is increased with prolonged use over 3 years.

      b. Denosumab:
         i. Monoclonal antibody to RANKL.
         ii. Given every 6 months.
         iii. Reduces risk of vertebral fractures by 68%, hip fractures by 40%, and nonvertebral fractures by 20%.
         iv. Can be associated with atypical femur fractures, osteonecrosis of the jaw, and rebound increased bone turnover.
         v. Indicated in patients with contraindication to bisphosphonate use.

    c.   Hormone replacement therapy:

        i.   Effective in reducing risk of all fractures.

        ii.   Not used commonly due to increased risk of cardiovascular disease, venous thrombosis, and breast cancer with prolonged use.

    d.   Raloxifene:

        i.   Selective estrogen receptor modulator (SERM).

        ii.   Estrogen agonist at bone and antagonist in other tissues (no increased risk of malignancy).

        iii.   Decreases risk of vertebral fractures only.

        iv.   Not commonly used.

    e.   Tibolone:

        i.   Partial agonist at estrogen, progesterone, and testosterone receptors.

        ii.   Reduces risk of vertebral fractures by 45% and nonvertebral by 26%.

2.   Anabolic medications—increase bone turnover, result in net positive bone deposition.

    a.   Parathyroid hormone 1–34 and 1–84:

        i.   Partial fragment (1–34), teriparatide, commonly used in cases of severe osteoporosis and failure of treatment.

        ii.   Increased risk of osteosarcoma in animal models has not been reported in humans.

        iii.   Nonetheless, contraindicated in patients with conditions of increased bone turnover (Paget's disease, open physes, unexplained elevation in alkaline phosphatase, previous external beam or implant radiation therapy).

3.   Initiation of pharmacotherapy following fracture:

    a.   Animal studies show a delay in callus maturation following administration of bisphosphonates.

    b.   No clinical evidence to suggest that bisphosphonates retard bone healing when administered in the perioperative period for the proximal femur and distal radius.

4.   Bisphosphonates should be stopped following treatment of atypical femur fractures.

VIII. Prevention

A.   Decreasing fall risk—use of proper ambulatory aids, correction of poor visual acuity (cataract surgery), proper illumination of rooms, removal of obstacles to ambulation (remove clutter), rubber soled shoes to improve grip, skid-proof backing on rugs and carpets, use of a bath mat, install bathroom bars, readily accessible flashlight in the bedroom.

B.   Dietary supplementation of calcium and vitamin D.

C.   Fragility fractures

   1.   Important to recognize that BMD is one data point used to assess risk of fracture.

   2.   Original studies correlating BMD with risk of fracture calculated relative risk.

   3.   The WHO Fracture Risk Assessment Tool (FRAX) is a 12 question survey assessing key risk factors that is used to predict the chance of one sustaining an osteoporosis-related fracture in the next 10 years.

   4.   Fragility fracture risk factors are listed in ▶ Table 10.1.

   5.   Following a fragility fracture (low-energy spine fracture, hip fracture, distal radius fracture, proximal humerus fracture, pelvic ring injury, sacral insufficiency fracture) the following labs should be ordered:

    a.   Serum calcium.

    b.   Parathyroid hormone.

    c.   Thyroid-stimulating hormone, free T4.

    d.   25-hydroxycholecalciferol (vitamin D).

Table 10.1 Risk factors for fragility fracture

- Age more than 65 years
- First-degree relative with fractured hip
- Current tobacco use
- Menopause prior to age 45 years
- Lifelong low calcium intake
- Poor vision despite correction
- Minimal weight-bearing exercise
- History of fragility fracture
- Self-report health as "fair" or "poor"
- Weight less than 127 pounds
- Amenorrhea

- Excess alcohol consumption (over 3 units/day)
- History of falls
- Glucocorticoid use
- Hyperthyroidism
- Chronic lung disease
- Endometriosis
- Malignancy
- Chronic hepatic or renal disease
- Hyperparathyroidism
- Vitamin D deficiency
- Cushing's disease

6. Consider a consultation to a dedicated metabolic bone clinic for ongoing management of bone health following discharge.

7. Order a physical therapy consultation for home safety evaluation to minimize the risk of falls.

Summary

The incidence of osteoporosis-related fragility fractures will most likely increase in the coming years. Focus has turned to prevention with use of calcium and vitamin D supplements and routine screening with dual-energy X-ray absorptiometry (DEXA) scans. Pharmacotherapy is indicated for patients with a T-score < −2.5, history of fragility fracture, or T-score in the osteopenic range (−1.0 to −2.5) coupled with a high risk of fracture according to the FRAX calculator. Several classes of medications are available for treatment. Bisphosphonates are considered first-line pharmacotherapy and have been shown to reduce the rate of hip and vertebral fractures. A coordinated approach involving the orthopaedic surgeon and primary care physician is necessary to initiate osteoporosis treatment and conduct appropriate follow-up.

Suggested Readings

Dell R, Greene D, Schelkun SR, Williams K. Osteoporosis disease management: the role of the orthopaedic surgeon. J Bone Joint Surg Am 2008;90(Suppl 4):188–194

Kates SL, Ackert-Bicknell CL. How do bisphosphonates affect fracture healing? Injury 2016;47(Suppl 1):S65–S68

Lagari V, Gavcovich T, Levis S. The Good and the Bad About the 2017 American College of Physicians Osteoporosis Guidelines. Clin Ther 2017 (November)

Miki RA, Oetgen ME, Kirk J, Insogna KL, Lindskog DM. Orthopaedic management improves the rate of early osteoporosis treatment after hip fracture. A randomized clinical trial. J Bone Joint Surg Am 2008;90(11):2346–2353

Molvik H, Khan W. Bisphosphonates and their influence on fracture healing: a systematic review. Osteoporos Int 2015;26(4):1251–1260

Tosi LL, Gliklich R, Kannan K, Koval KJ. The American Orthopaedic Association's "own the bone" initiative to prevent secondary fractures. J Bone Joint Surg Am 2008;90(1):163–173

11 Pathologic Fractures

Joel M. Post

Introduction

The incidence of pathologic fractures is rising and patients with metastatic disease are living longer. All orthopaedic surgeons providing trauma call coverage should have a sound knowledge of the principles and approach to the treatment of this subset of fractures. The approach to lesions of uncertain etiology should be systematic and complete starting with a detailed history and physical examination, laboratory evaluation, and imaging studies. Early return to maximal function by minimizing restrictions and surgical complications is paramount to provide patients with a meaningful quality of life. Most procedures are of palliative nature and an understanding of patient performance status, medical comorbidities, stage of disease, and establishing goals of care are most optimally provided through a co-management, team-based approach with internal medicine, palliative care, nutrition, medical oncology, radiation oncology, and physiotherapy services. A general knowledge of the behavior of tumor subtypes is vital for avoiding pitfalls. Construct stability must be durable and sustainable for the remainder of the patient's life expectancy. The purpose of this chapter is to review the approach and work-up for patients with an impending or actual pathologic fracture and provide management principles that can be employed by the general orthopaedic surgeon to avoid pitfalls, maximize functional recovery, and limit complications in the treatment of patients with bone metastases (▶Video 11.1).

Keywords: pathologic fractures, bone metastases, prophylactic fixation, surgical adjuvants, palliative treatment

I. History and Physical Exam

A. Include any personal or family history of malignancies, environmental exposures, and tobacco.

B. Constitutional symptoms, such as fever/chills, fatigue, malaise, or weight loss, can be suggestive of some tumor subtypes.

C. The physical exam should be more thorough than the typical focused musculoskeletal exam (lymphatics, abdomen, breast, rectal, integumentary).

II. Staging and Biopsy

A. Full staging studies are ideally obtained prior to any surgical interventions including biopsies.

1. Radiographs in orthogonal planes of the entire bone to ensure there are no additional lesions.

2. Localized advanced imaging, such as magnetic resonance imaging or computed tomography (CT), is sometimes helpful for characterization of the lesion, endosteal extent, or soft tissue extension.

3. CT chest, abdomen, and pelvis to assess the most common sources of osseous metastases (lung, breast, thyroid, renal, prostate).

4. Whole-body nuclear medicine scan for complete osseous assessment of metastatic disease.

5. Skeletal survey when myeloma is suspected or has been diagnosed.

B. Labs: complete blood count, comprehensive metabolic panel, serum/urine protein electrophoresis.

C. If multiple osseous lesions are noted or a primary mass is identified (i.e., lung/renal), tissue can be obtained for confirmation at the time of surgical stabilization.

D. A pitfall in the management of pathologic fractures is delay in definitive treatment by waiting for subspecialty services, such as interventional radiology and pathology, to obtain lesional and diagnostic tissue (▶Table 11.1).

Table 11.1 Pitfalls in the treatment of pathologic fractures

Inadequate imaging/staging studies prior to proceeding with surgical intervention	Delay in definitive treatment waiting for various subspecialty services (interventional radiology, pathology, etc.)
Lack of a "captain of the ship" directing care delivery and working with subspecialty teams	Not taking the time to understand patient goals of total care
Inadequate tissue obtained (hematoma, callus/fibrosis, bone which needs to be decalcified, medullary reamings, crushed cells) for diagnosis	Local disease progression after surgical intervention due to lack of tumor control or adjuvant treatment (radiation)

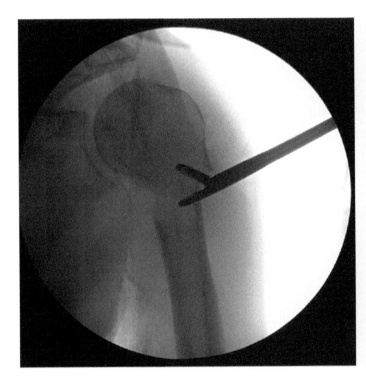

Fig. 11.1 A pituitary rongeur works well to obtain lesional (not bone or hematoma) biopsy tissue. Efforts should be made to not crush or smear the biopsy sample.

E. If the osseous lesion is solitary and staging studies reveal no clear site of primary disease, one should proceed with caution as a primary sarcoma of bone needs to be ruled out.

F. Biopsy tissue can be obtained at the time of definitive fixation, but lesional tissue must be obtained.

   1. Hematoma and cancellous/cortical bone have significant limitations in establishing an accurate diagnosis via frozen section. Decalcification of bone can be performed on permanent (formalin) samples only.

   2. Tissue is best obtained with an angled curette/pituitary rongeur (▶ **Fig. 11.1**).

   3. Do not crush or smear specimen; place on saline soaked nonadherent Telfa pad.

   4. Do not place in formalin if intraoperative frozen section is requested/desired.

   5. Medullary reamings are a poor source of tissue given crushing and distortion of cells.

III. Indications and Timing

A. A sound understanding of baseline performance status, medical comorbidities, and current disease state is vital in the multidisciplinary approach to patients with impending or completed pathologic fractures.

B. An active discussion with the medical oncology team is important in understanding immunosuppression, cytotoxic medications, and determining the most optimal time to surgery.

C. Involving palliative care or hospice services can be helpful in the decision-making and guiding expectations on operative risks and life expectancy, as many procedures are performed for pain palliation.

D. Decision to proceed with surgery should be a shared discussion with the patient, family or care givers, and the treating teams.

E. Several scoring systems have been used in attempt to predict fracture risk. The Mirels score is a widely used system factoring location, pain, type of lesion, and size. A score of 8 or higher often warrants prophylactic fixation (▶Table 11.2).

F. In general, lytic lesions of the peritrochanteric or diaphyseal region of the femur that are associated with functional weight-bearing pain and are greater than half the diameter of the bone, are at highest risk for fracture (▶Fig. 11.2).

G. Lytic lesions appear "dark" or radiolucent on radiographs as bone is destroyed/lost from the underlying destructive process. In contrast, blastic lesions appear "light," sclerotic, or radiopaque. Lytic lesions impart a higher risk for pathologic fracture as compared to blastic lesions as the flexural rigidity of the bone is lowered.

H. A multidisciplinary approach with the radiation and medical oncology teams is instrumental in management as radiation and bisphosphonate therapies play an important role in management.

Table 11.2 Mirels' criteria

Variable	1	2	3
Site	Upper limb	Lower limb	Peritrochanter
Pain	Mild	Moderate	Functional
Lesion	Blastic	Mixed	Lytic
Size	< 1/3	1/3–2/3	> 2/3

Source: Mirels H. Metastatic disease in long bones. A proposed scoring system for diagnosing impending pathologic fractures. Clin Orthop Relat Res 1989(249):256–264

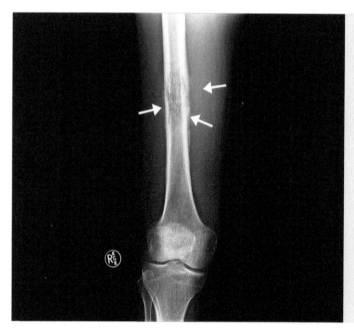

Fig. 11.2 Anteroposterior radiograph demonstrating a mid-diaphyseal aggressive, lytic, destructive lesion of the femur with periosteal reaction, cortical thinning, and associated soft-tissue mass (*arrows*) concerning for impending pathologic fracture. (Radiograph courtesy of Drew D. Moore, MD).

IV. Behaviors of Tumor Subtypes

A. A review of pathologic fractures would be remiss without discussion of tumor subtype behavior. Not all metastatic lesions behave the same and many vary in their response to adjuvant treatments such as radiation and chemotherapy.

B. These "personalities" directly affect oncologic approach, and not respecting these differences can impact construct survivorship, lead to pitfalls in management, and compromise quality of life.

C. Prostate metastases tend to be blastic and the role for prophylactic fixation is low in these cases.

D. Renal and thyroid metastases are notorious for their hypervascularity—liberal use of tourniquet control, when applicable, and strong consideration for preoperative embolization can significantly limit blood loss and assist with local hemostasis during procedures for these hypervascular lesions (▶ **Fig. 11.3**).

E. Plasma cell neoplasms (plasmacytoma and multiple myeloma) and lymphoma respond favorably to adjuvants such as radiation and chemotherapy.

F. Large extraosseous soft-tissue masses can impart significant alteration in normal anatomy. These tumor burdens will significantly decrease with radiation and chemotherapy, and there is little role for aggressively excising these masses unless arthroplasty is being performed for pathologic fracture.

G. Renal cell carcinoma and melanoma are classically less responsive to radiation therefore alternative strategies including the use of surgical adjuvants is helpful to decrease tumor burden and risk of local disease progression (▶ **Table 11.3**).

H. Neoplasms of mesenchymal lineage are termed sarcomas and their behavior, approach, and treatment greatly differs from that of carcinoma, myeloma, or lymphoma.

I. The extent of bone and soft-tissue sarcoma management is beyond the scope of this chapter, but a basic understanding of their presentation and management is instrumental to avoid complications when treating pathologic fractures.

    1. Any biopsy performed in the suspicion of a bone sarcoma should be carried out at an institution that is best suited for definitive management.

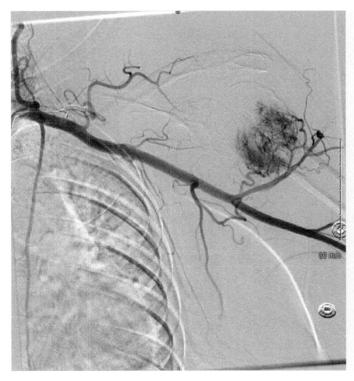

Fig. 11.3 Angiogram demonstrating a hypervascular proximal humerus renal metastases that was successfully embolized prior surgery.

Table 11.3 Surgical adjuvants

Mechanical	Chemical	Thermal
Curettage	Phenol	Argon beam coagulation
Burr	Sterile/distilled water	Electrocautery
	Hydrogen peroxide (H_2O_2)	Liquid nitrogen (cryotherapy)
		Polymethylmethacrylate

2. The biopsy tract should be in line with a future limb salvage approach and meticulous hemostasis should be used to avoid contamination. If clinical suspicion is high for a primary musculoskeletal malignancy, the biopsy should typically be referred to a musculoskeletal oncologist to perform.
3. Neurovascular structures and intermuscular planes should be avoided.

V. Treatment and Management

The principle goal is balancing quality of life and function with disease management. There is little role for restricted weight-bearing or prolonged recovery in the treatment of metastatic disease as median survivorship is often less than 12 months depending on tumor subtype. A sound understanding of disease stage, performance status, patient goals, tumor subtype, and anatomic location are paramount in successful management of these challenging situations.

A. Humerus
   1. Location in the bone often guides treatment options, as lesions proximally involving the humeral head or distally about the elbow are likely best managed with prosthetic replacement.
   2. Reverse total shoulder and alloprosthetic composite have gained favor in their ability to provide pain relief and return to function while balancing complications (▶ **Fig. 11.4**).
   3. Diaphyseal lesions are largely treated with intramedullary fixation or, in rare situations, an intercalary resection and reconstruction (renal cell).
   4. Metaphyseal lesions can be approached with internal fixation in the form of plates/screws or an intramedullary nail depending on location and extent of disease. Surgical adjuvants (▶ **Table 11.3**) play an important role in decreasing local tumor burden, limiting progression of disease, and increasing construct stability which can lead to longer implant survivorship.

B. Acetabulum
   1. The acetabulum is one of the most challenging anatomic locations in the treatment of bone neoplasms given critical locoregional anatomy and associated surgical morbidity.
   2. Complications such as instability, infection, and construct failure have to be weighed against tumor subtype, disease burden, and life expectancy.
   3. Nonoperative adjuvants such as radiation or bisphosphonate treatments or minimally invasive options such as interventional cryoablation, radiofrequency ablation, or cementoplasty play important roles in the options available to manage impending fractures.
   4. Completed fractures that involve the weight-bearing dome that are associated with debilitating pain and functional limitation are best approached with complex arthroplasty. Use of bone cement and Steinmann pins, porous metal augments, or large acetabular shells combined with antiprotrusio cages can be used to reconstruct large osseous defects.
   5. Tumor subtype and extent of disease will often dictate surgical timing as the treatment of periacetabular myeloma and lymphoma will largely be initiated with radiation, bisphosphonates, and chemotherapy followed by delayed surgical reconstruction (▶ **Fig. 11.5**).

C. Femur
   1. Pathologic fractures of the femoral head and neck are best served with arthroplasty.
      a. Various lengths of stem options (curved and straight) and proximal bodies should be available (calcar replacing, modular).

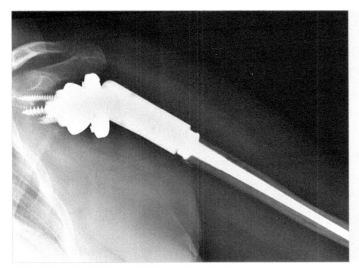

Fig. 11.4 Lateral radiograph of a humerus demonstrating a long stem cemented modular reverse proximal humerus replacement for reconstruction after en bloc resection of a solitary proximal humerus renal cell pathologic fracture.

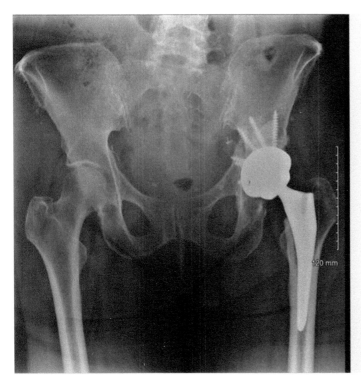

Fig. 11.5 Anteroposterior pelvis radiograph demonstrating multiple screws, cement, and a trabecular metal revision acetabular shell used to reconstruct a solitary plasmacytoma with associated pathologic fracture after neoadjuvant external beam radiation and initiation of systemic bisphosphonates.

    b. Cement is often advocated in the setting of metastatic disease as fixation does not rely on ingrowth and many patients will go on to receive adjuvant radiation.

    c. Caution should be used as intraoperative cardiopulmonary events have been reported with this technique.

    d. Low-viscosity cement, forgoing canal pressurization, and the use of cement restrictor as well as high fractions of inspired oxygen and/or a distal vent hole (i.e., 2.5-mm drill bit) can be various strategies employed to lower this risk.

2. The peritrochanteric area of the femur has received the most attention, given the mechanical stress and construct failure observed with both extramedullary and intramedullary devices.

    a. Extramedullary devices (plates) are associated with higher failure rates.

    b. A statically locked long cephalomedullary device allows immediate weight-bearing through its load sharing properties.

3. A high number of pathologic fractures will never obtain osseous union and therefore several technical considerations are important to consider as the mechanical properties and elastic modulus of the implants vary between traumatic and pathologic etiologies.

    a. Proximal nail diameter varies by manufacturer and using a larger-diameter (both proximally and distally) implant increases the bending rigidity of a cannulated implant by the radius to the third power.

    b. As a general principle, statically locked (often with more than one distal interlocking screw) antegrade intramedullary nails are recommended for diaphyseal lesions.

    c. Retrograde femoral nails should be avoided as they do not protect the femoral neck and risk intra-articular contamination and progression of disease.

    d. Implants with a lower radius of curvature (more bowed) can facilitate more distal fixation when performing antegrade fixation for quite distal fractures (i.e., extreme nailing).

    e. A dynamic interlocking hole can be used for "kissing screws" with both medial and lateral directed interlocking screws.

    f. Hybrid fixation with plate/nail can provide accurate and reliable spanning fixation and allow for immediate weight-bearing.

    g. The use of blocking screws to increase construct stability (▶ Fig. 11.6).

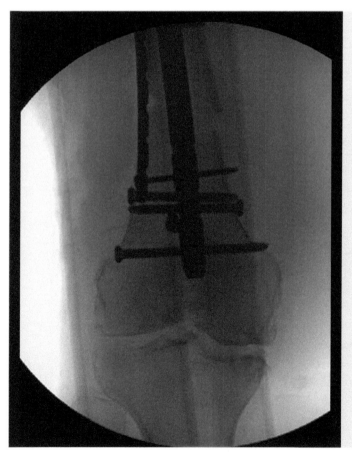

Fig. 11.6 A statically locked long antegrade intramedullary femoral nail with low radius of curvature allowing more distal placement for this metaphyseal metastatic lung carcinoma pathologic fracture. Note "kissing screws" through dynamic interlocking hole, blocking screw and plate augmentation to allow immediate weight-bearing and increase construct rigidity with relatively short working length.

4. Arthroplasty removes many of the limitations of internal fixation by replacing the diseased and fractured bone, but benefits must be balanced with risk.

5. Wound healing, infection, and instability remain challenges in the often nutritionally and immunocompromised hosts.

6. Disease stage, performance status, patient goals, and the plan for adjuvant treatments (timing of chemotherapy) need to be carefully considered when deciding between arthroplasty and internal fixation.

D. Tibia

1. Pathologic fractures of the tibia are less frequently encountered, but can provide unique management challenges.

2. En block resection/proximal tibia replacement presents functional challenges with extensor mechanism reconstruction and therefore the use of surgical adjuvants in addition to robust fixation and poly (methyl methacrylate) (PMMA) can often provide durable fixation while providing patients an early functional return with limited restrictions (▶ **Fig. 11.7**).

3. Intramedullary nail tenets as outlined for the femur have similar application to impending or completed pathologic fractures of the tibia.

   a. Large-diameter nails.

   b. Numerus interlocking screws in multiple planes of fixation.

   c. Adjuvant blocking screws to increase short working length stability (▶ Fig. 11.6).

   d. Extra-articular insertion technique.

   e. Meticulous respect for soft tissues.

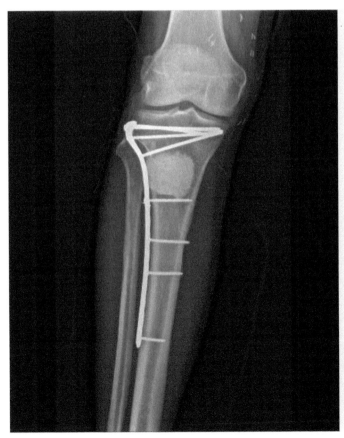

Fig. 11.7 Postoperative anteroposterior radiograph of a proximal tibia metastatic renal cell fracture treated with adjuvants including embolization, open curettage, argon beam thermal coagulation, cementation and internal fixation to allow minimal postoperative restrictions and initiate systemic chemotherapy in a timely fashion while preserving the extensor mechanism of the knee.

VI. Adjuvants

A. Surgical adjuvants are largely what separate the treatment of pathologic fractures from traumatic fractures. They are used strategically and intentionally to not only decrease tumor burden and chance for local disease progression or recurrence, but allow for safe and effective management while providing lasting and durable results.

B. Surgical adjuvants can be mechanical, chemical, or thermal in nature (▶Table 11.3). They are particularly useful in high stress, metaphyseal locations with significant bone loss from tumor destruction or comminuted fracture.

   1. An assortment of angled curettes, pituitary rongeurs, and various diameter round burrs are quite helpful for meticulous mechanical adjuvant treatment of an endosteal lesion.

   2. Argon beam thermal coagulation or monopolar electrocautery on a "fulgurate" setting work quite effectively to provide local thermal ablation and are more readily available.

   3. PMMA can serve as a thermal adjuvant as well as provide additional structural stability by serving to increase both bending and torsional rigidity as the stress modulus is similar to that of bone.

C. A multidisciplinary approach with referral to a radiation oncologist, medical oncologist as well as dedicated bone health provider (consideration for bisphosphonate or anabolic bone agent) is crucial in the management strategy beyond the technical aspects of the surgical procedure.

VII. Complications and Pitfalls

A. The treatment of pathologic fractures is not without complications. With the exception of prophylactic fixation, few procedures are elective and many patients present in a nutritionally depleted state.

B. Electrolyte imbalances, cytopenia, and immunosuppression from systemic treatment need to be corrected in a team fashion.

C. Complications

   1. Delayed/failure of wound healing: common in patients receiving antiangiogenic chemotherapeutic medications.

   2. Infection.

   3. Local disease progression.

   4. Mechanical fixation failure.

   5. Instability.

D. The majority of pathologic fractures will be treated by orthopaedic surgeons not specialized in orthopaedic oncology and the incidence of pathologic fractures continues to increase as life expectancy has increased with newer targeted agents and immune therapies. Diligence is vital to avoid pitfalls in management (▶Table 11.1).

Conclusion

Pathologic fractures are frequently encountered and a sound understanding of treatment principles is fundamental to every surgeon caring for these challenging patients (▶Table 11.4). Approach needs to vary from that of traditional traumatic fracture fixation principles, as many of these fractures will never go on to osseous union. An algorithmic approach to a lytic lesion of bone with an unknown primary origin is necessary to avoid pitfalls in diagnosis and treatment. Basic serum studies, CT of the chest, abdomen, and pelvis, and a whole-body nuclear medicine bone scan for staging should be initiated prior to biopsy or surgical intervention in general.

Understanding the basic behavior of certain tumor subtypes is helpful to avoiding pitfalls as several tumor subtypes are poorly radiosensitive, highly vascular, and prone to local progression despite surgical

Table 11.4 Take home points in the management and treatment of pathologic fractures

Perform a thorough and complete history and physical examination which includes abdomen, breast, rectal, lymphatic and integumentary systems	Staging studies including labs (CBC, CMP, SPEP/UPEP) and imaging (CT C/A/P and whole-body nuclear medicine bone scan) should be performed prior to surgical intervention
Obtain diagnostic/lesional tissue at time of procedure to confirm diagnosis and guide postoperative treatment	Radiographs including two orthogonal views of the entire bone are mandatory to avoid multifocal lesions
Renal and thyroid subtypes are often hypervascular (consider embolization), poorly sensitive to radiation, and en bloc resection can be considered in isolated disease	Liberal use of surgical adjuvants (mechanical: curettage, burr; thermal: argon beam coagulation, PMMA)
Robust and durable fixation constructs (large-diameter nails, locking screws, cement, hybrid fixation, etc.)	Low threshold for arthroplasty in periarticular locations
Goal for immediate and unrestricted weight-bearing postoperatively	Postoperative radiation referral for adjuvant control of localized disease

Abbreviations: CBC, complete blood count; CMP, comprehensive metabolic panel; CT C/A/P, computed tomography chest abdomen pelvis; PMMA, polymethylmethacrylate; SPEP/UPEP, serum/urine protein electrophoresis.

intervention. Most procedures performed for pathologic fractures are of palliative nature, but a subset of patients will have long-term survival so construct stability requires durability.

The threshold for arthroplasty for periarticular pathologic fractures should be low, as goals of treatment are to provide immediate and unrestricted activity. The use of surgical adjuvants such as chemoembolization, curettage, argon beam thermal coagulation, cryotherapy, PMMA and radiotherapy should be employed liberally to decrease tumor burden and progression of local disease.

By adhering to a principle-based approach for pathologic fractures, treating surgeons can return patients to optimal and timely function while providing durable local control of disease and lasting construct stability.

Suggested Readings

Mankin HJ, Lange TA, Spanier SS. The hazards of biopsy in patients with malignant primary bone and soft-tissue tumors. J Bone Joint Surg Am 1982;64(8):1121–1127

Mirels H. Metastatic disease in long bones. A proposed scoring system for diagnosing impending pathologic fractures. Clin Orthop Relat Res 1989(249):256–264

Nathan SS, Healey JH, Mellano D, et al. Survival in patients operated on for pathologic fracture: implications for end-of-life orthopedic care. J Clin Oncol 2005;23(25):6072–6082

Rougraff BT, Kneisl JS, Simon MA. Skeletal metastases of unknown origin. A prospective study of a diagnostic strategy. J Bone Joint Surg Am 1993;75(9):1276–1281

12 Principles of Pediatric Fracture Management

George Gantsoudes

Introduction

Children are not small adults. They have different anatomy (physes, thicker periosteum, etc.), different physiology (faster healing), and have the potential to remodel angulated fractures. This chapter will discuss the unique treatment of pediatric fractures about the elbow, forearm, knee, and ankle. The Salter–Harris classification is the most frequently used classification to describe physeal injury (▶Fig. 12.1; ▶Video 12.1, ▶Video 12.2).

Pediatric Elbow Fractures

I. Preoperative

A. Obtain a good history

1. These injuries often occur from falls greater than 6 feet (frequently from the monkey bars).
2. Make sure that there has not been any head or neck trauma or loss of consciousness that will require further work-up.

B. Physical exam

1. Check all four limbs for additional injury—remember that the most commonly missed fracture is "the second one."
2. Assess the antecubital fossa for puckering or hematoma—this indicates a more significant injury and should push for earlier surgical management.

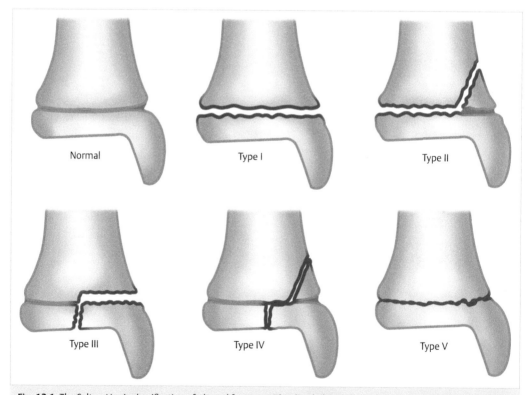

Fig. 12.1 The Salter–Harris classification of physeal fractures. The distal tibia is shown here as an example.

C. Neurologic exam

    1. Children in pain are often scared and can be uncooperative with a physician in a rush.

    2. A little bit of effort to make the child feel comfortable can go a long way.

    3. There are many simple exams to look for radial, median, ulnar, anterior interosseous (AIN) and posterior interosseous (PIN) nerve function.

        a. Minimize motion of the elbow and wrist, as these are frequently the most injured areas.

        b. A simplified approach is to check for:

            i. PIN: thumb interphalangeal (IP) extension, "thumbs up."

            ii. AIN: thumb IP and index distal IP flexion, "A-OK sign."

            iii. Ulnar: interosseous muscle function, "cross-fingers" or "scissors."

            iv. Median: isolate flexor digitorum superficialis function to middle finger.

    4. Sensory exam to light touch is acceptable, but this is a subjective exam.

        a. A frightened child may just tell you what you want to hear to make you go away.

        b. If there is sufficient concern that a nerve may be damaged and the child cannot or will not cooperate, a moist towel may be wrapped around the fingers for 5 minutes. There will not be any skin wrinkling to insensate fingers.

D. Vascular exam

    1. Check for pulses at the wrist.

    2. If the pulses cannot be palpated or cannot be auscultated with a Doppler, assess the capillary refill. There can be sufficient arterial flow to the hand even in cases of brachial artery disruption due to abundant collateral supply.

        a. Pink hand: the capillary refill matches that of the other side. It signifies sufficient flow and should be treated urgently.

        b. White hand: if there is no, or severely diminished, capillary refill:

            i. Signifies insufficient flow, should be treated emergently.

            ii. Consult vascular surgery immediately if flow does not return with reduction.

II. Anatomy and Imaging

A. The elbow has six secondary centers of ossification that ossify and fuse at different times. Knowledge of these can help an orthopaedist tell the difference between a normal and abnormal elbow radiograph (▶ Fig. 12.2).

    1. Below are average ages of *appearance* of secondary ossification centers—boys tend to lag behind girls by 1 to 2 years.

    2. Capitellum: 1 to 2 years.

    3. Radial head: 3 to 5 years.

    4. Medial epicondyle: 5 to 8 years.

    5. Trochlea: 7 to 10 years.

    6. Olecranon: 8 to 10 years.

    7. Lateral epicondyle: 11 to 13 years.

B. The "fat pad signs" can be seen on the lateral radiograph and especially the posterior fat pad sign can help identify an "occult" fracture that cannot be easily visualized on emergency department (ED) radiographs (▶ Fig. 12.3a, b).

C. Assess the angles on the anteroposterior and lateral views—if you are not sure if the angles are appropriate, obtain a radiograph of the normal limb for comparison.

D. Obtain oblique views (internal oblique) to visualize maximum displacement of lateral condyle fractures.

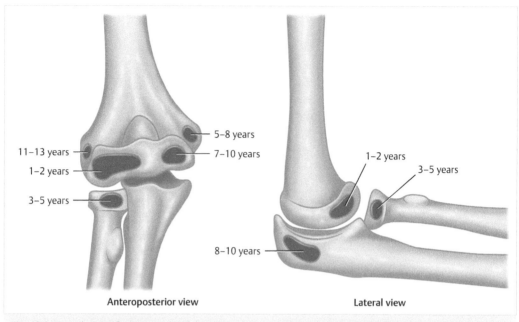

Fig. 12.2 Secondary ossification centers of the elbow with approximate ages of appearance.

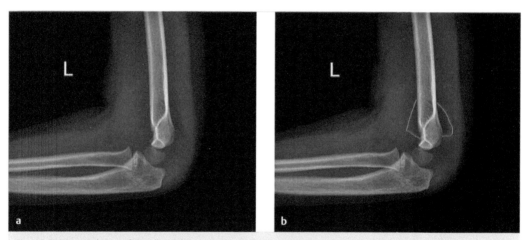

Fig. 12.3 (a) Lateral view of the elbow showing a type I supracondylar humerus fracture with anterior and posterior fat pads visible. (b) Lateral view of the elbow with fat pads outlined.

III. Classification

A. Supracondylar humerus fractures

   1. Gartland (extension type makes up 95%) (▶ **Fig. 12.4**):

      a. I—nondisplaced.

      b. II—angulated, but at least one cortex intact.

      c. III—no continuity between cortices.

      d. IV—this is an intraoperative assessment and is a type III without an intact periosteal hinge; can be iatrogenically created from hyperflexion of a malreduced type III.

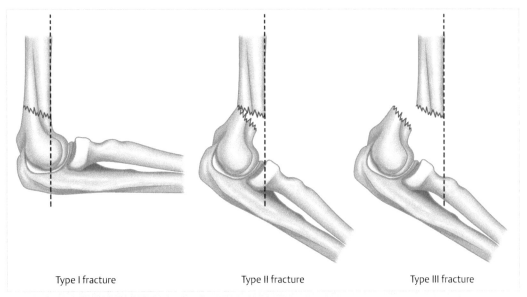

| Type I fracture | Type II fracture | Type III fracture |

Fig. 12.4 The Gartland classification of extension-type supracondylar distal humerus fractures; types I to III.

B. Lateral condyle fractures
    1. Most commonly used classification is Jakob.
        a. I—nondisplaced with intact articular cartilage hinge.
        b. II—complete fracture, but minimally displaced (2–4 mm).
        c. III—complete fracture and malrotated out of the joint.

IV. Initial Management

A. Supracondylar humerus fractures
    1. Type I—unless there is significant varus (type Ib) on the anteroposterior image, these are treated in a cast for 3 to 4 weeks.
    2. Type II—splint in the ED and should undergo closed reduction and percutaneous pinning (can be done electively).
    3. Type III—splint in a position of comfort and treat with closed (possible open) reduction and percutaneous pinning. The soft tissue and neurovascular status will determine if this is done same day or next day.
    4. Transphyseal fractures—can occur in the very young patients (usually less than 3 years old).
        a. Fifty percent of these patients present because of nonaccidental trauma (NAT).
B. Lateral condyle fractures
    1. Type I—placed into a long arm cast/splint and given weekly follow-up for 2 weeks to check for further displacement.
    2. Type II—closed (possible open) reduction and percutaneous pinning (electively); assess articular congruency with an arthrogram.
    3. Type III—splint position of comfort, followed by open reduction and percutaneous pinning (or screws, if fracture pattern allows). This should be done when the best team is available; not in an emergency.

V. Definitive Management

A. Supracondylar humerus fractures

1. Pinning technique is almost always done from the lateral side, unless the fracture pattern necessitates a medial pin.

2. Pin spread across the fracture site is crucial for stability.

3. A good rule of thumb is two pins are required for a type II and three (or more) are required for a type III (▶ **Fig. 12.5**).

4. Medial pins should be placed after initial stabilization is performed laterally and with the elbow in slight extension to protect the ulnar nerve—in meta-analyses, 3 to 4% patients had injury to the ulnar nerve with a medial pin technique.

5. Large C-arm positioning:
   a. Place the C-arm parallel to the long axis of the patient, and swing it around to check the lateral image prior to pinning.
   b. This prevents undesired rotation that may occur through the fracture site if one rotates the arm instead.

6. A long-arm cast (which is subsequently univalved/bivalved) is placed over sterile dressing.

7. Follow-up in 1 week to overwrap the cast.

8. Pin pull is done in the clinic after 3 to 4 weeks (longer for older children).
   a. Activity restrictions are in place for 6 to 8 weeks postoperatively.
   b. Further cast immobilization is rare.

B. Lateral condyle fractures

1. Pinning technique maximizes pin spread across the fracture site.

2. Stability is key to prevent nonunions (which can happen in lateral condyle fractures).

3. For open reduction, consider a head lamp to aid in visualization.

4. The goal is to reduce the articular surface; anatomic reduction of the articular surface with metaphyseal abnormalities typically will not result in adverse outcomes.

5. A long-arm cast (which is subsequently univalved/bivalved) is placed.

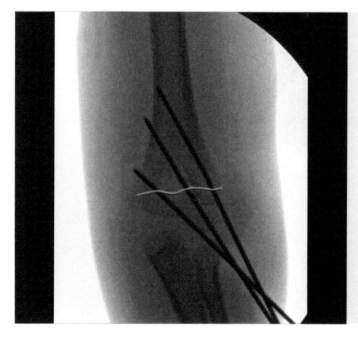

Fig. 12.5 Three lateral entry pins demonstrating good spread across the supracondylar distal humerus fracture site, crossing the lateral, middle, and medial columns.

6. Follow-up in 1 week to overwrap the cast.
7. Pins are pulled after 4 weeks, and **only** if there is sufficient bridging callus. Sometimes 6 weeks' time is required.

VI. Complications

A. Supracondylar humerus fractures
   1. Complications are almost always related to the nonosseous injuries.
   2. Nerve injuries are usually neuropraxias that can take months (but frequently just weeks) to resolve.
      a. AIN is most common.
      b. Radial nerve less common.
      c. Ulnar nerve more common with flexion type.
   3. Compartment syndrome is more frequent with ipsilateral radius/ulna fractures. Cases with a median nerve injury need to be very closely monitored, as the patient may not have sensation sufficient to alert the physician to worsening pain.
   4. Vascular injuries require close attention.
      a. A preoperative pink, pulseless hand that fails to regain pulses should be monitored for at least 24 hours postoperatively.
      b. A white pulseless hand that fails to revascularize after closed reduction should be opened (with the appropriate vascular staff available).
   5. Pin infection.
   6. Malunion.
B. Lateral condyle fractures
   1. Nonunion.
   2. Avascular necrosis.
   3. Stiffness (most common complication).
   4. Malunion.
   5. Lateral overgrowth.

VII. Rehabilitation

A. Very few children require therapy for these fractures.
B. Families should be counseled that it can take 6 to 12 months for range of motion to return to normal.

VIII. Outcomes

A. Supracondylar humerus fractures—children should be able to return to full activities within 2 to 3 months from the injury.
B. Lateral condyle fractures
   1. Children should be able to return to full activities within 3 months from the time of injury.
   2. These fractures can take longer for range of motion to return to normal; advise families appropriately.

Pediatric Forearm Fractures

I. Preoperative

A. See the elbow section above.

II. Imaging

A. In order to properly assess pediatric forearm fractures, it is imperative to adequately image the elbow and wrist. The dreaded "missed Monteggia" fracture is an unacceptable complication and difficult to treat late (see Chapter 25, Olecranon and Monteggia Fractures, for further discussion of Monteggia injury).

B. Order dedicated elbow and wrist X-rays if needed.

III. Classification

A. Pediatric forearm fractures are generally classified by location, fracture pattern, and positioning.

B. Other than fractures that involve the elbow (i.e., Monteggia) or the wrist (i.e., Galeazzi), forearm fractures do not have a routinely used classification system.

C. OTA/AO classifications are largely for research purposes and are not generally used.

IV. Initial Treatment

A. Closed forearm fractures should generally undergo an attempt at a closed reduction under sedation in the ED with fluoroscopy.

1. Exceptions:

   a. Angulation < 15 degrees in the midshaft and 10 degrees in the proximal radius is acceptable in children 9 years and under.

   b. Most open fractures are treated in the operating room; however, the treatment of type 1 open fractures is controversial.

   c. The setting of impending/ongoing compartment syndrome.

2. The greater the kinetic energy involved in the injury, the older the child, and the more complex fracture, the more are the chances that the patient will fail closed reduction and require operative treatment.

B. Forearm reduction should pay close attention to the fracture pattern.

C. It is imperative to have a focused assistant hold the arm, or use finger traps (+/– weights).

1. Greenstick fractures:

   a. Usually rotational injuries with at least one of the long bones intact.

   b. Reduction of rotational injuries **should not** use techniques that "recreate" the fracture pattern.

      i. This will render a largely stable fracture pattern unstable.

   c. Fractures with apex volar deformities can be reduced with a pronation maneuver, and those with apex dorsal deformities can be reduced with supination (▶Fig. 12.6a, b).

2. Complete fractures:

   a. All attempts should be made to restore the length of the forearm (via the ulna) and to restore the radial bow.

D. The author prefers to place all patients in a long-arm cast that is univalved (with spacers placed in the gap). The cast should have a good interosseous mold and a straight ulnar border.

E. Postreduction radiographs should be carefully assessed for alignment on anteroposterior and lateral images.

1. The axial plane can be assessed by making sure that the radial styloid is roughly 180 degrees of supination from the biceps tuberosity and that the ulnar styloid is roughly 180 degrees of supination from the coronoid process.

2. There is wide anatomic variation and contralateral radiographs may be of assistance.

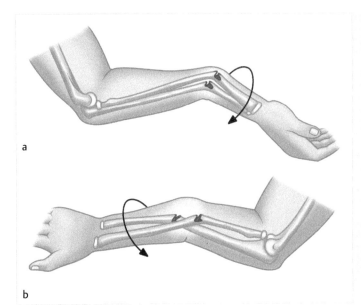

Fig. 12.6 The "rule of thumb" technique reduces the rotation and angulation in a forearm fracture. (a) Apex volar fracture created by excessive supination. This fracture is reduced using a pronation maneuver (rotating the thumb toward the apex of the deformity). (b) Apex dorsal fracture with a pronation deformity. A supination maneuver reduces this deformity.

F. Failure to achieve adequate reduction (variable by age and location in the bone) may be an indication to go to the operating room; this is almost always done electively.

G. If reduction is adequate, follow-up within 7 to 10 days to assess alignment and overwrap of the cast is mandatory—one of the reasons that the author prefers a cast to a long-arm splint is the availability to wedge a cast in clinic, if needed.

V. Definitive Treatment

A. Cast treatment is definitive for the majority of patients.

B. If operative treatment is indicated, choose age-appropriate implants.

1. Plates and screws are rarely the best choice for young children. Rigid fixation is not needed and retention and removal of plates has been associated with late refracture.

2. Relative stability provided by flexible nails (titanium or steel) or even K-wires has been shown to be effective with less operative morbidity.

C. When choosing relative stability, it is important to understand that there will often be slight translation or angulation; this is almost always acceptable.

1. Young children have a remarkable potential to remodel forearm translation and, to a lesser extent, angulation.

2. Remember: "If it's acceptable in the emergency room (ER), it's acceptable in the operating room." Also remember that remodeling potential relies upon remaining growth; a 12 year old may not be able to remodel what a 6 year old can.

VI. Complications

A. Malunion (malrotation is most common)

1. In order to prevent malunion, weekly imaging is mandatory until either bridging callus is seen or the fracture has not displaced since postreduction ER imaging. Forearm fracture alignment does not spontaneously improve; if loss of reduction is noted, an intervention (new cast, cast wedge, operative treatment, etc.) should be performed.

B. Missed ipsilateral injuries. Examples are Galeazzi or Monteggia fractures (see Chapter 25, Olecranon and Monteggia Fractures, and Chapter 28, Distal Radius and Galeazzi Fractures; respectively, for further reading).

C. Compartment syndrome

1. Rare complication for nonoperative fractures.

2. Reported increased risk after three or more false passages of flexible nails.

D. Refracture.

VII. Rehabilitation

A. Rarely indicated.

VIII. Outcomes

A. For well-reduced fractures, outcomes are excellent.

B. Poor outcomes largely come from "hoping" remodeling will occur, despite evidence to the contrary.

1. Older patients and those with rotational deformities will not remodel predictably.

2. The further away from the fast-growing distal radius/ulna physis the fracture is, the less the potential for remodeling.

Femoral Shaft

I. Preoperative

A. Obtain a good history.

1. Does the story make sense?

   a. Low-energy femoral fractures (especially proximally) do not occur in healthy pediatric bone.

   b. Look carefully for pathologic bone.

2. Ask for details.

   a. Discerning between child abuse and accidental trauma can be difficult and is often beyond the scope of the orthopaedist's practice.

   b. However, the ability of the parents to recall (and repeat) specific details of incident is inversely correlated with NAT.

   c. When in doubt, alert the appropriate personnel in the hospital if there are **any** questions about child abuse.

B. Physical exam

1. These patients are often in extreme pain; do a brief (but comprehensive) physical exam.

2. Assess for other injuries and distal neurovascular function.

   a. Scared, young patients may not even "wiggle" their toes; reassurance that you won't ask the patient to do anything painful often helps.

   b. Do a thorough neurologic and vascular exam.

   c. Compartment syndrome is rare in the thigh.

II. Anatomy and Imaging

A. Anteroposterior and lateral images are standard in the ER. High-energy injuries should also have dedicated hip images to assess for ipsilateral femoral neck injuries.

B. If the fracture pattern is obvious and a trip to the OR is planned, it is often ok to accept suboptimal orthogonal imaging rather than subjecting a child in pain to multiple trips to the X-ray suite.

III. Classification

A. Pediatric femoral shaft fractures are generally classified by location, fracture pattern, and positioning.

B. OTA/AO classifications are largely for research purposes and are not generally used.

IV. Initial and Definitive Treatment

A. Fracture management can be stratified into (roughly) four age groups:

1. Birth to 6 months—soft wrap or Pavlik harness.

2. Six months to 4–6 years—generally, closed reduction and spica cast.

3. 4–6 years to 8–10 years—flexible nails versus submuscular plate.

4. More than 10 years:

   a. Can treat with rigid intermeduallary fixation (lateral entry) or submuscular plate.

   b. Flexible nails should not be used in patients > 50 kg.

B. The youngest group can be definitively treated in the ED and sent home once cleared for risks of NAT. The orthopaedist should **not** be the clearing physician unless sufficiently trained to be so.

C. Patients going to the OR for definitive treatment should be made comfortable for their trip to the OR.

1. Only patients with neurovascular compromise require emergent or urgent fixation.

2. Most patients can be made comfortable in a posterior splint (younger) or Buck's traction (older).

3. Traction pins are **rarely** used, but if necessary, should be placed in the metaphysis of the distal femur (**avoid physeal injury!**).

V. Type of Immobilization or Fixation

A. Spica cast

1. It should be placed while on a spica table.

2. Femoral shaft fractures can be expected to drift 5 to 10 degrees in to varus and procurvatum. "Overcorrection" in anticipation of these drifts is part of the treatment plan.

3. The single-leg walking spica cast has been shown to be safe and effective without compromising outcomes (▶**Fig. 12.7**). Parental satisfaction is significantly greater.

4. The spica cast is generally worn for a time period determined by a "formula" of (age in years) + (3) = weeks in cast. Long oblique fractures generally can be removed earlier than short oblique/transverse diaphyseal fractures. It is rare to need a spica cast for longer than 5 weeks.

B. Flexible nails

1. Indications for this treatment have a range of starting age (4–6 years), but it is generally more acceptable after age 5.

2. The ideal patient is one less than 50 kg with a length stable fracture.

3. In general, two nails are placed with opposing concavity, the size of each nail can be estimated by measuring the canal at its narrowest part.

   a. A canal fill of ~80% is the goal.

   b. The diameter of each nail should be about 40% of the narrowest canal diameter.

4. Toe-touch weight bearing until callus forms.

5. Nail removal is electively scheduled about 1 year from surgery.

C. Submuscular plates

1. Generally for those patients who are not eligible for flexible or rigid nail.

2. Typically a bridge plate.

3. Toe-touch weight bearing until callus forms.

4. Plate removal is electively scheduled about 1 year from surgery.

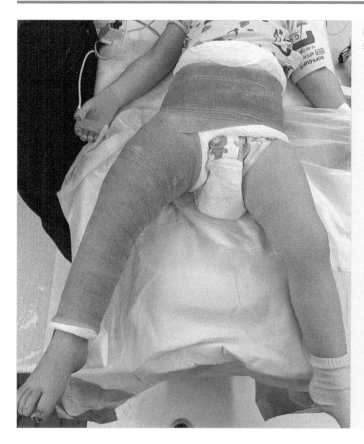

Fig. 12.7 Photograph of a walking single-leg hip spica cast.

D. Rigid intramedullary nail

1. Indications are any child ineligible for flexible nails older than age 9. The use of **lateral entry** rigid intramedullary nails has been shown to be safe in children > 9 years of age.

2. Advantages:

   a. Techniques are very familiar to all orthopaedists.

   b. Immediate weight-bearing is almost always possible.

3. A **lateral entry** nail designed for use in pediatric patients must be used to prevent avascular necrosis.

4. It is not necessary to remove the nail; author prefers to remove the distal interlock.

   a. In a child with substantial growth remaining, the distal interlock will migrate proximally with growth.

   b. An interlock that was once metaphyseal will become diaphyseal and become prominent medially.

VI. Complications

A. Malunion

1. It is important to understand the amount of angulation allowed for each age group.

   a. In infants, virtually all deformities will remodel.

   b. For spica casts, malalignment under 10 degrees of coronal plane and under 15 degrees in the sagittal plane is the goal.

   c. Anatomic alignment is the goal for fractures treated with internal fixation.

B. Infection

    1. Infection following operative treatment of femur fractures is very rare.

C. Symptomatic hardware

    1. Flexible nails—the quadriceps frequently become symptomatic if the entry point is made anterior to the midline of the femur.

    2. Submuscular plate—rare.

    3. Rigid nail—distal interlocks can become symptomatic with growth.

VII. Rehabilitation

A. Spica cast

    1. Therapy rarely indicated, but an option.

        a. The family needs to be prepared for weeks to months of "limping," especially for the younger child.

            i. Remember, the difference between an excuse and explanation is timing, and an ill-prepared family will worry unnecessarily and call your office frequently.

B. Flexible nails and submuscular plates

    1. Toe-touch weight bearing initially and advance to weight bearing as tolerated (WBAT) once callus forms.

C. Rigid intramedullary nail

    1. Almost all can start with WBAT.

VIII. Outcomes

A. Symptomatic malunion is rare.

B. Children should be followed for at least 1 year after injury to check for limb length inequality.

    1. Even in cases of anatomic reduction, an idiopathic ipsilateral overgrowth can be seen.

Pediatric Physeal Ankle Fractures

I. Preoperative

A. Perform a thorough neurologic and vascular exam.

    1. Check the function of the tibial, superficial peroneal, deep peroneal, sural, and saphenous nerves.

    2. Document pulses and capillary refill.

B. Check for skin tenting.

II. Anatomy and Imaging

A. Anteroposterior, lateral, and mortise films.

B. The distal tibia physis closes in a pattern that can cause specific fractures in adolescents (see below). The physis closes from central → anterior → medial → posterior → lateral.

C. Do not forget to look for intra-articular fractures. Following reduction (see below), further imaging with a computed tomography scan can determine the extent of intra-articular involvement.

III. Classification

A. The Salter–Harris classification of physeal fractures is generally used to describe these injuries (▶ Fig. 12.1).

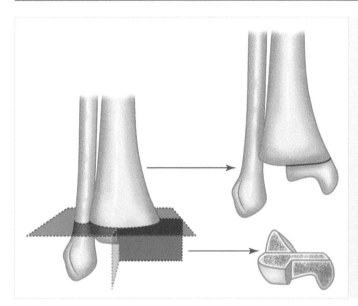

Fig. 12.8 An example of a triplane distal tibia fracture.

B. Fracture patterns that have been described in adolescents (largely due to the pattern of physeal closure).

1. Tillaux (Salter–Harris III): The anterior-lateral epiphyseal portion of the distal tibial physis can be avulsed via the anterior-inferior tibiofibular ligament. This pattern occurs because that segment of the distal tibial physis is the last to close, and thus the weakest link in the chain.

2. Triplane (Salter–Harris IV): This fracture pattern exits both through the metaphysis and the epiphysis. However, it is not always easy to identify this pattern looking at one image, and careful examination of multiplanar imaging is necessary (▶Fig. 12.8).

IV. Initial Treatment

A. Nondisplaced fractures should be immobilized in a bivalved cast or splint and definitive cast should be placed once the swelling recedes.

B. Almost all displaced fractures benefit from a closed reduction in the ER under sedation.

C. Multiple attempts of unsuccessful physeal fracture reduction should be avoided as physeal damage can occur.

D. Triplanes and Salter–Harris II fractures can avulse periosteum off of the metaphysis that can be entrapped in the fracture site and prevent reduction.

V. Definitive Treatment

A. Different fracture patterns require different methods of treatment.

1. Most extra-articular fractures can be treated with or without an open reduction and K-wires.

2. Open reduction of physeal fractures almost always involves removal of entrapped periosteum to aid in reduction.

   a. The indication for open reduction is malalignment, not the prevention of physeal arrest.

   b. Open reduction does not reduce the rate of premature physeal closure (PPC).

   c. Any growth arrest that occurs is felt to be due to the injury itself.

3. Typically, Salter–Harris III and IV fractures displaced ≥ 2 mm require anatomic open reduction, usually with rigid fixation.

    a. Fractures with 0 to 1 mm displacement require close follow-up.

    b. For the patient with growth remaining, avoid crossing the physis with screws.

B. Most children with bimalleolar ankle fractures do not require plate fixation of their fibula. Older adolescents with adult-pattern Weber B or C fractures should be assessed and treated similar to adults.

VI. Complications

A. Physeal arrest

1. Salter–Harris I and II patterns have a PPC rate of up to 40%, regardless of closed or open treatment.

2. Salter–Harris III and IV patterns have an increased rate of physeal arrest with closed treatment.

3. Due to the slow rate of growth of the distal tibia physis (4–5 mm/year), follow-up of at least 6 months is required to ensure physeal arrest does not occur.

VII. Rehabilitation

A. It is the author's opinion that patients recovering from ankle fractures benefit from a physical therapy program to work on strengthening and proprioception to prevent reinjury.

VIII. Outcomes

A. As long as PPC can be avoided, the outcomes are universally good.

B. There is controversy about whether or not to remove periarticular implants. The author removes the intraepiphyseal screws 6 to 12 months after implantation.

Suggested Readings

Badkoobehi H, Choi PD, Bae DS, Skaggs DL. Management of the pulseless pediatric supracondylar humeral fracture. J Bone Joint Surg Am 2015;97(11):937–943

Flynn JM, Garner MR, Jones KJ, et al. The treatment of low-energy femoral shaft fractures: a prospective study comparing the "walking spica" with the traditional spica cast. J Bone Joint Surg Am 2011;93(23):2196–2202

Keeler KA, Dart B, Luhmann SJ, et al. Antegrade intramedullary nailing of pediatric femoral fractures using an interlocking pediatric femoral nail and a lateral trochanteric entry point. J Pediatr Orthop 2009;29(4):345–351

Pennock AT, Charles M, Moor M, Bastrom TP, Newton PO. Potential causes of loss of reduction in supracondylar humerus fractures. J Pediatr Orthop 2014;34(7):691–697

Russo F, Moor MA, Mubarak SJ, Pennock AT. Salter-Harris II fractures of the distal tibia: does surgical management reduce the risk of premature physeal closure? J Pediatr Orthop 2013;33(5):524–529

Wilkins KE. Nonoperative management of pediatric upper extremity fractures or 'Don't throw away the cast'. Tech Orthop 2005;20(2):115–141

13 Acute Compartment Syndrome

Christopher Doro

Introduction

Acute compartment syndrome (ACS) remains a clinical emergency that occurs in orthopaedic trauma practice. ACS continues to present orthopaedic surgeons and other clinicians with diagnostic and treatment challenges. Evaluation of patients with suspected ACS must be prompt and fasciotomies, if needed, must be rapidly performed.

I. Preoperative

A. Risk factors for ACS

1. Tibia fractures are most commonly associated with ACS, followed by soft-tissue injuries and finally forearm/wrist fractures.

2. When looking at all the causes of ACS, sport-related injuries lead to the highest total number of ACS cases (~ 25%).

3. Many other causes of ACS have been reported including bleeding, burns, intravenous (IV) infiltrations, intraoperative positioning, compressive dressing or casts, reperfusion injury, high-pressure injection injuries, and drug overdoses (prolonged pressure on dependent compartment).

4. Incidence of ACS with specific injuries:

    a. Tibia shaft fracture: 3%–10%.
    b. Tibial plateau fracture: 12%.
    c. Bicondylar plateau fractures and medial condyle fracture-dislocations: up to 30%.

5. Multiple studies have shown younger age to be a major independent risk factor. Ages from 10 to 30 years tend to be the strongest predictor for ACS.

6. Civilian ballistic injuries have a reported low rate of ACS (~3%). However, isolated fibula and isolated tibia ballistic injuries have ~11% reported incidence of ACS. Proximal injury location accounted for nearly 90% of the cases.

7. Open fractures are not protected from ACS. Most series show an increase in ACS when open fractures are compared to closed.

B. Diagnosis

1. Diagnosis is difficult and rates of ACS diagnosis can vary from surgeon to surgeon within the same institution treating the same injuries (surgeons ranged from 2% to 24% in ACS diagnosis and treatment).

2. Exam in ACS

    a. Clinical exam is considered the gold standard for diagnosis, and unless a reliable exam is not possible (obtunded patient, head injury, intraoperative, etc.) other diagnostic modalities are not indicated.

    b. Classically, the five Ps have been incorrectly applied to ACS exam and diagnosis (pain, pallor, pulselessness, paresthesias, and paralysis). These were initially described for arterial insufficiency and are not very accurate for ACS. The vast majority of ACS patients have normal pulses.

    c. Typical exam findings include:

        i. Pain out of proportion.
        ii. Pain with passive stretch of the muscle in the affected compartment.
        iii. Paresthesias.
        iv. Anesthesia or decreased sensation.

     v. Muscle weakness or paralysis.

     vi. Tense compartment on palpation—be aware as palpation of compartments alone has a low sensitivity and specificity in diagnosis of ACS (24 and 55%, respectively).

3. Intracompartmental pressure measurements (ICP)

   a. ICP is the current standard for diagnosis when exam is questionable or not possible.

   b. Pressures have been shown to be highest at the fracture site and dissipate with increasing distance from the fracture.

   c. Most clinicians recommend measuring the ICP close to the fracture site.

   d. Classic dogma uses ΔP measurement < 30 mm Hg for diagnosis.

     i. ΔP is calculated by subtracting the ICP from the patient's diastolic blood pressure prior to anesthesia (if being done in the operating room). Theoretically as this number approaches 0, the perfusion decreases in the compartment.

     ii. ΔP > 30 mm Hg is a very conservative threshold. Clinical studies show this to be a safe threshold; however, it may lead to overtreatment.

     iii. False positive rates of 35% in operative tibia fractures (no ACS when ICP measured).

   e. Typical modern devices used for pressure measurement include slit catheter (▶ **Fig. 13.1a**), side port needle (▶ **Fig. 13.1b**), solid-state transducer intracompartmental catheter (STIC), electronic transducer tipped catheter, and arterial-line transducers.

     i. These methods are fairly similar in their pressure measurements (0.83 correlation). However, ~30% of the time the differences can exceed 10 mm Hg between these devices.

     ii. The invasive portion of the device (slit catheter, side port needle, 18-guage needle) in early literature showed the side port to be superior; however, more recent studies suggest that an 18-gauge was as accurate as the others.

   f. There is a concerning variability in pressure measurements clinically. In one study, 60% of clinicians measured ICP within 5 mm Hg of the control ICP.

   g. The use of continuous pressure monitoring is still being evaluated. To date, all studies that have compared continuous monitoring to clinical monitoring with noncontinuous ICP measurements have not shown a difference in outcome or delay in treatment.

4. Other diagnostic modalities

   a. Near-infrared spectroscopy (NIRS):

     i. NIRS relies on the difference in absorption of near-infrared wavelengths of light (600–1,000 nm) in biologic tissue. The wavelengths can pass through skin, soft tissue, and bone but are absorbed by hemoglobin and can determine its oxygenation state.

     ii. NIRS is a noninvasive and rapid assessment of tissue oxygenation that has future promise.

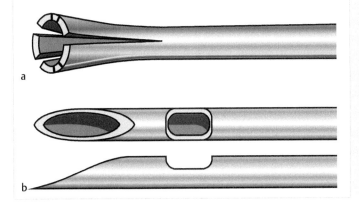

Fig. 13.1 Intracompartmental pressure measurement devices: (a) slit catheter; (b) side port needle.

        iii. To date, the literature is mixed on the accuracy in diagnosis of ACS.

        iv. Large trials are ongoing to determine its effectiveness.

    b. Biomarkers:

        i. Serum levels of creatine kinase (CK) > 4,000 U/L, Cl >104 mg/dL, and blood urea nitrogen (BUN) < 10 mg/dL have been shown to be significantly correlated to ACS; however, the ability to aid in diagnosis is unclear.

        ii. Lactate levels have been evaluated in vascular patients with an acute embolism, the relevance in ACS needs to be evaluated.

        iii. Intracompartmental glucose concentration and pH have been shown to be significant markers in experimental animal models only. Clinical data is lacking.

    c. Ultrasonography:

        i. Pulsed phase-locked loop ultrasound uses reflection off fascial planes to identify a characteristic waveform from local arterial pulsation that is altered in ACS.

        ii. Preliminary research shows this may be effective in the future.

    d. Other methods:

        i. MRI, scintigraphy, and laser Doppler flowmetry are some of the other diagnostic tools purposed for ACS diagnosis.

        ii. Drawbacks related to these modalities include decreased specificity, limited availability, cost and increased time required to evaluate patients.

        iii. As of now they have no role in diagnosis of ACS.

C. Radiographic correlations with ACS

    1. The odds of ACS in tibia fractures increases by 1.7 per 10% increase in the ratio of fracture length to total tibia length.

    2. Initial femoral displacement ratios (> 8%) (displacement with respect to the tibia divided by femoral condylar width) have a significant correlation with ACS in plateau fractures.

    3. Initial plateau widening (> 5%) after plateau fracture has been associated with ACS.

D. Compartment anatomy

    1. Leg—four compartments (▶Fig. 13.2)

        a. Anterior—tibialis anterior, extensor digitorum longus, extensor hallucis longus, peroneus tertius, anterior tibial artery, and deep peroneal nerve.

        b. Lateral—peroneus brevis, peroneus longus, and superficial peroneal nerve.

        c. Deep posterior—tibialis posterior, flexor digitorum longus, flexor hallucis longus, tibial nerve, peroneal artery, and posterior tibial artery.

        d. Superficial posterior—gastrocnemius, soleus, popliteus, plantaris, and sural nerve.

    2. Thigh—three compartments

        a. Anterior—sartorius, rectus femoris, vastus lateralis, vastus intermedius and vastus medialis, articularis genus, femoral nerve, and femoral artery.

        b. Posterior—biceps femoris, semitendinosus, semimembranosus, profunda femoris, and sciatic nerve.

        c. Adductor—pectineus, external obturator, gracilis, adductor longus, adductor brevis, adductor minimus, and adductor magnus.

    3. Gluteal—typically considered three compartments: (the compartment can also be considered the epimysium over these large muscles) tensor fascia lata, gluteus medius and minimus, and gluteus maximus.

    4. Foot—traditionally considered to be nine compartments. The medial, superficial, and lateral compartments run the length of the foot. The adductor and four interossi compartment are in the forefoot and calcaneal compartment is in the hindfoot.

        a. Four intraosseous compartments.

        b. Medial—abductor hallucis and flexor hallucis brevis.

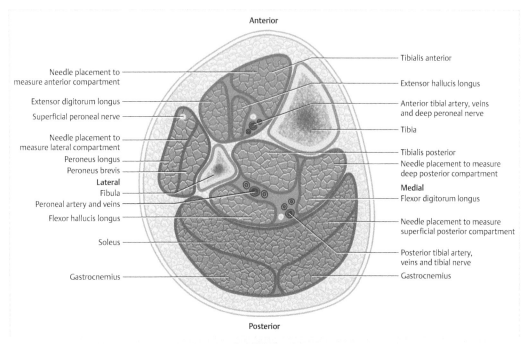

Fig. 13.2 Lower leg compartments with depiction of needle placement for pressure measurement.

Labels (left): Needle placement to measure anterior compartment; Extensor digitorum longus; Superficial peroneal nerve; Needle placement to measure lateral compartment; Peroneus longus; Peroneus brevis; **Lateral**; Fibula; Peroneal artery and veins; Flexor hallucis longus; Soleus; Gastrocnemius

Labels (top/right): Anterior; Tibialis anterior; Extensor hallucis longus; Anterior tibial artery, veins and deep peroneal nerve; Tibia; Tibialis posterior; Needle placement to measure deep posterior compartment; **Medial**; Flexor digitorum longus; Needle placement to measure superficial posterior compartment; Posterior tibial artery, veins and tibial nerve; Gastrocnemius; Posterior

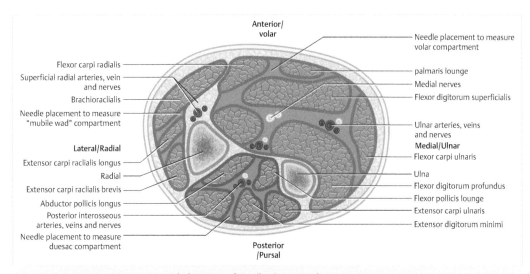

Fig. 13.3 Forearm compartments with depiction of needle placement for pressure measurement.

Labels (left): Flexor carpi radialis; Superficial radial arteries, vein and nerves; Brachioraclialis; Needle placement to measure "mubile wad" compartment; **Lateral/Radial**; Extensor carpi raclialis longus; Radial; Extensor carpi raclialis brevis; Abductor pollicis longus; Posterior interosseous arteries, veins and nerves; Needle placement to measure duesac compartment

Labels (top/right): Anterior/ volar; Needle placement to measure volar compartment; palmaris lounge; Medial nerves; Flexor digitorum superficialis; Ulnar arteries, veins and nerves; **Medial/Ulnar**; Flexor carpi ulnaris; Ulna; Flexor digitorum profundus; Flexor pollicis lounge; Extensor carpi ulnaris; Extensor digitorum minimi; Posterior /Pursal

     c. Superficial (or central) compartment—flexor digitorum brevis, flexor digitorum longus tendons, and four lumbricals.

     d. Calcaneal—quadratus plantae.

     e. Adductor—adductor hallucis.

     f. Lateral—flexor digiti minimi brevis and abductor digiti minimi.

5. Forearm (▶ **Fig. 13.3**)

     a. Anterior (volar)—flexor carpi radialis, palmaris longus, flexor carpi ulnaris (FCU), pronator teres, flexor digitorum superficialis (FDS), flexor digitorum profundus (FDP), flexor pollicis longus (FPL), pronator quadratus.

  b. Dorsal—extensor carpi ulnaris, extensor digitorum, extensor digiti minimi, abductor pollicis longus (APL), extensor pollicis longus (EPL), extensor pollicis brevis, extensor indicis, and supinator.

  c. Mobile wad—brachioradialis, extensor carpi radialis brevis (ECRB), and extensor carpi radialis longus (ECRL).

 6. Arm

  a. Anterior—coracobrachialis, biceps brachii, brachialis, brachial artery, ulnar and median nerve.

  b. Posterior—triceps, anconeus, and radial nerve.

 7. Deltoid.

 8. Hand (10 total).

  a. Hypothenar, thenar, adductor pollicis, dorsal interosseous (× 4), palmar interosseous (× 3).

  b. The carpal tunnel should be included in decompression.

II. Treatment

A. Surgical

 1. Muscle and tissue ischemia if untreated will lead to irreversible necrosis and contracture of the limb.

 2. Rapid and thorough decompression of the affected limb is the standard of care.

 3. Single incision and dual incisions are both acceptable for the lower leg.

 4. Incision should be almost the full length of the compartment. The dermis can contribute to increased pressure in the compartment.

 5. Lower leg fasciotomies—dual incision approach (▶ **Fig. 13.4**).

  a. Lateral incision halfway between the tibial crest and fibula extending approximately two-third of the leg.

   i. Elevate skin flaps and identify the intermuscular septum.

   ii. Release anterior compartment fascia throughout the length of the wound.

   iii. Release lateral compartment fascia.

   iv. Protect the superficial peroneal nerve as it emerges from deep to superficial between the peroneus longus and brevis, and courses from the lateral compartment in the middle one-third of the leg and pierces the deep fascia approximately 12 cm

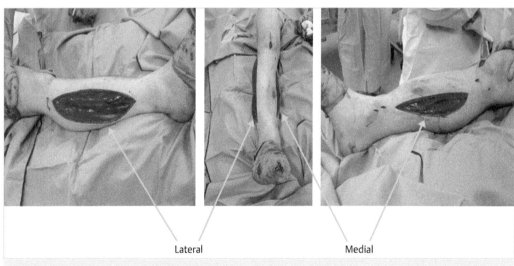

Lateral   Medial

Fig. 13.4 Clinical photo showing a two-incision technique for lower leg fasciotomy.

proximal to the tip of the lateral malleolus. It then courses distally in the anterior subcutaneous tissue. The nerve has considerable variation. The nerve can often run with the intermuscular septum and can pass into the anterior compartment before exiting the deep fascia.

   b. Medial incision 1 to 2 cm posterior to the posterior border of the tibia:

       i. Identify and protect the saphenous bundle.

      ii. Decompress the superficial posterior compartment by incising the fascia of the lateral head of the gastrocnemius and lateral soleus.

     iii. Carefully release soleus off the proximal posterior tibia to access the deep posterior compartment. Release fascia distally with an elevator to completely decompress the deep posterior compartment.

6.   Forearm fasciotomy (▶ **Fig. 13.5**)

   a. Volar forearm:

       i. There are many skin incisions that have been described. The most practical incisions should start lateral/radial proximally and should end medial/ulnarly. This allows the surgeon to extend proximally and cross the elbow crease lateral to medial, to expose brachial artery if needed and cross the wrist crease medial to lateral. This allows soft tissue coverage over the carpal tunnel if decompressed and protects the palmer cutaneous branch of the median nerve. The resultant incision is a "lazy S."

      ii. Identify the distal biceps and release the lacertus fibrosus. The artery can be identified here if needed.

     iii. Develop the plane between FDS and FDP decompressing and protecting the median nerve, and release the fibrous arch of the FDS and deep fascia over FDP.

     iv. Systematically evaluate and release any other muscle bellies, if needed.

      v. Proceed to carpal tunnel release if desired.

   b. Alternate volar forearm (ulnar):

       i. The ulnar approach has been described to cause the least amount of iatrogenic surgical injury.

      ii. The skin incision is made radial to FCU and extended to medial epicondyle.

     iii. Release the superficial fascia.

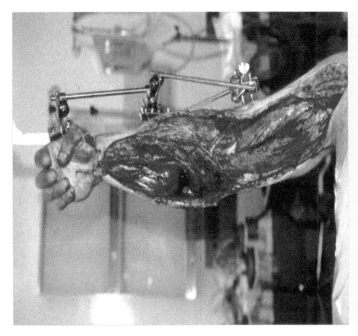

Fig. 13.5 Clinical photo showing volar forearm fasciotomy associated with arm fasciotomy.

      iv. Identify the interval between FCU and FDS.

      v. Identify and protect the ulnar bundle, and develop the plane between the ulnar bundle and FDS. The segmental branches from the ulnar artery to the FDS will need to be divided.

      vi. Elevate FDS to decompress the deep fascia (PQ, FDP, FPL).

  c. Dorsal forearm:

      i. If necessary, after volar release proceed to dorsal release.

      ii. Create a midline incision between EDC and ECRB.

      iii. Release the fascia/epimysium over extensors.

      iv. Avoid injury to the posterior interosseous nerve.

      v. Extend distally to include APL and EPL and deep for supinator, if necessary.

  d. Mobile wad (lateral compartment):

      i. If necessary, after volar release and or dorsal proceed to mobile wad release.

      ii. Usually the fascia over brachioradialis, ECRL, and ECRB can be accessed through the dorsal or volar incisions. If not, make additional incision directly over the mobile wad.

      iii. Release the fascia over the mobile wad and individual epimysium as needed.

B. Medical treatment

  1. The patient must be adequately resuscitated.

    a. Monitor renal function and myoglobinuria:

      i. Diuresis is critical in myoglobinuria treatment.

      ii. Raising the pH of the urine to 6.5 or higher may minimize the breakdown of myoglobin and formation of toxic metabolites. It is unclear if this technique is superior to aggressive hydration and diuresis.

  2. Anti-inflammatory treatment is being evaluated in animal models and may show some promise in decreasing muscle damage.

C. Other treatment methods

  1. Ultrafiltration is another proposed treatment of ACS that has been described. This technique requires inserting a catheter into the concerning compartment and removing excess fluid. This has been shown to be effective in some animal models. At this time more robust clinical data is needed before any recommendations can be made.

D. Outcomes

  1. Missed ACS can be devastating with significant loss of limb function and contractures.

  2. The sequelae of fasciotomies include sensory changes, swelling, possible decrease in muscle strength, muscle herniation, tethered scars, and cosmetic issues.

  3. Increased infection rates and nonunion/delayed union rates have been published in patients with ACS and tibia plateau or tibia shaft fractures.

  4. ACS more than doubles hospital stay and charges.

III. Special Considerations

A. Pediatric patients

  1. Traumatic cases causing ACS occur most commonly in children > 14 years of age.

  2. In younger children (< 10 years), vascular injuries and infection causes of ACS are more common.

  3. Examination can be difficult in the pediatric patient.

  4. The three As are more appropriate in children. Increasing anxiety, agitation, and analgesic requirement.

  5. Management is similar to adults.

B. Treatment of ACS in the foot

1. Traditionally, ACS in the foot has been treated with emergent fasciotomies.

2. Recently, some authors have suggested that delayed treatment of ACS in the foot (e.g., claw toes) may be easier to treat than managing fasciotomy wounds (especially in the setting of fractures requiring fixation).

3. Others have suggested dorsal dermal fenestrations ("pie crusting") as a possible treatment method instead of formal fasciotomies. The advantage of this technique is that is minimizes the need for secondary soft tissue procedures. However, it is unclear if this technique adequately decompresses all of the compartments in the foot.

4. Little data is available to guide surgeons on outcomes regarding delayed treatment versus fasciotomies. There is, however, literature demonstrating
an increased complication rate with increased time to fasciotomy for foot ACS. Many authors feel that the complications of delayed treatment are still greater than that of fasciotomies.

Suggested Readings

McQueen MM, Court-Brown CM. Compartment monitoring in tibial fractures. The pressure threshold for decompression. J Bone Joint Surg Br 1996;78(1):99–104

McQueen MM, Duckworth AD, Aitken SA, Court-Brown CM. The estimated sensitivity and specificity of compartment pressure monitoring for acute compartment syndrome. J Bone Joint Surg Am 2013;95(8):673–677

McQueen MM, Duckworth AD, Aitken SA, Sharma RA, Court-Brown CM. Predictors of compartment syndrome after tibial fracture. J Orthop Trauma 2015;29(10):451–455

Mubarak SJ, Owen CA. Double-incision fasciotomy of the leg for decompression in compartment syndromes. J Bone Joint Surg Am 1977;59(2):184–187

Shadgan B, Pereira G, Menon M, Jafari S, Darlene Reid W, O'Brien PJ. Risk factors for acute compartment syndrome of the leg associated with tibial diaphyseal fractures in adults. J Orthop Traumatol 2015;16(3):185–192

Whitesides TE, Haney TC, Morimoto K, Harada H. Tissue pressure measurements as a determinant for the need of fasciotomy. Clin Orthop Relat Res 1975(113):43–51

14 Amputations

Kevin Tetsworth and Vaida Glatt

Introduction

Relative roles of limb salvage and amputation after trauma remain controversial (▶ **Fig. 14.1**). Difficult choice reflects severity of the injury, patient's expectations and demands, surgeon's training and experience, and the capabilities and limitations of a particular institution. Many limbs can be saved with effort and huge investment (time and money); in some instances the patient would be better served with an early amputation. Amputation is an excellent reconstruction option and should never be considered a "failure of treatment." Decision to amputate involves many factors and it is carried out after a thorough discussion between patients, their families, prosthetists, rehabilitation physicians, and surgeons. Most often the final decision involves consultation between two or more senior surgeons regarding the indications, treatment alternatives, and patient-specific considerations.

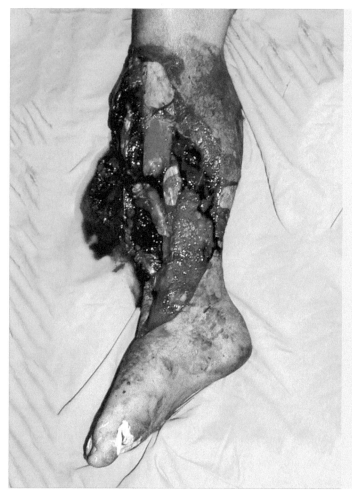

Fig. 14.1 Mangled extremity, type 3B open tibia fracture with significant diaphyseal bone and soft-tissue loss. Highly complex and difficult decisions are required in determining whether to perform an early amputation or to proceed with limb salvage and reconstruction.

I. Preoperative Assessment

A. History and physical examination

1. Consider all the aspects related to patient: employment, education level, psychiatric issues/personality disorders, compliance, patient motivation, and quality of their social support network.

2. These factors are more closely related to outcome than anything surgeons do.

3. History of the injury.

4. Systemic factors:

   a. Comorbidities—blindness, Parkinson's disease, obesity, dementia, stroke—consider end-bearing stump.

   b. Smoking.

5. Local factors—vascularity, scarring, and bony prominences.

6. Multiple limb involvement—introduces another level of complexity.

7. Pain—localized tenderness (neuroma, bursitis, or infection), dysesthesias or neurogenic pain that is characteristic of neuroma, suspicion of chronic regional pain syndrome (CRPS).

8. Medication use—opioid dependency and illicit drugs.

9. Range of motion (ROM) of knee, hip, elbow—assess for hip flexion and knee flexion contractures.

10. Strength of local muscles—knee flexion/extension, hip flexion/extension, hip abduction/adduction.

11. The single most important muscle for functional gait is hip extension.

B. Imaging

1. Routine radiographs are usually all that is necessary.

2. For vasculopaths, Doppler studies and an ankle–brachial index (ABI) can be used to assess vascular supply and the risk of wound healing insufficiency.

3. Computed tomography scans and magnetic resonance imaging both are useful when assessing tumors and chronic infections.

4. Nuclear medicine scans are generally not helpful.

5. Dual-energy X-ray absorptiometry scans to assess bone mineral density are very useful if osseointegration is an option.

C. Classification

1. **Acute injuries—**many classification systems exist but overall interobserver variability is poor and not typically helpful in prognosis. The extent of soft-tissue injury or loss may be the most predictive outcome regardless of which classification system is used.

2. **Amputations—**most often these are classified according to expected anatomic level:

   a. **Upper limb** (▶Fig. 14.2)—forequarter, shoulder disarticulation, transhumeral (above elbow), through elbow, transradial (below elbow), wrist disarticulation.

   b. **Lower limb** (▶Fig. 14.3 and ▶Fig. 14.4)—hip disarticulation, transfemoral (above knee), through knee (knee disarticulation), transtibial (below knee), Syme's, Boyd or Pirogoff (preserve a portion of the calcaneus and the attached heel pad; fuse this composite to the distal tibia), Chopart (through talonavicular and calcaneocuboid joints), Lisfranc (through the tarsometatarsal joints), transmetatarsal, metatarsophalangeal joint (▶Fig. 14.5).

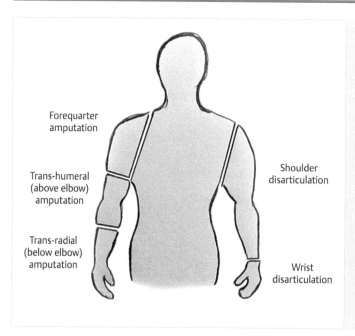

Fig. 14.2 Upper extremity amputation options.

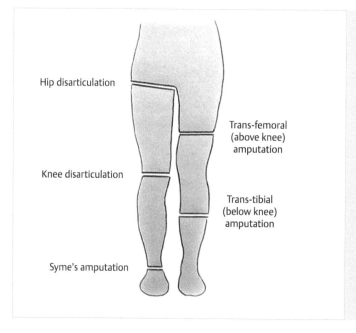

Fig. 14.3 Lower extremity amputation options.

II. Initial Management

A. Initial management steps

1. Polytrauma patients should follow advanced trauma life support (ATLS) principles (see Chapter 9, Polytrauma, for additional details on the ATLS protocol).

2. Thorough debridement and lavage in the operating room: evaluate the injury severity, hemostasis, remove all foreign or devitalized material, extend margins of wound for better visualization, and excise bone fragments completely stripped of soft tissue.

3. Assess for possible compartment syndrome.

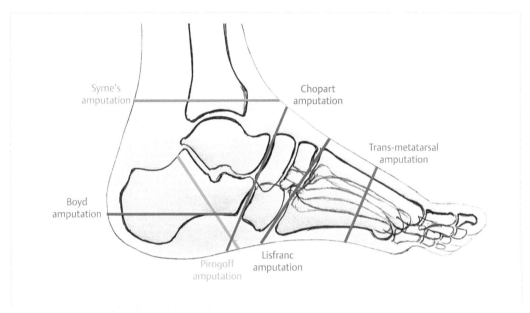

Fig. 14.4 Foot amputation options.

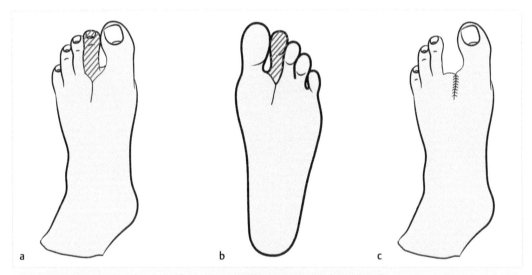

Fig. 14.5 (a–c) Racquet style incision for a toe amputation (metatarsophalangeal level).

4. Improve reduction and apply spanning external fixation and sterile dressings.

5. Consider consultation with Plastic Surgery, Vascular, and Trauma Units.

B. Limb salvage or early amputation

1. Preinjury status (education, income, social support) is more important than the injury or treatment.

2. Comparable outcomes with limb salvage or primary amputation.

3. Patients can confidently choose which route they prefer with the expectation of similar outcomes.

4. Delayed amputation can still lead to a good outcome and permits an initial attempt of limb salvage.

III. Definitive Management

A. Indications for immediate amputation

1. Traumatically amputated limb, or nearly so.

2. Severely injured limb beyond what could be reasonably reconstructed—subjective, and the "severity" reflects clinical acumen and experience of surgeons involved.

3. Limb completely avascular and vascular repair not possible.

4. Limb is the source of uncontrollable hemorrhage.

5. Limb is the source of life-threatening infection.

B. Relative indications for early amputation

1. Severe open injuries of the foot and ankle.

2. Degloving soft-tissue injuries of the foot with loss of the heel pad (▶Fig. 14.6).

3. Anticipated outcome will inevitably result in a stiff, painful, and nonfunctional foot or hand.

4. Extensive soft tissue and/or bone loss.

C. An insensate plantar surface is no longer considered a relative indication as long-term prospective studies have shown sensation may return and this does not appear to significantly affect functional outcome.

D. Indications for amputation for definitive late post-traumatic reconstruction

1. Recalcitrant nonunion.

2. Chronically/recurrently infected.

3. Dysvascular.

4. The focus of incapacitating neurogenic pain.

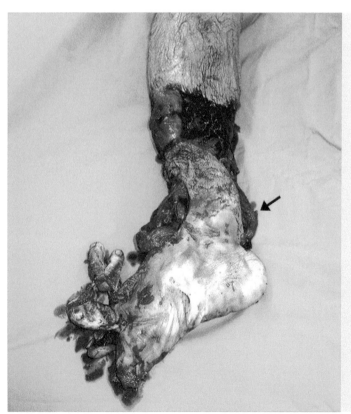

Fig. 14.6 Degloving injury, skin avulsed from entire foot (*arrow* indicates exposed calcaneus).

5. Significant neurologic deficit affecting the patient's function.

6. Stiff/painful/deformed foot or hand.

IV. Surgical Principles

A. Metabolic cost of gait after amputation

1. Metabolic demand is measured as energy expenditure or oxygen consumption.

2. Depends on the level—inversely proportional to the length of the residual limb.

3. General attempt is to preserve as much length as possible.

4. Increased energy consumption relative to baseline (intact lower limbs):

   a. Syme: 15%.

   b. Below knee amputation (BKA; transtibial): vascular 40%, traumatic 25% (short residuum 40% or long residuum 10–15%).

   c. Above knee amputation (AKA; transfemoral): vascular 100%, traumatic 70%.

   d. Bilaterals:

      i. BKA + BKA = 40%.

      ii. BKA + AKA = 120%.

      iii. AKA + AKA > 200%.

5. Almost 90% of bilateral above knee amputees are wheelchair bound within 2 years.

6. Unfortunately, stump length is most often dictated by soft tissues and local vascularity.

B. The ideal stump

1. Short stump lacks mechanical advantage necessary for gait and can slip out of the socket.

2. Long stump is also more difficult to fit with a prosthetic limb—adequate space is required to accommodate all the components necessary.

3. Optimum length (▶ **Fig. 14.7**):

   a. For AKA, 15 cm above the knee joint line.

   b. For BKA, 10 cm below tibial tubercle or 15 cm below knee joint line:

      i. A longer stump has mechanical advantages and length should be preserved when possible.

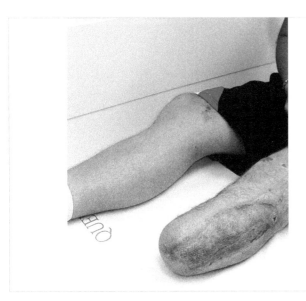

Fig. 14.7 Typical clinical appearance of a post-traumatic below knee amputation stump, 15 months after the injury. Extensive scarring and skin grafts complicate prosthetic fitting.

     ii. The fibula is more mobile in longer stumps and may become symptomatic (post-traumatic):
- Consider creating a formal tibiofibular synostosis (Ertl procedure).
- More difficult and technically demanding.
- It has been shown in military injuries to not affect outcome with higher complication rates.

    iii. Minimum of 25 cm clearance to fit components for a prosthetic foot/ankle—longer stump is easier to achieve in a tall patient, difficult when patient is short.

4. Smooth, firm, and round or conical-shape end best fits a socket-mounted prosthetic limb.

5. Minimal scar or prominent bone.

6. Opposing muscle groups sutured together over the bone end (myodesis).

7. Soft tissue covers bone end and provides effective cushion to local trauma.

8. Soft tissue coverage well vascularized; stable, not mobile.

9. For the lower limb, scars should be positioned away from the end of the residuum.

10. For upper limb amputations, the scar can be terminal.

11. Nerves transected short, buried in muscle away from the end of the residuum.

C. Transtibial (below knee) amputation after trauma

1. The operative techniques described here encompass the major principles of amputation surgery and can be generally applied to most other locations and different levels as required.

2. Incisions:

    a. Guillotine—used in an emergency situation to control hemorrhage or infection; in general, preserve as much good soft tissue as possible for later definitive amputation.

    b. "Fish mouth"—simplest and least technically demanding incision.

    c. Extended posterior flap—best applied for a BKA (▶ Fig. 14.8).

    d. "Racquet"—useful for amputation of digits (▶ Fig. 14.5).

3. Specific to transtibial (below knee) amputation (extended posterior flap):

    a. Supine, nerve block for pain control in perioperative period.

    b. Tourniquet to 250–275 Torr (mm Hg).

    c. Traditionally amputation site is hands breadth below the tibial tubercle:

        i. Now it is more common to do a mid-tibial amputation.

        ii. Prosthetists need 25 cm clearance from the ground to bottom of the stump.

        iii. Middle third length a good balance—better mechanics and more strength.

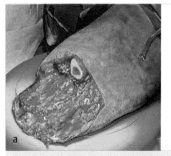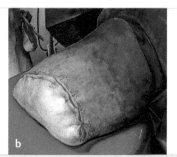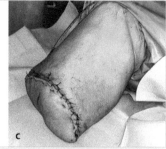

Fig. 14.8 Extended posterior flap: (**a**) intraoperative photograph of a completed transtibial amputation, prior to closure; (**b**) posterior flap trimmed of excess tissue and provisionally closed with subcuticular resorbable sutures; (**c**) postoperative photograph after closure completed with nylon sutures.

4. As residuum gets longer it "scissors" more and can be symptomatic, particularly when there is prior diastasis between the tibia and fibula (as in a displaced pilon fracture).

5. Controversial, but young trauma patients may be best candidates for a "bone bridge" (Ertl) procedure.

6. Based on soft tissues and other issues, select a level: examine limb from lateral view, and estimate width of limb with a ruler (e.g., 16 cm); distal margin posterior soft-tissue flap should lie at a point (n + 1) cm distal (i.e., 17 cm).

7. Surgical approach for a BKA:

   a. Incisions: straight transverse anterior at level of expected bone cut—extend distally medial/lateral posterior to equator—through skin, SQ, fascia.

   b. Distal posterior—straight transverse at calculated level—through skin, SQ, fascia.

   c. Medially isolate saphenous vein and nerve.

   d. Traction on nerves and cut sharply—saphenous is the least problematic (Chapter 13, Acute Compartment Syndrome, ►Fig. 13.2).

   e. Do not cut nerve at same level as prosthetic limb will rest—needs to be 1 to 2 cm proximal.

   f. On lateral side find interosseous membrane.

   g. Slide a clamp under it, then transect anterior and lateral compartments with knife.

   h. Retract muscle distally, then expose neurovascular bundle—ligate tibialis anterior vessels and then identify the deep peroneal nerve—traction on nerve, cut and allow it to retract proximally.

   i. Cut the tibia with a power saw under saline irrigation; cut fibula 1 to 2 cm shorter.

   j. Use a bone hook to control the tibia and use an amputation knife on posterior surface.

   k. Directly on back of tibia and fibula—complete amputation, remove foot and distal tibia.

   l. Dissect between deep and superficial posterior compartments; this plane is easier to find medially.

   m. Neurovascular bundle stays with fascia of the deep compartment—dissect out completely.

   n. Open the sheath distally, split longitudinally—take entire nerve out, do not injure vein.

   o. Traction on nerve, transect sharply independent of vessels—retract 8 to 10 cm proximal.

   p. Transect neurovascular bundle and isolate artery and two veins—suture ligate peroneal vessels.

   q. All named vessels get two ties with 0 silk suture—stick tie distal, free tie more proximal.

   r. Do not use free ties alone because the pulsatile motion could loosen the suture.

   s. In case of patients with "throbbing pain" after amputation possibly from ligating peroneal nerve with vessels of anterior compartment—separate them and cut nerve independently.

   t. Identify sural nerve in midline posteriorly—pull out 15 cm and then transect under tension.

   u. Ligate small saphenous vein adjacent to sural nerve—generally large, tendency to bleed.

   v. Remove soleus as needed to facilitate closure, but leave thick fasciocutaneous flap.

   w. Bevel end of exposed bone with a saw and then bevel the two corners created, rasp edges.

   x. Release tourniquet, get hemostasis—many venous bleeders in soleus—suture ties useful.

   y. Complete myodesis with heavy suture to close posterior fascia to anterior periosteum; the myodesis can be completed through drill holes in the anterior tibial cortex for a more secure repair.

   z. Close the superficial subcutaneous layer with 2-0 absorbable sutures and the skin with 2-0 non-absorbable sutures, using Steri-Strips to augment the closure between sutures; then apply sterile dressings, plus/minus a removable cast.

D.   Transfemoral (above knee) amputation
1.   Fish mouth incision.
2.   Transect anterior (quadriceps) and lateral musculature using principles described above.
3.   Identify and isolate the femoral artery and vein, suture ligate as described above.
4.   Apply traction to the femoral nerve, cut sharply and allow to retract proximally.
5.   Pull traction and sharply transect the saphenous nerve allowing it to retract proximally.
6.   Transect medial musculature (adductors, sartorius, gracilis) 5 to 10 cm distal to the anticipated femoral cut for later adductor myodesis.
7.   Cut the femur ~ 15 cm proximal to the knee joint.
8.   Transect the remaining posterior (hamstring) musculature.
9.   Identify the sciatic nerve and place a single suture ligature; apply traction and sharply transect the sciatic nerve, allowing it to retract proximally.
10. Complete the adductor myodesis with heavy suture through drill holes in the distal femoral residuum; suture the posterior hamstring fascia to the anterior quadriceps fascia for additional soft-tissue coverage of the stump.

V. Postoperative Care

A.   Some surgeons prefer a drain for several days.
B.   Elevate unless dysvascular to reduce edema.
C.   Early mobilization.
D.   Various options available for dressings:
1.   Rigid dressings—plaster of Paris (POP) rigid removable cast for first 4 to 6 weeks; decreases edema and postoperative pain, protects stump end from trauma, allows immediate mobilization, molds residuum into conical shape to accelerate prosthetic fitting, and prevents flexion contractures.
2.   Soft dressings—bulky cotton gauze wrapped with elastic crepe bandage. These decrease edema and mold residual limb into conical shape to accelerate prosthetic fitting.
3.   Elastic gauze—inexpensive, light weight, and readily available. Care must be taken or it may create a tourniquet, also it needs frequent reapplication.
E.   Suture removal at 3 to 4 weeks, wound often slow to heal (particularly in dysvascular and diabetic patients).

VI. Complications

A.   Early
1.   Wound hematoma.
2.   Infection and dehiscence.
3.   Soft-tissue necrosis.
4.   Anemia.
5.   Deep vein thrombosis.
6.   Pulmonary embolism.
7.   Phantom limb pain common early with approximately 30% long-term pain.
B.   Late
1.   Pain.
2.   Adherent scar.
3.   Heterotopic bone.

4. Ulceration/cellulitis/infection.

5. Contractures and limited joint motion.

C. Pain can have several different sources, and one must identify the etiology: neuromas, CRPS, "phantom limb."

D. Symptomatic neuroma

1. Very common; severed nerves will inevitably form a neuroma.

2. Transect nerves under tension, migrates proximally away from end of stump.

3. Localize by gentle percussion, local injections.

4. Try cortisone injections, but this often leads to revision surgery for formal neurectomy.

E. CRPS

1. Neuromas can be localized, but CRPS has a global response.

2. Can be extremely difficult to manage.

3. Phantom limb sensation (sense absent limb is still present).

4. Phantom limb pain (sense absent limb is still painful).

F. Potential etiologies—remaining nerves continue to generate signals; spinal cord initiates excessive spontaneous firing in the absence of expected sensory input, altered signal transmission/modulation/response within the somatosensory cortex.

VII. Rehabilitation

A. The rehabilitation steps include:

1. **Goals**—residual limb shrinkage, limb desensitization, maintaining joint ROM, strengthening residual limb, maximizing self-reliance, and reintegration into the workforce/society.

2. **Home modifications**—external ramps, stair lift/railings, doors widened for wheelchairs, kitchen work surfaces and sinks adjusted lower, shower with level entrance, shower seat, possible hoist for bath, adapted furniture/mirrors.

3. **Car modifications**—modify pedals/seat, lift to assist entry, consider hand controls.

4. Encourage socialization, vocational training, return to gainful employment.

5. Educate patient regarding future goals and prosthetic options.

B. Socket fitting

1. POP casting—make an initial mold of the residual limb.

2. Creation of a custom-fitted thermoplastic socket to best fit each unique residual limb.

3. Goal is to achieve an intimate fit with a very close match between socket and residuum.

4. Aim to minimize motion at the skin–socket interface.

5. Residual limb must be suitable—postoperative edema completely resolved, no prominent bone, clear of infection, scars pliable; contractures addressed; strength and ROM restored to maximal extent; pain, hypersensitivity, or neuromas have been addressed; "stump wrapping" has created a conical shape.

6. Socket-mounted prosthetic limbs (▶ **Fig. 14.9**)—critical interface between skin and prosthetic limb; socket transmits significant forces from the prosthetic limb and must be meticulously fitted to the residual limb, otherwise a source of potential irritation or damage to the skin or underlying tissues; soft liner is typically situated within the interior of the socket, and a patient might also wear a layer of one or more prosthetic socks to achieve a snug fit.

7. **Suspension system**—harnesses, such as straps, belts, or sleeves, are used to attach the prosthetic limb; currently far more common for upper limb amputations.

   a. Harness is sometimes still necessary with a short residuum after a high transfemoral amputation.

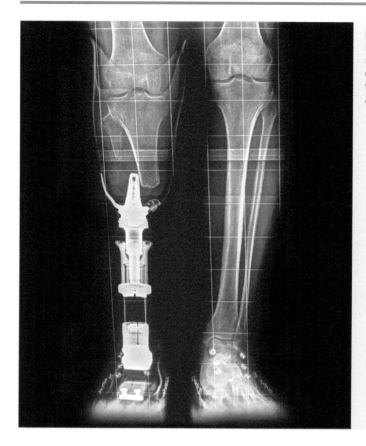

Fig. 14.9 Radiograph of below knee amputee in standard suction-mounted prosthetic socket. Note characteristic valgus of artificial limb, tibial residuum positioned medially and 2 cm LLD.

   b. For some types of amputations, the prosthetic is able to stay attached by fitting around the shape of the residual limb.

   c. One of the most popular types of suspension mechanisms relies on suction—the prosthetic limb fits snugly onto the residual limb and an airtight seal keeps it in place.

   d. After preparing a preliminary socket, multiple revisions and modifications are often necessary to achieve a satisfactory fit.

   e. Much of this process is empirical, and the prosthetist makes adjustments as necessary to satisfy the user.

C. Direct skeletal attachment—osseointegration (▶Fig. 14.10a–c)

   1. Highly promising alternative method for attachment of a prosthetic limb.

   2. Macroporous titanium implants fully incorporate directly into skeletal residuum, providing a solid, intimate bond between patient and prosthetic limb.

   3. Main indication is for amputees unable to use a socket-mounted prosthetic limb due to short stumps, scarred adherent skin, bony prominences, and recurrent ulcerations and infection.

   4. Transcutaneous implants protrude through skin with adapters for connections.

   5. Concerns regarding risk of infection—when using contemporary implants and improved techniques, infection is much less problematic than anticipated.

   6. Currently no Food and Drug Administration approved implants for use in the United States, but popular internationally.

   7. Best for transfemoral amputees (above knee): studies have confirmed dramatically better functional (TUG [Timed Up and Go] and 6MWT [6-minute walk test]) and subjective outcome measures (SF-36, Q-TFA [Questionnaire for persons with a Trans-Femoral Amputation]).

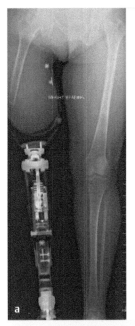 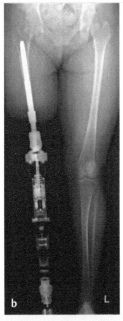 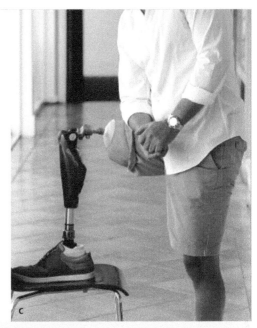

Fig. 14.10 (a) The femur is often markedly abducted in a traditional socket in a transfemoral amputee; (b) radiograph of an osseointegration prosthesis demonstrating anatomic alignment of the femur; (c) clinical photograph of a patient with an osseointegration prosthesis.

8. Role for transhumeral amputees evolving: combined with targeted muscle reinnervation and using the most advanced myoelectric prostheses; early results are promising.

9. May be suitable for BKA if unable to tolerate a socket-mounted prosthetic limb.

VIII. Outcome Measures for Amputees

A. Q-TFA (2004)—currently no comparable validated outcome measure for transtibial amputees.

B. The Short Form (SF-36 and SF-12) Health Survey.

C. TUG test and 6MWT.

D. Amputee Mobility Predictor (AMP-Pro or AMP-noPro).

E. Medicare Functional Classification Levels—"K Levels":

1. K 0—unable to use/benefit from a prosthetic limb—wheelchair bound or requires crutches.

2. K 1—uses a prosthetic limb for transfers or ambulation on a level surface—household ambulator.

3. K 2—only able to traverse low environmental barriers, limited community ambulator.

4. K 3—capable of variable cadence—able to traverse most environmental barriers, curbs or stairs—unlimited community ambulator.

5. K 4—higher-demand patients, few if any restrictions including running, jumping, sports (typical of children), active adults, athletes.

IX. Special Considerations for Pediatric, Geriatric, and Compromised Patients

A. **Pediatric patients**—BKA is less suitable in a growing child, prone to overgrowth and often needs reoperation; Syme's distally or through-knee amputation best proximally; allows almost immediate full-weight bearing on stump itself, especially useful for infants and toddlers (particularly bilateral cases).

B. **Geriatric patients**—Parkinson's, Alzheimer's, dementia, blindness all create issues; difficult or impossible to use a prosthetic limb, high risk of falls with possible fractures, amputation may leave them wheelchair bound; consider end-bearing stump (Boyd/Pirogoff amputation).

C. **Morbidly obese patients**—unlikely to use socket-mounted prosthesis if weigh > 150 Kg, difficult to fit socket, consider end-bearing stump (through knee, Boyd, or Pirigoff).

Suggested Readings

Al Muderis M, Tetsworth K, et al. The Osseointegration Group of Australia Accelerated Protocol (OGAAP-1) for two-stage osseointegrated reconstruction of amputees. Bone Joint J 2016;98B:952–960

Bosse MJ, MacKenzie EJ, Kellam JF, et al. An analysis of outcomes of reconstruction or amputation after leg-threatening injuries. N Engl J Med 2002;347(24):1924–1931

MacKenzie EJ, Bosse MJ, Castillo RC, et al. Functional outcomes following trauma-related lower-extremity amputation. J Bone Joint Surg Am 2004;86(8):1636–1645

Taylor BC, Poka A. Osteomyoplastic transtibial amputation: the Ertl technique. J Am Acad Orthop Surg 2016;24(4):259–265

Tintle SM, LeBrun C, Ficke JR, Potter BK. What is new in trauma-related amputations. J Orthop Trauma 2016;30(Suppl 3):S16–S20

15 Rib Fractures

Aaron Nauth

Introduction

Rib fractures are commonly encountered in polytrauma patients and are often seen in combination with orthopaedic injuries. A wide spectrum of injury can be encountered with rib fractures, ranging from single/nondisplaced rib fractures to multiple fractured/displaced ribs to flail chest injuries with mechanical instability of the chest wall. Increasing severity of rib injury is clearly correlated with increasing levels of morbidity and mortality. The traditional management of these injuries (including severe injuries such as flail chest) has been largely nonoperative with analgesia, supportive care of respiratory function as required, and chest tube placement for the management of associated pneumothorax/hemothorax. Recently, there has been increasing interest in the surgical management of more severe rib fractures and chest injuries (e.g., multiple displaced rib fractures or flail chest injuries).

I. Preoperative

A. History and physical exam

1. Substantial rib injuries typically occur as a result of high-energy blunt trauma (typically motor vehicle collisions, falls from 10 feet or greater, pedestrian hit by vehicle, etc.).

2. Patient assessment should proceed following Advanced Trauma Life Support (ATLS) protocol as these patients often suffer from multiple injuries and can present with imminently life-threatening injuries.

3. Specific physical examination of the chest should include assessment of cardiovascular function (heart rate, blood pressure, cardiac monitoring), respiratory function (tracheal deviation, oxygen saturation, air entry, percussion for dullness or hyper resonance, asymmetric or paradoxical chest movement), and physical findings of chest trauma (ecchymosis, seat-belt sign, open injuries, crepitus, subcutaneous emphysema).

4. Commonly associated orthopaedic injuries include clavicle and scapula fractures.

5. Commonly associated nonorthopaedic injuries include head injuries and intra-abdominal injuries such as spleen or liver lacerations.

B. Anatomy—in addition to the anatomy of the thoracic cage and its contribution to respiratory function, it is important to recognize the anatomic structures contained within the thorax and upper abdomen by the ribs, and the associated injuries which can occur to these structures.

1. Mediastinal structures including the heart (cardiac tamponade, cardiac contusion, laceration), great vessels (vascular injury), trachea (tracheobronchial injury), and esophagus (esophageal rupture).

2. Pleural space (tension pneumothorax, sucking chest wound, pneumothorax, and hemothorax).

3. Lungs (pulmonary contusion, laceration).

4. The diaphragm, liver, and spleen are contained by the lower ribs (10–12) and injury to these structures can be associated with rib fractures (diaphragmatic rupture, spleen or liver laceration).

5. Ribs and thoracic cage (increasing severity of rib injuries cause increasing impairments in ventilatory function due to both painful inspiration/expiration and compromised respiratory mechanics).

6. Intercostal vessels and nerves (neurovascular injury).

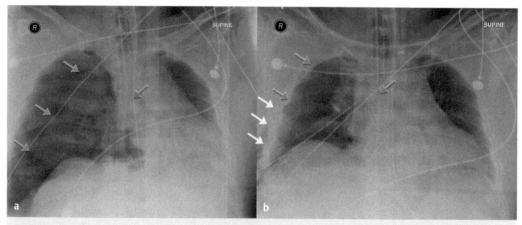

Fig. 15.1 (a) Anteroposterior (AP) chest radiograph of a 46-year-old male who sustained blunt trauma to his chest from a motor vehicle accident. He was transferred to our Level 1 trauma center with multiple suspected right-sided rib fractures after being intubated. He presented with hypoxia, tachycardia, and hypotension. His chest X-ray shows a large pneumothorax (*blue arrows*) and tracheal deviation (*red arrow*) consistent with a tension pneumothorax. (b) AP chest radiograph following urgent needle decompression and chest tube placement, showing resolution of the pneumothorax (*blue arrows*) and restoration of the trachea and mediastinal structures to the midline (*red arrow*). Multiple right-sided rib fractures are also evident (*yellow arrows*). The patient's clinical condition rapidly stabilized after placement of the chest tube.

C. Imaging

    1. AP chest X-ray:

        a. Per ATLS protocol, all patients with suspected chest trauma should undergo expedited imaging with an AP chest X-ray.

        b. This initial investigation is critical for the early detection of injuries representing an immediate threat to life, such as tension pneumothorax (see ▶ **Fig. 15.1a,b**), massive hemothorax, or mediastinal injury.

        c. Serves as the initial screening test for the identification of rib fractures, pneumo/hemothorax, and diaphragmatic rupture.

    2. Contrast-enhanced thoracic and abdominal computed tomography (CT):

        a. CT of the chest and abdomen with intravenous contrast is indicated for all patients with suspicion of these injuries based on injury mechanism, physical exam or initial imaging.

        b. CT scanning is the imaging modality of choice for identification and characterization of fractures of the ribs and sternum.

        c. Three-dimensional (3D) reconstructions are helpful for further characterization of fracture pattern and displacement, particularly in those instances where surgical treatment is being considered (see ▶ **Fig. 15.2b**). In addition, CT scan is the modality of choice for identifying the associated injuries outlined above.

D. Classification

    1. Although no widely recognized classification system exists for rib fractures or bony injuries to the thoracic cage, it is important to recognize that a wide spectrum of pathology exists.

    2. Injuries range from:

        a. Single and nondisplaced rib fractures.

        b. Multiple, displaced rib fractures.

        c. Flail chest injuries (an entire segment of the chest wall is free-floating).

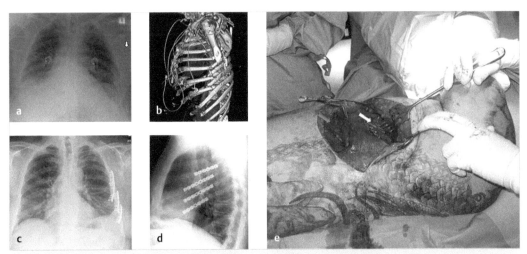

Fig. 15.2 **(a)** Anteroposterior chest radiograph in a 48-year-old male demonstrating a left-sided flail chest and multiple displaced/comminuted anterolateral rib fractures sustained from blunt trauma. **(b)** Three-dimensional computed tomography reconstruction in the same patient demonstrating multiple left-sided, anterolateral rib fractures with substantial displacement/comminution. **(c, d)** Postoperative and lateral chest radiograph in the same patient demonstrating fixation of multiple left-sided, anterolateral rib fractures performed through an anterolateral approach. **(e)** Intraoperative photograph demonstrating the **anterolateral approach** in this patient for fixation of anterolateral rib fractures. Muscle-splitting windows in the serratus anterior (*white arrow*) and external oblique (*blue arrow*) have been used to access rib fractures. Reproduced with permission from Nauth A. Surgical approaches for rib fracture fixation. In: McKee MD and Schemitsch EH, eds. Injuries to the Chest Wall: Diagnosis and Management. New York, NY: Springer; 2015:81–88.

3. The literature has clearly shown that as the severity of these injuries increases, there are substantial increases in both morbidity and mortality.

4. Flail chest injuries occur when multiple ribs have segmental fractures, creating a "flail segment" which moves paradoxically with respiration (inward during inspiration and outward during respiration). Flail chest injuries have been defined as:

   a. Three or more unilateral segmental rib fractures.

   b. Three or more bilateral rib fractures.

   c. Three or more unilateral rib fractures combined with sternal fracture or dissociation.

II. Treatment

A. Initial management

1. Initial management should follow ATLS protocol to allow for the rapid detection and treatment of life-threatening injuries that can be associated with rib fractures (▶ **Fig. 15.1**).

2. Initial management is often directed at the treatment of associated injuries and supporting ventilation with the goals of maintaining oxygenation and controlling hemorrhage.

3. Depending on associated injuries, this may require:

   a. Airway support.

   b. Chest tube placement.

   c. Mechanical ventilation

   d. Fluid resuscitation and/or blood product transfusion.

4. Both the initial and definitive treatment of patients with severe rib injuries often requires multidisciplinary assessment and treatment involving orthopaedic surgery, general surgery or thoracic surgery, and intensive care specialists.

B. Definitive management

1. Nonoperative treatment:

a. The traditional management of rib fractures (including flail chest injuries) has largely been nonoperative with analgesia, supportive ventilation, monitoring in the intensive care unit (ICU), and chest tube placement for the management of associated pneumothorax or hemothorax.

b. In severe patterns of rib injury, such as flail chest injuries, the chest wall is rendered mechanically unstable resulting in impaired mechanics of breathing and significant pain with respiratory efforts. As a result, a substantial portion of patients (> 50%) require mechanical ventilation and most (> 80%) require admission to the ICU.

c. Patients with nonoperatively treated flail chest injuries frequently require prolonged mechanical ventilation (average = 12 days) and are prone to complications such as ventilator-associated pneumonia (VAP), septicemia, and need for tracheostomy.

d. Mortality rates with nonoperative treatment in the literature have varied, but are generally significant (ranging 5–46%).

e. In addition, there has been concern regarding longer term complications with nonoperative treatment including malunion, nonunion, and persistent impairment in pulmonary function.

2. Operative treatment:

a. The poor results seen with nonoperative treatment, and the high morbidity and mortality encountered with these injuries has prompted substantial interest in the operative treatment of these injuries with open reduction and internal fixation (ORIF) of the fractured ribs in severe patterns of injury such as flail chest.

b. The goals of surgery are not dissimilar from other orthopaedic procedures and include restoration of thoracic anatomy and the stabilization of rib fractures to restore chest wall stability, thereby reducing pain with breathing and improving respiratory mechanics.

c. Several comparative series in the literature, including small randomized trials, have shown substantial benefits to surgery including reduced mortality, significantly fewer days requiring mechanical ventilation and reduced rates of pneumonia and tracheostomy.

d. There have been substantial increases in the rates of operative treatment, from < 1% prior to 2010 to approximately 10% in recent years, although the overall rates of surgical intervention remain low.

e. There are no absolute surgical indications for fixation of rib fractures.

f. Relative surgical indications are controversial but include:

i. Open injuries.
ii. Flail chest injuries with failure to wean from mechanical ventilation.
iii. Nonintubated patients with flail chest injuries who develop respiratory compromise.
iv. Severe deformities of the rib cage (e.g., > 25% loss of volume of the hemithorax or "caved-in" chest).
v. Rib fractures associated with other thoracic injuries requiring surgical intervention (e.g., thoracotomy for massive hemothorax, cardiovascular injury, tracheobronchial injury, diaphragm injury, pulmonary laceration).
vi. Multiple displaced rib fractures with intractable pain.

g. It is important to recognize that surgical indications, although controversial, are limited to severe patterns of injury with multiple segmental and/or grossly displaced rib fractures causing mechanical instability of the chest wall. Undisplaced or minimally displaced fractures of one or more ribs do not require surgery.

C. Surgical approaches

1. The surgical approach is selected based on the location and displacement of the rib fractures requiring fixation with the goal of restoring stability to the chest wall.

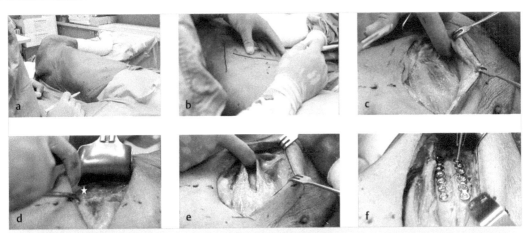

Fig. 15.3 Cadaver pictures demonstrating the anterolateral approach. **(a)** Patient positioning in lateral decubitus position with arm free draped over a padded mayo stand. **(b)** Anterolateral incision marked out anterior to the lateral border of the scapula. **(c)** Anterolateral incision exposing the serratus anterior. **(d)** Posterior retraction of the latissimus dorsi exposing the long thoracic nerve on the lateral border of serratus anterior (*white star*). **(e)** Blunt dissection is used to create a muscle-splitting window in the serratus anterior to expose anterolateral rib fractures. **(f)** Plating of multiple rib fractures through a split in the serratus anterior. Reproduced with permission from Nauth A. Surgical approaches for rib fracture fixation. In: McKee MD and Schemitsch EH, eds. Injuries to the Chest Wall: Diagnosis and Management. New York, NY: Springer; 2015:81–88.

2. Surgical planning is based on 3D reconstructions of the CT chest.
3. One of three main surgical approaches is used based on the above:
   a. Lateral thoracotomy (anterior or posterior):
      i. This approach is used for anterolateral (see ▸ **Fig. 15.2** and ▸ **Fig. 15.3**) or posterolateral fractures.
      ii. The patient is positioned lateral decubitus.
      iii. A thoracotomy-type incision centered over displaced rib fractures is used.
      iv. Dissection proceeds anterior to latissimus dorsi (anterolateral) or in the interval between latissimus, trapezius, and inferior scapula (posterolateral).
      v. Deep dissection involves splitting of serratus anterior fibers to access fractured ribs.
   b. Posterior paramedian approach (▸ **Fig. 15.4**):
      i. This approach is used for posterior fractures adjacent to the spine.
      ii. The patient is positioned lateral decubitus.
      iii. A vertical incision parallel the spinous processes is made directly over the fractured ribs.
      iv. Deep dissection is in the interval between latissimus, trapezius, and inferior scapula.
      v. The erector spinae is elevated toward the midline to access the fractured ribs.
   c. Inframammary approach (▸ **Fig. 15.5**):
      i. This approach is used for anterior fractures and costochondral dislocations.
      ii. The patient is positioned supine.
      iii. A horizontal incision inferior to pectoralis major is used along the inframammary crease.
      iv. Deep dissection is carried out underneath the pectoralis and/or breast tissue.
      v. Elevation of pectoralis minor and/or splitting of serratus anterior fibers is performed to expose fractured ribs.
D. Fixation techniques
   1. A variety of surgical fixation techniques have been described, although most modern series have described plate and screw fixation with either pelvic reconstruction plates (locking or

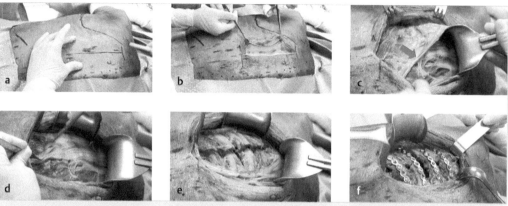

Fig. 15.4 Cadaver pictures demonstrating the posterior paramedian approach. **(a)** Patient positioning in lateral decubitus position with arm free draped over a padded mayo stand. The posterior paramedian incision is marked out parallel and lateral to the spinous processes. **(b)** The posterior paramedian incision. **(c)** The triangle of auscultation. The trapezius has been retracted superiorly, the inferior border of the scapula is just lateral to the retractor and the latissimus dorsi is inferior (*blue arrow*). **(d, e)** The underlying erector spinae is reflected laterally to expose the underlying posterior rib fractures. **(f)** Plating of exposed posterior rib fractures. Reproduced with permission from Nauth A. Surgical approaches for rib fracture fixation. In: McKee MD and Schemitsch EH, eds. Injuries to the Chest Wall: Diagnosis and Management. New York, NY: Springer; 2015:81–88.

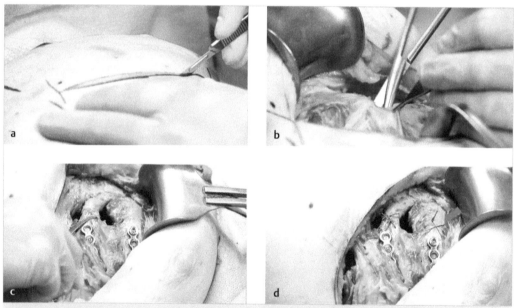

Fig. 15.5 Cadaver pictures demonstrating the inframammary approach. **(a)** The inframammary incision is made inferior to the pectoralis major in the inframammary crease. **(b)** The pectoralis major and breast tissue are elevated to expose the serratus anterior and pectoralis minor. A muscle split is performed in the serratus anterior to expose the anterolateral rib fractures and costochondral dislocations. **(c, d)** The exposed anterolateral rib fractures are plated and the costochondral dislocations are fixed with transosseous suture (*blue arrow*). Reproduced with permission from Nauth A. Surgical approaches for rib fracture fixation. In: McKee MD and Schemitsch EH, eds. Injuries to the Chest Wall: Diagnosis and Management. New York, NY: Springer; 2015:81–88.

nonlocking; 2.7 or 3.5 mm) or rib-specific plating systems (typically precontoured locking plates or specially designed intramedullary splints).

2. There is lack of comparative literature between implants and the current standard of care would involve either of these two strategies.

E. Complications
1. The literature on surgical fixation for rib fractures is relatively novel and complications following surgical treatment have been inconsistently reported.
2. General complications such as death, sepsis, tracheostomy, and pneumonia have been lower than those reported with nonoperative treatment.
3. Reported rates of surgery-specific complications have been very low in the available literature and likely underreported.
4. Reported surgery-specific complications have included wound infections (3%), symptomatic hardware (2%), loose hardware (1%), nonunion (1%), chest wall numbness (0.6%), empyema (0.1%), retained hemothorax (0.1%), and recurrent hemothorax (0.1%).

F. Rehabilitation
1. Postoperative treatment in the acute phase consists of supportive care in the ICU.
2. Chest tube placement is required for all patients subsequent to rib fixation.
3. Patients are mobilized as soon as they are able to be extubated and also receive chest physiotherapy and incentive spirometry.

G. Outcomes
1. Recent meta-analyses have been published comparing operative to nonoperative treatment for the management of flail chest injuries.
2. These reviews have consistently shown significant benefits to operative treatment including:
   a. Decreased mortality.
   b. Decreased days on mechanical ventilation/ICU days/hospital stay.
   c. Decreased pneumonia/sepsis/tracheostomy.
3. It is important to recognize that these reviews have compiled data from small, single-center studies with variable methods of rib fracture fixation and significant limitations.
4. Further research in this area is required to confirm the benefits surgery and better define surgical indications.

Summary

Rib fractures are common in polytraumatized patients. Isolated rib fractures are treated nonoperatively, however the indications for multiple rib fractures are evolving. There is growing evidence that operative management of flail chest injuries improves outcomes and decreases complications.

Suggested Readings

Coughlin TA, Ng JW, Rollins KE, Forward DP, Ollivere BJ. Management of rib fractures in traumatic flail chest: a meta-analysis of randomised controlled trials. Bone Joint J 2016;98-B(8):1119–1125

Dehghan N, Mah JM, Schemitsch EH, Nauth A, Vicente M, McKee MD. Operative stabilization of flail chest injuries reduces mortality to that of stable chest wall injuries. J Orthop Trauma 2018;32(1):15–21

Fowler TT, Taylor BC, Bellino MJ, Althausen PL. Surgical treatment of flail chest and rib fractures. J Am Acad Orthop Surg 2014;22(12):751–760

Lafferty PM, Anavian J, Will RE, Cole PA. Operative treatment of chest wall injuries: indications, technique, and outcomes. J Bone Joint Surg Am 2011;93(1):97–110

Slobogean GP, MacPherson CA, Sun T, Pelletier ME, Hameed SM. Surgical fixation vs nonoperative management of flail chest: a meta-analysis. J Am Coll Surg 2013;216(2):302–11.e1

16 Imaging of Orthopaedic Trauma

Kyle M. Schweser and Brett D. Crist

Introduction

Basic imaging concepts will be reviewed, including when to obtain specific imaging modalities, basic radiation safety, and anatomic specific imaging. The goal is to offer a quick reference for specific images. General trauma concepts include plain films as the typical initial study in evaluating fracture. Computed tomography (CT) scan is typically performed for periarticular fractures and fractures of the pelvic ring or acetabulum. Magnetic resonance imaging (MRI) is typically performed to further evaluate soft tissue injury or stress fracture if not seen on plain films when there is a high-clinical suspicion (▶Video 16.1).

Keywords: imaging, X-ray, Computed Tomography, Magnetic Resonance Imaging, specific imaging, radiation safety

I. Choice of Imaging

A. Several factors affect the imaging that can be performed.
   1. Patient condition—a patient may be unable to tolerate a CT or MRI based on current medical status.
   2. Tissue or area of the body one wishes to image.
   3. Radiation exposure—pregnancy may preclude a CT if other imaging is available.
   4. Cost.
   5. Availability of imaging modalities.
   6. Patient implants—i.e., pacemaker, shrapnel, orthopaedic implants, ports, etc.

II. Imaging Modalities

A. Conventional radiography
   1. Principles of image generation:
      a. X-rays are short wavelength electromagnetic radiations that can pass through objects.
      b. An X-ray source is aimed at a detector; the density and chemical composition of an object determines how much absorption occurs.
      c. Bone is dense and composed of calcium, which readily absorbs X-rays. The denser the object, the more absorption occurs. Dense objects appear white on imaging.
      d. Modern digital radiography facilitates instant electronic transfer of images through multiple media platforms and enhances portability of image capture.
   2. Indications and characteristics:
      a. Initial choice for imaging.
      b. Relatively low cost.
      c. Low-dose radiation.
      d. High specificity and lower sensitivity in comparison to other modalities.
      e. Produces a two-dimensional image.
   3. Orthogonal (typically anteroposterior [AP] and lateral) views should always be obtained.
      a. Additional specialized views can be obtained based on injury or clinical suspicion.
      b. Care should be taken to ensure that the imaging is adequate and that true AP and lateral images are obtained. Inadequate imaging can lead to misdiagnosis.

    c. Portable radiography is occasionally limited in acquiring appropriately oriented images.

    d. Adequate imaging may be unattainable due to:

        i. Physiologic instability (unsafe for patient transport).

        ii. Difficulty with mobilization of an injured limb due to pain.

4. Image the entire bone:

    a. Long bone fractures—the joint above and below the injury should be included to avoid missing other injuries.

        i. Approximately 5 to 10% of femoral shaft fractures have an associated femoral neck fracture. These injuries are missed 20 to 50% of the time.

        ii. Most missed injuries are due to a lack of appropriate imaging.

    b. Periarticular injury radiographs should include the entirety of the bones involved.

        i. Ankle fracture—tibia/fibula and ankle X-rays.

        ii. Radial head fracture—elbow and forearm X-rays.

B. Computed Tomography (CT)

1. Principles of image generation:

    a. Uses X-ray to build multiple cross-sectional images of an anatomic region.

    b. Cross-sectional images, or "slices," are reconstructed to create images that can be displayed in multiple planes and formats.

        i. Axial.

        ii. Sagittal.

        iii. Coronal.

        iv. Three-dimensional.

    c. Much higher contrast resolution than conventional radiography which permits enhanced distinction of tissue types.

    d. Displays images on a grayscale based on the physical density of the tissue type and measured by Hounsfield units (HU).

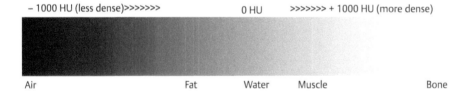

2. Indications and characteristics:

    a. Improved characterization of select injuries and also useful for preoperative planning.

        i. Periarticular fractures.

        ii. Pelvic ring injuries.

        iii. Limb alignment studies.

        iv. Three-dimensional CT reconstructions can further improve physician understanding of an injury pattern.

    b. Trauma scan (head, neck, chest, abdomen, and pelvis ± extremities) in multiple injured patients is primarily indicated for identification of life-threatening injuries.

        i. Allows diagnosis of injuries to the axial skeleton.

        ii. May aid in treatment decisions and preoperative planning for fracture surgery.

    c. Higher radiation dose than X-ray.

    d. Higher cost than X-ray but less than MRI.

    e. Highly sensitive and specific for bony injuries.

f. Soft tissue assessment, although better modalities are available.

    i. Computed tomography angiography (CTA).

    ii. The addition of contrast can aid in vascular/soft tissue assessment, but carries the risk of renal injury.

3. Limitations:

    a. Morbidly obese patients may not fit on the scanner.

    b. Metal inside or outside the patient can create "artifact" and obscure image detail.

    c. Relatively contraindicated in pregnant patients due to radiation risk. Pregnant patients presenting as trauma activations with potentially life-threatening injuries still undergo whole body CT scanning.

D. Magnetic Resonance Imaging (MRI)

1. Principles:

    a. Combines the use of strong magnetic fields and radiofrequency (RF) to create detailed images.

    b. Hydrogen protons (present in water and thus nearly all human tissue) both align with and absorb the energy from the magnetic field (behave similarly to the way a magnet pulls the needle of a compass).

    c. RF pulses disrupt proton alignment. When RF is turned off, protons realign at varying rates in different tissues and emit specific signals during this process.

    d. Detectors measure the energy released during proton realignment and the machine subsequently creates the image.

    e. RF pulse frequency can be manipulated:

        i. Repetition time (TR)—amount of time between RF pulses.

        ii. Time to Echo (TE)—time between RF pulse delivery and receipt of the signal.

    f. Imaging sequences:

        i. T1 images—short TE and TR times (▶Fig. 16.1).

         • Better for evaluating many anatomic structures.

         • Fat and bone marrow are bright; cartilage, tendon, and ligament are relatively darker.

         • Does not highlight edema or water content.

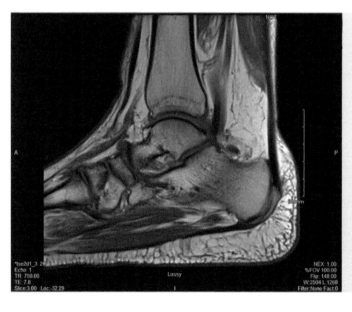

Fig. 16.1 Sagittal T1 ankle MRI. Notice the fat is the "lighter" or "brighter" structure on T1 imaging.

ii. T2 images—longer TE and TR times (▶Fig. 16.2).

- Better for assessing fluid (bright) such as swelling and bone edema.
- Surrounding anatomic structures are darker.
- Remember: T_2 and H_2O.

iii. Fluid-attenuated inversion recovery (FLAIR): very long TE and TR times. Can distinguish between cerebrospinal fluid (CSF) (dark) and pathologic inflammation (bright).

iv. STIR (Short T1 inversion recovery)–Suppresses fat.

2. Indications and characteristics:

a. Diagnosis and delineation of soft tissue injury, infection, and tumor. Trauma specific examples include:

i. Pathologic fracture and extent of tumor involvement (covered in chapter 11, Pathologic Fractures).

ii. Ligament and tendon injury.

iii. Chondral injury.

iv. Osteomyelitis.

b. Less useful for bony injury and is not the first-line imaging modality. Examples include:

i. Occult fractures (hip).

ii. Stress fractures (tibia, foot).

c. No radiation.

d. Highly sensitive and specific for soft tissue injuries–can be overly sensitive and should be interpreted with care.

3. Contrast-enhanced MRI—the addition of gadolinium can be helpful for studying tumors, inflammation, abscesses, and vascular pathology.–
enhances and delineates structures and tissue associated with fluid.

4. Limitations:

a. Patients may be unable to obtain secondary to implanted defibrillators, pacemakers, artificial heart valves, aneurysm clips, cochlear implants, shrapnel, or other metal implants that are magnetic and can lead to injury. Questionnaires are administered prior to obtaining the scan to avoid complications.

b. Most implanted metal and ballistic may be "MRI safe" but contributes to signal artifact and obscures image detail making interpretation difficult.

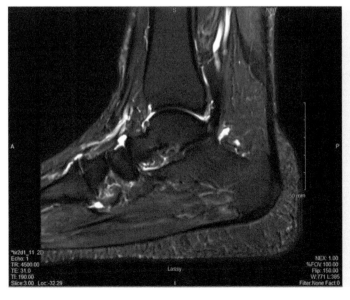

Fig. 16.2 Sagittal T2 ankle MRI. Notice the fluid is the "lighter" or "brighter" structure on T2 imaging

E. Ultrasound (US)

1. Effective in the evaluation of many soft tissue conditions.

   a. Tendon pathology such as rotator cuff tear and Achilles rupture.

   b. Fluid collection—intra-articular and soft tissue.

   c. US-guided injections—intra-articular and bursal.

   d. Identify deep vein thrombosis (DVT) utilizing Duplex technology.

F. Dual-energy X-ray Absorptiometry (DXA) scans

1. Measures bone density.

2. Used to diagnose and monitor treatment of osteoporosis.

3. T-score (calculated against the score for an average 35-year-old woman) and Z-scores (age-matched) are given.

   a. T-score:
      i. Less than −2.5 = osteoporosis.
      ii. Between −2.5 and 0 = osteopenia.
      iii. Greater than 0 = normal.

III. Radiation Safety

A. Orthopaedic surgeons are frequently exposed to radiation, and several precautions should be taken to minimize exposure.

B. Basic precautions

1. Wearing lead during times of imaging:

   a. Cover thyroid and reproductive organs, at the very least. Thyroid cancer is a major concern for orthopaedic surgeons.

   b. Pregnant women should wear wrap-around lead, and should also consider double lead during procedures.

   c. Lead should be inspected annually.

   d. The eyes are the most sensitive organ to radiation exposure. Cataracts are a major consequence of corneal exposure to radiation, and lead glasses can reduce that exposure by 90%.

   e. The surgeon's or assistant's hands typically receive the highest exposure.

2. Exposure should be limited whenever possible.

   a. Keep hands and other body parts out of the field.

   b. Leave the room if it is not necessary for you to remain.

   c. Scatter of X-ray is proportional to the inverse of the distance squared ($1/d^2$) from the X-ray source. Thus, doubling the distance from the X-ray source decreases the exposure by 4x.

C. C-arm function, positioning, and safety

1. ▶ Fig. 16.3 demonstrates a basic C-arm with different levels of patient positioning as well as associated scatter radiation.

2. Position of the C-arm and the surgeon is important in reducing radiation exposure.

3. The highest radiation and scatter occurs between the X-ray source and the patient.

   a. The surgeon should avoid standing next to the radiation source. The X-ray source should be positioned on the opposite side of the table from the surgeon, or beneath the patient. This will minimize scatter radiation exposure the surgeon receives.

   b. The image intensifier should also be placed as close to the patient as possible. This will not only provide the widest view of the patient, but also minimize scatter.

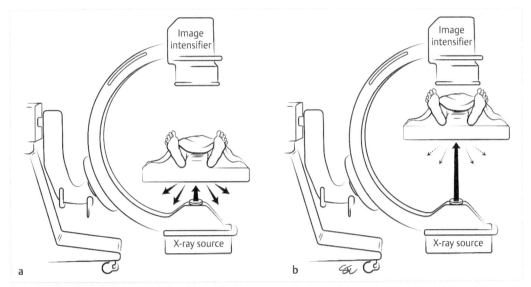

Fig. 16.3 (a, b) Graphic representation of a C-arm. Strength of radiation dose is indicated by the thickness of the arrow, with direction of the arrow indicating direction of X-ray beams.

4. The use of live fluoroscopy and magnification should be limited; however, collimating when possible and the use of low-dose settings should be utilized when applicable.

5. The larger the patient, or the thicker the area being X-rayed, the greater the amount of radiation necessary to obtain an adequate image. While little can be done, the surgeon should be aware and take all available precautions such as standing back from the imaging source.

IV. Imaging in a Trauma Patient

A. A basic trauma imaging series typically consists of an AP chest and pelvis X-ray. Recently, some trauma centers have described omitting the pelvis film in favor of a CT in select patients. However, the pelvis X-ray as part of the initial workup should still be considered as a gold standard for trauma patients.

B. CT of the head, cervical spine, chest, abdomen, and pelvis are all standard imaging modalities in a trauma patient and should be obtained as soon as the patient is physiologically stable. Historically, spine imaging for the trauma patient consisted of a lateral cervical spine image. However, due to difficulty in obtaining and interpreting an adequate image showing the C7/T1 segment, it has largely been abandoned in favor of CT.

C. The role of MRI in a trauma patient is typically reserved for patients with spinal cord injuries.

1. A patient with a cervical spine fracture/dislocation, who is awake and cooperative, can undergo reduction of his/her fracture dislocation prior to obtaining an MRI. However, an obtunded or uncooperative patient with a known cervical spine fracture/dislocation should undergo an MRI prior to a reduction attempt or surgical intervention.

2. Patients with a spine injury and neurological deficit (especially progressive) typically undergo an MRI prior to surgery.

D. CTA in a trauma patient is reserved for those cases where there is concern for vascular injury or continued hemodynamic instability.

V. Specific Imaging

A. Standard AP and lateral images should be obtained for all long bone injuries.

B. The following section will cover anatomic specific regions that have optional images for specific injuries. Radiographic parameters are covered in subsequent chapters.

C. Cervical spine
   1. AP and lateral views–adequate lateral views should include the occiput up to T1.
      a. Open-mouth odontoid view—AP view with beam aimed at patients' open mouth. Assesses:
         i. C2 injuries such as odontoid fractures.
         ii. C1 injuries such as burst fractures, transverse ligament injury, and basilar invagination.
   2. Flexion/extension radiographs—lateral C-spine image while the patient flexes and extends their neck.
      a. Assesses ligamentous injuries and chronic C-spine instability/disease.
      b. Should be ordered in all patients with rheumatoid arthritis prior to surgery.
D. Sternoclavicular joint
   1. AP chest.
   2. Serendipity view—40 degree of cephalic tilt.
      a. If the effected clavicle appears above/below the uninjured clavicle at the sternoclavicular joint, it is an anterior/posterior dislocation respectively.
E. Clavicle
   1. Upright/standing AP clavicle—measures true displacement and the effect of gravity.
   2. AP views of bilateral clavicles—usually viewed on a chest X-ray (CXR) or bilateral AC view without weights to measure accurate shortening through the fracture.
   3. Zanca—15 degree of cephalad tilt.
      a. Measure of true displacement.
      b. Can also assess AC joint displacement.
F. Shoulder
   1. Standard radiographs: AP, scapular Y, and axillary.
   2. An axillary view is the only image that can truly assess glenohumeral congruity. Multiple axillary views exist:
      a. Stryker Notch—affected arm on head, patient turned toward affected side 25 degree, beam centered on axilla, and aimed 10 degree cephalad. Example: Hill-Sachs lesions and coracoid fractures.
      b. West Point—patient positioned prone, beam centered on axilla, aimed 25 degree caudal from horizontal, and 25 degree medial. Example: Bony Bankart lesions.
      c. Velpeau—shoulder adducted/internal rotation (IR), patient leans back, and beam superior to inferior. Glenohumeral joint assessment in patients unable to position for axillary view.
      d. Trauma axillary–shoulder flexed and beam aimed toward shoulder from distal to proximal. Glenohumeral joint assessment in patients unable to position for axillary view.
G. Distal humerus and elbow
   1. Recommended—AP, lateral (▶Fig. 16.4).
   2. Acquiring a true lateral of the elbow is important.
   3. Traction radiographs for intra-articular fractures–Longitudinal traction is applied and radiographs are obtained to evaluate intra-articular fractures with ligamentotaxis.
   4. Oblique images can help determine displacement of condyle fractures.
H. Radial head/capitellum
   1. Greenspan—lateral elbow with beam aimed 45 degree toward the joint.
   2. Proximal radius fractures should receive wrist views and rule out Essex Lopresti injury (distal radial ulnar joint [DRUJ] disruption).

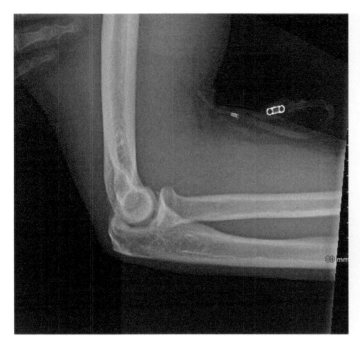

Fig. 16.4 Lateral view of an elbow. Notice the overlap of the distal humerus, limiting a "double bubble" sign, and forming two concentric circles.

I. Hand/Wrist
    1. Standard views:
        a. PA, lateral, and oblique views.
        b. Hand views should include carpal bones through the distal phalanges.
    2. Clenched fist view—bilateral PA projection of the wrist, with clenched fist. Helps in identifying Scapholunate dissociation.
    3. Ulnar-deviated wrist view:
        a. PA view with wrist in maximal ulnar deviation.
        b. Identifies—Scaphoid fracture.
    4. Scaphoid view:
        a. Partially supinated PA view with ulnar deviation.
        b. Identifies—scaphoid fracture.
J. Pelvis
    1. AP (▶**Fig. 16.5**).
    2. Inlet/outlet views—patient supine, beam tilted 20 to 40 degree cephalad/caudal. Helps in assessment of pelvic ring injuries.
    3. Iliac and obturator oblique "Judet" views—patient supine, beam centered over affected hip, and hips alternately titled 45 degree anterior. Helps in assessment of acetabular injuries.
K. Hip/proximal femur
    1. Recommended—AP hip and pelvis, lateral, and true AP. True AP of the proximal femur is obtained with 15 degree of IR.
    2. Traction view for proximal femur fractures for better visualization of comminution which may dictate treatment.
    3. Cross-table lateral hip X-ray—patient supine, unaffected hip/knee flexed 80 degree, affected limb internally rotated 15 degree, and beam is parallel to the patient and tilted 45 degree caudal.

    4. Frog leg—patient supine, affected hip abducted 45 degree with the knee bent, so the heel can rest against the contralateral knee, the beam is then directed toward the hip midway between the anterior superior iliac spine (ASIS) and pubic symphysis.

L. Knee

    1. Lateral knee in evaluation of patellar tendon rupture: the knee must be flexed 30 degree (▶Fig. 16.6).

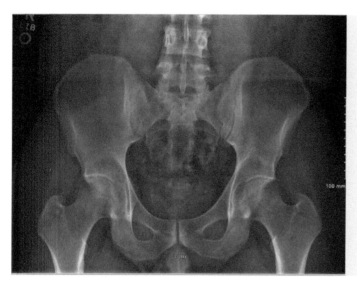

Fig. 16.5 Anteroposterior (AP) of the pelvis. A good AP should be demonstrated by symmetric obturator foramen, iliac wings, and a pubic symphysis that lines up with the midline of the sacrum.

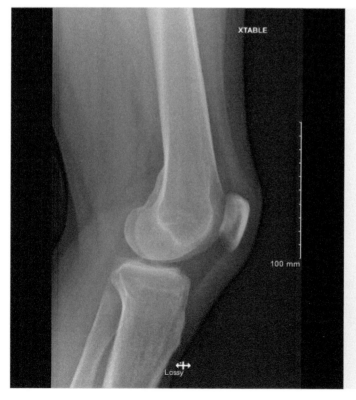

Fig. 16.6 Lateral view of a knee. The femoral condyles should line up in order to be a true lateral of the knee.

2. Sunrise view—knee flexed 45 degree, beam tilted 45 degree cephalad and directed at the knee.

   a. Evaluate patella dislocation.

   b. Should not be performed when a horizontal or comminuted patella fracture is present.

3. Plateau view—AP knee, with the beam titled 15 degree caudal. It can further assess tibial plateau fractures.

M. Ankle

1. AP, lateral, and mortise (▶ Fig. 16.7, ▶ Fig. 16.8, ▶ Fig. 16.9).

   a. Mortise view—beam centered over ankle joint with ankle internally rotated 15 degrees.

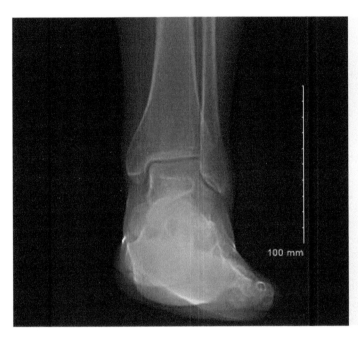

Fig. 16.7 Anteroposterior of the ankle. The lateral gutter is not typically visualized on a true AP and there is more overlap of the tibia on the fibula.

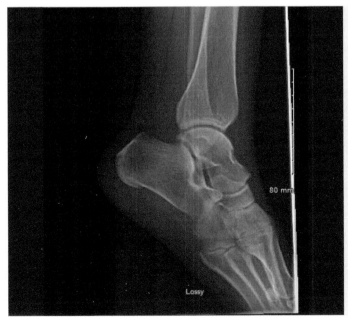

Fig. 16.8 Lateral of the ankle: A true lateral of the ankle demonstrates a smooth line on the dome of the talus. There should be no "double bubble" sign.

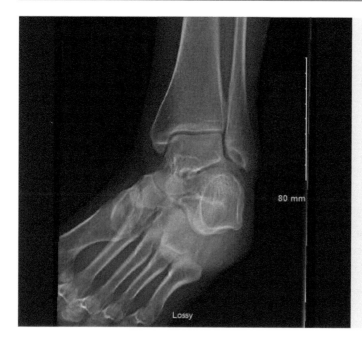

Fig. 16.9 Mortise view of the ankle. A true mortise will show the ankle joint, in its entirety (medial gutter, tibiotalar joint, and lateral gutter) with very little overlap of the tibia on the fibula.

2. When possible, ankle films should be weight bearing.
3. Stress views of the ankle.
   a. Manual stress—ankle internally rotated 15 degrees, and foot manually externally rotated while tibia is held static.
   b. Gravity stress—patient lies lateral with affected side down. A mortise view is obtained, and ankle is allowed to hang off the edge of the bed.
   c. Cotton test—intraoperative view. Mortise view achieved, then bone hook/clamp placed around the fibula with lateral traction applied.
   d. These stress views are used for evaluation of syndesmosis and/or deltoid incompetence. Typically obtained for all isolated lateral malleolus fractures at the level of the mortise (Weber B) or more proximal (Weber C) when nonoperative management is being considered to rule out an unstable injury.

N. Foot
1. AP, lateral, and oblique—weight-bearing films, when possible to evaluate ligamentous injuries evidence with the help of joint diastasis; for example, Lisfranc injury.
2. Talus
   a. Canale view—foot pronated 15 degrees and beam directed 75 degrees cephalad from horizontal. This has typically been replaced by CT to evaluate talus fractures but is still used intraoperatively to evaluate reductions.
3. Subtalar joint
   a. Broden's view—foot/ankle rotated 45 degrees internally, beam centered over lateral gutter, and sequential X-rays with 10, 20, 30, and 40 degrees of cephalic tilt are obtained.
4. Calcaneus
   a. Harris heel view—beam directed posterior to anterior, 45 degree cephalad from horizontal, and directed at the calcaneus.

Conclusion

Ordering the correct imaging in Orthopaedic trauma is critical. Missed diagnoses are often attributed to a lack of proper imaging. Several different modalities are at the disposal of orthopaedic surgeons, and choosing the correct one is critical. X-rays should always be the first choice, and a proper selection of specific images can aid in diagnosis. When clinical suspicion for injury goes beyond plain radiographs, then advanced imaging should be ordered. Care should be taken to weigh the benefits of cost and radiation exposure with necessity of advanced imaging. Computed Tomography is excellent for bony pathology, while MRI is better suited for soft tissue pathology. Practicing appropriate radiation safety is also critical for orthopaedic surgeons, as radiation exposure is linked to cancer, cataracts, and other pathology that can be mitigated by proper safety practices.

Suggested Readings

Clohisy JC, Carlisle JC, Beaulé PE, et al. A systematic approach to the plain radiographic evaluation of the young adult hip. J Bone Joint Surg Am 2008;90(Suppl 4):47–66

Kaplan DJ, Patel JN, Liporace FA, Yoon RS. Intraoperative radiation safety in orthopaedics: a review of the ALARA (As low as reasonably achievable) principle. Patient Saf Surg 2016;10:27

Pfeifer R, Pape HC. Missed injuries in trauma patients: A literature review. Patient Saf Surg 2008;2:20

Ricci WM, Gallagher B, Haidukewych GJ. Intramedullary nailing of femoral shaft fractures: current concepts. J Am Acad Orthop Surg 2009;17(5):296–305

Wolfe S, Pederson W, Kozin SH, Cohen M. Green's Operative Hand Surgery 2011; 18(1):643

Section II

Upper Extremity Trauma

II

17 Sternoclavicular and Acromioclavicular Dislocations

Raymond Pensy

Introduction

Sternoclavicular (SC) Dislocations

Dislocations of the SC joint are uncommon injuries which can result in significant complications. These injuries cross a wide range of age categories and injury mechanisms. In general, these dislocations occur either in an anterior or posterior direction, with the latter carrying more immediate risk and possibly warranting open treatment. Anterior dislocations carry less acute risk, but can result in significant functional impairment if recurrent instability ensues. Both injuries require vigilance, as the initial diagnosis is frequently delayed.

Acromioclavicular (AC) Dislocations

AC injuries are one of the most common injures in orthopaedics. These injuries are, by and large, treated nonoperatively. Injuries involving severe displacement, or comminution of the lateral clavicle, may require operative treatment to reduce the incidence of nonunion, symptomatic prominence, or in rare cases, stabilization of scapula–thoracic dislocation.

I. Preoperative Steps of Sternoclavicular Dislocations

A. History

  1. Typically, these injuries result from a lateral compression force: hockey, wrestling, football, and other contact sports can cause a significant compressive vector which forces the SC joint to dislocate anteriorly; a force applied to the medial clavicle directed posteriorly can also result in posterior dislocation.

  2. In high-energy trauma, T-bone motor vehicle collisions (MVCs) or roll-over accidents will similarly result in lateral compression of the chest, causing dislocation.

  3. The initial amount of displacement, reflective of the severity and magnitude of the imparted force, will manifest as varying degrees of soft tissue injury and stripping, represented by varying degrees of swelling, ecchymosis, and deformity.

B. Physical examination

  1. Swelling and deformity of the anterior, upper, and midline chest.

  2. Pain with attempted range of motion of the affected shoulder.

  3. Guarding against range of motion of the cervical spine, secondary to the injury to the origin of the sternal and clavicular heads of the sternocleidomastoids.

  4. A "fullness" or difficulty in swallowing or speaking, which is in severely displaced posterior dislocations (dysphagia, dysphonia).

  5. Rare neurologic compromise or swelling of the affected side, subsequent to neurologic compression and venous return.

  6. Associated chest wall tenderness and contusion, secondary to the lateral compression injury.

  7. Marked tenderness to palpation over the affected SC joint.

C. Anatomy

  1. In the axial plane, the SC joint is sloped in an oblique manner, such that in a pure compressive force, the clavicle tends to dislocate posteriorly (▶Fig. 17.1).

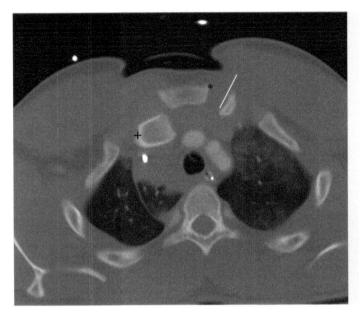

Fig. 17.1 '*' demonstrates the normal left sternoclavicular joint. Note the sloped nature of the joint in the axial plane. '+' demonstrates the right posteriorly dislocated sternoclavicular joint.

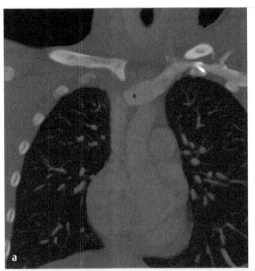
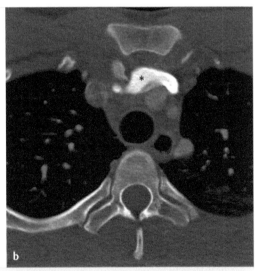

Fig. 17.2 (a, b) Effacement of the brachiocephalic vein by the posteriorly dislocated right sternoclavicular joint.

2. The joint is synovial, with an intra-articular disc, and described as a saddle joint. It is relatively flat and nonconstrained, lending to intrinsic instability without the support of the robust ligamentous capsule.

3. The medial clavicular epiphysis is the last to close, generally in the mid-to-late 20s. Physeal fractures are therefore common in young adults.

4. The SC joint lies immediately upon the brachiocephalic veins on the right and left. These structures pass behind the clavicles, but are anterior to the respective first ribs (▶ Fig. 17.2).

5. The relevant muscular anatomy includes the pectoralis major, sternocleidomastoids, and subclavius.

6. The SC joint itself is made of both extrinsic and intrinsic ligaments. The extrinsic ligaments include the costoclavicular and interclavicular ligaments, whereas the intrinsic ligaments are

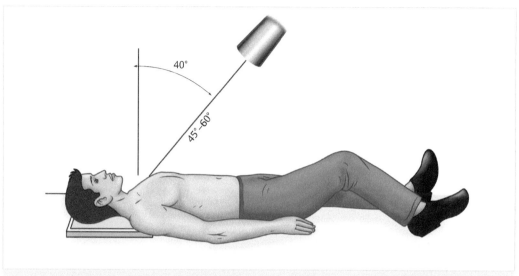

Fig. 17.3 Serendipity view.

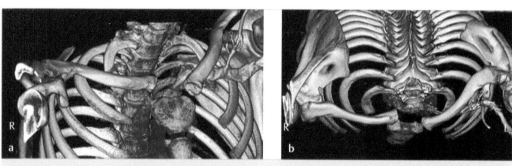

Fig. 17.4 (a, b) Three-dimensional CT reconstruction of the right posteriorly dislocated sternoclavicular joint.

part of the anterior and posterior joint capsule. The posterior capsular ligaments represent the strongest and most important of the SC joint stabilizers.

7.   The clavicle can rotate as much as 40 degrees along its axial plane throughout a full arc of shoulder rotation.

D.   Imaging

1.   Plain films of the chest demonstrate inadequate sensitivity for diagnosis. Asymmetry can, however, be recognized, and offers clues to the diagnosis.

2.   Although dedicated Serendipity or Henig views have been described, with any degree of suspicion, a computed tomography (CT) scan should confirm diagnosis. Serendipity views—with the patient supine, an anteroposterior (AP) of the medial clavicle is obtained with a 40-degree cephalic tilt of the X-ray beam (▶Fig. 17.3).

3.   CT scan should be used as the first line of imaging, which permits determination of the direction of displacement, as well as injury or effacement of retrosternal structures.

4.   Axial images will depict, in most cases, clear evidence of either anterior or posterior dislocation.

5.   Intravenous (IV) contrast can be helpful in discerning injury or effacement to the retrosternal structures particularly that of the brachiocephalic vein (▶Fig. 17.2).

6.   Three-dimensional imaging can be helpful in establishing additional vertical displacement (▶Fig. 17.4).

E. Classification

1. These injuries are broadly classified temporally as acute, subacute, or chronic. Chronic injuries may manifest as either of the following:

    a. Complete, irreducible dislocations.

    b. Recurrent instability, which in some cases can be voluntary or involuntary through muscle contraction, or shoulder range extremes.

II. Treatment of Sternoclavicular Dislocations

A. Initial and definitive management

1. The patient sustaining MVC or other high-energy mechanisms should be evaluated per advanced trauma life support (ATLS) guidelines (see Chapter 9, Polytrauma).

2. CT scan evaluation is very helpful in discerning accompanying frequent injuries, such as hemo/pneumo thorax, associated rib fractures, and injuries to the retrosternal structures. CT with IV contrast can be very helpful in identifying the proximity, and possible injury, to the posterior vascular structures.

3. Anterior dislocation:

    a. Anterior dislocations are generally treated closed through conscious sedation or general anesthesia.

    b. Traction and a posteriorly directed force is applied to the medial clavicle.

    c. When reduction is achieved, the arm is placed in a sling and graduated return to activity is permitted, but avoidance of contact sports is recommended for three months.

4. Posterior dislocation:

    a. These dislocations result in tracheal, esophageal, or neurovascular injury in up to 30% of cases if left untreated. Mortality has been reported in up to 4% of patients.

    b. Treatment is a topic of controversy with regard to open versus closed treatment. Consultation with cardiothoracic surgery is recommended prior to surgery. Some advocate for closed reduction under anesthesia, others advocate for open treatment.

    c. Reduction is difficult to confirm without CT scan, and redislocation can result in significant complication.

    d. Performing these procedures at a tertiary center is recommended, assuming the patient is not in distress with airway compromise and can tolerate transport, with the availability of cardiothoracic surgeons, in case of retrosternal venous, arterial, or cardiac complication.

B. Surgical approach and fixation techniques

1. Anterior dislocation—the patient is advised that recurrent dislocation is likely and a small percentage of patients will acquire symptomatic recurrent instability requiring operative treatment.

2. Posterior dislocation:

    a. The authors prefer operative treatment in order to confirm and maintain reduction. The patient is placed supine, with a horseshoe Mayfield headrest, to allow both the surgeon and the assistant access to the anterior chest and neck.

    b. Large bore intravenous access is recommended, as is type and cross match.

    c. A transverse linear incision is made, spanning the manubrium and the affected side.

    d. The sternocleidomastoid and pectoralis is lifted (if not already done so traumatically by the displacement) from the anterior aspect of the SC joint.

    e. The posterior dissection is generally completed by the injury.

    f. A malleable retractor is placed behind the manubrium, and two drill holes with a 3.2 or 4.5 mm drill are made in the sternum directed laterally, to facilitate placement of either suture or allograft tendon (Spencer et al, Petri et al).

g. The clavicle is grasped with a bone reduction clamp ("crab/lion" jaw) and presented to allow corresponding drill holes to be made in its medial aspect.

h. A 24 ga stainless steel wire is looped to act as a suture retrieval device, and an allograft tendon is placed in a figure of eight technique, crossing posteriorly, and sewn to itself in a Pulvertaft weave anteriorly.

i. The skin is closed over a drain and X-rays are obtained to verify no pneumothorax or other complications.

j. K-wire fixation, either smooth or threaded, of the SC joint is ABSOLUTELY CONTRAINDICATED subsequent to migration and fatal cardiac tamponade.

k. Closed reduction and treatment can be considered in those cases without evidence of mediastinal compression and acute recognition (< 7 days).

   i. These reductions should be performed under general anesthesia, and with appropriate consideration of the posterior vascular structures.

   ii. If closed reduction fails, the surgeon should be comfortable in completing open treatment.

   iii. Some authors suggest using a percutaneous tenaculum for reduction. Great care must be utilized, as, in the author's experience, significant swelling is common, and errant clamp placement can damage the juxtaposed brachiocephalic vein.

3. Reduction must be confirmed with postreduction CT imaging, as the existing literature reports a frequent redislocation rate.

C. Complications

1. Redisplacement and/or instability as described above.

2. Vascular injury with posterior dislocation can be fatal and precautions are taken as emphasized above.

3. Pneumothorax and/or airway compromise.

III. Preoperative Steps of Acromioclavicular Dislocations

A. History and typically, these injuries result from a direct blow to the shoulder, most commonly reported in sporting events, falls, motorcycle, or ejection MVC.

B. Physical examination

1. Swelling and pain are obvious about the lateral shoulder.

2. Pain with attempted range-of-motion is common.

3. Associated neurovascular injuries are common, but possible with higher energy mechanisms.

4. In subacute and chronic presentations, the distal clavicle will form an obvious prominence, which may or may not reduce with retraction of the shoulder and direct pressure upon the clavicle.

C. Anatomy

1. The AC joint is stabilized by the AC ligaments intrinsic to the joint (anterior, posterior, superior, and inferior).

1. It is also supported by the coracoclavicular ligaments which connect the corocoid to the lateral third of the clavicle (Chapter 18, Clavicle Fractures, ▶Fig. 18.1).

2. Conoid ligament medially.

3. Trapezoid ligament laterally.

4. The joint itself is synovial, diathrodial, and usually maintains an articular disc.

5. The muscles surrounding this articulation include the following: deltoid, trapezius, and pectoralis major.

D. Imaging

1. Standard chest X-rays will demonstrate significant displacement, but Zanca and dedicated clavicle views are important to demonstrate subtle. pathology. Zanca view—AP of the AC joint with a 15-degree cephalic tilt of the X-ray beam (▶Fig. 17.5).

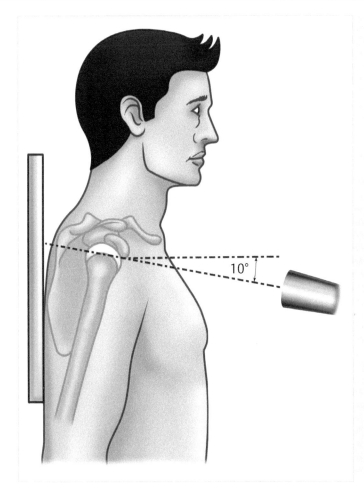

Fig. 17.5 Zanca view.

10°

2. As with any shoulder injury, orthogonal views of the shoulder are recommended, and Grashey and true axillary views are preferred.

3. CT and MRI scan, although rarely indicated, can be helpful to demonstrate significant displacement posteriorly or disruption of the soft tissues.

4. Regarding classification, vertical displacement shows reasonable inter-observer agreement, whereas horizontal displacement demonstrates significant variability.

5. No gold standard exists in imaging the injured AC joint beyond standard radiographs.

E. Injury (AC dislocation) classification (Rockwood) (▶ **Fig. 17.6**).

1. Type I—sprain of the AC ligaments without displacement.

2. Type II—disruption of the AC ligaments, with preservation of the coracoclavicular (CC) ligaments and minimal displacement.

3. Type III—disruption of both the AC and CC ligaments, with displacement of the lateral clavicle more than 100% in relation to the acromion.

4. Type IV—complete disruption of the AC and CC ligaments, with posterior dislocation of the lateral clavicle through the trapezius.

5. Type V—more than 100% displacement indicates significant soft tissue stripping of the trapezius and deltoid from the lateral clavicle and acromion.

6. Type VI—rare, with dislocation of the lateral clavicle inferior to the acromion or corocoid.

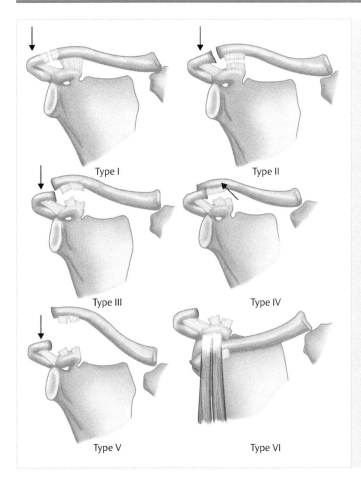

Fig. 17.6 Rockwood classification for AC dislocations.

Type I

Type II

Type III

Type IV

Type V

Type VI

F. Injury (lateral clavicle fractures) Classification (Neer) (▶**Fig. 17.7**). Fractures of the lateral end of the clavicle, which involve disruption of the corocaclavicular ligaments and have significant displacement, behave similarly to high-grade AC joint separations and are prone to nonunion (▶**Fig. 17.8 a–d**).

IV. Treatment of Acromioclavicular Dislocations

A. Initial and definitive management

1. Type I and Type II injuries:

   a. Nonoperative treatment with weight bearing and range of motion initiated immediately.

   b. Sling is provided and worn PRN for comfort only.

   c. Early motion is initiated once other shoulder pathology is ruled out by careful clinical examination and standard, orthogonal shoulder films.

2. Type III, IV, and V injuries are controversial in nature:

   a. Equivalent results have been found for nonoperative and operative treatment using a "hook" plate for fixation.

   b. There is a lack of evidence supporting operative treatment for type III AC dislocations initially. Typically, surgery is recommended for type III AC dislocations which undergo failed closed treatment.

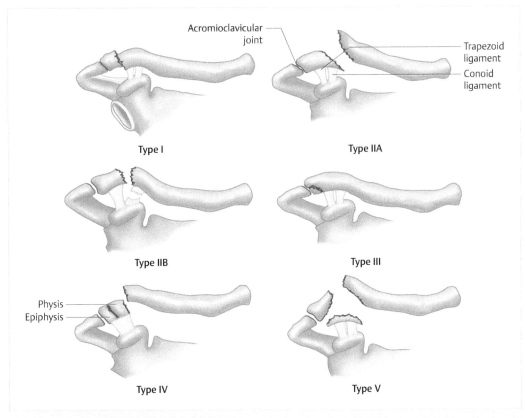

Fig. 17.7 Neer classification of lateral clavicle fractures.

    c.   Outcomes between operatively and non-operatively managed high-grade AC separations (III-V) are equivalent.

B.   Surgical approach and fixation techniques

    1.   The author prefers to position the patient supine, in a semi-beach chair position, on a Mayfield headrest, allowing the surgeon and the assistant appropriate access.

        a.   The AC joint and lateral clavicle is approached, in acute cases, from a direct superior exposure. Careful attention is paid in lifting the pectoralis and deltoid, as necessary, from the lateral clavicle and acromion, such that an accurate repair of these muscles can be completed.

        b.   The AC joint is reduced and held with a provision K-wire across the AC joint to then permit definitive fixation. No attempt is made to repair or reconstruct the torn CC ligaments in acute cases.

        c.   In chronic cases, the CC ligaments are reconstructed with allograft semitendinosis through an anterior exposure, which facilitates a proximal deltopectoral exposure of the corocoid.

        d.   If a "hook" plate is used, it is typically removed at 6 months post-operatively, as it may cause acromion erosion. It is also a common source of painful impingement (▶ Fig. 17.8c, d).

C.   Complications

    1.   Superior redisplacement of the distal clavicle can occur in up to 1/5 of surgically treated cases.

    2.   Pain and osteolysis may occur at the distal clavicle after reconstruction.

    3.   Peri-implant fracture can occur.

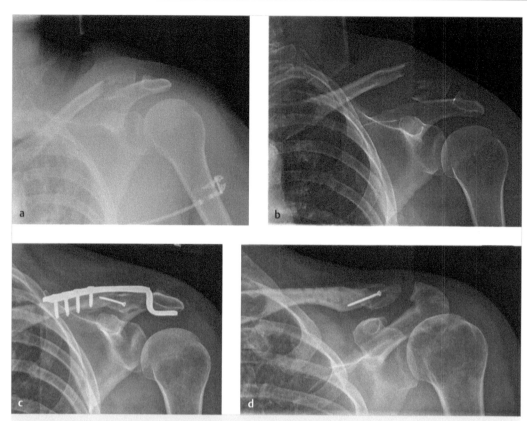

Fig. 17.8 (a–d) Nondisplaced fracture of lateral clavicle.

Conclusion

Injuries to the sternoclavicular joint, in particular, are difficult to diagnose and left untreated, may lead to significant morbidity. Operative treatment should be relegated to acute care settings where surgeons experienced in the anatomy and cardiothoracic surgeons are available. For acromioclavicular injuries, recent evidence suggests non-operative treatment is preferred for most injury patterns. Acromioclavicular injuries associated with lateral clavicle fracture may warrant operative treatment with implants that require eventual removal.

Suggested Readings

Sternoclavicular Dislocations

Lee JT, Campbell KJ, Michalski MP, et al. Surgical anatomy of the sternoclavicular joint: a qualitative and quantitative anatomical study. J Bone Joint Surg Am 2014;96(19):e166

Nettles JL, Linscheid RL. Sternoclavicular dislocations. J Trauma 1968;8(2):158–164

Petri M, Greenspoon JA, Horan MP, Martetschläger F, Warth RJ, Millett PJ. Clinical outcomes after autograft reconstruction for sternoclavicular joint instability. J Shoulder Elbow Surg 2016;25(3):435–441

Spencer EE Jr, Kuhn JE. Biomechanical analysis of reconstructions for sternoclavicular joint instability. J Bone Joint Surg Am 2004;86(1):98–105

Spencer EE, Kuhn JE, Huston LJ, Carpenter JE, Hughes RE. Ligamentous restraints to anterior and posterior translation of the sternoclavicular joint. J Shoulder Elbow Surg 2002;11(1):43–47

van Tongel A, MacDonald P, Leiter J, Pouliart N, Peeler J. A cadaveric study of the structural anatomy of the sternoclavicular joint. Clin Anat 2012;25(7):903–910

Acromioclavicular Dislocations

Canadian Orthopaedic Trauma Society. Multicenter randomized clinical trial of nonoperative versus operative treatment of acute acromio-clavicular joint dislocation. J Orthop Trauma 2015;29(11):479–487

Chang N, Furey A, Kurdin A. Operative versus nonoperative management of acute high-grade acromioclavicular dislocations: a systematic review and meta-analysis. J Orthop Trauma 2018;32(1):1–9

Longo UG, Ciuffreda M, Rizzello G, Mannering N, Maffulli N, Denaro V. Surgical versus conservative management of Type III acromioclavicular dislocation: a systematic review. Br Med Bull 2017;122(1):31–49

Rockwood CA. Acromioclavicular joint injuries Rockwood classification. In: Rockwood CA, ed. Fractures in Adults. Philadelphia, PA: Lippincott-Raven; 1996

Rockwood CA Jr, Williams GR, Young D. Disorders of the acromioclavicular joint. In: Rockwood CA Jr, Matsen F, eds. The Shoulder. Philadelphia, PA: Saunders; 1998;483–553

18 Clavicle Fractures

Robert Andrew Ravinsky, David H. Campbell, and Michael D. McKee

Introduction

The clavicle is one of the most commonly fractured bones, representing up to approximately 5% of all fractures. There is a growing body of evidence that select middle 1/3 clavicle shaft fractures in adults may benefit from operative management. Fractures of the medial 1/3 and lateral 1/3 of the clavicle are recognized as distinct clinical entities and deserve unique consideration (▶Video 18.1).

I. Preoperative

A. History and physical examination

1. The most common mechanism for sustaining clavicle fractures involves a fall directly onto the lateral aspect of the shoulder, followed by bicycle accidents, direct blow to the clavicle, motor vehicle accidents, and motorcycle accidents.

2. The distribution of this injury follows a bimodal distribution:
    a. One peak found in young, predominantly male, adults as a result of high-energy injuries.
    b. Second peak in individuals over the age of 70 years, primarily as a consequence of low-energy falls.

3. In patients having sustained high-energy mechanisms of trauma:
    a. Systematically assess the patient using the advanced trauma life support (ATLS) protocol to rule out associated occult and potentially life-threatening injuries.
    b. Scapular fractures or rib fractures my herald the presence of pneumothorax or pulmonary contusion. In this setting, an upright chest radiograph is indicated.
    c. Evaluate neurologic and/or vascular compromise.
    d. Scapulothoracic dissociation:
        i.   Often indicated by distraction, rather than shortening, at the clavicle fracture site.
        ii. High rate of neurologic and vascular injury.

4. Physical examination:
    a. Inspection of the shoulder girdle may reveal abnormalities in the soft tissue envelope such as abrasion, ecchymosis, swelling, skin tenting, or open fracture.
    b. Open fracture is uncommon.
    c. Skin tenting may be common but skin compromise due to displaced fracture ends is rare. Skin at risk of necrosis due to fracture displacement may necessitate more expeditious management.
    d. Palpation of the shoulder girdle may elicit focal tenderness, and gentle manipulation may result in appreciable crepitation at the fracture site.
    e. Perform a thorough neurologic and vascular examination.

B. Anatomy

1. Osteology:
    a. It is the last bone in the body to fuse, as its medial physis closes between 20 and 25 years of age.
    b. The clavicle is a tubular S-shaped bone, whose round and stout medial end articulates with the sternum via a synovial joint.
    c. The lateral end of the clavicle is flat and wide, and articulates via the synovial acromioclavicular (AC) joint with the acromial process of the scapula.

d. Medially, the clavicle has an anterior bow that curves near its midpoint to form a posterior bow laterally.

e. The central, tubular portion of the clavicle represents a weak, transitional area, making it more prone to fracture. This explains why most clavicle fractures are middiaphyseal.

f. The intramedullary canal begins 7 mm from the sternoclavicular joint and ends 20 mm from the AC joint.

2. Ligamentous anatomy (▶ Fig. 18.1):

a. There are several important ligamentous structures which attach to the clavicle and support shoulder function.

b. The coracoclavicular (CC) ligament, composed of the conoid ligament medially and the trapezoid ligament laterally, plays a role in suspending the scapula and supporting the weight of the arm.

c. Medially, the sternoclavicular ligaments and costoclavicular ligaments affix the upper extremity to the axial skeleton.

d. Laterally, the AC ligaments, strongest posterosuperiorly, prevent displacement of the lateral clavicle in the anteroposterior (AP) direction.

3. Muscular structures attaching the clavicle (▶ Fig. 18.2):

a. Knowledge of the muscular attachments to the clavicle are critical in understanding the deforming forces, and subsequent patterns of displacement seen in clavicle fractures.

b. The muscles that attach to the clavicle include—sternocleidomastoid, trapezius, deltoid, pectoralis major, sternohyoid, plastysma and subclavius.

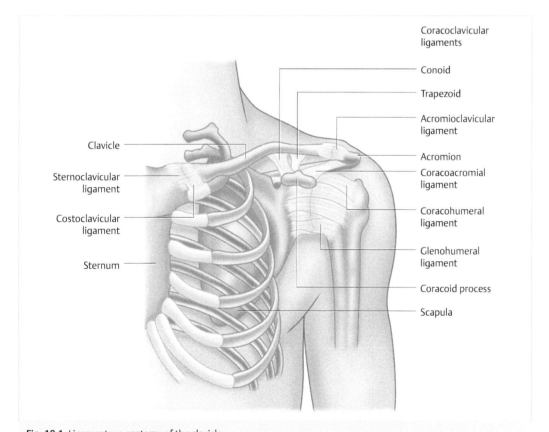

Fig. 18.1 Ligamentous anatomy of the clavicle.

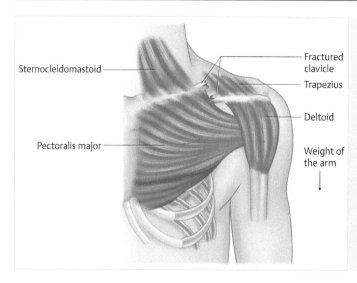

Fig. 18.2 Deforming forces affecting a fractured clavicle.

Sternocleidomastoid

Fractured clavicle

Trapezius

Deltoid

Pectoralis major

Weight of the arm

    c. Resultant forces lead to:
        i. Superior displacement of the medial fragment.
        ii. Medial (shortening), inferior, and anterior displacement (rotation) of the lateral fragment.

  4. Adjacent structures of relevance:
    a. Subclavian vessels—lie posterior to the medial clavicle and pass underneath the middle one-third of the clavicle. Subclavian artery lies posterior and superior to the subclavian vein.
    b. Brachial plexus—anterior and posterior divisions (continuation of the superior, middle, and inferior trunks) pass under the middle one-third of the clavicle.
    c. Lung—inferior to the medial half of the clavicle.
    d. Injury to these structures has been described in the course of injury to the clavicle, during the surgical approach, and from insertion of hardware.

  5. Clavicle function: The clavicle functions as both a strut and a suspension for the upper extremity.
    a. Strut function—the musculature of the shoulder girdle and thorax are maintained at their optimal working length due to the presence of the clavicle, thus optimizing their mechanical advantage.
    b. Suspensory function—dynamic suspension is achieved through the upward pull of the trapezius, and static suspension is achieved via the sternoclavicular (SC), AC, and coracoclavicular (CC) ligaments.

C. Imaging
  1. Although a clavicle fracture can usually be diagnosed on a standard plain chest radiograph, initial imaging for clavicle fractures should include AP and apical oblique radiographs. The latter involves 25 degrees of cephalic tilt of the beam, and allows unobscured view of the clavicle.
  2. For fractures of the medial and lateral ends of the clavicle, special films are occasionally needed:
    a. Medial clavicle fractures displace in the axial plane, and injuries of the sternoclavicular joint can be best viewed on a Serendipity view (X-ray centered on the SC joint and angled 40 degrees cephalad with the patient supine).
    b. Lateral clavicle fractures and injuries of the acromioclavicular joint may be best appreciated on a Zanca view (X-ray beam angled 20 degrees cephalad).

3. Cross-sectional imaging in the form of computed tomography (CT) scan is beneficial in delineating the fracture pattern for more complex, comminuted injuries. CT scanning is the imaging modality of choice for medial fractures.

D. Classifications

1. The Allman classification of clavicle fractures is the one most commonly used. It divides fractures based on anatomic region:

   a. Group 1: middle one-third.

   b. Group 2: lateral one-third.

   c. Group 3: medial one-third.

2. Group 2 (lateral) was further classified by Neer, based on the relationship between the fracture line and the CC ligaments. This classification was further modified by Rockwood to the classification in use today.

3. Another classification of clavicle fractures exists within the Arbeitsgemeinschaft für Osteosynthesefrage/Orthopaedic trauma association (AO/OTA) classification, which categorizes clavicle fractures first based on fracture location, followed by fracture characteristics and morphology.

II. Treatment

A. Initial management

1. After completing a clinical evaluation of the patient, initial management of clavicle fractures involves immobilization in a sling for comfort and appropriate analgesia.

2. In the setting of high-energy injuries, or polytrauma, it is recommended that the patient undergo a full trauma evaluation, including the ATLS protocol.

B. Definitive management

1. Nonoperative treatment is recommended for the majority of minimally displaced clavicle fractures:

   a. Two to four weeks of immobilization in a sling with initiation of motion as pain subsides.

   b. Figure-of-8 swathe has been associated with patient discomfort and skin issues and does not improve fracture reduction compared to a sling.

   c. Strengthening and resistance exercises are initiated following fracture union.

2. Generally accepted indications:

   a. Open fractures.

   b. Displaced fractures with significant tenting, leading to skin compromise.

   c. Medial clavicle fracture with posterior displacement and compression of mediastinal structures.

3. Relative indications:

   a. Floating shoulder (clavicle and glenoid neck fracture).

   b. Clavicle fracture with associated brachial plexus injury.

   c. Symptomatic nonunion.

   d. Symptomatic malunion that has failed conservative treatment.

   e. Middle one-third fracture with 2 cm of shortening or > 100% displacement (▶ Fig. 18.3a).

   f. Clavicle fracture in a polytraumatized patient (especially if upper extremity weight bearing is required).

   g. Multiple associated ipsilateral rib fractures.

   h. Multiple, associated upper extremity fractures.

   i. Bilateral clavicle fractures.

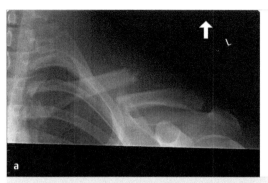 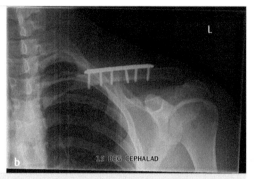

Fig. 18.3 (a) An isolated, completely displaced midshaft fracture of the clavicle. There was an obvious associated clinical deformity. (b) Anatomic reduction and plate fixation resulted in rapid return to activity and solid bony union at six weeks post-operatively.

C. Positioning and surgical approaches

 1. The patient should be positioned on the beach chair in semi-seated position, or supine with the injured extremity draped free. Prep to the contralateral chest and high onto the neck.

 2. Choice of surgical incision depends on the desired method of fracture fixation, with the superior approach being used for superior plate application, and a direct anterior approach reserved for anteroinferior plate fixation.

 3. Superior approach:

 a. Skin incision is made longitudinally along the length of the clavicle, and subcutaneous tissues are split in line with the incision.

 b. Platysma and clavipectoral fascia is incised.

 c. The deltotrapezial muscle layer is developed laterally, and the layer between the pectoralis major and sternocleidomastoid is developed medially.

 d. Efforts should be made to preserve the branches of the supraclavicular nerve, as they run in the surgical field.

 i. To prevent chest numbness and dysesthesia.
 ii. It is prudent to warn the patient of the probability of peri-incisional numbness preoperatively.

 e. Medial clavicle—subperiosteal dissection of the pectoralis anteriorly, as needed, to expose the fracture site and facilitate implant fixation.

 f. Lateral clavicle—subperiosteal dissection of the deltoid anteriorly and trapezius posteriorly, as needed, to expose the fracture site, mobilize the fragment, and allow implant placement.

 g. Care should be taken to preserve soft-tissue attachments and accompanying blood supply to promote fracture healing.

 4. Direct anterior approach:

 a. The superficial and deep dissection is similar to the superior approach.

 b. However, the incision is not centered over the clavicle, but rather at the anterior border of the clavicle.

 c. Shifting the incision anteriorly facilitates exposure of the anterior clavicular surface for eventual anteroinferior plating.

D. Fixation techniques

 1. Intramedullary fixation:

 a. Cannulated screw.

 b. Precontoured, lockable intramedullary nails.

 c. Elastic, titanium intramedullary nail.

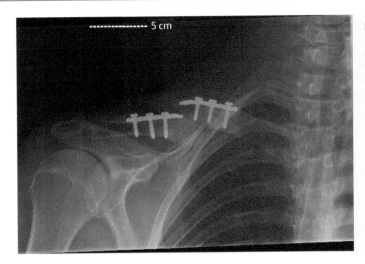

Fig. 18.4 Early failure of a 3.5 mm pelvic reconstruction plate in an active male patient who weighed over 220 pounds. This plate is not as strong as precontoured or compression plates, and may break prior to union in larger, active, or noncompliant patients.

2. Plate and screw fixation:

    a. For surgical fixation of the clavicle, the use of precontoured plates with three points of fixation (for simple fracture patterns) both proximal and distal to the fracture site is recommended (▶ **Fig. 18.3a, b**). While 3.5 mm pelvic reconstruction plates have also been used with reasonable results, when used in isolation, they have a higher mechanical failure rate than compression or precontoured plates, especially in physically larger (North American) patients (▶ **Fig. 18.4**).

    b. For comminuted fractures, a relative stability construct, employing a bridge plating technique with minimal soft-tissue stripping is preferred to preserve the biology of the fracture site. It is important to restore length and rotation accurately if this technique is used.

    c. Both superior and anteroinferior plating have been used for internal fixation of the clavicle.

        i. Results of the two techniques are similar in terms of rates of union, nonunion, malunion, implant failure, and functional outcome scores.

        ii. Superior plating is associated with a higher load to failure in biomechanical studies.

        iii. Superior plating, in contrast to anteroinferior plating, is associated with a higher incidence of symptomatic hardware, and higher reoperation rates for implant removal.

        iv. There is no good clinical evidence to suggest locking plates are superior to nonlocking plates; however, precontoured locking plates with nonlocking screws are routinely used.

E. Complications

    1. Nonoperative treatment:

        a. Nonunion: Several risk factors contributing to nonunion have been discussed in the literature. These include increased fracture displacement, smoking, comminution, advanced age, female gender, and shortening of the fracture.

        b. Malunion: Increased fracture displacement has been shown to be a predictor for increased pain and dysfunction after midshaft clavicle fracture.

    2. Surgical treatment:

        a. Symptomatic or prominent hardware: Symptomatic hardware is the most commonly reported sequelae of internal fixation of the clavicle. As many as one quarter of patients who have undergone open reduction and internal fixation (ORIF) of the clavicle will later undergo reoperation for hardware removal. This can be minimized by using a precontoured plate (▶ **Fig. 18.5a, b**) and waiting a minimum of two years before removing hardware.

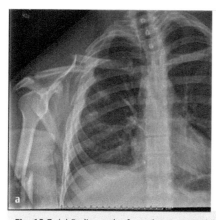 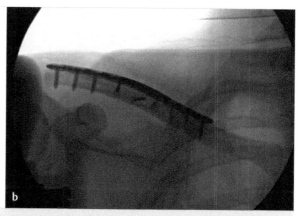

Fig. 18.5 (a) Radiograph of a pedestrian struck by a car. In addition to the clavicle fracture, there were ipsilateral rib, humeral, and radial fractures. This represents a good indication for fixation. (b) Intraoperative fluoroscopic image following open reduction and internal fixation (ORIF) with a precontoured plate. The patient also had ORIF of the humeral shaft and radial fractures. An excellent clinical result ensued despite the severity of the injuries.

    b. Infection: Risk factors contributing to infection after clavicle ORIF include diabetes mellitus, intravenous (IV) drug use, and revision surgery/previous shoulder surgery. When infection is suspected, it is recommended that cultures be held for a minimum of 10 days in order to recognize the presence of fastidious organisms such as c. acnes.

    c. Neurovascular injury: Neurovascular injury is a rare and severe complication of clavicle ORIF. This complication can be avoided by ensuring that drills, taps, and screws do not penetrate into the subclavicular space.

    d. Pneumothorax: Another rare complication of clavicle ORIF. It is the result of violation of the pulmonary pleura during exposure, or drilling of the clavicle. It can occur in thin, small, female patients among whom the distance between the clavicle and pleura is limited.

    e. Nonunion: Underlying infection, especially with c. acnes, should be suspected if there is failure of plate or nail fixation of a clavicle fracture.

    f. Malunion: This complication is very rare. Corrective osteotomy and revision fixation may be indicated.

    g. Hardware failure: This may result from plate/screw breakage, due to excessive motion at the fracture site, or may occur at the screw-bone interface as screw pullout.

    h. Adhesive capsulitis: Although a rare complication of clavicle ORIF, both prolonged immobilization of the upper extremity and recent surgical intervention are known risk factors for adhesive capsulitis.

F. Rehabilitation

  1. After nonoperative treatment:

    a. Many surgeons will allow immediate weight bearing as tolerated (WBAT) with range of motion (ROM), although other surgeons may take a more conservative approach with delayed weight bearing and ROM at 2 to 4 weeks.

    b. At six weeks, if the patient is pain free and there is radiographic evidence of progressive union of the fracture, the patient may begin strengthening exercises.

    c. Return to full, unrestricted activity occurs at three months postoperative; however, the patient must be pain free, with full strength and full ROM.

  2. After surgical treatment:

    a. Most surgeons will allow immediate WBAT and ROM, although some surgeons will take a more conservative approach with immobilization for 7 to 10 days.

    b. At six weeks postoperative, if the patient is pain free and there is radiographic evidence of progressive union of the fracture, the patient may begin strengthening exercises.

    c. Return to full, unrestricted activity occurs when the patient is pain free with full strength and ROM, typically by 3 months postoperative.

G. Outcomes

  1. With respect to displaced, midshaft fractures of the clavicle, there is a substantial body of literature demonstrating improved outcomes with surgical intervention over nonoperative treatment.

  2. This includes improved pain scores, as measured by the Visual Analog Scale (VAS), improved functional outcomes, as measured by the Disabilities of the Arm, Shoulder and Hand (DASH) score, and lower rates of nonunion and symptomatic malunion.

  3. Although studies have shown improved functional outcomes, some consider the improvements to be of minimal clinical relevance.

  4. Most surgeons tailor surgery to the specific patient, with more healthy, active patients typically undergoing surgery and less active patients or those with comorbidities typically being treated conservatively.

  5. There is data to support a more rapid return to function and athletic pursuits with primary fixation, and this treatment has become routine in most professional sports leagues where time to return to play is critical.

III. Special Considerations

A. Open fracture

  1. Open fracture of the clavicle necessitates early administration of IV antibiotics, and tetanus prophylaxis if tetanus status is unknown or not up to date. The antibiotic of choice is a third-generation cephalosporin.

  2. Following assessment and stabilization of the patient, he or she should be taken for urgent operative irrigation and debridement, and open reduction internal fixation of the fracture.

B. Clavicle fracture in the elderly

  1. While in recent years, there has been an increase in the proportion of clavicle fractures in patients above 65 years of age undergoing ORIF, it has been suggested that not all displaced fractures in this patient population require surgical fixation.

  2. Patients of very advanced age, especially those whom are infirm or very low demand, should be considered for nonoperative treatment in the absence of an absolute indication for surgery.

C. Adolescent clavicle fracture

  1. Traditionally, clavicle fractures in children and adolescents have been treated nonoperatively and the union rate is high.

  2. However, not all adolescents treated in this fashion are satisfied with their outcome, and there are cases of nonunion and symptomatic malunion.

  3. Plate fixation can be performed in this age group with a high degree of success; although it is controversial, there are surgeons who feel that primary fixation may be an option for older adolescents with severely displaced fractures.

D. Pathologic fracture

  1. Surgical treatment of pathologic fractures of the clavicle are indicated to establish a tissue diagnosis of the pathologic lesion. This will aid in guiding medical management, whether the etiology of the lesion is benign, neoplastic or infectious. Furthermore, pathologic lesions may not possess the biologic capability or mechanical stability to heal without surgical intervention; thus, ORIF may be necessary to stabilize these lesions.

Conclusion

The midshaft clavicle fracture is a commonly encountered orthopaedic injury. Indications for surgical fixation continue to change as the significant morbidity of nonoperative treatment in displaced fractures and patterns associated with related injuries becomes more readily understood. Precontoured plates provide ease of implantation and hardware resiliency in larger patients. The utility of fixation in adolescent patients and the elderly continues to be controversial. Continued research is essential in determining the ideal patient and injury factors predictive of a superior postoperative functional outcome in these groups.

Suggested Readings

Hill JM, McGuire MH, Crosby LA. Closed treatment of displaced middle-third fractures of the clavicle gives poor results. J Bone Joint Surg Br 1997;79(4):537–539

Lenza M, Buchbinder R, Johnston RV. Surgical Versus Conservative Interventions for Treating Fractures of The Middle Third of The Clavicle. The Cochrane. Database of Systematic Reviews. 6th ed. Hoboken, NJ: Wiley; 2013

McKee RC, Whelan DB, Schemitsch EH, McKee MD. Operative versus nonoperative care of displaced midshaft clavicular fractures: a meta-analysis of randomized clinical trials. J Bone Joint Surg Am 2012;94(8):675–684

McKee MD, Wild LM, Schemitsch EH. Midshaft malunions of the clavicle. J Bone Joint Surg Am 2003;85(5):790–797

Nordqvist A, Petersson CJ, Redlund-Johnell I. Mid-clavicle fractures in adults: end result study after conservative treatment. J Orthop Trauma 1998;12(8):572–576

Canadian Orthopaedic Trauma Society. Nonoperative treatment compared with plate fixation of displaced midshaft clavicular fractures. A multicenter, randomized clinical trial. J Bone Joint Surg Am 2007;89(1):1–10

Robinson CM. Fractures of the clavicle in the adult. Epidemiology and classification. J Bone Joint Surg Br 1998;80(3):476–484

Simpson NS, Jupiter JB. Clavicular Nonunion and Malunion: Evaluation and Surgical Management. J Am Acad Orthop Surg 1996;4(1):1–8

19 Scapular Fractures

Brian Buck

Introduction

Scapula fractures comprise approximately 1% of all fractures and 3-5% of upper extremity fractures. 90% of scapula fractures are associated with concomitant injury to the thorax/chest including: pneumothorax, hemothorax, pulmonary contusion, cardiac contusion, aortic injury, rib fracture, flail chest, clavicle fracture, and spine fracture. They are typically due to a high-energy mechanism of injury with a lateral impact to the shoulder girdle and/or traction injury to the arm. Up to 15% of scapula fractures are diagnosed late due to incomplete examination or precedence given to life-threatening injuries. The vast majority of scapula fractures are treated nonoperatively and this chapter will explore indications for surgical consideration.

I. Preoperative

A. History and physical examination
   1. Mechanism of injury—high-energy trauma to chest wall and shoulder girdle.
   2. Location of pain:
      a. Patients complain of shoulder pain/posterior scapular border pain.
      b. Distinguish between chest wall trauma and scapula/shoulder girdle pain.
   3. Associated injuries:
      a. Chest wall injuries to thoracic cage.
      b. Ipsilateral clavicle/upper extremity fractures.
      c. Neurovascular injury.
   4. Inspection:
      a. Asymmetry compared to contralateral shoulder girdle.
      b. Soft tissue swelling/ecchymosis over posterior scapular border.
      c. Associated soft tissue swelling over clavicle/shoulder girdle with associated trauma.
      d. Documentation of dermal abrasions with location, depth, and degree of contamination.
      e. Identification of associated trauma wounds and location of chest tube placement/intravenous (IV) lines.
   5. Palpation:
      a. Crepitus over posterior shoulder girdle and scapula border.
      b. Tenderness to palpation over fracture site.
      c. Late detection of injury with missed fractures is not uncommon, highlighting the importance of correlation of examination findings with radiographic analysis.
   6. Motor function:
      a. Difficult to fully assess motor function based on injury pattern and associated life-threatening injuries.
      b. Patients typically demonstrate significantly limited shoulder function.
      c. Careful evaluation of the brachial plexus and sound knowledge of peri-scapular muscular innervation are required to accurately diagnose neurological deficits.
      d. Associated extremity injury or deficits should alert physician to more extensive injury.

7. Sensory function:

   a. Assess and document dermatomal sensory function.

   b. Assessment of brachial plexus.

8. Vascular status:

   a. Identification of palpable pulses.

   b. Documentation of capillary refill.

   c. Auscultation over proximal vascular tree for audible bruits or palpation of thrills.

B. Anatomy (▶ **Fig. 19.1**)

1. Supraspinatus fossa:

   a. Origin of supraspinatus muscle.

   b. Suprascapular artery and nerve travel through suprascapular notch over superior border.

2. Infraspinatus fossa—origin of infraspinatus muscle in fossa and origin of teres major and minor over inferior and lateral border.

3. Subscapularis fossa—origin of subscapularis muscle.

4. Glenoid—articular component of scapula enveloped by joint capsule and labrum.

5. Acromion process:

   a. Termination of spine of scapula.

   b. Contributes to acromioclavicular (AC) joint complex.

   c. Articulates with distal clavicle.

6. Coracoid process:

   a. Bony prominence anteriorly over scapula, with base lateral and cranial to lateral scapular border.

   b. Attachment of short head of biceps brachii and coracobrachialis muscle.

   c. Attachment of coracoacromial and coracoclavicular (CC) ligament complex.

7. Spine:

   a. Begins over medial border and terminates as acromial arch and acromion.

   b. Suprascapular artery and nerve enters into infraspinatus fossa, as spine becomes acromial arch.

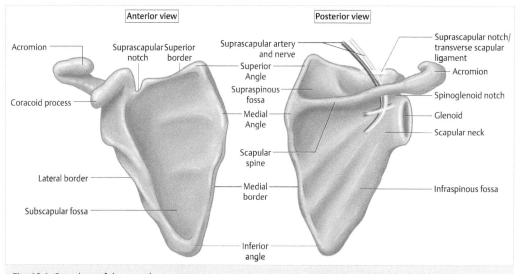

Fig. 19.1 Osteology of the scapula.

8. Lateral border:
   a. Superficial border posterior deltoid muscle.
   b. Glenoid and glenohumeral joint centrally and superiorly, and quadrangular and triangular space laterally and inferiorly.
      i. Quadrangular space defined superiorly by teres minor, medially by long head of triceps, laterally by humerus and lateral head of triceps, and inferiorly teres major.
      ii. Contents of quadrangular space include axillary nerve and posterior humeral circumflex artery.
      iii. Triangular space bordered superiorly by teres minor, inferiorly by teres major, and laterally by long head of triceps.
      iv. Content of triangular space circumflex scapular artery.
9. Medial border:
   a. Superficial border trapezius muscle.
   b. Deep border levator scapulae superiorly, and rhomboids centrally and inferiorly.

C. Imaging
1. Chest radiograph.
2. Anteropoterior (AP)/lateral/axillary radiographs shoulder.
3. Clavicle radiographs when indicated.
4. CT scapula/shoulder girdles: Three-dimensional reconstruction.

D. Classification
1. Classifications are used mainly for research purposes and to guide surgical decision planning.
2. Ideberg classification with Goss modification describes glenoid fracture patterns with extension into scapular body.
3. AO/OTA classification distinguishes separately glenoid, body, and process fracture patterns.
4. Anatomic:
   a. Anatomic description can be used to describe coracoid, acromion, and spine of scapula fractures.
   b. Location description can be used to identify body fractures involving supra (superior body) or infraspinatus fossae (inferior body).
   c. Extra-articular fractures involve the body or neck, but do not involve the glenoid.
      i. Peripheral margins of scapula are thicker than fossae, which are thin and associated with comminution.
      ii. Important to identify extent of medial involvement, which is often best interpreted or assessed on three-dimensional computed tomography (CT) reconstruction.
   d. Intra-articular (glenoid) fractures:
      i. Posterior glenoid fractures can be associated with posterior fracture-dislocation patterns.
      ii. Anterior glenoid fractures can be associated with anterior fracture-dislocation patterns.
   e. Superior shoulder suspensory complex injuries (SSSC):
      i. Osseoligamentous ring contributing to stability about the shoulder.
      ii. Bone contribution: clavicle, coracoid, acromion, and glenoid.
      iii. Soft tissue contribution: CC, coracoacromial, and AC ligaments.
      iv. Disruption of two of these structures is referred to as "double disruption".
   f. Scapulothoracic dissociation:
      i. Limited published data owing to injury rarity.
      ii. Results from high-energy traction injury to upper extremity.
      iii. Can present as flail, anesthetic, and pulseless upper extremity.
      iv. Internal degloving injury with closed forequarter amputation.

     v. Bone injury:
- Laterally displaced scapula.
- Sternoclavicular (SC) subluxation/dislocation.
- AC dislocation.
- Displaced, distracted clavicle fracture.

    vi. Vascular injury:
- Subclavian/axillary artery injury.
- Dense collateral vascular network rarely results in ischemia.
- May require urgent/emergent ligation in cases of severe hemorrhage and hemodynamic instability.
- Revascularization with saphenous vein interposition grafting when indicated.

   vii. Neurologic injury:
- Tend to be proximal root and cord injuries.
- Result in complete or partial brachial plexopathies.
- Poor outcome with complete plexus injury despite attempts at nerve grafting.
- Outcome following TSD depends on extent of neurologic injury.
- Recommendation for acute above elbow amputation in the setting of complete plexus injury.

II. Treatment

A. Initial management
1. Advanced trauma life support (ATLS) protocols.
2. Sling/immobilizer.
3. Address soft tissue injuries and debride grossly contaminated dermal abrasions.
4. Non-weightbearing through affected extremity.
5. Identification and provisional treatment of associated injuries.

B. Definitive management
1. Nonoperative management:
   a. Large majority of extra-articular scapular fractures meet nonoperative criteria.
   b. No evidence based guidelines exist for operative criteria.
   c. Sling or immobilizer for pain control.
   d. Restoration of early range of motion (ROM) with pendulum exercises and active assist/passive ROM.
   e. As pain subsides, progressive ROM protocol to increase glenohumeral and scapulothoracic motion.
   f. Strengthening and release to full to activities between 3 to 6 months in most cases.

2. Operative management:
   a. Indications for operative fixation are relative and depend on fracture pattern.
   b. Extra-articular fractures:
      i. More than 40 to 45 degrees angular deformity.
      ii. Shortening > 2.5 cm.
      iii. Medial displacement of lateral scapular border > 2.5 cm.
      iv. Glenopolar angle < 20 degrees.
   c. Intra-articular fractures (▶ Fig. 19.2a–c):
      i. Historically, > 5 mm articular displacement; however, several recent studies narrow considerations to 2 to 4 mm step off.
      ii. Involving 25% of glenoid with resulting subluxation of humeral head.
      iii. Glenoid fracture with persistent or episodic subluxation/dislocation of glenohumeral joint.

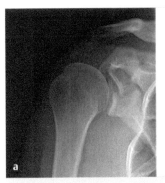 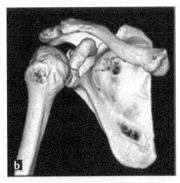 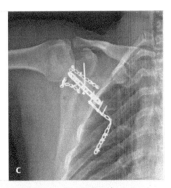

Fig. 19.2 (a) Anteropoterior (AP) shoulder demonstrating displaced glenoid fracture. (b) Three-dimensional reconstruction detailing scapula fracture with glenoid, coracoid component, and superior body fracture extension exiting medial border. (c) AP scapula after operative fixation.

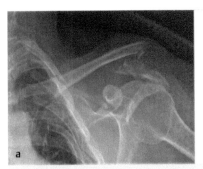 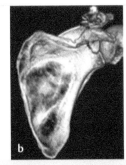 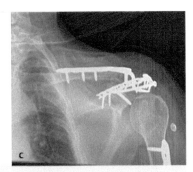

Fig. 19.3 (a) Left shoulder superior shoulder suspensory complex injuries (SSSC) injury with displaced distal clavicle, coracoid, acromion, spine of scapula and associated humerus fracture. (b) Three dimensional reconstruction of unstable SSSC injury. (c) Postoperative anteropoterior shoulder with stable reconstruction of SSSC.

  d. Double disruptions of the SSSC "floating shoulder" (▶Fig. 19.3a–c):

    i. Each disruption indicated when unstable and/or greater than 1 cm displacement.

  e. Coracoid, acromion, and spine fractures:

    i. Consideration for fixation when associated with ipsilateral scapula fracture or SSSC disruption.

    ii. Relative indication with displacement > 1 cm.

    iii. Signs/symptoms indicative of painful nonunion.

C. Surgical approaches

 1. Anterior:

  a. Deltopectoral approach to address isolated coracoid fractures (Chapter 21, Proximal Humerus Fractures, ▶Fig. 21.3 a–c).

  b. Access to anterior glenoid fractures.

  c. Can be used when associated with combined SSSC injuries to address ipsilateral clavicle fixation/AC joint injuries/ipsilateral upper extremity fracture fixation.

 2. Posterior:

  a. Straight posterior approach (▶Fig. 19.4 a, b):

    i. Provides access to posterior glenoid and/or glenoid neck fractures.

    ii. Straight posterior skin incision in line with the glenohumeral joint.

    iii. Dissect between the posterior one-third and middle one-third of the deltoid in line with its fibers. Alternatively, detach the posterior one-third of the deltoid off the scapular spine.

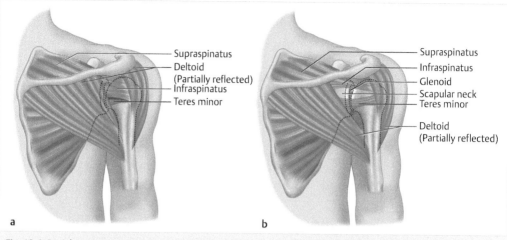

Fig. 19.4 Straight posterior approach to the glenoid and scapular neck: **(a)** superficial dissection and **(b)** deep dissection.

    iv. The deep interval is between the infraspinatus (suprascapular nerve) cranially and the teres minor (axillary nerve) caudally.

    v. Perform a posterior arthrotomy if indicated.

  b. Judet approach/modified Judet approach:

    i. More traditional extensile approach.

    ii. Allows for access to acromion, spine, peripheral medial and lateral borders, scapular neck, and glenoid.

    iii. Visualization of glenoid and glenoid neck may be limited by vascular pedicle soft tissue tension.

    iv. Horizontal limb beginning 1 cm caudal to acromion paralleling spine and extending medially to superomedial angle (SMA) of scapula.

    v. Vertical limb just lateral to medial border of scapula, extending inferiorly while paralleling medial border of scapula.

    vi. Full thickness elevation to expose fascia over posterior muscular shoulder girdle.

    vii. Posterior deltoid retracted/released from infraspinatus superolaterally and spine of scapula.

    viii. Infraspinatus and posterior deltoid elevated from medial to lateral off infraspinatus fossa, and spine of scapula on neurovascular pedicle or interval between infraspinatus/teres minor (modified Judet approach).

  c. Minimally invasive approaches:

    i. Requires experience and preoperative planning combined with knowledge of fracture personality.

    ii. Strategic incisions expose fracture personality, providing windows for fracture exposure along with corridors for secure fracture fixation.

  d. Combined approaches:

    i. Anterior and posterior approaches for double disruptions of the SSSC.

    ii. Scapula body fractures with associated separate acromion or coracoid fractures.

D. Fixation techniques

  1. Fixation strategy determined by fracture personality, and principles of fixation and goals of surgical reconstruction.

  2. Scapula has osseous corridors to achieve reduction and apply fixation.

  3. Lateral border, medial border, spine of scapula, and caudal base of glenoid neck not only provide best points for bone fixation but also allow for assessment of reduction.

4. Anatomic reduction indicated for intra-articular glenoid fracture.

5. Reconstruction of medial border/lateral border may be indicated without attempt to reconstruct fossa body comminution, depending on fracture personality.

6. Fixation typically consists of minifragment (2.0–2.7 mm) and/or small fragment (2.7–3.5 mm) plates/screws. Provide more screw holes per plate length available for fixation opportunities.

7. Precontoured plates also available for certain fracture patterns and surgeon preference.

8. Locking plate may provide improved fixation for thin bone of scapula.

E. Complications

1. Nonoperative management:

   a. Progressive deformity—unstable patterns associated with multiple rib fractures and double/triple disruptions of SSSC.

   b. Shoulder dyskinesia.

   c. Pain.

   d. Symptomatic nonunion/malunion.

2. Operative management:

   a. Infection—rate of 4% following open reduction and internal fixation (ORIF) in large systematic review of the literature.

   b. Nerve palsy:

      i. Two percent in systematic review.

      ii. Suprascapular nerve palsy due to superior dissection or excessive cranial traction on the infraspinatus with Judet approach/modified Judet approach.

      iii. Axillary nerve palsy rare complication from superolateral retraction over posterior deltoid/teres minor or heterotopic ossification.

      iv. Differentiating etiology of nerve injury from original injury or surgical complication can present difficulties secondary to limited preoperative examination.

   c. Hematoma/seroma—2% in systematic review.

   d. Symptomatic hardware—most common complication, requiring removal in 7% of systematic review.

   e. Wound dehiscence.

   f. Muscle atrophy.

F. Rehabilitation

1. Nonoperative management:

   a. Sling immobilization from 2 to 4 weeks.

   b. Initial active assist and passive progressive ROM.

   c. Full active ROM at 2 to 4 weeks postinjury.

   d. Strengthening and scapular stabilization training begins between 6 to 10 weeks postinjury.

2. Operative management:

   a. Sling immobilization.

   b. Postoperative active and passive ROM immediately following fixation.

   c. Postoperative strengthening from 5 to 6 weeks.

   d. Postoperative resistance training and sport specific training from 8 to 9 weeks.

G. Outcomes

1. Good to excellent outcomes are expected for most nonoperatively and operatively treated scapula fractures.

2. Analysis of operative versus nonoperative treatment of scapular body and neck fractures.

   a. No difference in fracture union rate, ability to return to work, and pain relief between groups.

   b. Polytrauma is a major determinant of function and result.

   c. No recommendation for operative management of minimally displaced scapula fractures.

3. Functional outcome following scapulothoracic dissociation:

   a. Extent of neurologic injury most predictive of outcome.

      i.   All complete plexus avulsions resulted in flail upper extremity or required amputation.
      ii. Improvement variable with partial plexus injury.
      iii. Little functional improvement detected with operative repair.

   b. Mortality rate > 10% related to overall trauma.

   c. Up to 25% result in a transhumeral amputation.

III. Special Considerations for Pediatric Patients

A. The vast majority of pediatric scapula fractures are treated nonoperatively.

B. Similar indications for operative management to adult patients.

Suggested Readings

Ada JR, Miller ME. Scapular fractures. Analysis of 113 cases. Clin Orthop Relat Res 1991;(269): 174–180

Goss TP. Double disruptions of the superior shoulder suspensory complex. J Orthop Trauma 1993;7(2):99–106

G. Zlowodski M. Bhandari M, Zelle B, Kregor P, Cole P. Treatment of scapular fractures: systematic review of 520 fractures in 22 case series. J Orthop Trauma 2006;20:230–233

Jones CB, Sietsema DL. Analysis of operative versus nonoperative treatment of displaced scapular fractures. Clin Orthop Relat Res 2011;469(12):3379–3389

Judet R. Surgical treatment of scapular fractures. Acta Orthop Belg 1964;30:673–678

Lantry JM, Roberts CS, Giannoudis PV. Operative treatment of scapular fractures: a systematic review. Injury 2008;39(3):271–283

Lantry JM, Roberts CS, Giannoudis PV. Operative treatment of scapular fractures: a systematic review. Injury 2008;39(3):271–283

Zelle B, Pape HC, Gerich T, et al. Functional outcome following scapulothoracic dissociation. J Bone Joint Surg Am 2004;86(A):2–8

20 Shoulder Dislocation

Scott R. Bassuener

Introduction

The glenohumeral joint of the shoulder has minimal anatomic constraint and a high degree of mobility. It is the most commonly dislocated large joint, with injury patterns including both high- and low-energy mechanisms (▶ **Video 20.1**).

I. Preoperative

A. History

    1. Either high-energy or low-energy trauma mechanisms.

    2. Pain and inability to actively move the shoulder joint.

B. Physical examination

    1. Arm position:

        a. Anterior dislocation—painful, mildly abducted, and externally rotated arm with inability to reach the hand across to the opposite shoulder.

        b. Posterior dislocation—adducted and internally rotated arm with inability to actively externally rotate.

        c. Inferior dislocation (Luxatio Erecta)—shoulder fixated in a flexed or abducted position following a forced traumatic hyperabduction episode.

    2. Neurovascular examination—axillary nerve sensation on lateral aspect of the upper arm typically decreased, and there was difficulty in assessing motor function before or after reduction.

C. Anatomy

    1. Convex humeral head articulates with the concave glenoid fossa of the scapula–Static soft tissue constraints (see Chapter 18, Clavicle Fractures, ▶ **Fig. 18.1**).

        a. Superior glenohumeral ligament—resists anterior translation/dislocation of the humeral head, while the shoulder is in a neutral position.

        b. Middle glenohumeral ligament—primary restraint to anterior dislocation when the shoulder is externally rotated with abduction to approximately 45 degrees.

        c. Anterior–inferior glenohumeral ligament—anterior restraint with shoulder abduction up to 90 degrees.

        d. Posterior–inferior glenohumeral ligament—primary static restraint to posterior dislocation.

        e. Fibrocartilaginous glenoid labrum—increases the contact area for the glenohumeral articular surface. Attachment surface for the capsule and glenohumeral ligaments.

        f. Musculotendinous rotator cuff—applies stabilizing counter forces on the humerus to maintain glenohumeral alignment during active shoulder motion.

D. Imaging

    1. Orthogonal radiographs:

        a. Grashey or Neer anteroposterior (AP) image (▶ **Fig. 20.1a**):

            i. Taken in the coronal plane of the scapula.

            ii. No overlap between the reduced humeral head and the glenoid.

        b. Scapular Y lateral image:

            i. Shows anterior or posterior displacement of the humeral head.

            ii. Can be difficult to assess due to overlapping structures.

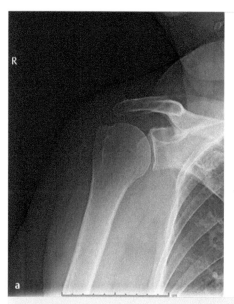 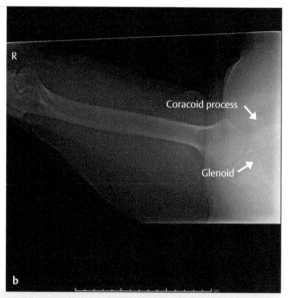

Fig. 20.1 (a, b) Grashey anteroposterior and axillary lateral radiographs of a well-reduced glenohumeral joint.

    c. Axillary lateral (▶ **Fig. 20.1b**) or Velpeau image:

        i. Eliminates overlapping structures.

       ii. Improves lateral visualization of the glenohumeral articulation.

      iii. In Velpeau image, there is easier patient positioning for painful shoulder.

  2. Advanced imaging—not routinely necessary for acute dislocation management:

    a. Computed tomography (CT) scan—assesses bone integrity in fracture dislocations.

    b. Magnetic resonance imaging (MRI)—evaluation of soft tissue damage for reconstruction/ stabilization.

        i. Increasing acute utilization following traumatic dislocations due to high incidence of associated ligamentous or labral injuries.

E. Classification

  1. Anatomic—direction of humeral dislocation:

    a. Anterior, posterior, and inferior.

    b. 95% of dislocations are anterior.

  2. Descriptive classification of anterior glenohumeral dislocations:

    a. "**TUBS**" injuries:

        i. Traumatic mechanism.

       ii. Unidirectional instability episodes.

      iii. Bankart lesion—resultant disruption of the glenoid labrum.

      iv. Surgical management—frequently necessary for addressing significant associated injuries with this type of dislocation.

    b. "**AMBRI**" injury pattern:

        i. Atraumatic injury.

       ii. Multidirectional shoulder instability.

      iii. Bilateral shoulder instability issues are commonly identified.

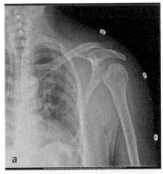 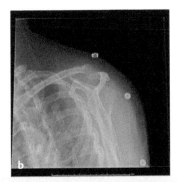 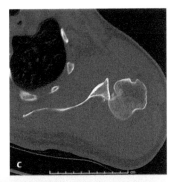

Fig. 20.2 Subtle radiographic appearance of a posterior shoulder dislocation on (a) anteroposterior and (b) scapular Y lateral image. (c) Posterior shoulder dislocation with anterior Hill-Sachs impaction injury engaging the posterior glenoid rim.

      iv. Rehabilitation—expected to respond favorably to dynamic stabilization physical therapy protocols.

      v. Inferior capsular shift—shoulder stabilization procedure for multidirectional instability after exhausting all therapy options.

3. Posterior shoulder dislocations:

    a. Occur with shoulder adducted and internally rotated—associated with seizure and electrocution. Inability to externally rotate the shoulder on physical examination.

    b. Less than 5% of all glenohumeral dislocations.

    c. Subtle radiographic appearance (▶ **Fig. 20.2 a, b**)—up to 50% are missed on initial presentation.

4. Inferior glenohumeral dislocation (Luxatio Erecta):

    a. Shoulder fixed in significant flexion or abduction.

    b. Highest rates of associated fractures and neurologic injuries.

F. Coexisting Injuries—best differentiated by MRI with intra-articular contrast.

1. Bankart lesion:

    a. Detachment of the anterior–inferior glenohumeral ligament and labrum.

    b. Possible avulsion fracture of the glenoid rim.

    c. Present in approximately 90% of traumatic anterior shoulder dislocations.

2. Posterior Bankart lesion:

    a. Detachment of the posterior capsulolabral complex and the posterior band of the inferior glenohumeral ligament.

    b. Common in posterior shoulder dislocations.

3. Humeral avulsion of the glenohumeral ligament (HAGL) lesion—higher rates of recurrent instability than a glenoid Bankart injury.

4. Anterior labral periosteal sleeve avulsion (ALPSA) injury:

    a. Medial disruption of the static anterior stabilizing structures.

    b. Tissues heal aberrantly along the anterior glenoid neck.

5. Hill-Sachs defect:

    a. Impaction fracture of the humeral head from contact with the glenoid rim.

    b. Posterior impaction is present in approximately 80% of anterior dislocations. Anterior humeral head defect—posterior shoulder dislocations (▶ **Fig. 20.2c**).

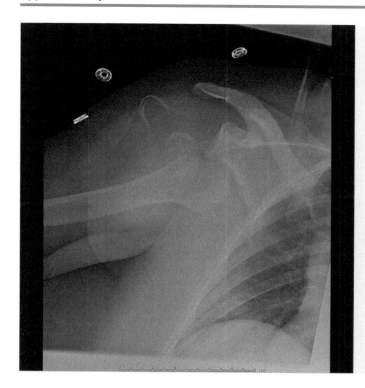

Fig. 20.3 Anterior–inferior shoulder dislocation with fracture of the greater tuberosity and intact humeral neck.

6. Rotator cuff tear:
   a. Most commonly supraspinatus tears or subscapularis avulsion injuries.
   b. Incidence increases with patient age at the time of injury:
      i. First three decades of life rarely tear the rotator cuff.
      ii. Age > 40 years—approximately 30% will have a rotator cuff tear.
      iii. Age > 60 years—approximately 80% will have a rotator cuff tear.
7. Fractures of the proximal humerus:
   a. Occur in up to 25% of acute shoulder dislocations.
   a. Isolated greater tuberosity fracture (▶ **Fig. 20.3**)—most common.
   b. Lesser tuberosity fracture—associated with posterior dislocations.
   c. Humeral neck fracture—typically require open surgical techniques for joint reduction.

II. Treatment

A. Initial Management
   1. Closed reduction of anterior glenohumeral dislocation
      a. General anesthesia with muscle relaxation:
         i. Physically, the easiest to achieve reduction; minimal musculoskeletal risk.
         ii. Elevated cost, time consumption, and physiologic risk to the patient.
         iii. Reserved for specific high-risk cases: Humeral neck fracture dislocations, engaged Hills-Sachs lesions, and subacute or chronic neglected dislocations.
      b. Procedural sedation or intra-articular anesthetic—successful reduction rates reported range from 70 to 96%.
      c. Milch glenohumeral reduction technique:
         i. Patients with palpable humeral head and minimal muscle spasm.
         ii. Supine patient with arm near their side.

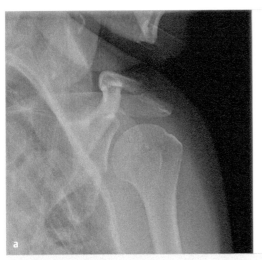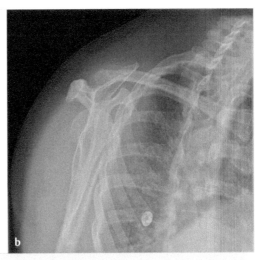

Fig. 20.4 (a, b) Grashey anteroposterior and scapular lateral orthogonal postreduction images confirming reduction after the posterior shoulder dislocation from ▶Fig. 20.2a–c.

      iii. Passively externally rotate, abduct, and elevate the arm overhead.

      iv. Provider pushes the humeral head with his or her thumb; anterior lateral pressure to elevate it over the rim of the glenoid.

  d. Spaso technique:

      i. Patient body and arm manipulation similar to Milch technique.

      ii. Addition of manual traction applied to the arm as it advances overhead.

  e. Traction techniques:

      i. Supine patient, mildly abducted arm, providers pull manual longitudinal traction with countertraction through a folded sheet wrapped around the patient's lateral chest wall. Requires multiple providers, commonly used in clinical settings.

      ii. Eskimo technique with patient in lateral lying position.

      iii. Stimson technique of hanging weight from the arm of a prone patient.

  f. Scapular manipulation technique—patient upright, manual anterior–inferior longitudinal traction applied to the affected arm, medial manipulation of the inferior pole of the scapula.

  g. Historic techniques—abandoned due to elevated risk of iatrogenic injury:

      i. Kocher rotational leverage, Hippocratic manual traction.

      ii. Fractures, musculotendinous tears, and neurovascular injuries.

2. Closed reduction of posterior dislocation

  a. Traction technique—with the patient in the supine position, pull manual traction on the arm, apply a posterior to anterior directed force on the humeral head, and gently rotate the arm.

3. Orthogonal postreduction radiographs (▶Fig. 20.4 a, b)

  a. Confirm articular reduction.

  b. Evaluate missed or iatrogenic fractures.

4. Sling immobilization

  a. Standard versus abduction slings—improved labrum positioning in abduction and external rotation slings.

  b. Clinical benefit not conclusive.

5. Nonsurgical management
    a. Repeat clinical evaluation within 1 to 2 weeks of reduction.
    b. Physical therapy protocols for strengthening the muscular dynamic stabilizers.
    c. Avoidance of provocative instability positions—Ranges from 3 to 6 weeks.
    d. Recurrent instability rates increase with shorter immobilization intervals.
B. Definitive Management
    1. Absolute surgical indications
        a. Irreducible joint by closed methods.
        b. Vascular disruption.
        c. Open injury with traumatic arthrotomy.
    2. Relative surgical indications
        a. Associated displaced fractures.
        b. Recurrent instability episodes including recurrent dislocation.
        c. Coexisting injuries with high risk of recurrent instability among young active patients.
    3. Bankart lesion repair and capsulorrhaphy (arthroscopic or open technique)
        a. Labrum and ligamentous reattachment to the glenoid.
        b. Minimum of three suture anchors recommended to secure the repair.
    4. Inferior capsular shift or capsular imbrication—addresses multidirectional laxity of the primary static stabilizers.
    5. Bony Bankart lesion/glenoid deficiency reconstruction
        a. Typically open procedures, arthroscopic options for smaller bony avulsions.
        b. > 20% glenoid deficit: Critical lesion indicated for bone-restoring procedures:
            i. Latarjet/Bristow procedures: Partial coracoid transfer to the glenoid.
            ii. Bone grafting of the glenoid using allograft or tricortical iliac autograft: Reserved for salvage after failed coracoid transfer.
    6. Hill-Sachs humeral lesion management
        a. Lesion involving approximately 25% of the humeral head can contribute to instability.
        b. Remplissage—suturing infraspinatus tendon and posterior capsule into the lesion.
        c. Bone grafting, or rotational osteotomies, to realign or fill humeral head defect.
    7. Reconstruction of sequela of shoulder dislocation
        a. Rotator cuff repair, total shoulder arthroplasty, and reverse shoulder arthroplasty.
        b. Rarely used in acute instability settings.
C. Complications
    1. Recurrent instability
        a. 80 to 90% lifetime recurrence risk with first anterior dislocation in the teens—20s.
        b. 40% recurrence risk for dislocations in patients aged between 25 to 40 years.
        c. 15% risk in patients with their first dislocation after age 40 years.
    2. Neurologic deficits
        a. Complete neuroevaluation before and after any shoulder reduction attempt.
        b. Neurologic dysfunction identifiable by electromyography (EMG) in approximately 45% of shoulder dislocations.
        c. Neuropraxia to the axillary nerve—most common clinical finding.
        d. Lateral shoulder numbness and shoulder abduction weakness.

D. Outcomes
1. Near normal shoulder functional outcomes can be achieved—minimal expected loss of shoulder external rotation.
2. Prevention of recurrent instability episodes is critical to positive outcomes.:
   a. Recurrent instability—reconstructive surgical procedures.
   b. Lower functional outcome scores anticipated if surgical stabilization is required.
3. Conflicting primary goals of treatment
   a. Early functional return to activities versus prevention of long-term instability.
      i. Trend toward more frequent acute surgical management of dislocations.
      ii. Accelerated rehabilitation protocols and decreased immobilization times.
   b. Evidence to support a universal treatment protocol remains insufficient: Patient's goals and priorities must be considered.

Summary

Diagnosis of shoulder dislocations is made on standard radiographs: AP, Grayshey, and Scapular Y lateral imaging. Diligence is required during radiographic analysis to avoid the common pitfall of a missed posterior shoulder dislocation. The vast majority of shoulder dislocations are able to be close reduced in the Emergency room with conscious sedation/relaxation. Axillary or Velpeau radiograph views are helpful in confirming glenohumeral reduction. Indications for surgical management include: irreducible dislocation, associated vascular injury and open fracture. Surgery should also be considered in patients with associated displaced proximal humerus or glenoid fractures and those with episodes of recurrent instability.

Suggested Readings

Dala-Ali B, Penna M, McConnell J, Vanhegan I, Cobiella C. Management of acute anterior shoulder dislocation. Br J Sports Med 2014;48(16):1209–1215

Federer AE, Taylor DC, Mather RC. Using evidence-based algorithms to improve clinical decision making: the case of a first-time anterior shoulder dislocation. Br J Sports Med 2014;48(16):1209–1215

Handoll HH, Almaiyah MA, Rangan A. Surgical versus non-surgical treatment for acute anterior shoulder dislocation. Cochrane Database Syst Rev 2004(1):CD004325

Robinson CM, Howes J, Murdoch H, Will E, Graham C. Functional outcome and risk of recurrent instability after primary traumatic anterior shoulder dislocation in young patients. J Bone Joint Surg Am 2006;88(11):2326–2336

Thomas SC, Matsen FA III. An approach to the repair of avulsion of the glenohumeral ligaments in the management of traumatic anterior glenohumeral instability. J Bone Joint Surg Am 1989;71(4):506–513

21 Proximal Humerus Fractures

Laurence B. Kempton

Introduction

Fractures of the proximal humerus are common injuries with outcomes primarily dependent on the severity of the initial injury. Outcomes range from full recovery to significant loss of shoulder function. Scientific literature includes many retrospective series and few prospective studies (many with small numbers of patients), and shows similar clinical outcomes between compared treatments, with more complications arising from surgical treatment. Therefore, surgeons are forced to make treatment recommendations based on limited evidence, anecdote, and opinion.

I. Preoperative

A. History and physical examination

1. Age, activity level, and comorbidities—help to define patient goals for recovery and influence treatment plan.

2. Mechanism of injury—low energy versus high energy and associated injuries.

3. Incidence increased in elderly females secondary to osteoporosis and falls.

4. Open proximal humerus fracture uncommon.

   a. Soft tissue envelope requires substantial displacement with high-fracture energy.

   b. Usually result from penetrating trauma.

5. Neurovascular examination:

   a. Axillary artery injury rare.

   b. Axillary nerve:

      i. Difficult to assess motor function (teres major and deltoid) due to pain.
      ii. Can test sensory function in skin over lateral shoulder.

6. Associated injuries:

   a. Other fragility fractures (e.g., distal radius and femoral neck).

   b. Glenohumeral dislocation with or without glenoid fracture ("Bony Bankart" lesion).

B. Anatomy (▶ Fig. 21.1 a–d)

1. Bone:

   a. Humeral head:

      i. Majority of blood supply from branches of the anterior and posterior humeral circumflex arteries.
      ii. Retroverted 25 to 35 degrees relative to epicondylar axis.

   b. Greater tuberosity—attachment for supraspinatus, infraspinatus, and teres minor tendons, which displace tuberosity proximally and posteriorly.

   c. Lesser tuberosity—attachment for subscapularis tendon, which displaces tuberosity medially.

   d. Humeral shaft—extension of proximal humerus fracture distally to the humeral shaft is common with high-energy fractures.

   e. Anatomic neck:

      i. Plane defined by the distal/lateral edge of the proximal humeral articular surface which separates head from tuberosities.
      ii. Fracture here increases the risk of humeral head avascular necrosis.

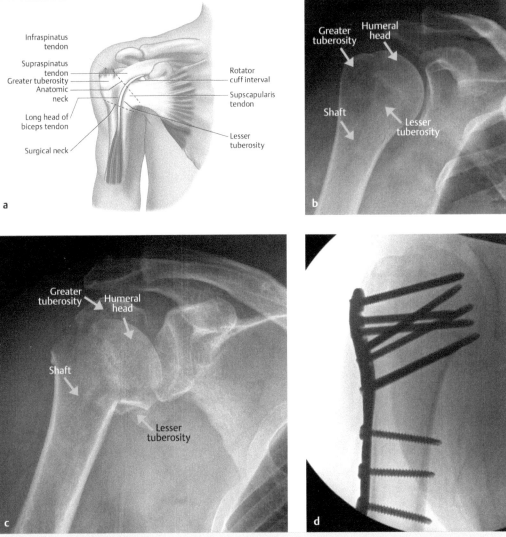

Fig. 21.1 Proximal humerus anatomy. A drawing (**a**) depicting normal anatomic relationships and sources of deforming force in the proximal humerus, followed by a Grashey view of a normal shoulder for comparison (**b**) and a typical 4-part proximal humerus fracture (**c**). (**d**) Figure depicting the fracture reconstructed with a locking plate. Note the plate positioning with the screws in the inferior humeral head.

     f. Surgical neck—plane separating the humeral head and tuberosities from the shaft.

     g. Bicipital grove:

         i. Separates tuberosities—lesser tuberosity medial, and greater tuberosity lateral.

         ii. Helps to judge axial plane rotation of the shaft—the long head of the biceps tendon passes deep to the pectoralis major tendon, and the bicipital grove lies proximal to this landmark.

2. Tendons:

     a. Rotator cuff tendons:

         i. Not usually injured acutely with proximal humerus fractures but should be evaluated intraoperatively.

         ii. Sutures through tendons are useful for tuberosity manipulation and fixation during surgery as the bone quality of the tuberosities is usually poor.

b. Long head of biceps tendon:

    i. Helpful in judging rotational reduction as described above.

    ii. Can dislocate from the bicipital grove through a greater tuberosity fracture and become entrapped behind the humeral head.

    iii. Potentially, a pain generator in the long-term; therefore, tenodesis or tenotomy may be considered depending on intraoperative findings.

c. Shoulder capsule—usually torn when humeral head is dislocated from glenoid and could act as a barrier to glenohumeral reduction.

d. Pectoralis major and deltoid muscles.

    i. Can contribute to medial displacement and abduction, respectively.

    ii. In high-energy injuries, pectoralis major tendon may be avulsed from the humerus.

C. Imaging

  1. Radiographs:

    a. Anteroposterior (AP), scapular-y, and axillary views necessary for fracture evaluation and glenohumeral articulation.

    b. Velpeau view may substitute for axillary view if patient is unable to tolerate abduction:

      i. Patient leans backward (hip/back extension) over a horizontal X-ray cassette.

      ii. X-ray source is positioned above the shoulder and aimed directly downward.

    c. Grashey view:

      i. "True AP" of the scapula with X-ray beams tangential to the glenoid surface.

      ii. Patient is rotated 40 degree in axial plane with affected side away from X-ray source.

      iii. Often better for evaluation of fracture morphology than AP due to less superimposition of greater tuberosity, humeral head, and glenoid.

      iv. No superimposition of humeral head and glenoid can confirm that humeral head is not dislocated; however, anterior or posterior subluxation cannot be ruled out.

  2. Computed tomography (CT):

    a. Not always necessary—useful for more complex fractures or when radiographs do not provide sufficient evaluation.

    b. May affect preoperative planning compared to radiographs alone.

    c. Useful to evaluate glenohumeral articulation when patients cannot tolerate positioning for axillary or Velpeau views.

    d. Can define fragment size and location better than radiographs in complex fractures.

    e. Smaller humeral head fragment size and/or lower bone density may influence decision in favor of arthroplasty instead of ORIF in surgically treated patients.

  3. Findings:

    a. Radiographic considerations for preferred treatment and preoperative planning include fragment location, size, displacement, glenohumeral articulation, and bone quality.

    b. Pseudosubluxation:

      i. Humeral head inferiorly translated relative to glenoid, but not superimposed on the glenoid on a proper Grashey view.

      ii. Thought to occur secondary to hemarthrosis, with expanded joint space and humeral head shifting away from glenoid.

      iii. Differs from dislocation in that head fragment does not displace through the capsule or get impacted on the edge of the glenoid.

D. Classification

  1. Neer classification (▶**Fig. 21.2**):

    a. Four parts—humeral head, greater tuberosity, lesser tuberosity, and humeral shaft.

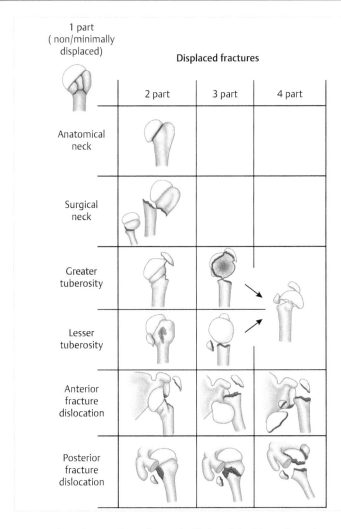

b. The number of parts is distinguished by at least 1 cm of displacement of one part relative to another part or > 45 degrees of angulation.

2. Orthopaedic trauma association (OTA) classification—example is 11-C3.3:

   a. Location (bone and segment)—first digit "1" for humerus; second digit "1" for proximal.

   b. Type:

      i.   A—extra-articular, unifocal (e.g., 2-part fracture).
      ii. B—extra-articular bifocal (e.g., 3-part fracture).
      iii. C—articular fracture or 4-part fracture.

   c. Groups and subgroups—1 to 3 for each digit (last two digits).

      i. Description considers fracture location and morphology, direction of displacement (impaction vs. dissociation), and comminution.
      ii. Varies depending on type.

II. Treatment

A. Initial management

   1. Shoulder immobilizer or sling and swath for comfort.

   2. Closed reduction of fracture fragments generally not helpful.

B. Definitive management

1. Nonsurgical treatment:

    a. Fractures with an acceptable degree of displacement (controversial and depends on patient age and activity level).

    b. Limit weight bearing and no overhead activity for 6 weeks (no studies support this common practice).

    c. Start Codman's (pendulum) exercises within a few days and advance to passive range of motion (ROM) within the first few weeks.

    d. Greater tuberosity fractures associated with a shoulder dislocation often reduce to an acceptable position when the glenohumeral joint is reduced.

2. Surgical treatment:

    a. Indications controversial and not necessarily literature supported as many studies have shown high-complication rates and similar functional outcomes with nonsurgical treatment, especially among elderly, low-demand patients.

        i. "Accepted" historical indications including fracture displacement > 1cm or greater tuberosity displacement of 5 mm are not literature supported.

        ii. Open reduction internal fixation (ORIF):

            • Open fracture.
            • Neurological or vascular injury.
            • Associated glenohumeral dislocation not reducible closed.
            • Head split (usually treated with arthroplasty for older patients).
            • Displacement to a degree that the surgeon believes reduction would improve final outcomes.

        iii. Hemiarthroplasty—surgeon believes surgical treatment is warranted for any of the above indications but that reduction or fixation will not be adequate; most often head-splitting fractures and 4-part fracture dislocations.

        iv. Reverse arthroplasty—older patient (varies by surgeon and patient medical comorbidities, but usually > 60–70 years of age) in whom surgeon believes that surgical treatment is warranted, that reduction or fixation will not be adequate, AND that patient's final function will be more predictable and/or better than with hemiarthroplasty

    b. Goals: ORIF (▶ Fig. 21.1 c, d):

        i. Restore anatomic relationship of fracture fragments:

            • Avoid head-shaft varus—can increase risk for subacromial impingement and mechanical failure of fixation.
            • Tuberosity-head relationship—restores rotator cuff length for optimal function and reduces risk of subacromial impingement.

        ii. Stable fixation:

            • Calcar fixation: screws along the inferior humeral head and head/shaft junction provide optimal resistance to failure.
            • Fixation of tuberosities with sutures (or a soft tissue washer on intramedullary nail interlock) in the rotator cuff tendons: tuberosity bone quality is generally poor, and screw fixation alone may not prevent failure.
            • Allograft strut to support humeral head is an option with osteoporotic bone to decrease risk of screw cutout.

    c. Goals: Hemiarthroplasty:

        i. Restoration of humeral head height—in the absence of other keys to reduction, the top of the humeral head should be approximately 5.6 cm above the proximal pectoralis major tendon.

    ii.   Fixation and bone grafting of tuberosities:

- Most important—cerclage suture around both tuberosities and prosthesis to compress tuberosities in place.
- Also, fix tuberosities to shaft, to each other, and to prosthesis.

  d. Goals: Reverse arthroplasty:

    i.   Tension soft tissues to maintain shoulder stability.

    ii. Reduce and fix tuberosities similar to hemiarthroplasty.

- Tuberosity fixation is unnecessary for stability.
- Tuberosity fixation and successful healing can improve functional outcomes, likely due to rotator cuff function, especially external rotation.

C. Surgical approaches

  1. Deltopectoral (▶ **Fig. 21.3 a–c**):

    a. Useful for ORIF, hemiarthroplasty, and reverse arthroplasty.

    b. Provides better access to lesser tuberosity than deltoid split.

    c. Description of the approach:

      i.   Anterior incision from the coracoid process extending distally.

      ii. Identify the cephalic vein which marks the interval between the deltoid (retract laterally) and the pectoralis major (retract medially). The cephalic vein can be mobilized medially or laterally.

     iii. Incise the deltopectoral fascia and continue in the deltopectoral interval until the long head of the biceps is identified in the bicipital groove on the anterior proximal humerus between the lesser and greater tuberosities.

     iv. Deeper dissection may be required (e.g., develop subacromial space to mobilize greater tuberosity, or incise clavipectoral fascia lateral to conjoined tendon to get access to lesser tuberosity).

  2. Deltoid split:

    a. Useful for ORIF, especially when lesser tuberosity is not a separate fragment.

    b. Often preferred for isolated greater tuberosity fractures.

    c. Reverse arthroplasty possible with this approach, but tuberosity fixation is more difficult.

    d. Description of the approach:

      i.   Lateral 5 cm incision extending from the acromion distally.

      ii. Split deltoid in line with its fibers.

     iii. Must protect the axillary nerve which passes posterior to anterior, just deep to deltoid muscle, approximately 4 to 5 cm distal to lateral edge of acromion.

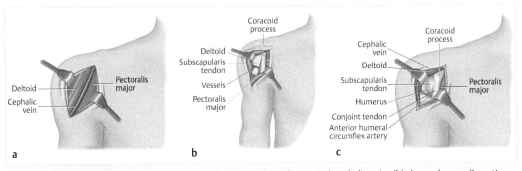

Fig. 21.3 Deltopectoral approach **(a)** depicts initial dissection with exposed cephalic vein, **(b)** shows deeper dissection as cephalic vein is retracted, and **(c)** deep exposure of the anterior shoulder.

D. Fixation techniques

1. Closed reduction percutaneous pinning (CRPP).

2. Plate and screw fixation:

   a. Precontoured locking plates usually used to "suspend" humeral head in the appropriate position relative to the humeral shaft.

   b. Modern studies of plate fixation for proximal humerus fractures use locking plates.

3. Intramedullary nail fixation.

4. Modern literature does not support specific indications for operative versus nonoperative treatment for proximal humerus fractures, nor does it support specific indications for various types of surgical fixation.

5. Surgical versus nonsurgical treatment—the highest quality studies have found no clinically significant difference in outcomes, especially among elderly, low-demand patients. It is not clear whether they show that proximal humerus fractures should be treated without surgery or that it is simply difficult to predict which subsets of patients will benefit from surgery.

6. Hemiarthroplasty versus nonsurgical treatment (randomized control trial of 50 patients with 4-part fractures)—similar clinical outcomes except more abduction strength in nonop group.

7. Reverse arthroplasty versus nonsurgical treatment—literature limited and does not favor either.

8. ORIF versus arthroplasty—not good literature to support either.

9. Hemiarthroplasty versus reverse arthroplasty—limited data supports better forward elevation and abduction with reverse arthroplasty, but hemiarthroplasty outcomes may be similar if tuberosities heal.

E. Complications

1. Intra-articular screw placement—the humeral articular surface is convex; therefore, screws that appear to be within the humeral head on fluoroscopy or radiographs may still perforate articular surface.

2. Loss of fixation—may lead to varus collapse of humeral head (inferomedial head displaces laterally) and screw perforation of humeral head articular surface.

3. Avascular necrosis of humeral head—likelihood increases with more severe fractures; often not symptomatic, but may lead to symptomatic glenohumeral arthritis.

4. Malunion is typical for closed treatment but typically asymptomatic (or at least well tolerated) in elderly, low-demand patients. Most common symptomatic malunion is observed with greater tuberosity displacement. Patient satisfaction is dependent on expectations.

5. Nonunion uncommon in proximal humerus fractures.

6. Stiffness can occur with surgical or nonsurgical treatment.

7. Resorption or loss of fixation of tuberosities with hemiarthroplasty significantly worsens outcomes.

8. Reverse shoulder arthroplasty—postoperative dislocation—usually from a position of shoulder adduction and extension (e.g., pushing up from a chair).

F. Rehabilitation

1. Weight bearing is limited for the first 6 weeks and then gradually progressed.

2. Start early ROM including Codman's exercises within 2 weeks.

3. Limit active internal rotation and passive external rotation after fixation of lesser tuberosity, especially with arthroplasty.

G. Outcomes

1. Most important factor is injury severity.

2. Loss of shoulder ROM (depending on severity) and strength are common with both surgical and nonsurgical treatment, but surgical treatment to restore anatomy and allow early ROM may improve final ROM (patient and fracture dependent).

III. Special Considerations

A. Pediatric patients

1. Vast majority are Salter-Harris I or II fractures.

2. Management depends on displacement and age (capacity to remodel) but typically treated closed in a sling or hanging arm cast, as the patient has significant potential to remodel.

3. If reduction is performed (not typically indicated), usually closed reduction with or without percutaneous pin fixation is successful; however, open reduction may be needed in cases of open fractures, neurological or vascular injury, or soft tissue interposition (biceps tendon or periosteum).

Summary

Treatment of proximal humerus fractures typically includes nonsurgical, open reduction with internal fixation, hemiarthroplasty, or reverse total shoulder arthroplasty depending on patient factors, fracture morphology and displacement, and surgeon opinion. Current literature has many limitations and often suggests similar outcomes between various treatment types.

Suggested Readings

Bernstein J, Adler LM, Blank JE, Dalsey RM, Williams GR, Iannotti JP. Evaluation of the Neer system of classification of proximal humeral fractures with computerized tomographic scans and plain radiographs. J Bone Joint Surg Am 1996;78(9):1371–1375

Gupta AK, Harris JD, Erickson BJ, et al. Surgical management of complex proximal humerus fractures—a systematic review of 92 studies including 4500 patients. J Orthop Trauma 2015;29(1):54–59

Iyengar JJ, Devcic Z, Sproul RC, Feeley BT. Nonoperative treatment of proximal humerus fractures: a systematic review. J Orthop Trauma 2011;25(10):612–617

Neer CS II. Displaced proximal humeral fractures I. Classification and evaluation. J Bone Joint Surg Am 1970;52(6):1077–1089

Neer CS II. Displaced proximal humeral fractures II. Treatment of three-part and four-part displacement. J Bone Joint Surg Am 1970;52(6):1090–1103

Rangan A, Handoll H, Brealey S, et al; PROFHER Trial Collaborators. Surgical vs nonsurgical treatment of adults with displaced fractures of the proximal humerus: the PROFHER randomized clinical trial. JAMA 2015;313(10):1037–1047

22 Humeral Shaft Fractures

Lisa K. Cannada and Ugochi Okoroafor

Introduction

Humeral shaft fractures comprise approximately 3% of extremity fractures and 20% of humerus fractures. This chapter will explore the indications for nonoperative versus operative management of humerus fractures. Several surgical approaches are described in detail. Advantages and disadvantages are different fixation methods, most commonly plates and nails, are discussed.

I. Preoperative

A. History and physical examination

    1. Mechanism of injury:

        a. Fall from standing more common in elderly.

        b. High-energy trauma more common in younger patients.

    2. Physical examination:

        a. Perform thorough sensory, motor, and vascular examination to identify any deficits.

        b. Pain, swelling, and deformity.

    3. Radial nerve palsy most common:

        a. Holstein Lewis—spiral distal third shaft fracture. Commonly associated with radial nerve palsy.

B. Anatomy

    1. Deforming forces—deltoid, pectoralis major, brachialis, coracobrachialis, brachioradialis, biceps, and triceps (▶**Fig. 22.1 a–c**):

        a. Fracture proximal to pectoralis major insertion—external rotation and abduction of the proximal fragment due to rotator cuff. Adduction of distal fragment by pectoralis major and deltoid.

        b. Fracture between pectoralis major and deltoid—adduction and internal rotation of proximal fragment by pectoralis major, teres major, and latissimus dorsi; abduction of distal fragment by deltoid.

        c. Fracture distal to deltoid—abduction and flexion of proximal fragment by deltoid, and shortening of distal fragment due to pull from triceps, biceps, and coracobrachialis.

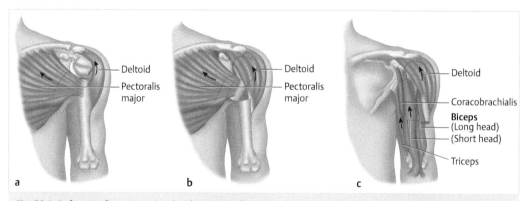

Fig. 22.1 Deforming forces associated with a proximal humerus fracture **(a)** proximal to the pectoralis major insertion; **(b)** between the deltoid and pectoralis insertion; **(c)** and distal to the deltoid insertion.

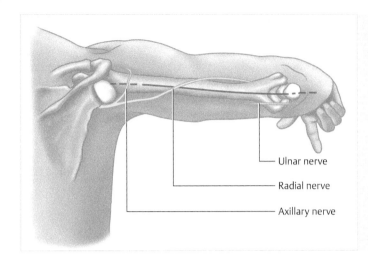

Fig. 22.2 Structures at risk associated with a posterior approach (*red line*) to the humerus.

Ulnar nerve

Radial nerve

Axillary nerve

2. Neurologic (▶ **Fig. 22.2**):

    a. Radial nerve—courses along spiral groove, and crosses from medial to lateral approximately 20 cm proximal to medial epicondyle.

    b. Ulnar nerve travels posterior to the medial epicondyle.

    c. Axillary nerve wraps around the proximal humerus from medial to lateral.

C. Imaging

    1. Radiographs—anteroposterior (AP) and lateral of the humerus.

    2. Always obtain X-rays of the joint above and below—shoulder and elbow AP and lateral.

    3. Computed tomography (CT) not indicated in fractures of the humeral shaft.

    4. Magnetic resonance imaging (MRI) typically not necessary, unless suspect pathologic fracture and trying to identify lesion.

D. Classification: There is not a commonly used "named" fracture classification for humeral shaft fractures.

    1. Arbeitsgemeinschaft für osteosynthesefrage/orthopaedic trauma association (AO/OTA) classification:

        a. Type 12A—simple fractures:

            i. A1—simple spiral.

            ii. A2—simple oblique.

            iii. A3—simple transverse.

        b. Type 12B—wedge fracture:

            i. B2—intact wedge.

            ii. B3—fragmented wedge.

        c. Type 12C—multifragmentary:

            i. C2—intact segmental fracture.

            ii. C3—fragmentary segmentalfracture.

II. Treatment

A. Initial management

    1. Coaptation splint for initial management—U-shaped splint splint extending from axilla to the neck laterally and sling.

    2. Parameters for acceptable reduction limited by small retrospective studies without correspondence to the following validated functional outcome scores: < 20 degrees anterior-posterior (sagittal) angulation, < 30 degrees varus valgus angulation, and < 3 cm shortening.

B. Definitive management

1. Nonoperative management

   a. Sarmiento functional brace—typically converted from a splint to brace approximately one-week postinjury when pain and swelling improve:

      i. Affects reduction through tissue compression.

      ii. Fracture heals by secondary bone healing.

      iii. Indications—most closed diaphyseal fractures. Patient must be able to maintain semi-upright position during early treatment phase.

      iv. Contraindications to bracing—axial distraction between fracture fragments, open fractures with significant soft tissue injury, bilateral humeral fractures, fractures with associated vascular injuries, ipsilateral brachial plexus injury, and nonambulatory polytrauma patients.

      v. Radial nerve palsy is NOT a contraindication to bracing.

      vi. Risk contributing to failure of nonoperative management—simple, transverse fractures, distal one-third fractures, proximal one-third fractures (conflicting evidence), distraction at fracture site, brachial plexus injury, large body habitus, pendulous breasts, and unbraceable arm.

      vii. Best results with midshaft fractures, and spiral and oblique patterns.

      viii. Need close follow-up, and follow-up radiographs should include upright films.

      ix. Instructions to patients must be clear—tighten brace daily, some surgeons recommend sleeping upright initially until the fracture begins to heal, and physical therapy ordered for range of motion (ROM) of shoulder, elbow, wrist and hand.

2. Absolute surgical indications:

   a. Vascular injury.

   b. Floating elbow.

   c. Failure of trial of nonoperative management.

   d. Open fracture.

3. Relative surgical indications:

   a. Polytrauma patient—provides ability to bear weight.

   b. Segmental fracture.

   c. Intra-articular extension.

   d. Pathologic fracture.

   e. Brachial plexus injury.

   f. Bilateral humeral shaft fracture.

   g. Obese patient.

   h. Large breasts.

   i. Soft tissue interposition.

4. Indications for radial nerve exploration in the setting of radial nerve palsy:

   a. Open fracture.

   b. Penetrating injury.

   c. High-energy gunshot wound (rifle or close-range shotgun).

   d. Vascular injury.

   e. Nerve deficit after closed reduction, although this is controversial.

C. Surgical approaches

1. Anterior approach:

   a. Proximally, dissect between the deltoid (axillary nerve) laterally and the pectoralis major (medial and lateral pectoral nerves).

   b. In the midshaft and distally, mobilize the biceps medially (musculocutaneous nerve).

   c. Deep dissection continues by splitting the brachialis to expose the humerus. The brachialis has dual innervation, allowing it to be safely divided down the center (musculocutaneous nerve medially and radial nerve laterally).

2. Anterolateral approach (▶Fig. 22.3 a–c):

   a. Preferred for proximal third fractures, and can also be used for midshaft fractures.

   b. Interval between biceps/brachialis medially (musculocutaneous nerve) and brachioradialis laterally (radial nerve).

   c. Advantages—supine, can extend proximally via deltopectoral approach, no direct nerve exposure, and good for positioning in polytrauma patient.

   d. Disadvantages—less direct exposure of radial nerve, and not ideal for distal humerus fractures.

3. Posterior approach—triceps splitting or triceps sparing (▶Fig. 22.4 a–c):

   a. No internervous plane.

   b. Preferred for midshaft and distal third fractures.

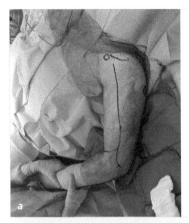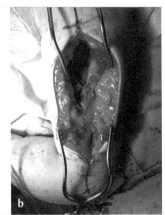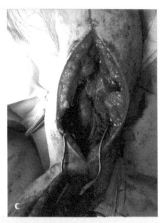

Fig. 22.3 Anterolateral approach to the humerus: **(a)** planned skin incision; **(b)** superficial dissection; **(c)** deep dissection between the biceps and brachialis medially, and the brachioradialis laterally, to expose the humerus.

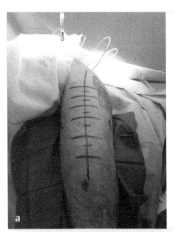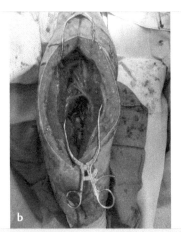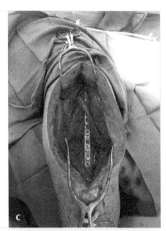

Fig. 22.4 Posterior approach to the humerus: **(a)** planned skin incision; **(b)** deep dissection with mobilization of the triceps and clear depiction of the radial nerve; and **(c)** plate fixation of the humerus fracture with radial nerve lying posterior to the implant.

    c. Advantages—direct exposure of the radial nerve, and can be applied a broad plate to flat surface of distal humerus for distal fractures.

    d. Disadvantages—not ideal for proximal fractures, prone or lateral positioning required, and requires mobilization of radial nerve for plate application (▶ Fig. 22.5 a, b).

4. Lateral approach:

    a. Can be used for distal one-third fractures. This also represents an alternative approach in revision surgery.

    b. Interval between triceps and brachioradialis.

    c. Advantages—allows radial nerve exposure, extensile approach can be used, and supine positioning.

    d. Disadvantage—not commonly used, and risk to posterior antebrachial cutaneous nerve.

D. Fixation techniques

1. External fixation:

    a. Indications—burns, extensive soft tissue injury, grossly contaminated open fracture, associated neurovascular injury, and infected nonunion.

    b. Advantages—good for cases with extensive soft tissue compromise, and shorter operative time in setting of damage control orthopaedics.

    c. Disadvantages—nonanatomic reduction.

2. Open reduction and internal fixation (ORIF):

    a. Recommend a nonlocking large fragment (4.5 mm) narrow compression plate in most instances.

    b. Orthogonal dual plating with small fragment (3.5 mm) fixation has also been described. This provides an alternative in small patients with a narrow humerus.

    c. Minifragment plates assist with reduction.

    d. Advantages—direct visualization of fracture reduction and radial nerve, avoid shoulder pain associated with antegrade nail or elbow pain associated with retrograde nail, allows nerve exploration if needed, more predictable healing, anatomic reduction, and literature supports weight bearing in polytrauma patients fixed with plates.

    e. Disadvantage—longer incision, greater potential for iatrogenic nerve injury compared to intramedullary nail (IMN), load bearing, and greater risk of infection compared to IMN.

3. IMN:

    a. Relative indications—segmental fractures, osteopenic bone, pathologic fractures, fractures with extension to surgical neck, and comminuted fractures.

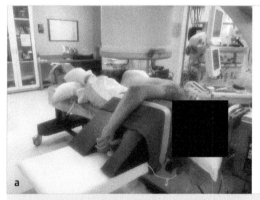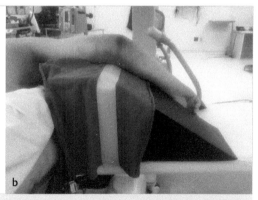

Fig. 22.5 Lateral positioning in preparation of a posterior approach to the humerus: (a) Fluoroscopy is located at the head of the bed; and (b) positioning aids may facilitate reduction and imaging.

  b. Antegrade—proximal third or midshaft fracture.

   i. Entry point—medial to the greater tuberosity through rotator cuff and typically just lateral to the articular surface.

   ii. Historically, higher incidence of shoulder pain or impingement compared to ORIF. Seat nail deep to cuff to avoid impingement.

   iii. Recent studies have shown equivalent shoulder and elbow function, union rates, and complications between nails and plates.

  c. Retrograde—distal third or midshaft fracture.

   i. Technically difficult, especially with commercially available locked IMNs.

   ii. Entry point proximal to olecranon fossa.

   iii. Higher incidence of elbow pain compared to ORIF and iatrogenic fracture at insertion site.

  d. Advantages—smaller incision, immediate weightbearing, does not require direct fracture exposure, smaller bending loads compared to plate, and load sharing.

  e. Disadvantages—higher complication rate, higher risk of reoperation, risk to radial nerve with lateral to medial screws distally, risk to musculocutaneous nerve with AP screws distally, and higher incidence of shoulder or elbow pain.

E. Complications

 1. Nonunion:

  a. Historical reports demonstrated nonunion rates of 2 to 7% with closed treatment and bracing; however, recent literature has reported nonunion rates of up to 20%.

  b. Higher rate for open fractures compared to close.

  c. Five percent rate reported with operative management.

  d. Risk factors—transverse fracture, elderly, osteoporosis, endocrine disorder, radiation therapy, and steroid use.

 2. Malunion:

  a. Most commonly observed with transverse fracture pattern.

  b. More often associated with nonoperative treatment—There is conflicting evidence as to whether proximal one-third fractures have a higher rate of nonunion when treated nonoperatively.

 3. Radial nerve palsy:

  a. Reported incidence from 1 to 34% (average of 12%).

  b. Increased rate of radial nerve laceration or entrapment observed with spiral distal third (Holstein-Lewis fracture).

  c. Increased incidence of neuropraxia with transverse middle third fractures.

  d. Increased rate with higher energy injuries.

  e. Overall recovery rate of 88%.

  f. Spontaneous recovery in 99% of patients managed with Sarmiento bracing.

  g. Consider a baseline electromyogram/nerve conduction velocity (EMG/NCV) after 6 weeks but average nerve recovery time is 3 to 6 months.

 4. Infection after surgical fixation—Higher rate with ORIF (3%) compared to IMN (1.5%).

 5. Loss of shoulder ROM—6 to 36% incidence after antegrade humeral nail.

F. Rehabilitation

 1. Protocol for nonoperative management:

  a. Initial coaptation splint in emergency department.

  b. Change to Sarmiento functional brace within 1 to 2 weeks.

  c. May recommend upright position for sleeping initially (may sleep in chair or elevate head of bed [HOB]).

      d.   Initial pendulum exercises and active elbow motion.

      e.   Active shoulder exercises delayed until fracture is stable.

2.   Postop protocol for ORIF:

      a.   Dry dressing postoperatively or Sarmiento brace.

      b.   Edema glove.

      c.   Immediate shoulder and elbow ROM.

      d.   Avoid shoulder abduction > 90 degrees for 4 weeks.

      e.   Weightbearing per surgeon preference based on fracture pattern and plate used, typically weight bearing as tolerated (WBAT) in awake and alert patient with good fixation of an extraarticular fracture.

3.   Postop protocol for IMN fixation:

      a.   Dry dressing postoperatively.

      b.   Edema glove.

      c.   Immediate shoulder and elbow ROM.

      d.   WBAT immediately postop.

G.   Outcomes

1.   Nonoperative management successful in approximately 90% of cases, especially isolated fractures.

2.   Transverse and short oblique humeral shaft fractures most likely to fail nonoperative management.

3.   No evidence from randomized controlled trials (RCTs) to determine whether outcome is better with surgical versus nonsurgical management.

Summary

Humeral shaft fractures may be associated with radial nerve injuries due to its location along the posterior humerus. Up to 90% of radial nerve palsies ultimately recover. Most humerus fractures can be successfully treated nonoperatively with initial splinting followed by functional bracing. Absolute indications for surgery include open fracture, vascular injury, floating elbow, and failure of nonoperative management. Plates and IMN are both effective treatment methods for most diaphyseal fractures.

Suggested Readings

Carroll EA, Schweppe M, Langfitt M, Miller AN, Halvorson JJ. Management of humeral shaft fractures. J Am Acad Orthop Surg 2012;20(7):423–433

Chapman JR, Henley MB, Agel J, Benca PJ. Randomized prospective study of humeral shaft fracture fixation: intramedullary nails versus plates. J Orthop Trauma 2000;14(3):162–166

Denard A Jr, Richards JE, Obremskey WT, Tucker MC, Floyd M, Herzog GA. Outcome of nonoperative vs operative treatment of humeral shaft fractures: a retrospective study of 213 patients. Orthopedics 2010;33(8)

Ekholm R, Adami J, Tidermark J, Hansson K, Törnkvist H, Ponzer S. Fractures of the shaft of the humerus. An epidemiological study of 401 fractures. J Bone Joint Surg Br 2006;88(11):1469–1473

Koch PP, Gross DFL, Gerber C. The results of functional (Sarmiento) bracing of humeral shaft fractures. J Shoulder Elbow Surg 2002;11(2):143–150

McCormack RG, Brien D, Buckley RE, McKee MD, Powell J, Schemitsch EH. Fixation of fractures of the shaft of the humerus by dynamic compression plate or intramedullary nail. A prospective, randomised trial. J Bone Joint Surg Br 2000;82(3):336–339

Sarmiento A, Zagorski JB, Zych GA, Latta LL, Capps CA. Functional bracing for the treatment of fractures of the humeral diaphysis. J Bone Joint Surg Am 2000;82(4):478–486

23 Distal Humerus Fractures

John Michael Yingling, Richard S. Yoon, and Frank A. Liporace

Introduction

Distal humerus fractures comprise 7% of all fractures and 30% of all elbow fractures. Approximately 7% are open fractures due to their subcutaneous location. Bimodal distribution includes young, accident-prone patients and elderly individuals with osteopenic bone. Highest incidence is observed among elderly women who are > 60 years of age (▶ **Video 23.1**).

Keywords: distal humerus fracture, elbow fracture, elbow dislocation

I. Preoperative

A. History and physical examination

1. Mechanism of injury:

   a. Low-energy falls (common in the elderly).

   b. High-energy trauma with extensive comminution and intra-articular involvement. Gunshot wound, motor vehicle accident, and fall from a height

   c. Typically results from an axial load.

2. Clinical evaluation

   a. Present with elbow pain, swelling, and crepitus or gross instability with attempted range of elbow motion.

   b. Perform a careful neurovascular examination, especially radial nerve, ulnar nerve, and distal arterial flow.

   c. Assess compartment syndrome; serial compartment examinations may be required to avoid resultant Volkmann contracture.

B. Anatomy

1. The elbow is a constrained hinge composed of two joints:

   a. Ulnohumeral—flexion and extension of the forearm.

   b. Radiocapitellar—forearm pronosupination.

2. Two columns—orientation in reference to the shaft (▶ **Fig. 23.1**):

   a. Medial—45 degree in coronal plane.

   b. Lateral—20 degree in coronal and 35 to 40 degree in sagittal plane.

   c. Valgus alignment is 4 to 8 degree.

   d. Internal rotation is 3 to 8 degree.

   e. Carrying angle is 10 to 17 degree in full extension.

C. Imaging

1. Radiographs:

   a. Anteroposterior (AP) and lateral of the humerus and elbow.

   b. Forearm and wrist when concomitant injuries are present.

   c. Oblique—useful in diagnosing condylar fractures and degree of displacement.

   d. Traction radiographs—improved delineation of fracture fragments and aid in preoperative planning.

2. Computed tomography (CT) scan—particularly useful for preoperative evaluation of intra-articular fractures with comminution. Three-dimensional CT reconstruction improves the inter- and intraobserver reliability of classification.

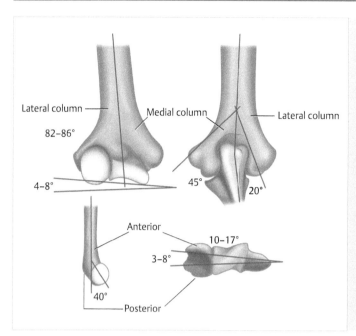

Fig. 23.1 In the coronal plane, the lateral column projects approximately 20 degrees and the medial column projects nearly 45 degrees from the shaft with a net carrying angle of about 15 degrees of the elbow. Due to the capitallar facet, the forearm rest in 3 to 8 degrees of internal rotation in the frontal plane and 40 degrees in the sagittal plane. (Adapted from Rockwood and Green's Fractures in Adults, Eighth Edition, Volume 1, Section 2, Ch. 35 pg. 1239 Figure 35–8.)

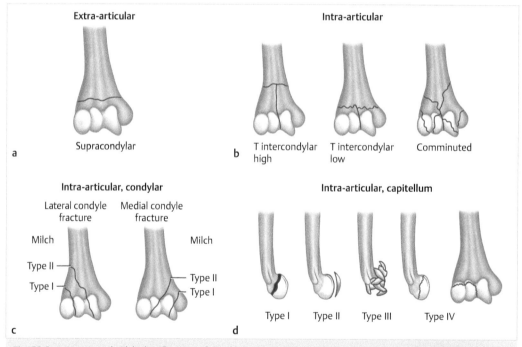

Fig. 23.2 Anatomic and Milch classifications of distal humerus fractures: **(a)** Extra-articular, supracondylar fracture; **(b)** Intra-articular fractures including high T intercondylar, low T intercondylar, and comminuted intercondylar; **(c)** Milch classification of lateral and medial condylar fractures; **(d)** Capitellum fracture types I–IV. (Adapted from Milch H. Fractures and fracture-classifications of the humeral condyles. J Trauma. 1964;4:592–607.)

D. Classification

    1. Anatomic—based on the number of columns involved, the location of the fracture, and rotational displacement:

        a. Supracondylar—extra-articular and extra-capsular (▶ **Fig. 23.2a**).

    b. Transcondylar—extra-articular and intra-capsular.

    c. Columnar—intra-articular, lateral or medial condylar fracture, and capitellum/trochlea fracture (▶ **Fig. 23.2b, c**).

    d. Intercondylar—intra-articular (▶ **Fig. 23.2d**).

2. Orthopaedic trauma association (OTA) classification—13-X:

    a. 13-A (extra-articular).

    b. 13-B (partial articular).

    c. 13-C (complete articular).

3. Specific types of intra-articular fractures:

    a. Condylar—involving a single column (▶ **Fig. 23.2b**):

        i. Milch type I fractures—lateral trochlear wall is attached to the shaft of the humerus, and forearm maintains alignment with humerus; therefore, more stable.

       ii. Milch type II fractures—lateral wall of the trochlea is attached to the displaced fracture fragment, and forearm follows fragment; therefore, less stable.

    b. Capitellum fractures—coronal shear (▶ **Fig. 23.2c**):

        i. Type I (Hahn-Steinthal)—involves most of the capitellum and may include part of the trochlea.

       ii. Type II (Kocher-Lorenz)—separation of articular cartilage with minimal attached subchondral bone.

      iii. Type III—severely comminuted multifragmentary fractures.

      iv. Type IV—McKee modification—significant extension of the fracture into the trochlea.

II. Treatment

A. Initial management

1. Bicolumnar fracture—typically splinted in a position of comfort, general guidelines are a posterior splint 45 to 90 degrees of elbow flexion, 30 degrees of wrist extension, forearm in neutral rotation, and allow full metacarpophalangeal (MCP) range of motion (ROM).

2. Isolated lateral column fracture—splint forearm in supination.

3. Isolated medial column fracture—splint forearm in pronation.

B. Definitive management

1. Nonsurgical treatment indications:

    a. Nondisplaced or minimally displaced fractures.

    b. Displaced fractures in elderly, low-demand patients and/or patients with extensive comorbidities:

        i. Splint 1 to 2 weeks before initiation of ROM exercises.

       ii. Wean out of removable splint by 6 weeks if there is progressive evidence of healing.

      iii. May accept 20 degree loss of condylar shaft angle.

    c. Comminuted osteoporotic fractures in elderly "bag of bones":

        i. Immobilization for 2 weeks in 90 degree of elbow flexion.

       ii. After 2 weeks, begin gentle ROM.

      iii. Goal is to ultimately achieve a minimally painful, functional pseudoarthrosis.

2. Surgical fixation:

    a. Indications—displaced fractures and for those associated with an open or vascular injury.

    b. Supracondylar fractures; OTA type A:

        i. Open reduction and internal fixation (ORIF)—plate and screws placed on the medial and lateral columns (▶ **Fig. 23.3a,b**):

          • Ninety-degree plating (orthogonal direct medial and posterolateral).

          • Parallel plating (parallel direct medial and lateral).

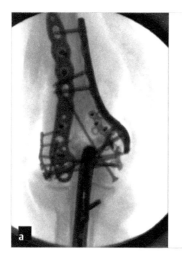
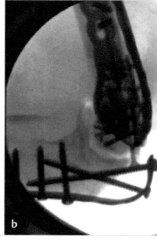

Fig. 23.3 Demonstrates orthogonal plating oriented 90 degrees from each other supplemented with bicolumnar, minifragment plate and screw fixation using an olecranon osteotomy. (a) Intra-operative fluoroscopic posterior-anterior (PA); (b) Intra-operative fluoroscopic lateral

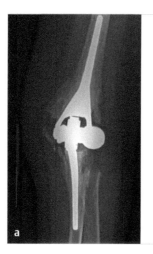
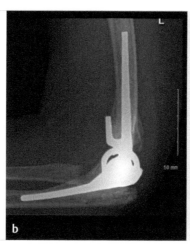

Fig. 23.4 Total elbow arthroplasty, (a) Anteroposterior; (b) Lateral postoperative radiographs.

  c. Transcondylar fractures—Consider total elbow arthroplasty (TEA) for elderly patients with distal, comminuted fractures and poor bone quality (▶ **Fig. 23.4a, b**).

  d. Condylar fractures, partial articular; OTA type B—ORIF, lag screws with unilateral plating.

  e. Capitellum fractures:

    i. ORIF

- Minifragment screw fixation from posterior to anterior.
- Countersunk minifragment screws from anterior to posterior.
- Headless screws.
- Minifragment plate fixation supplementation.

    ii. Excision for nonreconstructible parts of type II and III fractures as a last resort.

    iii. Consider replacement among elderly.

  f. Trochlea fractures:

    i. ORIF for displaced fractures often repaired with minifragment or headless screw constructs similar to strategies for fixation of capitellum fractures.

  g. Epicondylar fractures:

    i. ORIF if markedly displaced or evidence of elbow instability with ROM. Repair with small or minifragment screws.

    ii. Late presentation as a painful nonunion and unreconstructable fragment can be treated by excision.

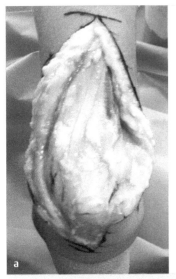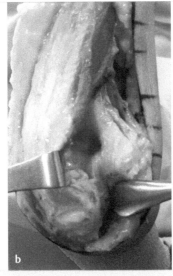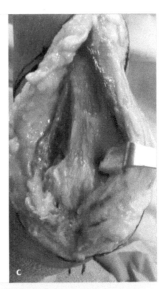

Fig. 23.5 Direct posterior approach. (**a**) Midline incision with large full thickness medial and lateral flaps developed. (**b**) Ulnar column exposure after ulnar nerve was identified and transposed anteriorly. (**c**) Radial column exposure after radial nerve was identified and protected in proximal extent of exposure.

    h. Supracondylar process fracture:
        i. A congenital variant, and the supracondylar process is a bony protrusion on the antero-medial surface of the distal humerus.
       ii. Excision if there is evidence of arterial injury or nerve compression.
    i. Intercondylar fractures, OTA type C fractures:
        i. ORIF for displaced fractures—minifragment and small fragment articular fixation combined with bicolumnar plates (orthogonal versus parallel) (▶ **Fig. 23.3a, b**).
       ii. TEA for elderly patients with severe comminution and/or nonreconstructible fractures with poor bone quality (▶ **Fig. 23.4a, b**).

C. Surgical approaches
    1. Most supracondylar and intercondylar distal humerus fractures are treated through one of several described posterior approaches. The deep interval varies based upon fracture pattern and surgeon preference.
    2. Superficial dissection is the same for the various deep interval approaches described below (▶ **Fig. 23.5a**):
      a. Posterior skin incision.
      b. Develop medial and lateral subcutaneous flaps.
      c. Identify the ulnar nerve as it emerges between intermuscular septum beneath Osbourne ligament, approximately 2 cm proximal to medial epicondyle or distally between the two heads of flexor carpi ulnaris (FCU) at the origin of the first motor branch. Mobilize it anteriorly.
      d. There is conflicting evidence surrounding anterior subcutaneous transposition of the ulnar nerve versus in-situ decompression and return of the nerve to its normal anatomic location.
      e. Develop a more anterior interval for single column, capitellum, or trochlea fractures through same posterior skin incision.
    3. Deep dissection:
      a. Paratricipital (Alonso-Llames) (▶ **Fig. 23.5b, c**):
        i. Indications—extra-articular or simple partial articular fractures.
       ii. Create medial and lateral windows between the intramuscular septae and triceps.

      iii. Identify and protect the ulnar and radial nerves.

      iv. Pros—does not disrupt the extensor mechanism and it can be converted into an olecranon osteotomy.

      v. Cons—lack of visualization of the entire articular surface.

  b. Triceps reflecting (Bryan-Morrey):

      i. Reflect extensor mechanism from a medial interval.

      ii. Subperiosteally dissect the extensor mechanism off the olecranon and take as a flap in continuity with the extensor compartment of the forearm.

      iii. Pros—more extensile and promotes increased visualization.

      iv. Cons—disrupts the extensor mechanism.

  c. Triceps reflecting anconeus pedicle (TRAP):

      i. Reflect entire triceps along with anconeus off of olecranon as one flap.

      ii. Pros—improved articular visualization.

      iii. Cons—less extensile and disrupts the extensor mechanism.

  d. Triceps splitting:

      i. Sharply dissect interval between long and lateral heads of triceps.

      ii. Identify the radial nerve which can be found:

- Crossing the lateral border of the posterior humerus at an average distance of 11 cm proximal to the proximal extent of the olecranon fossa (range 8–14 cm).
- Crossing the medial border of the posterior humerus at an average distance of 15 cm proximal to the proximal extent of the olecranon fossa (range 10–20 cm).
- Alternatively, the lateral brachial cutaneous nerve can be traced proximally to where it branches from the radial nerve proper at the level of the deltoid insertion near the lateral intermuscular septum.

      iii. Distally, it can be carried to the ulnar insertion and reflected off the olecranon but left in continuity with the fascia.

      iv. Pros—does not disrupt extensor mechanism.

      v. Cons—limited visualization of anterior surface.

  e. Olecranon osteotomy:

      i. Indications—extensive articular involvement.

      ii. Contraindications—planned TEA.

      iii. Create a chevron-style osteotomy pointing distally at the level of the bare area of the olecranon approximately 2 to 2.5 cm distal to the proximal tip.

- Some surgeons prefer to drill and tap the proximal ulna for an intramedullary screw or plate prior to osteotomizing the olecranon to facilitate later fixation.
- Drill a small 2.0 mm hole at the distal apex of the planned osteotomy to prevent unwanted fracture propagation.
- Make initial cuts with an oscillating saw followed by osteotomes to prevent the kerf of the saw blade from removing articular cartilage that will lead to step off after final fixation.
- Reflect entire extensor mechanism proximally to allow visualization of the entire distal humerus.
- Repair the osteotomy:
    - Kirschner wires and a tension band type construct.
    - Long, large-fragment intramedullary screw fixation with a tension band.
    - Plate fixation.
    - Two small-fragment lag screws.
- Pros—best visualization of articular surface.
- Cons—risk of osteotomy nonunion and hardware prominence.

4. Lateral approach for lateral condyle and capitellar fractures:

  a. Superficial dissection—direct lateral or posterior skin incision.

    b. Deep interval:

       i. Most common—Kaplan interval between extensor carpi radialis brevis (ECRB) and extensor digitorum comminus (EDC).

      ii. Rarely used—Kocher interval between anconeus and extensor carpi ulnaris (ECU).

  5. Medial approach for medial condyle, trochlea, and coronoid fractures—FCU splitting approach:

       i. Identify the ulnar nerve between the two heads of the FCU. Protect the nerve and allow it to retract posteriorly.

      ii. Incise the flexor—pronator muscle mass from the medial epicondyle distally toward the sublime tubercle and elevate the anterior head of the FCU off the anteromedial coronoid and proximal ulna.

     iii. Take care not to disrupt the underlying medial collateral ligament.

     iv. Elevate the anterior portion of the flexor pronator mass off of the medial supracondylar ridge as necessary.

D. Fixation techniques

  1. Anatomic articular reduction:

    a. Use of K-wires and clamps.

    b. Avoid decreasing the dimensions of the trochlea.

  2. Stable internal fixation of the articular surface—minifragment and small fragment fixation.

  3. Restoration of axial alignment.

  4. Fixation of the articular segment to the metaphysis and diaphysis:

    a. Orthogonal plating versus parallel plating (▶ **Fig. 23.6**).

    b. Locking plates are often recommended in osteoporotic fractures and/or extensive articular comminution.

    c. Avoid ending plates at the same level to prevent a stress riser.

  5. Early ROM of the elbow.

E. Complications

  1. Fixation failure.

  2. Malunion and nonunion.

  3. Infection (0–6%)–most commonly with type 3 open fractures.

  4. Ulnar nerve palsy/neuritis—10 to 30%.

  5. Post-traumatic arthritis

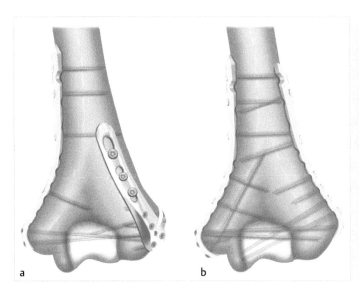

Fig. 23.6 (a) Orthogonal plating where the constructs are oriented 90 degrees from each other with the medial plate lying within the coronal plane and the lateral plate lying posterior in the sagittal plane. **(b)** Parallel plating where both constructs are oriented 180 degrees from each other in the coronal plane.

a   b

F. Rehabilitation
   1. ORIF:
      a. Postoperatively nonweight bearing with the elbow immobilized at 90 degrees of flexion.
      b. Initiate elbow motion at 3 to 7 days postoperatively. Consider delay in mobilization for 2 to 4 weeks if stable fixation cannot be achieved and in noncompliant patients.
      c. Two weeks postop—allow progression to full active, active-assisted, and passive elbow ROM if the wound has healed.
      d. Six to twelve weeks postop—allow progression to WBAT if there is clinical and radiographic evidence of healing.
   2. TEA:
      a. Postoperatively immobilize with an anterior splint in near full extension to protect the wound.
      b. Begin ROM when the skin has healed.
G. Outcomes
   1. ORIF:
      a. The goal of treatment is a functional arc of elbow motion from 30 to 130 degrees and pronosupination of 150 to 160 degrees.
      b. Greater than 90% rate of union.
      c. Seventy five percent of flexion and extension strength.
   2. TEA:
      a. Average range of postoperative elbow motion is 25 to 130 degrees and good for excellent functional outcomes.
      b. Good pain relief.
      c. Must be able to abide by the lifelong weight bearing restrictions.

Summary

Intra-articular distal humerus fractures often require surgical treatment to yield consistent results and adequate function. This chapter outlines the usual presentation, how to diagnose, classify, and treat, along with traditional surgical approaches and outcomes of distal humerus fracture management.

Suggested Readings

Caravaggi P, Laratta JL, Yoon RS, et al. Internal fixation of the distal humerus: a comprehensive biomechanical study evaluating current fixation techniques. J Orthop Trauma 2014;28(4):222–226

Doornberg J, Lindenhovius A, Kloen P, et al. Two and three-dimensional computed tomography for the classification and management of distal humeral fractures. Evaluation of Reliability and Diagnostic Accuracy. J Bone Joint Surg Am 2006;88(8):1795–801

Ek ET, Goldwasser M, Bonomo AL. Functional outcome of complex intercondylar fractures of the distal humerus treated through a triceps-sparing approach. J Shoulder Elbow Surg 2008;17(3):441–446

Erpelding JM, Mailander A, High R, Mormino MA, Fehringer EV. Outcomes following distal humeral fracture fixation with an extensor mechanism-on approach. J Bone Joint Surg Am 2012;94(6):548–553

McKee MD, Wilson TL, Winston L, Schemitsch EH, Richards RR. Functional outcome following surgical treatment of intra-articular distal humeral fractures through a posterior approach. J Bone Joint Surg Am 2000;82(12):1701–1707

Milch H. Fractures and fracture-classifications of the humeral condyles. J Trauma 1964;4:592–607

Sanchez-Sotelo J, Torchia ME, O'Driscoll SW. Complex distal humeral fractures: internal fixation with a principle-based parallel-plate technique. J Bone Joint Surg Am 2007;89(5):961–969

Seigerman DA, Choung EW, Yoon RS, et al. Identification of the radial nerve during the posterior approach to the humerus: a cadaveric study. J Orthop Trauma 2012;26(4):226–228

Schildhauer TA, Nork SE, Mills WJ, Henley MB. Extensor mechanism-sparing paratricipital posterior approach to the distal humerus. J Orthop Trauma 2003;17(5):374–378

24 Elbow Dislocation

Jodi Siegel

Introduction

Simple elbow dislocations involve dislocation of the ulnohumeral and radiocapitellar joints with no associated fractures. The elbow joint is typically stable after closed reduction. Older patients, patients with higher-energy mechanisms, and fracture-dislocations have a higher risk for residual instability which may require operative intervention.

Keywords: Elbow instability, terrible triad, posterolateral rotatory instability, posteromedial rotatory instability, coronoid fracture

I. Preoperative

A. History and physical exam

1. The typical mechanism is fall on an outstretched hand. Patients present with obvious deformity and pain.

2. Inspect the skin for open wounds.

3. A thorough distal neurovascular examination must be performed and documented for both sensory and motor functions. Radial and ulnar pulses should be evaluated and compared to the contralateral extremity.

4. Ipsilateral upper extremity injuries occur in up to 20% of patients with elbow fracture-dislocations and most commonly these injuries are in the wrist.

B. Anatomy

1. Elbow stability is conferred by the surrounding soft tissues and the bony articulations.

2. Static soft-tissue stabilizers (capsule, collateral ligaments):

   a. Joint capsule contributes to stability in full flexion and full extension.

   b. Lateral collateral ligament (LCL), which has three components (the radial collateral ligament, annular ligament, and lateral ulnar collateral ligament [LUCL]), is the primary varus and posterolateral rotational stabilizer.

   c. Medial collateral ligament (MCL) is composed of two bundles—the anterior bundle is the main valgus stabilizer; the posterior bundle is a secondary restraint to valgus forces.

3. Dynamic soft-tissue stabilizers (muscles crossing the elbow):

   a. Muscular contraction loads the elbow joint creating joint reaction forces which contribute to stability, most importantly when the static constraints are disrupted.

   b. Biceps, brachialis, and triceps provide compressive force while common extensor muscle group supplies valgus stability.

   c. As such, pronation will help to stabilize the LCL-deficient elbow.

4. The stabilizing structures of the elbow can also be divided into primary and secondary stabilizers.

5. Primary stabilizers:

   a. MCL.

   b. LCL.

   c. Coronoid: primary stabilizer to varus stress.

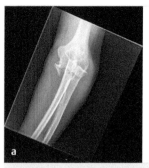
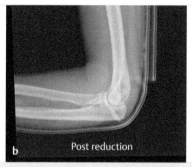
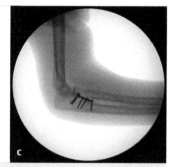

Fig. 24.1 Anteroposterior radiograph showing an elbow dislocation with a large anteromedial coronoid fragment (**a**). Post reduction (**b**) and postsurgical (**c**) lateral images show the ulnohumeral and radiocapitellar joints reduced and the coronoid fragment stabilized. Surgical treatment was through a medial flexor carpi ulnaris splitting approach with a mini-fragment buttress plate.

6. Secondary stabilizers:
   a. Capsule.
   b. Radiocapitellar articulation: the radial head is a secondary valgus stabilizer.
   c. Common extensor and flexor origins.
7. Pathoanatomy:
   a. Simple dislocation typically results in disruption of the LCL, MCL, and capsule.
   b. Muscular origins may also be disrupted.
   c. In the general population, most residual instability is due to incompetence of the LCL as most activities of daily living (ADLs) result in varus stresses across the elbow.
   d. In overhead throwing athletes who repeatedly have valgus stresses across the elbow, the MCL is the more important stabilizer and more likely to be compromised.
8. Coronoid fractures occur in up to 15% of elbow dislocations (▶ **Fig. 24.1**).
   a. The size and location of the fragment and the associated soft-tissue injury dictates treatment.
   b. Coronoid plays an important role in providing varus stability and acts as an anterior and varus buttress.
   c. It also helps to resist axial and posterolateral and posteromedial rotatory forces.
   d. The sublime tubercle is on the anteromedial facet of the coronoid and serves as the insertion site of the anterior bundle of the MCL. The MCL acts as a restraint to valgus and posteromedial rotatory instability.
9. The ulnar nerve is the most commonly injured nerve with elbow dislocation.

C. Imaging
1. Anteroposterior, lateral, and oblique plain radiographs of the elbow are used to diagnose a dislocation and to confirm a concentric reduction.
2. Computed tomography scan and magnetic resonance imaging are rarely indicated unless there are concerns for associated fractures or nerve entrapment for which management would be altered.
3. Completion plain radiographs of the injured extremity are obtained as they are clinically necessary.

D. Classification
1. Simple dislocations are named according to the direction of the distal segment: posterior, posterolateral, posteromedial, medial, lateral, and anterior.
2. The most common dislocations are posterior or posterolateral.

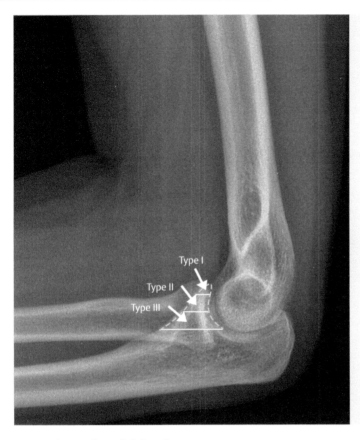

Fig. 24.2 Regan and Morrey classification of coronoid fractures. Type I: tip of coronoid fracture; Type II: coronoid fracture less than 50% of the height; Type III: coronoid fracture greater than 50% of the height.

3. Posterolateral dislocations:

   a. Occur due to a valgus, axial, and posterolateral forces.

   b. Soft-tissue injury is thought to begin on lateral side with disruption of LCL and proceed through the capsule to medial side with the MCL injured last.

4. Posteromedial dislocations:

   a. Less common; they occur due to a varus, axial, posteromedial force.

   b. The force runs medial to lateral and frequently results in small anteromedial coronoid fracture.

5. 'Terrible triad':

   a. Elbow dislocation.

   b. Radial head fracture.

   c. Coronoid fracture.

   d. Typically a posterolateral rotatory mechanism that shears off the anterolateral radial head and tip of the coronoid while dislocating the elbow joint.

6. Coronoid fractures—Regan and Morrey classification (▶ **Fig. 24.2**).

II. Treatment

A. Initial management

   1. Closed reduction:

      a. After adequate pain control and relaxation, gentle steady traction is applied to the forearm while stabilizing the humerus.

205

      b.   The elbow is placed in approximately 30 degrees of flexion while supinating the forearm for most successful reductions.

      c.   Typically the reduction of the joint is palpable.

  2. Post reduction examination:

      a.   The elbow should then be ranged through a full flexion-extension arc of motion in pronation, neutral, and supination to assess for blocks to motion and ulnohumeral stability.

  3. Immobilization:

      a.   The elbow is then splinted at 90 degrees to allow for soft tissue rest and pain control.

      b.   Pronation of the forearm may assist with maintaining the reduction if the elbow is unstable.

      c.   Post reduction plain radiographs are required to confirm a concentric reduction.

B.   Definitive management

  1. Most simple elbow dislocations can be treated nonsurgically.

  2. Although some residual coronal plane instability may be appreciated, this is not an indication for surgical treatment.

  3. Instability with extension beyond 30 degrees, especially once the patient has regained normal muscle tone, must be noted and requires continued close monitoring.

  4. Surgical management of simple elbow dislocations is required in following cases:

      a.   Nonconcentric reductions.

      b.   Irreducible dislocations.

      c.   Open dislocations.

      d.   Vascular disruption.

      e.   If prolonged immobilization is required.

  5. Surgical management of elbow fracture dislocations is required in the following cases:

      a.   Most terrible triad injuries due to residual instability after a closed reduction—successful repair of a terrible triad requires a systematic plan to address the radial head, the coronoid fragment, the LCL, and possibly the MCL.

      b.   Also, any block to forearm rotation or incarcerated joint fragments indicates surgery.

C.   Surgical approaches

  1. Posterior midline approach:

      a.   It allows medial and lateral access through full thickness flaps.

      b.   Laterally, option of working through the soft tissue disruption or use the Kocher interval (between extensor carpi ulnaris and anconeus).

      c.   Deep dissection requires identification of the LCL and/or the radial head fracture (terrible triad).

      d.   If an extended Kocher approach is necessary, take care to keep the forearm pronated to protect the posterior interosseous nerve (PIN).

      e.   Caution when dissecting more than 2 cm distal to the joint as the PIN can be in close proximity to the proximal radius.

      f.   If the medial structures need to be addressed, the ulnar nerve must be identified and protected after raising the medial flap.

      g.   The MCL can be repaired through the traumatic injury or the extensor-pronator mass can be elevated to allow access for ligament repair.

  2. Lateral approach:

      a.   Kocher interval and deep dissection as described above.

b. Work through the soft tissue disruption.

c. Alternatively, use a Kaplan interval between extensor carpi radialis brevis and extensor digitorum communis—this interval is more anterior taking your dissection farther from the LUCL, but closer to the PIN.

3. Medial approach:

   a. Flexor carpi ulnaris (FCU) split:

      i. Work between the two heads of the FCU.

      ii. It provides access to large coronoid fragments, the sublime tubercle, and the MCL.

   b. Detaching the entire flexor-pronator mass will provide excellent access to the coronoid and the MCL.

4. The best approach for repair of a coronoid fracture is unknown with many options available to access it.

   a. It can be accessed laterally through a radial head fracture (terrible triad).

   b. Medial access will depend on the size and location of the fragment.

D. Fixation techniques

   1. Direct repair of the ligaments, capsule, or muscle origins may be necessary.

   2. The LCL and the extensor fascia can be repaired with transosseous bone tunnels or suture anchors placed at the center of the flexion–extension axis—the sutures are tensioned with the elbow at 90 degrees of flexion and full pronation.

   3. Range the elbow including full extension in pronation, neutral, and supination verifying the reduction clinically and fluoroscopically.

   4. Overtensioning can cause medial joint space widening if the MCL is deficient.

   5. In rare cases, the MCL and the flexor-pronator mass will also need to be repaired; drill holes or suture anchors can be used.

   6. Small coronoid fractures (type I and II):

      a. Rarely require fixation in terrible triad injuries if elbow stability is achieved by radial head fixation/replacement and ligament repair.

      b. If repair is necessary to increase stability: pass suture around the tip, through the anterior capsular, and then through bone tunnels in the proximal ulna.

   7. Large coronoid fracture (type III):

      a. Posterior to anterior lag screws.

      b. Buttress plating from a medial approach (▶ Fig. 24.1).

   8. Static or hinged elbow spanning external fixation can be used for cases with persistent instability.

      a. Hinged devices require precise placement of the axis pin as maltracking or dislocation may occur.

      b. Ulnar nerve may be injured when placing the axis pin.

      c. Radial nerve is at risk when placing the humerus shaft pins.

      d. If hinged external fixators are not available or the surgeon is not familiar with them, static fixators can be used.

         i. Two pins are placed in the humerus using an open technique while the elbow is reduced and held at 90 degrees.

         ii. Two ulnar pins are then placed and a static frame is assembled.

   9. In very rare salvage situations, cross pinning the joint with a large Steinman pin or cortical screw or spanning the joint with a plate may also be necessary.

      a. When placing transarticular cortical screws, be sure to penetrate the posterior cortex of the humerus so they can be removed later if broken.

    b. If a plate is chosen, a large fragment locking plate, which is bent to 90 degrees, can be placed through a triceps sparing approach over the tip of the olecranon on to the ulna leaving the triceps insertion intact.

E. Complications

  1. Stiffness can be avoided with early range of motion protocols—residual stiffness may require elbow release procedures or excision of any heterotopic bone to improve motion.

  2. Persistent instability, although rare, must be recognized early, as late treatment of subluxated elbows is very difficult.

  3. Nerve injuries are uncommon.

    a. The ulnar nerve is the most commonly injured due to the injury.

    b. The radial and ulnar nerves are at risk surgically with placement of external fixator pins, aggressive retraction, or MCL repair.

F. Rehabilitation

  1. Begin elbow motion within one week of injury.

  2. Patients with simple elbow dislocations can begin active range of motion exercises.

  3. Active motion is preferred as muscle contraction tends to stabilize the elbow.

    a. Full elbow flexion-extension with the forearm in full pronation only.

    b. Supination exercises are limited to 90 degrees of flexion.

  4. Normal activities can be resumed at 6 weeks including gentle strengthening.

  5. Varus and valgus stresses should be avoided until 12 weeks.

  6. Some patients with simple dislocations may have mild residual posterolateral instability/subluxation.

  7. Bracing with an extension block may be necessary for a few weeks.

  8. Patients who require surgical repair should have a defined fluoroscopic safe range which will guide the postoperative course.

  9. Potential modifications for surgically repaired terrible triad fracture dislocations:

    a. Active and active-assisted elbow flexion/extension 30 to 130 degrees in pronation only for 2 weeks.

    b. Full pronation/supination with the elbow at 90 degrees of flexion.

    c. Two to four weeks postoperatively—advancement to full elbow flexion/extension as tolerated in pronation only.

    d. Avoid varus stress to the elbow and avoid shoulder abduction.

  10. If external fixation is necessary, the frame is maintained for 4 weeks and then an active range of motion protocol is started as described above.

  11. Similarly, if joint spanning screws, pins, or plates are necessary, these are removed at 4 weeks and a similar protocol is initiated.

G. Outcomes

  1. Less than 10% of patients have residual instability after simple elbow dislocation.

  2. Rarely patients will complain of residual stiffness or pain.

  3. Patients with medial instability have worse radiographic and clinical outcomes.

  4. Prolonged immobilization is associated with a worse result.

  5. Terrible triad outcomes, including both persistent stiffness and residual instability, have improved as knowledge of the pathoanatomy and surgical techniques and implants have improved.

a. However, stable internal fixation of radial head fractures and coronoid fractures continues to present challenges.

b. The optimal surgical approach as well as ideal management of the ulnar nerve also remains elusive.

III. Special Considerations

A. Geriatric patients with elbow dislocations are more frequently unstable and require careful follow-up.

B. Throwing athletes may benefit from early direct repair of MCL injuries, as their mechanism of injury and functional requirements differ from the remainder of the population.

C. "Isolated" anteromedial fractures of the coronoid are rare when compared to terrible triad injuries, however their outcomes are notoriously poor because they are often missed.

1. They are associated with LCL and posterior bundle of the MCL injuries resulting in posteromedial rotatory instability.

2. The radial head is usually intact, which is the key differentiating factor.

D. Transolecranon fracture-dislocation (▶ Fig. 24.3)

1. Anterior elbow dislocation with a complex olecranon fracture typically including a large coronoid fragment.

2. The differing characteristic from a Monteggia fracture-dislocation is the proximal radioulnar joint remains relatively preserved.

3. Essential to recreate the contour and dimensions of the trochlear notch.

4. Collateral ligaments of the elbow are usually spared with this injury as compared to elbow dislocations without bony injury.

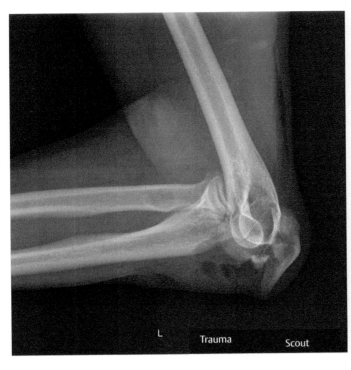

Fig. 24.3 Lateral radiograph of a transolecranon fracture-dislocation. The trochlea dislocated through the proximal ulna, a so-called anterior elbow dislocation. The proximal radioulnar joint (PRUJ) remains intact. This pattern differs from Monteggia variants in which there is a fracture-dislocation of the forearm with the PRUJ dislocated.

Summary

Simple elbow dislocations are typically stable after closed reduction and associated with good outcomes. Less than 10% of patients have residual pain or stiffness. In few cases, instability persists which requires surgical repair of well-established associated soft-tissue disruptions. Fracture-dislocations can be more difficult to treat and usually require surgical stabilization to allow early elbow motion. Accurate diagnosis, methodical surgical planning and execution, and close follow-up to identify early instability are vital. Elbow stiffness is a frequent complication that is best avoided by starting motion early.

Suggested Readings

Adolfsson LE, Nestorson JO, Scheer JH. Extensive soft tissue lesions in redislocated after simple elbow dislocations. J Shoulder Elbow Surg 2017;26(7):1294–1297

Huh J, Krueger CA, Medvecky MJ, Hsu JR. Skeletal Trauma Research Consortium. Medial elbow exposure for coronoid fractures: FCU-split versus over-the-top. J Orthop Trauma 2013;27(12):730–734

McKee MD, Pugh DM, Wild LM, Schemitsch EH, King GJ. Standard surgical protocol to treat elbow dislocations with radial head and coronoid fractures. Surgical technique. J Bone Joint Surg Am 2005;87(Pt 1, Suppl 1):22–32

O'Driscoll SW, Jupiter JB, Cohen MS, Ring D, McKee MD. Difficult elbow fractures: pearls and pitfalls. Instr Course Lect 2003;52:113–134

Pugh DM, Wild LM, Schemitsch EH, King GJ, McKee MD. Standard surgical protocol to treat elbow dislocations with radial head and coronoid fractures. J Bone Joint Surg Am 2004;86(6):1122–1130

Ring D, Jupiter JB, Sanders RW, Mast J, Simpson NS. Transolecranon fracture-dislocation of the elbow. J Orthop Trauma 1997; 11(8):545–550

25 Olecranon and Monteggia Fractures

Edward A. Perez and Eric A. Barcak

Introduction

Fractures of the olecranon occur commonly in both young and elderly patients. This chapter will review important preoperative considerations as well as tactics employed in surgery. Monteggia fracture-dislocations are fractures of the ulna (usually proximal) associated with dislocation of the proximal radioulnar joint that pose unique treatment challenges.

Fractures of the Olecranon

I. Preoperative

A. History and physical exam

1. Direct injuries, such as a fall on the olecranon, can result in comminution along with ligamentous instability.

2. Indirect injuries, such as a fall on an outstretched hand, can result in tension failure of the olecranon. This often creates more simple fracture patterns.

3. A complete exam of the injured extremity should be performed. Nerve as well as vascular status should be documented.

4. A thorough inspection of the skin (especially in elderly patients) surrounding the injury should be performed to rule out open fractures and degloving injuries.

B. Anatomy

1. The semilunar notch (greater sigmoid notch) of the proximal ulna is composed of both the olecranon and the coronoid process (▶ **Fig. 25.1**).

2. Articulation of the semilunar notch with the distal humerus (trochlea) creates a hinge with approximately 180 degrees of motion.

3. A central groove in the semilunar notch interdigitates with the trochlea to assist with stability.

4. The bare area is a transverse ridge separating the distal cartilage of the coronoid from the proximal cartilage of the trochlear notch.

5. The radial notch laterally articulates with the radial head.

C. Imaging

1. Three radiographic views (anteroposterior, oblique, lateral) are necessary to assist with fracture identification.

2. Unfortunately, obtaining quality imaging can be difficult secondary to the patient's pain and altered anatomy.

3. A computed tomography scan can be useful in evaluating high-energy fracture patterns associated with instability or comminution.

4. Additionally, preoperative fluoroscopic imaging can be of use.

D. Classification

1. No universally accepted classification system.

2. Descriptive: Transverse, oblique, and comminuted.

3. The Mayo classification categorizes olecranon fractures based on three factors that affect the treatment (i.e., displacement, comminution, and stability; ▶ **Fig. 25.2**).

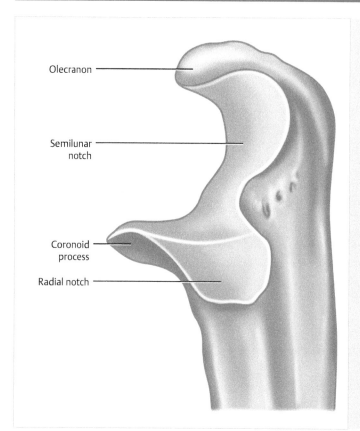

Olecranon

Semilunar
notch

Coronoid
process

Radial notch

Fig. 25.1 Osseous anatomy of the proximal ulna.

Mayo type I
Undisplaced

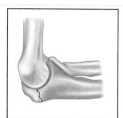

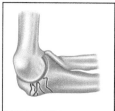

Mayo type II
Displaced

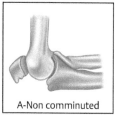

A-Non comminuted

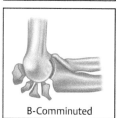

B-Comminuted

Mayo type III
Accompanying
lesions-Instability

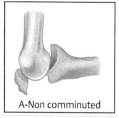

A-Non comminuted

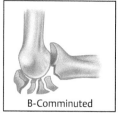

B-Comminuted

Fig. 25.2 Mayo classification of olecranon fractures.

II. Treatment

A. Initial management

    1. Initial treatment of olecranon fractures should be the placement of a well-padded posterior long-arm splint with the elbow in 45 to 90 degrees of flexion.

    2. Reduction maneuvers should be performed for fractures associated with elbow instability.

B. Definitive management

    1. Nonoperative:

        a. Nonoperative treatment is rare, but reserved for patients with stable minimally displaced fractures, low functional demands, or injuries and comorbidities that may preclude surgery.

        b. The stability of minimally displaced fractures can be determined by assessing displacement on flexion radiographs.

        c. Patients amenable to nonoperative management should have a long-arm cast applied at 45 to 90 degrees of flexion for 3 to 4 weeks, followed by advancement of motion.

    2. Operative:

        a. Most patients with displaced olecranon fractures will benefit from operative treatment.

        b. Evaluation of the fracture pattern along with the patient's clinical picture assists with determining appropriate fixation.

    3. Surgical approaches:

    Direct posterior approach is most commonly used to treat olecranon fractures.

        a. Positioning.

            i. Supine:

                • Arm adducted across the body.

                • Difficult without an assistant.

                • Beneficial in patients who must be supine for other reasons (multiple procedures).

           ii. Lateral—arm rested over an arm holder ("hockey stick"), roll of blankets, or rested on a sterile, padded mayo stand.

           iii. Prone—arm rested over an arm holder or on a table extension.

        b. An incision is made along the subcutaneous border of the ulna and extended proximally to the olecranon.

        c. A gentle lateral curve can be made when approaching the olecranon to avoid a potential site for skin irritation.

        d. Full-thickness skin flaps are created to expose the underlying fascia. There is often a traumatic rent in the fascia at the level of the fracture.

        e. Utilize the interval between flexor carpi ulnaris and extensor carpi ulnaris (ECU).

C. Reduction techniques

    1. Reduction of the fracture is determined by the fracture morphology.

    2. Simple fracture patterns with minimal comminution:

        a. Direct healing can be achieved by obtaining compression at the fracture site.

        b. The dorsal cortex can often provide an indirect read for the articular reduction.

        c. Pointed bone reduction clamp can be used to reduce the fragments.

        d. Crossing Kirschner (K) wires can be placed from proximal to distal to assist with reduction.

        e. Lag screw fixation is used when the fracture is amenable; otherwise, compression can be obtained by eccentrically drilling through a plate.

    3. Comminuted fractures present more of a challenge:

        a. The plate is often used as a template in this scenario.

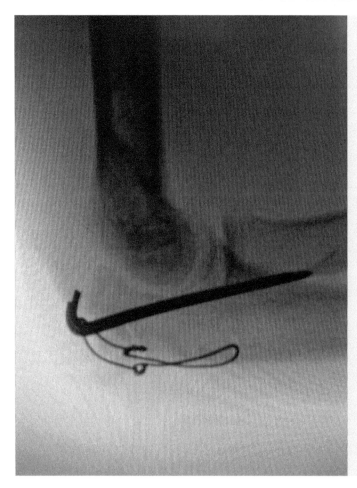

Fig. 25.3 Tension band fixation of an olecranon fracture.

    b. Length and rotation can often be judged radiographically and also by identifying bony landmarks such as the crest of the ulna.

    c. Mini-fragment fixation can assist with temporary and/or definitive stabilization of smaller fragments.

D. Fixation techniques

   1. Tension band (▶ **Fig. 25.3**):

    a. One of the most common techniques used for fixation of olecranon fractures.

    b. Must meet the following criteria:

      i. A relatively transverse fracture pattern.
      ii. Minimal articular comminution.

    c. Tension band constructs are variable and can consist of K wires, cannulated screws, wire (18 gauge), and heavy suture—Some studies have suggested that using cannulated screws or heavy suture provides similar mechanical benefits with less hardware irritation than traditional constructs (K wires and 18 gauge wire).

    d. When used in appropriate fractures, tension band fixation is a dependable, cost effective treatment option. ˙

   2. Plate and screws:

    a. Typically used for fractures that are oblique, comminuted, or associated with elbow instability.

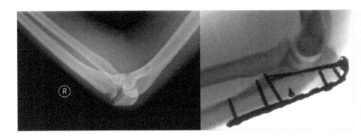

Fig. 25.4 Comminuted fracture of the olecraon treated with a precontoured locking plate.

    b. Precontoured locking plates, semitubular plates, and mini-fragment plates can be used for fixation (▶ **Fig. 25.4**).

    c. Plates can be used as neutralization devices (when accompanied with lag screw fixation), as templates in comminuted fracture patterns, and as reduction tools to prevent displacement of proximal fracture segments.

  3. Intramedullary nail or cancellous screw:

    a. Biomechanical evidence demonstrates superior strength when compared to plates or tension band, however clinical data is limited.

    b. Cannulated cancellous screw fixation:

      i. Obtain the correct starting point on an anteroposterior and lateral image.

      ii. Ensure the guidewire is inserted down the intramedullary canal.

      iii. Following drilling, consider tapping prior to screw insertion.

  4. Fragment excision and triceps advancement—typically used when extensive bone loss or poor bone quality prevents adequate fixation.

E. Complications

  1. Hardware prominence—occurs in up to 85% of patients.

  2. Loss of motion.

    a. Common after any surgery around the elbow.

    b. Can result from malreduction of the olecranon that results in a size mismatch with the trochlea.

    c. Loss of pronation and supination can be caused by screws or K wires that are too long and abut the radius.

  3. Failure of fixation—escape of the proximal fragment is most common and has been reported in locked plating constructs as well as tension bands.

  4. Nonunion is rare.

F. Rehabilitation

  1. Typically, early range of motion (ROM) can begin within 2 to 3 days if stable fixation has been obtained.

  2. Consider a period of posterior splint immobilization of 7 to 10 days for comminuted fractures or in patients with osteopenia.

  3. Non-weight-bearing of the injured extremity is usually maintained for 4 to 8 weeks. Progressive weight-bearing is permitted once signs of radiographic healing are observed.

G. Outcomes

  1. Union rates up to 98% have been reported.

  2. Often patients lose some strength and ROM compared to the contralateral side.

III. Special Considerations

A. Elderly patients with poor bone quality have been successfully treated with nonoperative management.

Monteggia Fractures

I. Preoperative

A. History and physical exam

    1. Typically occurs with a fall on a pronated outstretched hand.

    2. A complete exam of the injured extremity should be performed. Nerve as well as vascular status should be documented.

B. Imaging

    1. Anteroposterior and lateral imaging of the forearm along with orthogonal imaging of the elbow and wrist (▶ **Fig. 25.5**).

    2. Careful evaluation of the elbow must be performed with any proximal ulna shaft fracture. The radial head should bisect the capitellum on lateral imaging.

C. Classification

    1. Bado classification based on direction of dislocation of radial head (▶ **Fig. 25.6 a–d**).

       a. Type I—anterior dislocation of the radial head (most common in children).

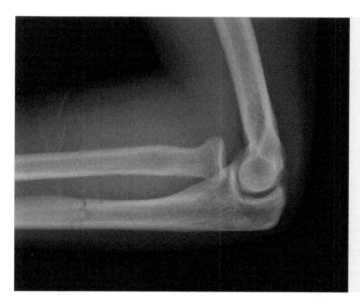

Fig. 25.5 Lateral radiograph of the elbow demonstrating a Monteggia fracture dislocation (ulna fracture with associated anterior radial head dislocation).

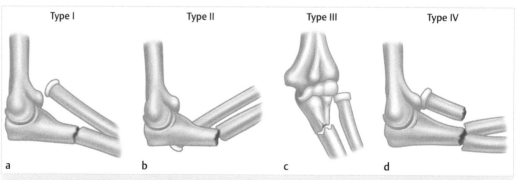

Type I   Type II   Type III   Type IV

a   b   c   d

Fig. 25.6 Bado classification of Monteggia fracture-dislocations is based on the direction of radial head dislocation. (**a**) Anterior dislocation of the radial head; (**b**) Posterior dislocation of the radial head; (**c**) Lateral dislocation of the radial head; (**d**) Fracture of both the radius and ulna associated with dislocation of the radial head.

    b. Type II—posterior dislocation of the radial head (most common in adults and is associate with radial head fracture, elbow instability, and worse outcomes).

    c. Type III—lateral dislocation of the radial head.

    d. Type IV—fracture of both the radius and ulna associated with dislocation of the radial head.

II. Treatment

A. Initial management

1. Application of a well-padded long-arm posterior splint can assist with making the patient more comfortable.

2. Closed reduction of the ulna fracture is often performed in pediatric patients. Anatomic reduction will often reduce the proximal radioulnar joint.

3. Maintenance of a closed reduction in adults is more difficult and surgical treatment is often required.

B. Definitive management

1. Application of a long arm bivalved cast with the wrist in supination can serve as definitive treatment in many pediatric patients.

2. Surgical treatment is recommended if the radial head cannot be reduced via closed means in pediatric patients.

3. Most adult Monteggia fracture-dislocations are treated operatively.

C. Surgical approach

1. Direct posterior approach as described above.

2. Lateral approach to the proximal radius.

    a. In cases of concomitant radial head fracture or irreducible proximal radioulnar joint (PRUJ) dislocation after ulna reduction, an additional deep interval may facilitate reduction.

    b. Work through the same posterior skin incision.

    c. Deep dissection between anconeus and ECU (Kocher interval) or extensor carpi radialis brevis and extensor digitorum communis (Kaplan interval) to access the radial head and PRUJ.

D. Fixation techniques

1. Similar fixation strategies to olecranon fractures as described above.

2. Open reduction and internal fixation of the proximal ulna is often performed with a plate construct.

    a. Anatomic reduction is necessary to ensure appropriate length and rotation to allow for reduction of the radial head.

    b. The size and type of plate is determined by the patient's size and bone quality. Often a 3.5 mm small fragment plate is sufficient.

    c. If comminution is present, contralateral imaging can be used to assist with judging the reduction.

3. Intramedullary implants can also be used for Monteggia fractures—flexible nails, in pediatric patients where periosteum remains intact.

4. After ulnar fixation, ROM of the elbow in flexion, extension, supination, and pronation should be performed to ensure that the radial head remains reduced.

5. Reevaluate the ulna reduction if the radial head continues to dislocate.

    a. If the ulna reduction is correct and the radial head will not reduce, then an open approach to the radial head should be performed.

    b. Case reports have described interposition of the annular ligament and capsule that preclude reduction.

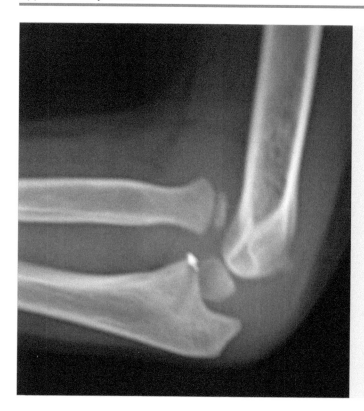

Fig. 25.7 Chronic radial head dislocation in a pediatric patient.

E. Complications

    1. Nerve palsy—most commonly posterior interosseus nerve, often transient.

    2. Chronic radial head dislocation (▶ **Fig. 25.7**).

F. Rehabilitation

    1. Active ROM is encouraged early within 2 to 3 days after surgery if stable fixation has been achieved and the PRUJ is stable throughout a full arc of flexion, extension, and pronosupination.

    2. Posterior splint immobilization until soft tissues and fracture stability permit ROM.

    3. Initial non-weight-bearing for 4 to 8 weeks. Progression of weight-bearing can begin once evidence of healing is present on radiographs.

G. Outcomes

    1. High union rates are common.

    2. Good functional outcomes can be expected in most patients.

    3. Chronic radial head dislocations can be treated with ulna osteotomy followed by open reduction of the radial head or radial head excision (▶ **Fig. 25.7** and ▶ **Fig. 25.8**).

Summary

Olecranon fractures are common in patients of all ages. Fracture morphology and degree of comminution are important considerations when executing reduction manuevers and deciding on fixation constructs. Early motion is advocated postoperatively to avoid elbow stiffness. Monteggia fracture-dislocations pose unique challenges. Persistent dislocation of the PRUJ following ORIF of the ulna warrants confirmation of anatomic reduction of the ulna.

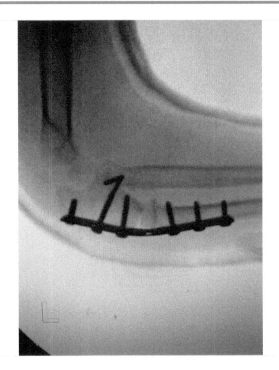

Fig. 25.8 Ulna osteotomy for treatment of a chronic Monteggia fracture- dislocation in a pediatric patient.

Suggested Readings

Fractures of the Olecranon

Duckworth AD, Bugler KE, Clement ND, Court-Brown CM, McQueen MM. Nonoperative management of displaced olecranon fractures in low-demand elderly patients. J Bone Joint Surg Am 2014;96(1):67–72

Duckworth AD, Court-Brown CM, McQueen MM. Isolated displaced olecranon fracture. J Hand Surg Am 2012;37(2):341–345

Weigand L, Bernstein J, Ahn J. Fractures in brief: olecranon fractures. Clin Orthop Relat Res 2012;40(12):3637–3641

Wilkerson JA, Rosenwasser MP. Surgical techniques of olecranon fractures. J Hand Surg Am 2014;39(8):1606–1614

Monteggia Fractures

Degreef I, De Smet L. Missed radial head dislocations in children associated with ulnar deformation: treatment by open reduction and ulnar osteotomy. J Orthop Trauma 2004;18(6):375–378

Jupiter JB, Leibovic SJ, Ribbans W, Wilk RM. The posterior Monteggia lesion. J Orthop Trauma 1991;5(4):395–402

26 Radial Head and Neck Fractures

Stephen Matthew Quinnan, Nikola Lekic, and Steven P. Kalandiak

Introduction

Radial head and neck fractures are the most common elbow fractures (33%) with an incidence of 2.5 to 2.9 per 10,000 people per year. Most radial head fractures are minimally displaced, isolated injuries that can be treated nonoperatively with a good functional outcome. Fractures can be associated with lateral collateral ligament (LCL), sometimes medial collateral ligament (MCL) injury, proximal ulna fracture, or a "terrible triad." A "terrible triad" includes radial head and coronoid process fractures and posterior elbow dislocation. The LCL is usually detached from its humeral origin. Axial load can cause interosseous membrane and distal radioulnar joint ligament injury resulting in axial forearm instability, known as an Essex–Lopresti injury. This chapter will discuss indications for nonoperative versus operative management as well as fixation options.

I. Preoperative

A. History and physical exam

   1. Most common mechanism is a fall onto an outstretched hand.

   2. Elbow swelling, pain, stiffness, and ecchymosis may be present.

   3. Lateral elbow tenderness suggests radial head and/or LCL injury.

   4. Medial elbow tenderness suggests MCL or sublime tubercle injury.

   5. Deformity suggests elbow subluxation or dislocation.

   6. The shoulder and wrist, especially the distal radioulnar joint, should be examined for associated injuries.

   7. It is important to evaluate for instability and mechanical block to elbow motion.

   8. An intra-articular elbow joint injection of local anesthetic is helpful in reducing pain and guarding for an accurate motion exam.

      a. Injection is usually performed from a lateral approach between the tip of the olecranon and the lateral epicondyle (▶ **Fig. 26.1**).

      b. After injection, forearm rotation and elbow flexion/extension are evaluated.

         i. A hard block to forearm rotation with a displaced fracture is a strong indication for surgery.
         ii. Complete elbow extension may not be possible due to hemarthrosis.
         iii. Document any crepitus or clicking.

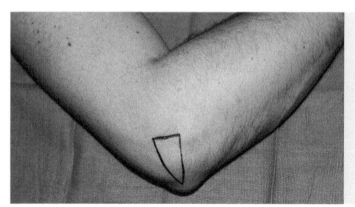

Fig. 26.1 An elbow injection can be safely performed through the "soft spot" of the lateral elbow. The "soft spot" is located within a triangular zone between the lateral epicondyle, radial head, and olecranon tip with the forearm in neutral position.

    c. Evaluate for significant ulnohumeral instability with elbow extension.

    d. Consider fluoroscopy to detect more subtle instability.

9. Perform neurovascular exam.

B. Anatomy

1. The radial head has a concave, elliptical dish shape at the radiocapitellar articulation with a flattened outer border that articulates with the ulna at the lesser sigmoid notch (radial notch).

2. The proximal radius "safe zone" for internal fixation is a 110-degree arc centered directly lateral with the forearm supinated 10 degree from neutral (▶ **Fig. 26.2**).

3. The radiocapitellar articulation is a strong stabilizer against valgus forces as is the MCL.

4. Posterolateral rotatory instability is the most common type of elbow instability that occurs secondary to disruption of the LCL.

    a. LCL origin: lateral epicondyle of the humerus.

    b. LCL insertion: crista supinatoris of the proximal ulna.

5. A "terrible triad" injury usually occurs as the result of an elbow fracture-dislocation associated with posterolateral rotatory elbow instability. LCL repair is required to restore rotational stability in a "terrible triad."

6. Longitudinal stability of the elbow is provided by the radial head articulation with the capitellum and the interosseous membrane, which transmits longitudinal forces from the distal radius to the ulna.

    a. The distal radius bears 80% of the load at the wrist.

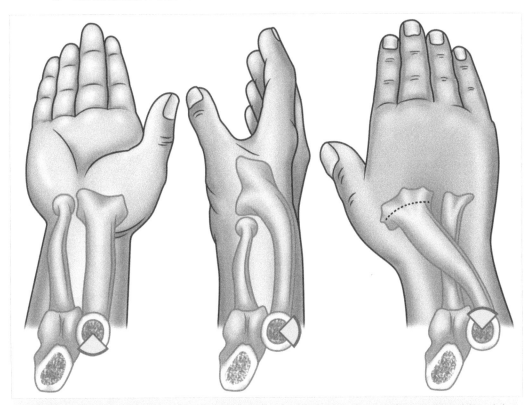

Fig. 26.2 The "safe zone" for internal fixation of the radial head/neck. There is a nonarticulating portion of the radial head (highlighted in *yellow*) in which it is safe to place hardware without the risk of impingement. This safe zone is centered straight lateral with the forearm supinated 10 degrees from neutral.

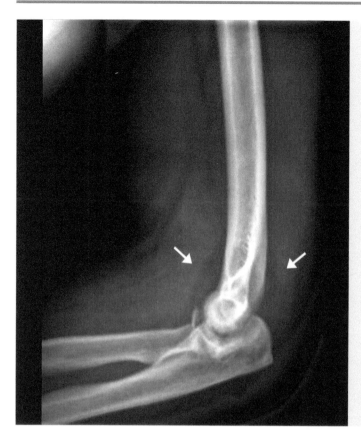

Fig. 26.3 Lateral X-ray of an elbow demonstrating a comminuted radial head fracture with *arrows* pointing to anterior and posterior "fat pads." A "fat pad" sign is a radiographic finding of lucency between the bone and the adjacent soft tissue. This is caused by soft tissue displacement due to underlying hematoma. Note that an isolated anterior fat pad in the absence of a posterior fat pad may be a variation of normal.

    b. Force transmission varies with rotational position of the elbow, but generally 60% of longitudinal forces pass through the radiocapitellar articulation.

    c. Fractures of the radial head or neck disrupt longitudinal load sharing causing all forces to be concentrated in the ulnohumeral articulation.

C. Imaging

    1. Anteroposterior and lateral X-rays should be obtained and are usually sufficient to diagnose displaced radial head fractures.

    2. Radiocapitellar or "Greenspan" view may help identifying less displaced fractures This modified lateral X-ray is obtained in neutral forearm rotation and 90 degree of elbow flexion by angling the X-ray beam 45 degree to eliminate coronoid process overlap.

    3. Nondisplaced radial head fractures can be difficult to diagnose, but are suspected when hemarthrosis causes anterior and posterior fat pad signs (▶ **Fig. 26.3**). An anterior fat pad sign alone is common in the normal population and is not a reliable marker of injury.

    4. When wrist pain is noted bilateral wrist X-rays should be obtained to evaluate for axial instability (Essex–Lopresti injury).

    5. Computed tomography (CT) scan may be required for surgical planning or if X-rays are not sufficient to visualize the location of fracture fragments. CT is especially helpful for evaluating osteochondral fragments, radial head fragment number and position, and associated fractures of the capitellum, coronoid, and proximal ulna.

    6. Magnetic resonance imaging is rarely necessary for isolated radial head fractures.

D. Classification

    1. Modified Mason classification is most commonly used as shown in ▶ **Table 26.1**.

Table 26.1 Modified Mason classification of radial head fractures

Mason classification modified by Hotchkiss and Broberg–Morrey	
Type I	Nondisplaced or minimally displaced (< 2 mm), no mechanical block to rotation
Type II	Angulated or displaced > 2 mm, may have mechanical block to forearm rotation
Type III	Comminuted and displaced, mechanical block to motion
Type IV	Radial head fracture with associated dislocation

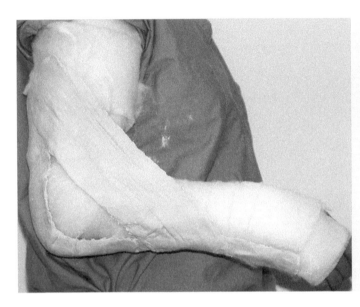

Fig. 26.4 Long arm, posterior slab splint with an "A-frame" oblique component for additional support. The splint should cross the wrist to control forearm rotation.

II. Treatment

A. Initial management

1. Reduce elbow if dislocated and immobilize with posterior slab and A-frame splint (▶ **Fig. 26.4**). Position elbow at 90 degrees with neutral forearm rotation.
2. If no displacement, dislocation or instability, only a sling for comfort is needed.
3. Ice and elevate the extremity to limit swelling and for pain control.

B. Definitive management

1. Nonoperative treatment:
   a. Indications:
      i. Less than 25% of radial head and no mechanical block to forearm rotation.
      ii. More than 25% of radial head with < 2 mm of displacement and no mechanical block to forearm rotation.
   b. Treatment course:
      i. Initial sling immobilization for comfort.
      ii. Begin active elbow and forearm range of motion after 5 to 7 days with sling reapplication between exercises for comfort.
      iii. Advance weight-bearing through elbow as tolerated by the patient.
      iv. Close clinical and radiographic follow-up to monitor fracture displacement and elbow motion.

2. Operative treatment:
    a. Surgical indications:
        i. Mechanical block to flexion/extension or forearm rotation secondary to fracture.
        ii. Intra-articular fracture fragments.
        iii. Associated elbow injuries that require surgery.
        iv. Elbow joint incongruity.
        v. Displacement > 2 mm (controversial).
    b. Treatment options:
        i. Fracture fragment excision (arthroscopic or open).
            • Usually Mason type II.
            • Indicated when fracture involves < 25% of radial head, is nonreconstructable, and displaced fragment is causing block to motion or joint incongruity.
        ii. Radial head excision.
            • Usually Mason types II and III.
            • Isolated fractures of radial head that are displaced and nonreconstructable.
            • If properly selected (no longitudinal or ulnohumeral instability), it may provide good results for many years.
            • Use with caution: in cases of lateral, medial or interosseous ligament injury, radial head excision may alter kinematics leading to pain, longitudinal instability, osteoarthritis, and valgus deformity.
        iii. ORIF:
            • Most are Mason type II, and some types III, IV.
            • Preferred treatment when technically possible.
            • Patients with good bone quality and with three or fewer fracture fragments are good candidates.
        iv. Radial head arthroplasty:
            • Usually Mason types III and IV.
            • Indicated when > 33% radial head involved, comminuted (≥3 fragments), and/or deemed nonreconstructable.
            • Provides greatest improvement to elbow stability.
C. Lateral surgical approaches
    1. May be done through a direct lateral incision or posterior skin incision with lateral and medial flaps as needed.
    2. Exploit any disruption of soft tissue encountered—extend proximal and distal as needed.
    3. Posterolateral (Kocher) approach (▶ Fig. 26.5):
        a. Skin incision (5 cm)—distal oblique incision from lateral epicondyle along anconeus/ extensor carpi ulnaris (ECU) interval.

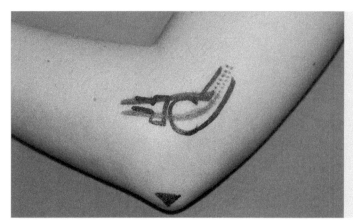

Fig. 26.5 Skin incision markings for the Kaplan and Kocher approaches. The Kaplan approach (red) is anterior to the Kocher approach (green). However, both of the deep dissection intervals can be reached through either of the two skin incisions. Both incisions can be extended up the lateral column of the humerus as necessary (dotted lines).

   b. Proximal incision along lateral supracondylar ridge.

   c. Deep interval—internervous plane between anconeus (radial nerve) and ECU (posterior interosseous nerve [PIN]). Release extensor carpi radialis brevis (ECRB) and anterior capsule to visualize anterior radial head.

   d. Create full-thickness skin flaps, expose and incise muscular fascia and deep capsule.

   e. With intact capsule and LCL, incise anterior to equator of radiocapitellar joint to protect the LCL.

   f. With forearm pronated, supinator may be incised for radial neck exposure.

   g. Posterior flap is maintained for joint stability.

   h. Pearls—protect PIN by pronating the forearm, which moves the nerve anteriorly away from radial neck (annular ligament should be repaired).

   i. Pitfalls—while exposure with a pronated forearm is relatively safe, caution is necessary distal to the annular ligament to avoid PIN injury.

4. Anterolateral (Kaplan) approach (▶ Fig. 26.5):

   a. Skin incision (5 cm), nearly straight incision from lateral epicondyle toward Lister's tubercle with arm in neutral position.

   b. Deep interval—intermuscular plane between extensor digitorum communis and extensor carpi radialis longus (ECRL)/ECRB. Release ECRB origin and anterior capsule to visualize radial head.

   c. Create full-thickness skin flaps, expose and incise muscular fascia and capsule.

   d. With intact capsule and LCL, incise anterior to equator of radiocapitellar joint to protect the LCL.

   e. With forearm pronated, supinator may be incised for radial neck exposure.

   f. Pearls and pitfalls are similar to Kocher approach above.

   g. Kaplan approach allows more direct exposure of the shaft for ORIF.

5. Posterior ("global") approach:

   a. Advantages—versatile approach with exposure to the medial and lateral elbow.

   b. Allows for fixation of virtually all fractures about the elbow.

   c. Disadvantages—long incision with large skin flaps that increase seroma/hematoma risk.

   d. A 15- to 25-cm skin incision starting in the midline proximal to the olecranon then passing just lateral to the olecranon tip and returning to midline distal to the tip.

   e. Raise full-thickness lateral and/or medial flaps as needed.

   f. Deep interval—same as Kocher or Kaplan for radial head exposure.

   g. Alternatively, may elevate anconeus and ECU off ulna and incise along crista supinatoris for direct posterior exposure of the proximal radius. Repair the LCL insertion on the crista supinatoris if released.

D. Fixation techniques

   1. ORIF:

      a. Reconstruct articular surface with provisional Kirschner wires (K-wires).

      b. Replace K-wires with mini-fragment screws (1.5, 2.0, or 2.4 mm), headless compression screws, and/or threaded K-wires as definitive fixation.

      c. If there is an associated radial neck fracture, consider using a mini-fragment or precontoured radial neck plate.

         i. Plate must be in "safe zone" (nonarticular portion) of radial head (▶ Fig. 26.2).
         ii. Plate fixation with three screws distal to the fracture is recommended.
         iii. Distal limit of plate placement is due to PIN.

   2. Radial head arthroplasty (▶ Fig. 26.6):

      a. Multiple implant options.

      b. Goal of implant selection is to replicate native head size and radial length.

c. After excising radial head, estimate size of implant by grossly reassembling pieces and measuring diameter of the radial head.

d. Care must be taken not to "overstuff" radiocapitellar joint by placing an implant that is too long or large.

   i. "Overstuffing" causes an incongruent joint and can cause lateral radiocapitellar and/or medial ulnohumeral wear.

   ii. An anteroposterior X-ray of an "overstuffed" elbow (▶ **Fig. 26.7**) will demonstrate widening of the lateral end of the medial ulnohumeral joint compared to its medial side. Excessive implant length can also cause varus deformity at the elbow.

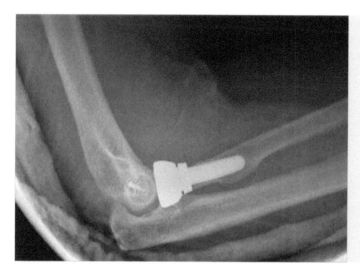

Fig. 26.6 Radial head arthroplasty with a lateral collateral ligament repair using a suture anchor.

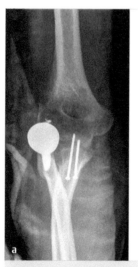 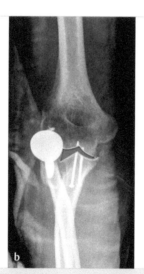 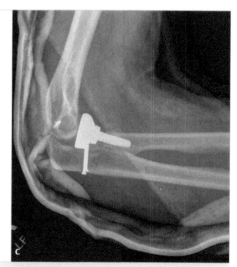

Fig. 26.7 (**a**) Anteroposterior radiograph of an elbow following radial head arthroplasty. (**b**) Ulnohumeral joint incongruity (*red*) is seen due to radial head overstuffing. The radial aspect of the ulnohumeral joint has greater gapping than the ulnar side. (**c**) Lateral radiographic view of the same elbow—note the incongruity of the ulnohumeral joint also seen on this view.

E. Complications

1. Surgical approach—injury to PIN when working distal to the annular ligament.

2. Radial head excision—joint laxity, early arthritis at the ulnohumeral joint.

3. Radial head fixation—hardware penetration into radiocapitellar joint due to concave radial head anatomy or ulnohumeral joint if screws are too long.

4. Radial head replacement:

   a. Large implants cause joint "overstuffing," incongruity and early degenerative change.

   b. Small implants can permit both longitudinal or valgus instability, and laxity due to suboptimal soft-tissue tensioning.

   c. In a recent large literature review:

      i. Overall revision rate for radial head arthroplasty is 8%.
      ii. High rate of implant osteolysis (50% of press-fit stems).
      iii. Most cases of osteolyses are asymptomatic.
      iv. No discernible benefit to any particular type of implant material, means of stem fixation, or polarity of prosthesis.

F. Rehabilitation

1. Postoperatively, the elbow is splinted in 90 degree of flexion.

2. Early range of motion within a safe arc is determined by elbow stability in surgery.

3. When instability is present, patient's elbow extension is blocked just short of point instability begins, and is gradually increased in 10 to 20 degree increments to full extension over several weeks.

4. Nonsteroidal anti-inflammatory drugs (NSAIDs) or radiation therapy may be used if the patient is thought to be at high risk of heterotopic ossification.

5. Radiation therapy and NSAIDs may increase risk of nonunion for fractures undergoing ORIF.

G. Outcomes

1. Results of poorly selected radial head excision show less strength, and worse function, compared to ORIF (except in a few select cases as discussed above).

2. Mason type II fractures treated with ORIF may have good-to-excellent functional outcomes.

3. Mason type III fractures treated with radial head arthroplasty may have good-to-excellent outcomes.

   a. However, ORIF can have good-to-excellent outcomes in Mason type III fractures if *stable* anatomic reduction, articular congruity, and early motion protocol can be achieved.

   b. Patient age, bone quality, number of fracture fragments, and presence of instability are all considerations when choosing to repair or replace the radial head.

III. Special Considerations For Pediatric and/or Geriatric Patients

A. Radial neck fractures in children

1. Children more often fracture through the physis or metaphysis of the proximal ulna than through the radial head.

2. The most common mechanism is a fall on an outstretched hand.

3. Up to 30 degree of angulation is generally accepted for nonoperative treatment of the fracture.

4. Greater than 30 degree of angulation is usually an indication for operative intervention, which may be performed by percutaneous (preferable) or open methods.

B. Pulled elbow syndrome (nursemaid's elbow)

1. Radial head subluxation.

2. Mean age 2 to 3 years, rare after age 7.

3. Mechanism of injury—longitudinal traction on extended elbow.

   a. Most commonly occurs when parents hold the hand of a child who is falling (e.g., during a misstep).

   b. Allows for partial slippage of annular ligament past radial head, into radiocapitellar joint.

   c. Forearm pronation renders elbow particularly vulnerable to this pathology due to the asymmetric anatomy that allows the round, narrow region of the radial head to slide past the annular ligament.

   d. In children less than 5 years, the radial epiphysis is not ossified which allows the relatively soft chondral epiphysis to slip past the annular ligament.

C. History and physical exam

   1. A traction event is important for diagnosis.

   2. If unwitnessed fall is the reason for elbow pain, other elbow pathologies including fractures should be higher on the differential.

   3. On exam, the affected extremity is not utilized and there is tenderness over radial head region.

D. Imaging—anteroposterior and lateral X-rays

   1. Evaluate radiocapitellar line: drawn down center of proximal radial shaft, passing through center of capitellum.

   2. X-ray technicians often unintentionally reduce the subluxation when the forearm is supinated for X-ray positioning.

E. Treatment

   1. Closed reduction is preferred and reliable. The maneuver follows: supinate forearm, flex elbow, often an audible snap is heard. If supination fails, hyperpronation may be attempted.

   2. Open reduction—only if chronic radial head subluxation and pain (very rarely indicated).

   3. Usually no immobilization necessary, but sling may be applied for comfort for 2 to 3 days.

Summary

Most minimally displaced and nondisplaced radial head fractures can be treated nonoperatively. Surgical indications include mechanical block to motion, intra-articular fragment(s), elbow subluxation/incrongruity, associated elbow injuries, and significant displacement (commonly cited at >2 mm but is controversial). Potential surgical options include partial excision, ORIF (commonly for Mason II), and radial head arthroplasty (commonly for comminuted fractures).

Suggested Readings

De Mattos CB, Ramski DE, Kushare IV, Angsanuntsukh C, Flynn JM. Radial neck fractures in children and adolescents: an examination of operative and nonoperative treatment and outcomes. J Pediatr Orthop 2016;36(1):6–12

Pike JM, Athwal GS, Faber KJ, King GJ. Radial head fractures—an update. J Hand Surg Am 2009;34(3):557–565

Ruchelsman DE, Christoforou D, Jupiter JB. Fractures of the radial head and neck. J Bone Joint Surg Am 2013;95(5):469–478, 23467871

Tejwani NC, Mehta H. Fractures of the radial head and neck: current concepts in management. J Am Acad Orthop Surg 2007;15(7):380–387, 17602027

27 Radius and Ulna Shaft Fractures

Robert J. Wetzel

Introduction

Fractures of the shaft of the radius and ulna (both bone forearm fractures) often occur from high-energy trauma, axial load injuries such as falls from height, and direct blows from protecting one's face and head. Open injuries are also common and even small poke holes should be investigated to ensure an open injury is not missed. Tenets of treatment are anatomic restoration of the radius and ulna to restore the radial bow and forearm motion. Rigid internal fixation obviates the need for immobilization and allows for immediate motion to avoid stiffness (▶ **Video 27.1**).

Keywords: radius, ulna, fracture, diaphysis, both bone forearm

I. Preoperative

A. History and physical exam

1. Low energy—fall onto an outstretch arm.

2. High energy—motor vehicle collision, pedestrian struck.

3. Often seen when defending one's face or head from oncoming trauma.

B. Anatomy

1. Osteology:

   a. Forearm rotation—axis of rotation is from the radial head at the elbow to the ulnar head at the wrist (effectively the radius rotates around the ulna).

   b. Radial bow and integrity of the interosseous membrane (IOM) are critical to maintain rotation of the forearm—central band, most important component of the IOM, if injured requires reconstruction. It acts as a "joint" in terms of importance of maintaining and restoring motion after an injury.

2. Soft tissue:

   a. Mobile wad.

   b. Dorsal compartment.

   c. Volar compartment.

C. Imaging

1. Orthogonal views of the elbow, forearm, wrist.

2. Consider computed tomography scan if there is extension into the elbow or wrist to evaluate the intra-articular involvement.

D. Classification

1. No widely accepted classification scheme is utilized.

2. Based most commonly on diaphyseal location (proximal one-third, mid one-third, distal one-third).

3. AO/OTA (anatomic) classification:

   a. Bone – 2.

   b. Midshaft – 2.

      i. A – simple.
      ii. B – wedge.
      iii. C – complex.

4. Nightstick fracture—isolated ulnar shaft fracture.

    a. Two categories—less than 50% displaced and more than 50% displaced. It can be successfully treated in a fracture brace if < 50% displaced.

5. Isolated radius fractures:

    a. These are rare, and can be ballistic or a direct blow.

    b. Not easily treated nonoperatively due to need for maintenance of the radial bow and preservation of forearm motion.

    c. Beware of the "isolated" radius fracture as it may be a subtle Galeazzi injury.

6. Galeazzi injury (see Chapter 28, Distal Radius and Galeazzi Fractures, for additional information). Typically distal one-third radius shaft fracture with distal radioulnar joint (DRUJ) subluxation or dislocation.

7. Essex–Lopresti injury:

    a. Longitudinal injury to the IOM seen with radial head fractures and DRUJ injuries.

    b. Associated with other injuries due to falls from height (i.e., lumbar spine injuries, calcaneus fractures, and femoral neck fractures).

    c. Highly unstable injury.

II. Treatment

A. Initial management

1. Full primary survey.

2. Assessment of soft-tissue envelope.

3. Open versus Closed.

4. Assess for compartment syndrome:

    a. Clinical exam is most reliable in an alert patient.

    b. Consider compartment pressure monitoring in an obtunded patient (see Chapter 13, Acute Compartment Syndrome).

5. Evaluate for associated or distracting injuries.

6. Temporizing plaster splint immobilization.

    a. Midshaft, distal third—sugar-tong splint.

    b. Proximal third—sugar-tong splint and consider adding long arm extension.

B. Definitive management

1. Vast majority of forearm fractures are treated operatively due to the importance of maintaining forearm motion and preventing prolonged immobilization resulting in elbow and wrist stiffness.

2. Nondisplaced bony injuries with intact IOM can be treated nonoperatively, nightstick fractures < 50% displacement.

C. Surgical approaches

1. Dual incision approaches are preferred in both bone forearm fractures to avoid radioulnar synostosis.

2. Volar approach of Henry (▶ **Fig. 27.1**)—utilitarian to radial shaft; can be extended proximally to the shoulder and distally to the wrist.

    a. Incision can be extended from lateral to biceps tendon at the elbow flexion crease to the wrist lateral to flexor carpi radialis (FCR) tendon.

    b. Incise fascia and develop the superficial interval by dissecting between brachioradialis (BR) and FCR distally, BR and pronator teres (PT) more proximally. Alternatively, the FCR tendon subsheath can be incised distally and FCR and flexor policis longus (FPL) are retracted ulnarly, giving access to pronator quadratus (PQ) and the distal radial shaft.

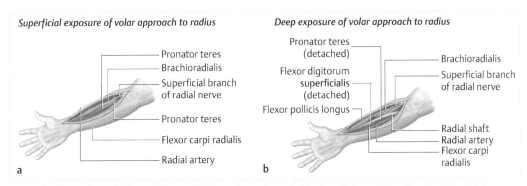

Superficial exposure of volar approach to radius

- Pronator teres
- Brachioradialis
- Superficial branch of radial nerve
- Pronator teres
- Flexor carpi radialis
- Radial artery

a

Deep exposure of volar approach to radius

- Pronator teres (detached)
- Flexor digitorum superficialis (detached)
- Flexor pollicis longus
- Brachioradialis
- Superficial branch of radial nerve
- Radial shaft
- Radial artery
- Flexor carpi radialis

b

Fig. 27.1 **(a)** Incision and superficial interval of the volar approach of Henry. **(b)** Deep interval and exposure of the volar surface of the radial shaft.

    c. Internervous plane is BR (radial nerve) and PT (median nerve) proximally and FCR (median nerve) distally.

    d. Superficial sensory branch of the radial nerve is on the undersurface of the BR and multiple recurrent leash vessels from the radial artery will need to be ligated or cauterized. The radial artery can be mobilized radially or ulnarly in the distal one-third of the forearm and is retracted ulnarly in the proximal two-third of the forearm.

    e. Proximally—follow the biceps tendon to the biceps tuberosity to expose the proximal shaft.

    f. Midshaft—pronate the forearm to expose the lateral insertion of the PT and release if needed to expose the midshaft of the radius.

    g. Distally sweep FPL ulnarly and release PQ from the radial border of the radius and expose the distal shaft.

3. Dorsal approach of Thompson (▶ **Fig. 27.2**)—often used for very proximal radial shaft exposure and open fractures.

    a. Incision landmarks are from lateral epicondyle to Lister's tubercle.

    b. Incise fascia between extensor carpi radialis brevis (ECRB) and extensor digitorum communis (EDC).

    c. Distally, the dissection plane changes to ECRB and abductor policis longus (APL).

    d. Internervous plane is ECRB (radial) and EDC (posterior interosseous nerve [PIN]) and APL (PIN) distally.

    e. Deep dissection focuses on finding and protecting PIN.

        i. It is easiest to find the PIN distally as it exits the supinator muscle and dissect it proximally, protecting branches that innervate the supinator itself.

        ii. Can also dissect from the proximal origin of the supinator and find the PIN proximally.

        iii. PIN can be easily mobilized dorsally (ulnarly) and protected by supinating the forearm for midshaft and distal exposure.

        iv. Pronate the forearm and mobilize the PIN volar (radial) when exposing the far proximal radius.

    f. Full access to the dorsal radius is then achieved with subperiosteal dissection.

4. Direct approach to the ulnar shaft:

    a. Skin incision along the subcutaneous border of the ulna.

    b. Interval is between extensor carpi ulnaris (ECU) and flexor carpi ulnaris (FCU).

    c. Internervous plane is ECU (PIN) and FCU (ulnar nerve), respectively.

    d. Subperiosteal dissection or submuscular dissection is then performed to expose the ulna.

    e. Of note, the dorsal or, less commonly, the volar aspect of the ulna shaft is typically exposed for plate location to avoid subcutaneous hardware prominence.

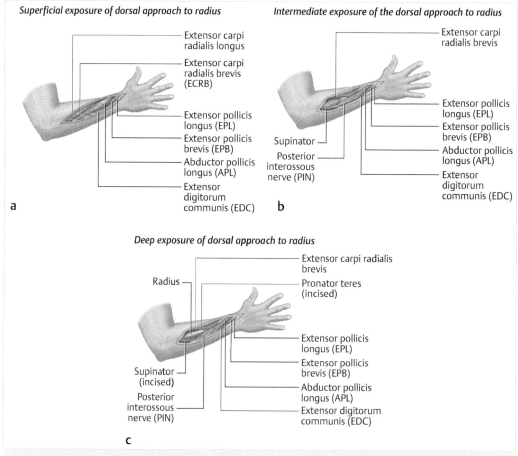

Superficial exposure of dorsal approach to radius

- Extensor carpi radialis longus
- Extensor carpi radialis brevis (ECRB)
- Extensor pollicis longus (EPL)
- Extensor pollicis brevis (EPB)
- Abductor pollicis longus (APL)
- Extensor digitorum communis (EDC)

a

Intermediate exposure of the dorsal approach to radius

- Extensor carpi radialis brevis
- Extensor pollicis longus (EPL)
- Extensor pollicis brevis (EPB)
- Abductor pollicis longus (APL)
- Extensor digitorum communis (EDC)
- Supinator
- Posterior interossous nerve (PIN)

b

Deep exposure of dorsal approach to radius

- Extensor carpi radialis brevis
- Pronator teres (incised)
- Radius
- Extensor pollicis longus (EPL)
- Extensor pollicis brevis (EPB)
- Abductor pollicis longus (APL)
- Extensor digitorum communis (EDC)
- Supinator (incised)
- Posterior interossous nerve (PIN)

c

Fig. 27.2 (**a**) Incision and superficial interval of the dorsal approach of Thompson. (**b**) Intermediate exposure with the course of the posterior interossus nerve identified. (**c**) Deep interval with mobilization of PIN and exposure of the dorsal surface of the radial shaft.

D. Fixation techniques (▶**Fig. 27.3**)

1. Compression plating:

   a. Anatomic reduction with lag screw fixation followed by volar neutralization plating.

   b. Alternatively, primary compression plating without lag screw can be performed to achieve primary bone healing by creating an axilla in the plate.

   c. 3.5 mm compression plates are recommended and smaller or weaker plates should typically be avoided so as not to lose reduction with postoperative early motion.

   d. Initial flexible fixation may be utilized with mini-fragment plates to hold reductions anatomic, if the proper trajectory for an independent lag screw is not feasible.

2. Bridge plating:

   a. Useful if the injury cannot be reconstructed anatomically.

   b. Avoid stripping in zone of injury.

   c. Radial bow must be restored to allow for proper forearm motion.

      i. Plate must sit eccentric if bow is properly restored (i.e., straight plate on a curved bone).

      ii. Alternatively, precontoured plates that have a built in radial bow can be used. These can be helpful in highly comminuted injuries.

   d. Ulnar bridge plating can be done percutaneously with small incisions away from the zone of injury.

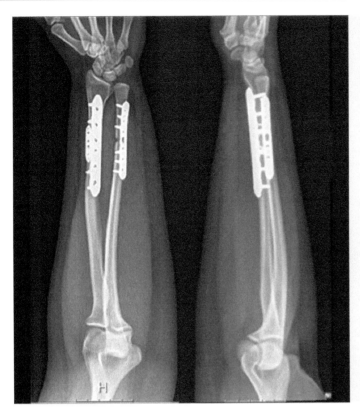

Fig. 27.3 Anteroposterior and lateral view demonstration of rigid internal fixation with compression plating and restoration of the radial bow. Note the example of mini-fragment flexible fixation used as a reduction aide on the radial shaft.

3. Locking fixation—generally not necessary in the diaphysis of the forearm unless bone quality is poor or a short segment requires fixed-angle fixation (i.e., small radial neck fragment).

4. Open fractures:

   a. Devitalized bone should be thoroughly debrided and excised to avoid an infectious nidus.

   b. Typically, acute bone grafting of bone defects in open fractures should be avoided due to risk for infection, although no definitive evidence supports this.

   c. Antibiotic cement spacers or beads should be considered for planned staged bone grafting once the wound is sterile.

E. Complications

1. Compartment syndrome:

   a. Most serious complication that can lead to Volkmann's contracture.

      i. Flexion contracture of the hand and wrist.
      ii. Results in a claw-like deformity of the hand and digits.

   b. Must have high clinical suspicion in closed and open injuries.

2. Fasciotomy should be performed from the carpal tunnel distally (including a carpal tunnel release) to the lacertus fibrosus proximally.

   a. Vital structures at risk—radial artery, median nerve, lateral antebrachial cutaneous nerve, and superficial sensory branch of the radial nerve.

   b. A volar compartment release may be sufficient in the majority of cases. Recheck dorsal and mobile wad compartments after volar release.

3. Radioulnar synostosis:

   a. Seen most frequently in high-energy injuries with significant injury to the IOM, and injuries where both bones are approached through one incision.

   b. Loss of forearm motion is the result.

    c.   Should be followed until maturity in a similar fashion as heterotopic ossification.

    d.   Can be resected (once mature) if symptomatic or limits function. Postoperatively, administer heterotopic ossification prophylaxis (radiation therapy or nonsteroidal anti-inflammatory drugs).

4.   Forearm stiffness:

    a.   Most frequently seen in supination.

    b.   Initially treat with aggressive physical and occupational therapy.

    c.   Can be avoided if early motion is initiated.

5.   Malunion/nonunion:

    a.   Malunion can be avoided reliably if, after fixation is complete, intra-operative range of motion is compared to the contralateral forearm. If malreduction is suspected, the fracture length and rotation should be meticulously inspected to avoid permanent loss of motion.

    b.   Nonunion is rare (▶ **Fig. 27.4**).

        i.   Nonunion repair success rates are high.

       ii.   Treated with autogenous bone grafting and revision compression plating.

      iii.   If bone loss is present, induced membrane technique can be utilized with a staged approach using a cement spacer with subsequent autogenous cancellous or structural autografting.

    c.   Infection workup with inflammatory markers should be performed to rule out occult infection.

6.   Infection:

    a.   Adequate debridement should be performed and initiation of culture-directed antibiotic therapy.

    b.   Hardware can be retained if less than 6 weeks from surgery. Alternatively, hardware exchange can be performed to increase eradication of biofilm from the wound.

7.   Bone loss:

    a.   Seen mainly in open fractures.

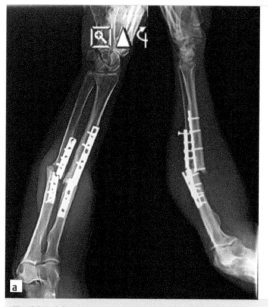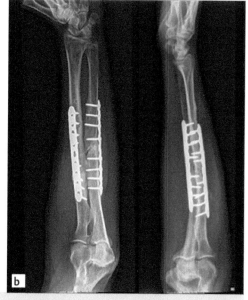

Fig. 27.4 **(a)** Anteroposterior (AP) and lateral views of a nonunion of the radial and ulnar shaft resulting in refractures and hardware failure after a fall. **(b)** AP and lateral views post-repair of the nonunion with rigid internal fixation with compression plating and autogenous bone grafting.

b. Acute bone grafting is recommended as an option for comminution greater than one-third the diaphyseal circumference—no definitive data regarding safety of acute grafting in open fractures is available.

c. Staged bone grafting is an effective treatment option by utilization of the induced membrane technique.

F. Rehabilitation

1. If stable fixation is achieved and the soft-tissue envelope is amenable, only a soft dressing is necessary.

2. Immediate shoulder, elbow, forearm, wrist, and hand/finger motion should be initiated.

3. Immobilize in a splint for soft tissue rest if deemed necessary. Motion should be initiated as soon as the soft tissues allows.

4. Lifting restrictions are at the discretion of the surgeon:

a. Typically, weight-bearing as tolerated; although, some surgeons might limit weight-bearing for 4 to 8 weeks until there is radiographic evidence of healing.

b. Consider immediate weight-bearing for mobilization purposes in polytrauma patients.

G. Outcomes

1. Union rates are approximately 98%.

2. Functional outcomes are not well reported in large groups and highly dependent on type and severity of injury.

3. Studies with smaller groups have shown some degree of loss of grip and forearm strength, and a 10-degree loss of rotational forearm motion compared to contralateral forearm.

III. Special Considerations for Pediatric Patients

A. Incomplete fractures: most commonly treated conservatively with closed reduction and casting.

1. Greenstick: Incomplete cortical disruption.

2. Plastic deformation:

a. It can be difficult to reduce.

b. May have to complete the fracture.

c. Can cause persistent radial head dislocations (in Monteggia injuries) if deformation not corrected.

3. Buckle fractures:

a. More common in metaphyseal region.

b. Incomplete compression injury.

c. Stable injuries that heal with cast immobilization.

B. Acceptable parameters for nonoperative treatment in pediatric patients.

1. Operative indications:

a. Less than 10 years old:

i. More than 15 degrees angulation in coronal or sagittal plane.
ii. More than 45 degrees malrotation.
iii. Bayonet apposition > 1 cm.
iv. Open injury.

b. Ten years of age or older:

i. More than 10 to 15 degrees angulation.
ii. Any malrotation; cannot remodel in the plane of rotation.
iii. Any shortening.
iv. Open injury.

2. Casting techniques:

   a. Short-arm versus long-arm casting. No difference in loss of reduction or outcomes is seen.

   b. Must obtain 3-point bend.

   c. Cast index (width of cast on lateral view/width of cast on anteroposterior view) should be less than 0.8; if more than 0.8, then high association with loss of reduction.

   d. Can remodel residual angulation ~10 to 12 degrees per year.

3. Fixation techniques:

   a. Intramedullary flexible nail fixation.

      i. Ulna—start point at the olecranon process.
      ii. Radius—can start at Lister's tubercle or radial styloid.

         • Must be proximal to the physis.
         • Mini open approach avoids injury to extensor tendons or superficial sensory branch of the radial nerve.

   b. Open reduction and internal fixation with plates and screws:

      i. Similar union and alignment results to flexible intramedullary nails.
      ii. Should be considered in the case of refractures (can be seen in up to 5% of cases).
      iii. Typically 3.5-mm plates.

Summary

Radius and ulna shaft fractures are common and usually operative injuries. Typically, a volar approach to the radius is performed in addition to a direct approach to the ulna. A dorsal approach to the radius is sometimes utilized in rare circumstances, but it comes with a significant risk to the posterior interosseous nerve. The forearm itself can be considered a joint and restoration of the radial bow is needed to allow for proper range of motion. Rigid internal fixation should be utilized along with immediate postoperative mobilization to prevent stiffness. Two incisions should be used to avoid a radioulnar synostosis, and there should be a high suspicion for compartment syndrome in high-energy injuries (closed and open). Pediatric fractures in patients younger than 10 years of age can be treated nonoperatively despite some residual deformity due to the remodeling potential. Operative pediatric injuries can be performed with flexible intramedullary nails in addition to plate fixation.

Suggested Readings

Anderson LD, Sisk D, Tooms RE, Park WI III. Compression-plate fixation in acute diaphyseal fractures of the radius and ulna. J Bone Joint Surg Am 1975;57(3):287–297

Baldwin K, Morrison MJ III, Tomlinson LA, Ramirez R, Flynn JM. Both bone forearm fractures in children and adolescents, which fixation strategy is superior - plates or nails? A systematic review and meta-analysis of observational studies. J Orthop Trauma 2014;28(1):e8–e14

Bot AGJ, Doornberg JN, Lindenhovius ALC, Ring D, Goslings JC, van Dijk CN. Long-term outcomes of fractures of both bones of the forearm. J Bone Joint Surg Am 2011;93(6): 527–532

Jones JA. Immediate internal fixation of high-energy open forearm fractures. J Orthop Trauma 1991;5(3):272–279

McQueen MM, Gaston P, Court-Brown CM. Acute compartment syndrome. Who is at risk? J Bone Joint Surg Br 2000;82(2):200–203

Weinberg DS, Park PJ, Boden KA, Malone KJ, Cooperman DR, Liu RW. Anatomic investigation of commonly used landmarks for evaluating rotation during forearm fracture reduction. J Bone Joint Surg Am 2016;98(13):1103–1112

28 Distal Radius and Galeazzi Fractures

Nicholas E. Crosby and Jue Cao

Introduction

Distal radius fractures are common orthopaedic conditions and these represent a large percentage of injuries treated in the emergency room, office, and operating room settings. The distal radius articular surface and its alignment require special attention, as does the ligamentous stability of the distal radioulnar joint (▶Video 28.1, ▶Video 28.2).

Keywords: distal, radius, wrist, galeazzi, fracture

I. Preoperative

A. History

    1. The mechanism of injury dictates the degree of injury severity. Attempts must be made to quantify both the amount of energy transmitted through the distal radius as well as the direction of the force transmitted.

    2. Associated injuries more proximal to the distal radius should be assessed. The surgeon must ask about pain in the forearm, elbow, and shoulder.

B. Physical exam

    1. Always search entire extremity for signs of direct trauma, such as open wounds, bruising, or lacerations. Open fractures often include small skin lacerations that can be found on the ulnar wrist where the ulna styloid has penetrated through the skin.

    2. Functional evaluation and point tenderness is noted on the entire extremity.

    3. Thorough neurological examination of the median, ulnar, and radial nerves is imperative. This includes fine sensation and carpal tunnel syndrome findings.

    4. Complete vascular examination is necessary but frequently normal.

C. Anatomy

    1. Osseous:

        a. The radius bows laterally allowing for rotation around the straight ulna.

        b. Articular surfaces include scaphoid and lunate facets separated by an interfacet prominence (sagittal ridge), and the sigmoid notch as part of the distal radioulnar joint (DRUJ; ▶Fig. 28.1).

        c. The radial bow and DRUJ relationships are necessary for proper forearm rotation.

    2. Soft tissue:

        a. Brachioradialis tendon inserts on the radial side of the styloid as the floor of the first dorsal compartment. It often acts as a deforming force in unstable fractures.

        b. Pronator quadratus covers the volar distal surface of both the radius and ulna.

        c. The triangular fibrocartilagenous complex (TFCC) stabilizes the DRUJ through superficial, and more important, deep ligaments.

            i. The superficial ligaments attach to the ulnar styloid, which is often fractured with distal radius fractures.

           ii. Deep ligaments run from the fovea of the ulna to the volar and dorsal rims of the sigmoid notch.

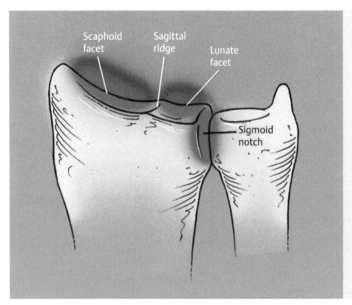

Fig. 28.1 Articular facets of the distal radius.

In figure: Scaphoid facet, Sagittal ridge, Lunate facet, Sigmoid notch

  d. The radius and ulnar are strongly connected by the interosseous membrane ligaments.

  e. Multiple extrinsic wrist ligaments stabilize the carpus. The dorsal radiocarpal ligament is a potential deforming force in comminuted intra-articular fractures.

 3. Nerve and artery:

  a. Anterior interosseous nerve (AIN) enters the pronator quadratus muscle proximally.

  b. The median nerve runs volar to the distal radius with the profundus tendons between the two.

  c. Ulnar nerve runs the length of the forearm deep to the flexor carpi ulnaris (FCU) muscle and tendon to just proximal to the wrist flexion crease where is passes into Guyon's canal radial to the tendon and the pisiform.

  d. Radial artery runs along the side of the forearm in close proximity to the radial metaphysis. A volar accessory branch crosses over the flexor carpal radialis (FCR) at the wrist flexion crease.

D. Imaging

 1. Radiographs—these are mainstay in assessment of distal radius fractures.

  a. It is imperative that adequate wrist X-rays are obtained. If possible, obtain a zero-rotation posterior-anterior (PA) view, a lateral view, and a fossa lateral view.

  b. Normal distal radius parameters:

   i. Radial height: 13 mm.
   ii. Radial inclination: 23 degrees.
   iii. Volar tilt: 11 degrees.
   iv. Teardrop angle: 70 degrees. A 45 degree pronated oblique view may help assess the dorsal ulnar cortex of the dorsal lunate fossa and the dorsal margin of the sigmoid notch.

  c. Contralateral X-rays may help identify normal variant anatomy.

  d. Fracture of the distal radius within 7.5 cm of the articular surface has been shown to be associated with a higher incidence of Galeazzi fracture and DRUJ injury.

 2. Computed tomography (CT) scans—although not always necessary, CT can be useful (after closed reduction) for assessment of intra-articular involvement and surgical planning purposes.

3. Magnetic resonance imaging (MRI) studies—usually not necessary for most distal radius fractures but MRI can be useful in evaluating soft-tissue injuries including TFCC and scapholunate ligament injuries.

E. Classification: Intraobserver and interobserver reliability is variable in most systems, so treatment indications based on classifications alone are difficult. Specific fracture-type eponyms are commonly utilized. Priority should focus on stable versus unstable patterns that require fixation.

1. AO/OTA classification:

   a. Typically higher inter/intraobserver reliability than most other systems.

   b. Good for description, but prognosis and treatment are not easily addressed.

2. Eponyms:

   a. Volar/dorsal Barton fractures—partial articular fractures through oblique shear force. The carpus displaces with the fracture fragment making this an unstable fracture amenable to buttress plate fixation (▶Fig. 28.2).

   b. Chauffeur's fracture—shear fracture line through the scaphoid facet exiting the radial metadiaphyseal cortex (▶Fig. 28.3).

      i. Longitudinal load and pull of the brachioradialis often displace the main radial styloid fragment.

      ii. Buttress or interfragmentary fixation is necessary.

   c. Colles' fracture (▶Fig. 28.4)—metaphyseal fracture with dorsal angulation and displacement.

      i. Often fragility fracture and cortical comminution present a significant concern for fracture stability.

   d. Smith's fracture—metaphyseal fracture with volar angulation and displacement (▶Fig. 28.5).

   e. Galeazzi fractures are fractures of the radius with an associated DRUJ disruption. These fractures can be of either distal radius or the radial shaft (▶Fig. 28.6).

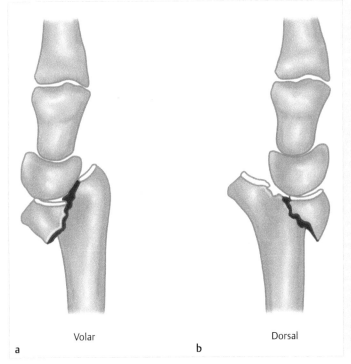

Fig. 28.2 (a) Volar Barton fracture and **(b)** dorsal Barton fracture.

Volar

Dorsal

a

b

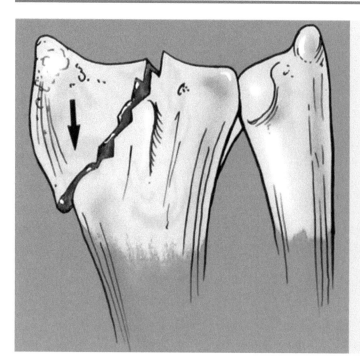

Fig. 28.3 Chauffeur's fracture of the radial styloid.

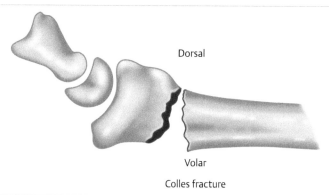

Dorsal

Volar

Colles fracture

Fig. 28.4 Colles' fracture: extra-articular fracture of the distal radius metaphysis with dorsal angulation.

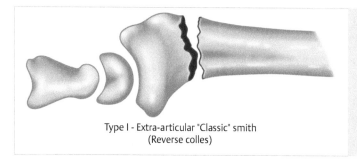

Type I - Extra-articular "Classic" smith
(Reverse colles)

Fig. 28.5 Smith's fracture: extra-articular fracture of the distal radius metaphysis with volar angulation.

3. Column theory:
   a. Characterization of fracture patterns that reference three columns (▶ **Fig. 28.7**).
   b. Stabilization must be evaluated and treated appropriately for all three columns. Particular attention is given to the intermediate column consisting mostly of the lunate facet and its supportive bone.

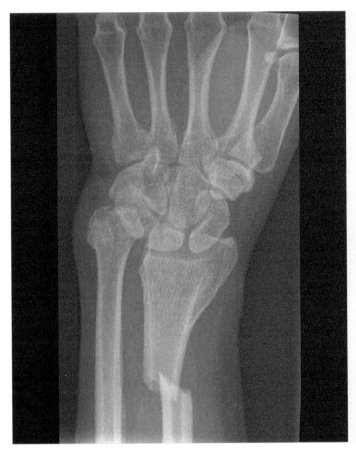

Fig. 28.6 Galeazzi fracture-dislocation: fracture of the distal radial shaft with associated distal radioulnar joint dislocation.

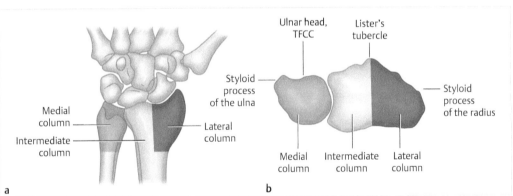

Fig. 28.7 (a, b) Three columns of the distal radius and ulna.

II. Treatment

A. Initial management—depends on location and timing of presentation.

1. Emergency department: Attempts should be made to perform a closed reduction of distal radius fractures that are displaced.

2. Office: Attempts should be made to proceed with closed reduction if the surgeon thinks the fracture is amendable to nonoperative management.

3. Open fractures require urgent antibiotics and debridement.

4. Hematoma block versus sedation—sedation might be indicated in pediatric patients or those with median nerve dysfunction (hematoma block may cause analgesia to the median nerve, precluding or delaying accurate post-eduction neurologic exam).

5. After hematoma block or during sedation, finger traps and weight for 5 to 15 minutes can provide traction to aid in reduction via ligamentotaxis.

6. Acceptable reduction criteria in an adult population:

   a. Radial height: < 3 mm shortening.

   b. Articular step-off: < 2 mm.

   c. Volar tilt: < 10 degree dorsal angulation.

   d. Radial inclination: < 5 degree change.

   e. Teardrop angle: 70 degree.

7. Geriatric population: In patients > 65 years of age and/or of low demand, greater degrees of deformity can be accepted.

8. A well-molded sugar-tong splint or a volar/dorsal splint should be applied with minimal cast padding and good three-point mold should be applied.

B. Definitive management

Several criteria determine the need for surgical or nonsurgical treatment. In 2009, the American Academy of Orthopaedic Surgeon (AAOS) developed guidelines of moderate strength for surgical treatment and in 2013, a large panel of treating physicians provided appropriate use criteria (AUC) for a variety of specific clinical fracture scenarios (216 cases) to determine treatment scores.

1. Indication for surgery if acceptable reduction criteria noted above are not met.

2. Criteria of Lafontaine et al provides five gravity factors for fractures prior to reduction. More than or equal to three gravity factors indicate a high likelihood of instability after reduction and relative necessity of surgical fixation.

   a. Initial dorsal angulation > 20 degree.

   b. Dorsal comminution.

   c. Radiocarpal intra-articular involvement.

   d. Associated ulna fracture.

   e. Age > 60 years.

3. Potentially unstable fracture patterns should be followed weekly for the first 3 weeks to monitor for unacceptable instability and displacement.

C. Surgical approaches are dictated by the fracture pattern

1. Volar approach (distal extent of the volar Henry approach to the forearm) can be used for stand-alone volar locked plating or part of the fragment-specific approach.

   a. Internervous plane—between brachioradialis (radial nerve) and FCR (median nerve).

   b. Between FCR and radial artery.

2. Trans-FCR approach: Similar to the traditional volar approach, except the FCR fascia is incised and the FCR tendon is retracted ulnarly.

3. Volar-extensile approach (extended carpal tunnel approach):

   a. Incision is made between palmaris longus and FCR and extended into the carpal tunnel.

   b. Allows direct visualization and reduction of the volar-ulnar corner of the distal radius as well as the DRUJ, radiocarpal, and the mid carpal joint.

   c. The median nerve and palmar cutaneous branch can be retracted ulnar or radial.

4. Dorsal approach—used for dorsal plating or a fragment-specific approach.

   a. Multiple intervals may be utilized to approach specific fragments.

   b. Trans-extensor pollicis longus (EPL) approach—"universal dorsal approach": Longitudinal incision made just ulnar to Lister's tubercle in line with the third metacarpal distally.

5. Dorsal ulnar approach—it can be used to visualize and reduce dorsal ulnar fracture fragments as well as surgical management of the DRUJ.

   a. Longitudinal incision is made over the DRUJ.

   b. The fifth extensor compartment is entered to gain access to the distal dorsal ulnar corner/DRUJ.

6. Radial approach—used for radial plate fixation or fragment-specific fixation.

   a. Longitudinal incision is made over the radial styloid.

   b. Identify and protect the radial sensory nerves.

   c. Release the first extensor compartment or elevate it subperiosteally to expose the styloid.

   d. Brachioradialis is released to gain access to the entire radial column and eliminate the deforming force.

D. Fixation techniques

1. Spanning external fixation—often utilized in open or severely comminuted fractures. Do not overdistract the wrist joint as it may result in permanent stiffness.

2. Nonspanning external fixation—fixation of distal radius fractures without crossing the wrist joint.

3. Spanning internal bridge plate fixation—gaining popularity in open and comminuted articular fractures. Requires limited dissection, provides stable fixation without exposed hardware, and can augment nonspanning fixation (▶ **Fig. 28.8**).

4. Volar locked plating: There has been a significant increase in popularity of this technique over past 20 years.

   a. Despite its popularity, outcome data have yet to consistently show superiority over other common fixation techniques (▶ **Fig. 28.9a, b**).

   b. It provides excellent fixation with a perceived limited risk to soft-tissue irritation.

   c. Proximal fixation plates sit on the volar metaphyseal flare and provide fixation for standard patterns (including intra-articular).

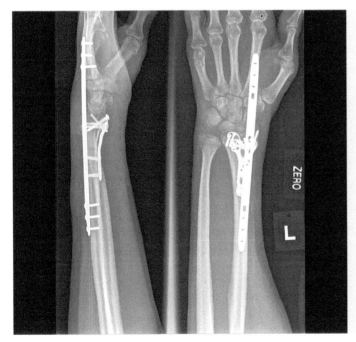

Fig. 28.8 Lateral and anteroposterior wrist radiographs after spanning internal bridge plate fixation.

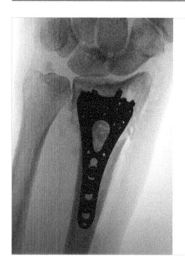 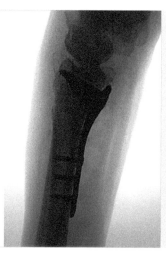

Fig. 28.9 Intra-articular distal radius fracture repaired with a volar locking plate.

d. Distal-bearing plates are becoming more common as attempts are made to provide fixation of far distal fragments.

  i. Plates either pass over or abut the watershed line (volar-most prominence of the distal radius).

  ii. Provide fixation of difficult distal fragments and limited subchondral bone.

  iii. Significant concern related to tendon irritation as assessed in the Soong classification.

5. Dorsal plating—occasionally used alone for dorsal buttress plating, but more commonly is used as an adjunct in combined volar/dorsal plating and fracture specific fixation. Extensor tendon irritation is a risk, but this might be reduced with the use of a retinacular flap reconstruction for plate coverage.

6. Fracture-specific fixation—multiple small plates, screws, wires, and constructs that independently stabilize fragments. Outcomes are similar to volar plate fixation.

7. Percutaneous pin fixation: Often used in pediatric fractures or in conjunction with plaster-style embedding in fragility fractures.

8. Intramedullary nail or cage fixation—represented with a variety of commercially available implants.

   a. Often utilize smaller dissection approaches.

   b. Have demonstrated variable results.

9. DRUJ assessment and fixation:

   a. After anatomic reduction and rigid fixation has been accomplished, intraoperative examination must be performed to assess the integrity of the DRUJ in neutral, supination, and pronation.

   b. If unstable, K-wire transfixation of the radius and ulna +/– TFCC repair may be required.

E. Complications

1. Malunion (most common)—nonoperative management: 35% malunions.

2. Complex regional pain syndrome (CRPS): 1 to 37% (increased with the severity of the fracture).

3. Infection:

   a. K-wire fixation: up to 33% (lower when pins are buried beneath the skin).

   b. External fixation: 10 to 20%.

   c. Open reduction and internal fixation: 1%.

4. Tendon ruptures:
   a. Extensor tendon ruptures following nonoperative or operative management are 3 to 5% (EPL being the most common).
   b. Flexor tendon ruptures: Flexor pollicis longus is the most common. These ruptures are directly related to the position of the plate (distal to the volar watershed line).

F. Rehabilitation
   1. Postoperative rehabilitation varies widely depending on fixation type.
   2. Plate fixation often provides sufficient stability to allow for early range of motion.
   3. Less stable pin or fragment-specific fixation may require longer periods of supportive immobilization.
   4. Once motion has started (typically within 1–2 weeks), the patient is provided with a removable splint to wear when active for comfort and protection.
   5. Edema control and scar care are also started shortly after surgery.
   6. Hand strengthening is started around 4 to 6 weeks, and wrist strengthening follows once significant fracture healing is noted on examination and radiography (typically 8–10 weeks postoperatively).

G. Outcomes: objective and subjective
   1. Objective: Range of motion, grip strength, and radiographic parameters.
   2. Subjective: Disabilities of the arm, shoulder, and hand (DASH) score or Quick DASH and visual analogue scale (VAS).
   3. Overall functional results of distal radius fractures are good despite not having anatomical alignment. However, anatomical restoration of the distal radius does correlate with excellent functional outcomes.
   4. Even in patients with excellent or good outcomes, mild deficits in range of motion and grip strength may be present.
   5. There is a difference between outcomes of younger patients compared to older patients.
      a. Patient age < 65 years:
         i. Less tolerance to malunion of the distal radius when compared to older or lower-functional-demand patients.
         ii. Restoration of volar tilt, radial inclination, and especially radial height seem to strongly correlate with clinical outcomes.
      b. Patient age > 65 years: No statistically significant relationship between typical radiographic parameters and pain/disability.
   6. Radiographic changes exhibiting post-traumatic arthritis may occur following distal radius fracture, especially if there is joint incongruity. However, patients with these radiographic changes may remain asymptomatic for long periods of time.

III. Special Considerations

A. Pediatric patients
   1. Depending on the age of the patient, remodeling potential is greater in the pediatric patients, especially those who are in their prepubescent stage.
   2. Most distal radius fractures in children can be managed with closed reduction and splinting or closed manipulation and percutaneous pinning.
   3. Remodeling potential in children is greatest in the plane of motion (sagittal plane: flexion/extension) and least in the plane of rotation.

4. Distal radius physeal fractures should not undergo manipulation when it has been longer than 10 days since injury because of increased risk of physeal arrest.

5. Most pediatric distal radius fractures have excellence outcomes including those with physeal involvement.

B. Geriatric patients

1. There is no consensus regarding the appropriate treatment of unstable distal radius fractures in the elderly patient as there are only minor differences between operatively and nonoperatively managed distal radius fractures.

2. There is no difference in function or pain between operatively treated and nonoperatively treated distal radius fractures in low-demand geriatric patients.

Suggested Readings

http://www.aaos.org/research/Appropriate_Use/DRF_AUC.pdf

Alluri RK, Hill JR, Ghiassi A. Distal radius fractures: approaches, indication and techniques. J Hand Surg Am 2016;41(8):845–854

Arora R, Lutz M, Deml C et al. A prospective randomized trial comparing nonoperative treatment with volar locking plate fixation for displaced and unstable distal radial fractures in patients sixty-five years of age and older. J Bone Joint Surg Am 2011;93:2146–53

Mathews AL, Chung KC. Management of complications of distal radius fractures. Hand Clin 2015;31(2):205–215

Medoff RJ. Essential radiographic evaluation for distal radius fractures. Hand Clin 2005;21:279–288

29 Hand Fractures and Dislocation

David Ring and Claire B. Ryan

Introduction

One-third of all injuries involve the upper extremity. Phalangeal and metacarpal fractures comprise a significant portion of upper extremity injuries. These are the second and third most common injuries of the hand/forearm, after distal radius fractures. Etiology in young patients includes sports injuries, in middle-aged patients work-related injuries, and in elderly patients falls. These injuries more commonly occur on the border digits.

Keywords: hand fracture, finger fracture, phalangeal/metacarpal fracture, carpal dislocation/fracture

I. Preoperative

A. History

    1. Age.

    2. Hand dominance.

    3. Pain:

        a. Onset.

        b. Location.

    4. Activity/occupation:

        a. Baseline function.

        b. Occupation.

        c. Valued hobbies.

    5. Mechanism of injury:

        a. Time of injury:

            i. Infection risk with open wounds.

            ii. Finger fractures heal quickly.

        b. Crush injury? Direct trauma (e.g., punch)? Torsional or axial load injury? Open laceration?, etc.

        c. Specific injuries—animal or human bite (tooth injury in punch).

        d. Soft-tissue injury.

        e. Potential for malalignment—originally malaligned and reduced?

    6. Neurologic symptoms:

        a. Baseline neurologic function.

        b. Any neurologic deficits after injury?

        c. Vascular compromise?

    7. Exposure:

        a. Especially important in open fractures.

        b. Concerned about exposure to human/animal oral flora, injuries occurring in a barnyard or in dirty water, industrial exposure, etc.

    8. Relevant past medical/surgical history:

        a. History of rheumatoid or osteoarthritis?

        b. Bone quality?

    c. Skeletally mature?

    d. History of diabetes mellitus or vascular disease?

    e. Previous injuries to affected hand?

B. **Physical examination**

    1. Inspection:

        a. Skin quality:

            i. Note ecchymosis, swelling, wounds, etc.

            ii. Warm, red—consider infection.

            iii. Cool, dry—consider vascular compromise.

        b. Deformity:

            i. Angular.

            ii. Rotational.

            iii. Shortening.

    2. Palpation:

        a. Tender areas merit greater attention and, potentially, radiographs.

    3. Range of motion:

        a. Note how close the tip of the fingernail gets to the distal palmar crease.

        b. Note any extensor lags.

    4. Neurovascular examination—important in both open and closed injuries.

        a. Test individual muscle groups in the radial, ulnar, and median distributions:

            i. Radial nerve/posterior interosseous nerve (C7):

- Test wrist extension.
- Test metacarpophalangeal (MCP) joint extension.
- Test thumb interphalangeal (IP) hyperextension and retropulsion.

            ii. Median nerve/anterior interosseous nerve (C8):

- Test thumb IP joint flexion.
- Motor recurrent branch → test thumb palmar abduction.

            iii. Ulnar nerve (T1)—test index finger abduction (first dorsal interosseous).

        b. Vascular examination:

            i. Test capillary refill (< 2 seconds).

            ii. Allen's test—occlude both radial and ulnar arteries, then release one:

- If arches are patent—hand should reperfuse with only one artery occluded.
- If reperfusion does not occur, suspect arterial injury or occlusion.

        c. Test sensation in the digits and in the radial, ulnar, and median nerve distributions (▶Fig. 29.1).

            i. Radial (C6)—dorsal thumb.

            ii. Median nerve (C6–C7)—palmar surface of index and middle fingers.

            iii. Ulnar nerve (C8)—dorsal surface of the fourth and fifth fingers.

            iv. Two-point discrimination test—ability to determine two separate points of sensation. Use 6 mm as minimum distance.

C. Anatomy

    1. Metacarpals:

        a. Comprise the longitudinal and transverse arches of the hand.

        b. Second and third carpometacarpal (CMC) joints are fixed.

        c. First, fourth, and fifth CMC joints are mobile.

        d. Dorsal and palmar interosseous muscles originate from metacarpals.

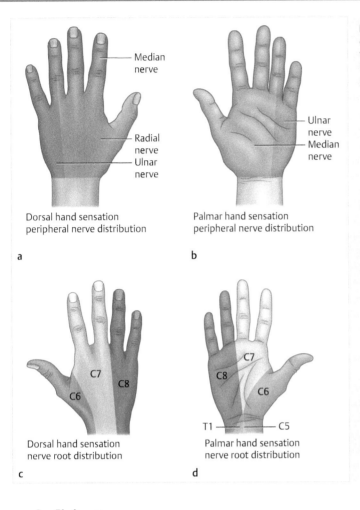

Fig. 29.1 **(a, b)** Sensory nerve distribution in the hand. **(c, d)** Depict the dermatomal distribution in the hand, indicating which nerve roots provide sensory function.

2. Phalanges:
   a. Proximal, middle, and distal phalanges.
   b. Ligaments of fingers important for distal IP (DIP) and proximal IP (PIP) joint stabilization. They contribute to deforming forces in the setting of fracture along with tendons at attachment sites.
3. Vascular:
   a. Radial and ulnar arteries supply superficial and deep palmar arch.
   b. Rich collateral blood supply.
   c. Deep arch predominantly supplied by radial artery.
   d. Superficial arch predominantly supplied by ulnar artery.

D. Imaging
   1. Radiographs:
      a. Anteroposterior (or posteroanterior), lateral, and oblique.
      b. Oblique X-rays are more difficult to interpret, but may help resolve doubt about subtle findings on the anteroposterior or lateral radiographs.
   2. CT:
      a. Assess articular pattern and alignment.
      b. Limit use to injuries where it might affect treatment options or prognosis.

3. MRI:

   a. Rarely used for fractures.

   b. Role for ligament injuries debated. Also, it can often be misleading.

E. Classification

   1. Descriptive classification:

      a. Open versus closed.

      b. Location—bone involved, specific area of bone involved in injury.

      c. Pattern, deformity, and displacement.

      d. Extension into surrounding structures—articular involvement, soft-tissue involvement, etc.

   2. Open hand fractures: Swanson et al classification:

      a. Type I—clean wound, no significant delay in treatment, no systemic signs of infection.

      b. Type II—includes one or more of human or animal bite and open injury in fresh water.

         i. Open injury occurring in a barnyard setting.
         ii. Contamination of open wound with gross debris.
         iii. Delay in treatment of over 24 hours.
         iv. Significant systemic illness that would impact healing/infection risk, such as rheumatoid arthritis, diabetes, etc.

II. Treatment

A. Initial Management

   1. Surgical indications:

      a. Open fractures.

      b. Some malaligned fractures.

      c. Rotational malalignment that cannot be corrected and maintained with nonoperative treatment methods.

      d. Associated nerve, vessel, or tendon injuries benefiting from treatment.

   2. Adequately aligned fractures that are unlikely to cause problems:

      a. Includes any fracture that is adequately aligned and stable (unlikely to move), a fracture that was initially displaced, but able to be reduced and remain aligned thereafter.

      b. Fractures with deformity consistent with good function, such as small finger metacarpal neck fractures and small finger proximal phalanx base fractures.

      c. Buddy taping, splinting, or casting.

      d. Selective repeat radiographs based on potential for problematic loss of alignment (routine repeat radiographs not necessary).

      e. Optional return visit for fractures with a good prognosis.

   3. Other considerations:

      a. Fight bite injuries:

         i. Any small crescent-shaped wound near an associated fracture site (particularly MCP) should be considered for possible contamination with oral flora.
         ii. Needs irrigation and debridement.
         iii. Consider antibiotic coverage to cover for aerobic and anaerobic bacteria.

      b. Animal bites:

         i. Consider antibiotic coverage for *Pasteurella*.
         ii. Leave wounds open—do not suture.

      iii. Wounds with exposed joints, tendons, or nerves should be debrided and irrigated in the operating room.

B. Definitive Management

  1. Carpal fractures and dislocations:

    a. Scaphoid:

      i. Most commonly fractured carpal bone:
- Most common location of fracture: waist.
- Less common—distal tubercle and proximal pole.

      ii. Limited blood supply of scaphoid:
- Risk of osteonecrosis.

      iii. Suspected fracture (fall, tender scaphoid, normal radiographs):
- Splint and re-examine in 1 to 2 weeks.
- MRI best for ruling out (high negative predictive value, low positive predictive value), so perhaps useful for return to sport or work.

      iv. Nonoperative management:
- Nondisplaced fractures.
- Immobilization for 10 weeks is standard, but as little as 6 weeks may be adequate for CT verified, nondisplaced fractures. A cast or splint is preferred. Evidence suggests no benefit to immobilizing the thumb or the elbow.

      v. Operative management:
- Option for nondisplaced fracture in order to avoid a cast or splint: percutaneous screw fixation.
- Also indicated for fractures with greater than 1 mm gap or any translation or angulation (seen on CT scan). Open or arthroscopic assisted open reduction and internal fixation (ORIF).

    b. Lunate/perilunate injuries:

      i. The lunate is known as the "carpal key stone" because of its well-seated location in the lunate fossa, securely attached to the distal radius via volar ligaments.

      ii. Most common traumatic pathologies are perilunate fracture dislocations:
- Carpal bones dislocate around the lunate, which stays in place. The most common is a trans-scaphoid perilunate fracture dislocation. Injury often occurs through the greater or lesser arc of the wrist secondary to an axial load (▶ Fig. 29.2a, b). Capitate, triquetrum, and radial styloid can also be involved. Pure lunate dislocation can also occur.
- Often dislocates volarly.
- High association with median neuropathy. Typically acute carpal tunnel syndrome.
- Reduction is attempted when experts are available.
- In the absence of acute carpal tunnel syndrome, arrangements can be made for later definitive care even if the wrist cannot be reduced.
- Operative treatment consists of reduction, realignment, fixation of any fractures, repair, and protection of interosseous ligament injuries. Treatment often consists of CRPP versus open reduction with screw fixation.

      iii. Clinical evaluation:
- Often present with generalized swelling to wrist.
- Can sometimes detect dorsal carpal bones in case of perilunate dislocation.

      iv. Lateral radiograph is important for assessing dislocation:
- "Spilled tea cup sign" = volar dislocation of lunate (▶ Fig. 29.3).

      v. CT scan useful for defining injury pattern and ligamentous injury.

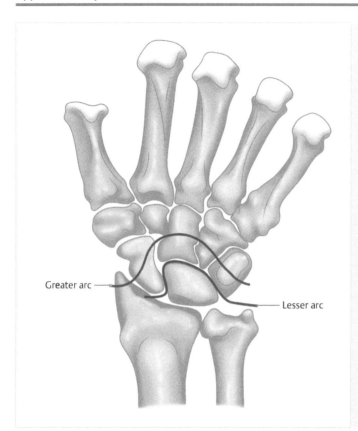

Fig. 29.2 Anatomical diagram depicting the greater and lesser arcs of the wrist. Perilunate dislocations often occur in a purely ligamentous manner (through the lesser arc) or via fracture through surrounding carpal bones (greater arc).

Greater arc

Lesser arc

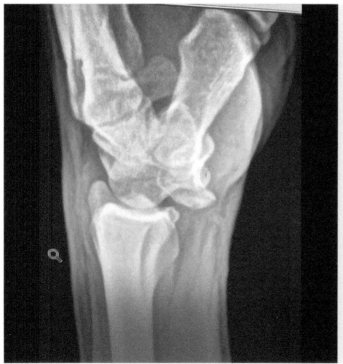

Fig. 29.3 Radiographic example of spilled tea cup sign, depicting a volarly dislocated lunate.

      vi. Treatment:
- Attempt timely closed reduction to limit risk of median neuropathy. It is important to obtain sedation. Longitudinal traction is helpful to relax forearm muscles. Maneuver includes hyperextending wrist with longitudinal traction applied with volar pressure to lunate. Subsequent flexion of wrist over restrained lunate.
- Prompt surgical intervention is necessary in cases of acute carpal tunnel syndrome.

  c. Trapezium:
     i. Fractures often involve articular surface.
    ii. Commonly associated with trapeziometacarpal (TMC) joint dislocation/subluxation.
   iii. Result from an axial blow to an adducted thumb.
   iv. Thumb spica splinting indicated for nondisplaced fractures.
    v. Surgery for fractures with substantial articular incongruity.

  d. Hamate:
     i. Articular surface with CMC fracture-dislocation:
- Displaced fractures and fractures with subluxation or impaction are treated operatively.
- Small marginal fragments associated with dislocation can be ignored and the joint reduced and pinned for a month.
- Others treated with ORIF.

    ii. Hook of the hamate:
- Direct blow to palm.
- Athletic activities such as golf or baseball. Deep branch of ulnar nerve closely associated with hook of the hamate.

   iii. CT scan often best visualizes hamate fractures.
   iv. Nondisplaced fractures can be treated nonoperatively with activity restriction and cast immobilization for 6 weeks.
    v. Patients with displaced hook of hamate fractures and established nonunions causing substantial symptoms are offered surgical excision.

2. Metacarpal head fractures:
     i. Range from epiphyseal fractures to metacarpal shaft fractures that extend into the MCP joint.
    ii. Minimally displaced, stable fractures lead to splint in MCP flexion of greater than 70 degrees:
- Shearing pattern—monitor radiographs each week for loss of reduction.

   iii. Displacement greater than 2 mm leads to open ORIF.

3. Metacarpal neck fractures:
  a. Often angulate apex dorsal given force exerted by interosseous muscles.
  b. Closed reduction and casting:
     i. Fracture redisplacement common after reduction.
    ii. Small finger malalignment is mostly aesthetic:
- "Lump in palm" feeling.
- Malrotation extremely uncommon.

   iii. Immobilize in extension or flexion for 4 weeks.
  c. Operative:
     i. Open fractures.
    ii. People willing to take the risks of surgery for potentially improved aesthetics.
   iii. Operative techniques:
- Closed reduction and percutaneous pinning (CRPP) either antegrade or retrograde.
- ORIF with plating generally reserved for fractures that cannot be reduced using CRPP.

4. Metacarpal shaft fractures:
   a. Closed reduction and splinting:
      i. Indications: acceptable angulation:
         • Less than 10 to 20 degrees in index and metacarpals.
         • Less than 30- to 40-degree angulation in the fourth and fifth metacarpals.
      ii. Little or no malrotation.
      iii. Shortening is aesthetic.
      iv. Most are treated symptomatically (removable splint or wrap).
   b. Operative:
      i. Considered for malrotation and angulation more than 10 to 20 degrees.
      ii. Techniques include CRPP and open reduction with screw or plate and screw fixation.

5. Metacarpal base fractures:
   a. Index through small metacarpals:
      i. May be associated with CMC joint dislocation.
      ii. Sometimes overlooked.
      iii. Common mechanisms: punch or fall.
      iv. Carpal bones can obscure fracture pattern on standard radiographs
          → 30-degree anterior oblique radiographs can be helpful.
      v. CT may aid in diagnosis and delineate intra-articular involvement.
      vi. Treatment includes CRPP if articular alignment is adequate and ORIF for articular malalignment.
   b. Thumb:
      i. Extra-articular fracture treatment:
         • Closed reduction and spica splint or cast. Quite a bit of angulation consistent with good function (e.g., 30 degrees).
         • CRPP greater angulation.
      ii. Intra-articular fractures:
         • Type I: Bennett's fracture—fracture/dislocation of TMC joint with variable sized volar lip fragment with attached volar oblique ligament. Metacarpal fragment is displaced by adductor and abductor pollicis longus and extensor pollicis longus.
         • Type II: Rolando's fracture—fragmented articular fracture of the base of thumb metacarpal (▶Fig. 29.4a, b). Both fracture patterns are unstable and usually treated operatively: closed reduction/percutaneous pinning versus ORIF.

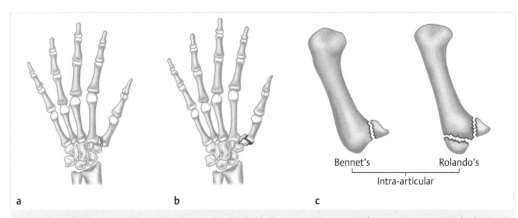

Bennet's   Rolando's
Intra-articular

a   b   c

Fig. 29.4 (a, b) Anatomical depiction of Bennet and Rolando fractures. (c) A Bennet fracture is an intrarticular fracture at the base of the first proximal phalanx with a palmar radial fragment. A Rolando fracture is a T or Y shaped intra-articular fracture at the base of the first proximal phalanx.

6. Fractures of the proximal and middle phalanges:

   a. Very common injury across all age groups.

   b. Proximal phalanges often apex volar:

      i. Deforming force—interosseous muscles.

   c. Middle phalanges can displace apex volar or apex dorsal:

      i. If fracture is proximal to flexor digitorum superficialis (FDS) insertion, it will displace the apex dorsal.

      ii. If fracture is distal to FDS tendon insertion, it will displace the apex volar.

   d. Closed reduction and buddy taping:

      i. Fractures with acceptable alignment and not likely to lose alignment (either without reduction or after reduction).

      ii. Extension block casting can work for some fractures at risk for loss of alignment (Burkhalter; ▶ Fig. 29.5).

      iii. Movement limits stiffness and prevents rotational malalignment.

   e. ORIF versus CRPP:

      i. Substantially angulated, rotated, or shortened fractures.

      ii. CRPP preferred for closed fractures.

      iii. ORIF for fractures with wounds or extensive soft-tissue crush. Also for some articular fractures.

7. PIP fracture dislocations:

   a. Dorsal PIP fracture dislocation:

      i. Volar lip fractures.

      ii. Treatment based on amount of joint surface involvement:

         • If less than 40% of joint is involved, it can be treated with closed reduction and splinting. It leads to reduction in flexion. Dorsal extension block splint is commonly used.

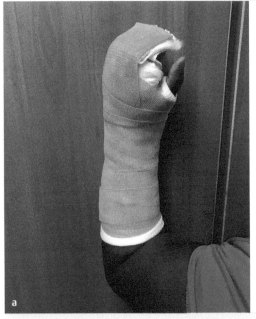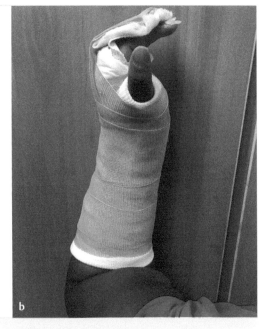

Fig. 29.5 (a, b) Example of an extension block cast.

- If greater than 40% of joint surface is involved, surgery is indicated. Extension block pin and transarticular pin are used. ORIF is difficult due to impacted articular fragments. Hemihamate arthroplasty is preferred for much damaged volar lip or for delayed treatment.

b. Volar fracture dislocation:

   i. Uncommon.

   ii. Associated with avulsion of central slip.

   iii. ORIF with disimpaction of articular fragments and replacement of central slip attachment.

8. Fractures of the distal phalanges:

a. Intra-articular fractures:

   i. Mallet's fracture (▶ Fig. 29.6a):

- Extensor digitorum avulsion with fracture of the dorsal lip.
- Commonly treated nonoperatively with dorsal splinting for 6 weeks.
- Surgery considered for subluxation.
- Not clear that surgery outperforms nonoperative treatment in the short or long term.

   ii. Jersey finger (▶ Fig. 29.6b):

- Flexor digitorum profundus avulsion.
- Most commonly involves the ring finger.
- Bone injury is often an avulsion fragment at the tendinous insertion site.
- Treatment is generally operative via tendon repair and repair of bony fragment if large.

b. Extra-articular fractures:

   i. Stellate crush fractures are treated nonoperatively:

- Splinting of DIP for comfort (should leave PIP joint free so as to promote maximum motion).

   ii. Operative indications:

- Displaced shaft fracture (at risk for nonunion).
- Concomitant wound and some nail bed injuries that might benefit from surgery.

   iii. Severely comminuted fractures or open fractures with significant soft-tissue injury may warrant amputation of distal phalanx.

9. MCP joint dislocations:

a. Dorsal dislocations are more common.

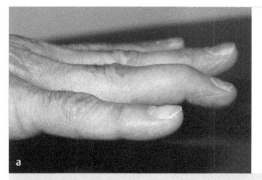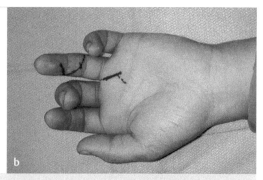

Fig. 29.6 (a) Example of mallet finger deformity. (b) Example of Jersey finger deformity—Rupture of FDP tendon disrupts normal finger cascade.

b. They can be seen on radiographs as joint space widening. It often requires lateral radiograph to adequately assess them.

c. Simple dislocations:

   i. Closed reduction after infiltration of local.
   ii. Usually stable after reduction.

d. Complex dislocations:

   i. Volar plate interposition into the joint or other soft-tissue involvement.
   ii. Irreducible closed.
   iii. Open reduction: dorsal—split the volar plate to allow it to go around the metacarpal head.

e. Volar dislocations are often unstable.

f. Thumb MCP dislocation is usually stable after closed reduction. Ligaments usually heal without surgery.

10. PIP joint dislocations:

a. Dorsal dislocations are common.

b. Volar and rotational dislocations are uncommon and more difficult to reduce from interposition of ligament.

c. Closed reduction under digital block:

   i. Active motion.
   ii. Buddy taping for 3 weeks.

d. ORIF for rare collateral ligament interposition.

11. DIP joint dislocations:

a. Often associated with tendon rupture or wound.

b. Generally easy to reduce under digital block.

c. Surgery is not helpful if reduction is stable, wound is adequately treated, and tendons are intact.

C. Surgical Approaches

1. Finger:

a. Dorsal approach—split extensor tendon in the midline or between the central slip and lateral band.

b. Volar approach:

   i. Brunner's (zigzag) incisions. Cross-flexion creases obliquely.
   ii. A1, A3, and A5 are expendable.
   iii. Flexor tendons can be retracted.

c. Lateral approach:

   i. Midaxial incision: make points at the end of flexion creases in flexion. These indicate incision line.
   ii. Important structures:

      • Digital nerve and artery are volar to incision.
      • Lateral bands need to be retracted or excised when approaching the proximal phalanx.

2. Metacarpals:

a. Dorsal approach:

   i. A straight, longitudinal incision is made between the adjacent metacarpal bones.
   ii. Interosseous muscles are elevated to expose the metacarpal.

3. MCP joint:

   a. Dorsal approach:

      i. Straight or curved incision over the MCP joint.

      ii. Extensor apparatus is incised longitudinally or sagittal band is detached.

      iii. Repair upon closure.

      iv. Longitudinal capsulotomy is performed to gain direct access to the joint.

D. Fixation Techniques

   1. Kirschner's wire fixation:

      a. Perpendicular to fracture line.

      b. Intramedullary.

   2. ORIF.

   3. Screws or plate and screws, depending on fracture pattern, fragmentation, and bone quality.

E. Complications

   1. Infection:

      a. Pin track infection caused often due to pin–skin motion.

      b. Deep infection—purulence, abscess, or osteomyelitis.

   2. Malunion/nonunion:

      a. Malalignment combined with dysfunction can be considered for osteotomy.

      b. Nonunion:

         i. Very uncommon.

         ii. Infection, technical deficiencies, devitalized bone.

   3. Stiffness:

      a. Joint contracture.

      b. Tendon adhesion.

      c. Most common with wounds, crush, or open treatment.

      d. Stretching after injury can be counterintuitive.

   4. Post-traumatic osteoarthritis—articular deformity, damage, or subluxation.

Summary

Hand trauma represents a significant portion of musculoskeletal trauma treated in emergency departments nationally. This text should serve as a guide to diagnosis and management of common hand fractures and dislocations. Most injuries are appropriate for nonoperative management. However, open injuries, significantly angulated/malrotated fractures and irreducible dislocations necessitate surgical intervention.

Suggested Readings

Cheah AE-J, Yao J. Hand fractures: indications, the tried and true and new innovations. J Hand Surg Am 2016;41(6):712–722

Freeland AE, Orbay JL. Extraarticular hand fractures in adults: a review of new developments. Clin Orthop Relat Res 2006; 445(445):133–145

Henry MH. Fractures of the proximal phalanx and metacarpals in the hand: preferred methods of stabilization. J Am Acad Orthop Surg 2008;16(10):586–595

Meals C, Meals R. Hand fractures: a review of current treatment strategies. J Hand Surg Am 2013;38(5):1021–1031, quiz 1031

Suh N, Ek ET, Wolfe SW. Carpal fractures. J Hand Surg Am 2014;39(4):785–791, quiz 791

Wong VW, Higgins JP. Evidence-based medicine management of metacarpal fractures. Plast Reconstr Surg 2017;140(1):140e–151e

Section III

Pelvis or Lower Extremity Trauma

30 Pelvic Ring Injuries

Raymond D. Wright, Jr. and Brandon R. Scott

Introduction

The successful management of pelvic ring injuries requires understanding of complex pelvic anatomy, determinants of stability, mechanism of energy, and host factors. High-energy unstable pelvic ring injuries may be associated with hemodynamic instability upon presentation to the trauma bay, and the treating practitioner must be able to function as an effective member of the resuscitating team when such a clinical presentation occurs (▶ **Video 30.1**).

I. Preoperative

A. History

1. Frequently results from a high-energy mechanism of injury in young patients (motor vehicle crash, motorcycle crash, bicycle crash, pedestrian struck, or fall from height).

2. May result from low-energy mechanism in elderly patients (fall from standing).

3. Multiple injuries are common in patients with high-energy pelvic ring disruptions.

B. Physical exam

1. Pain.

2. Hip, flank, perineal ecchymosis, and labial and scrotal swelling are common.

3. Subtle open injuries may be detected by careful examination of gluteal folds, perineum, genitalia, rectum, and flank.

   a. Blood at meatus of urethra may be a sign of urethral or bladder injury.

   b. Vaginal or scrotal tears can be subtle.

   c. Fracture may be open into vagina or rectum necessitating digital exam of both.

4. Nerve palsy:

   a. Lumbosacral plexus is in close proximity to the posterior pelvic ring.

   b. Peripheral nerve exam of lower extremities may detect injuries.

C. Anatomy

1. Osteology (▶ **Fig. 30.1**):

   a. Osseous pelvic ring comprises two innominate bones linked anteriorly at the symphysis pubis and posteriorly at the sacroiliac (SI) joints bilaterally.

   b. The bony connections are stabilized by ligamentous attachments—there is no inherent bony stability.

   c. Anatomic osseous variety in the sacrum (sacral dysmorphism) as well as in the anterior pelvic ring must be appreciated and understood if successful and safe operative fixation is to be performed. Sacral dysmorphism:

      i. Failure of segmentation in the upper sacral segment.
      ii. Osseous variation leads to radiographic findings (▶ **Fig. 30.2**):

      - Alar regions that have a cranial and anterior slope.
      - Mamillary processes.
      - Irregular upper segment nerve root tunnels.
      - Non-recessed upper segment on outlet view.
      - Tongue-in-groove SI joints.
      - Persistence of the S1 disc.

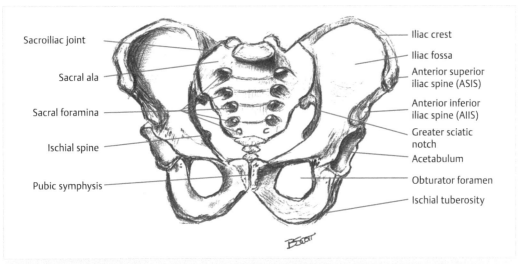

Fig. 30.1 Pelvic ring osteology. The osseous pelvic ring is made up of two innominate bones articulating with the sacrum posteriorly and the symphysis pubis anteriorly. Stability relies on ligamentous connections, as there is no inherent osseous stability in the pelvic ring.

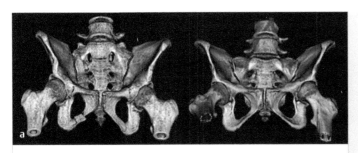
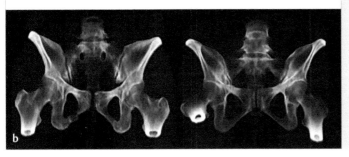

Fig. 30.2 Three-dimensional surface-rendered reconstructions of pelvic computed tomography scans of a dysmorphic upper sacral segment (a) and a "normal" upper sacral segment (b). The associated volume-rendered images are shown below and mimic the differences seen in dysmorphic versus "normal" sacral segments in pelvic radiographs.

2. Soft tissue:
   a. Posterior ligaments—anterior, intra-articular, and posterior SI ligaments, as well as sacrospinous and sacrotuberous ligaments.
   b. Anterior ligaments—symphyseal ligaments.
3. Neurologic:
   a. Lumbosacral plexus (▶ **Fig. 30.3**).
   b. Sacral nerve roots exit at the bottom of the corresponding vertebral body foramina. For example, S1 roots exit at the bottom of S1.
   c. L5: runs along cranial anterior surface of bilateral sacral alae.

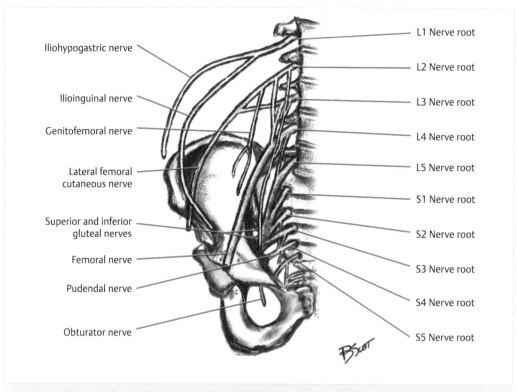

Fig. 30.3 Lumbosacral plexus. The proximity of the lumbosacral plexus to the posterior pelvic ring makes the plexus susceptible to injury when there is fracture displacement through the posterior pelvic ring.

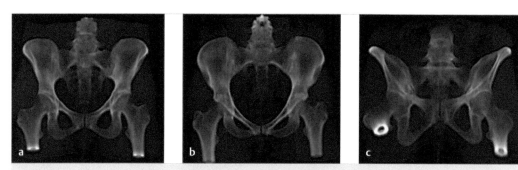

Fig. 30.4 Anteroposterior pelvis (a), inlet pelvis (b), and outlet pelvis (c).

D.   Imaging:
    1.   Radiographs—anteropoterior (AP), inlet, and outlet (▶**Fig. 30.4**).
        a.   Anterior-posterior:
            i.   Patient is placed supine, and beam is directed anterior to posterior.
            ii.   Tip of coccyx should be at the symphysis pubis.
            iii.   Lumbar spinous processes should be in line with pubic symphysis.
            iv.   Evaluates cranial and caudal displacement (in conjunction with outlet view).

b. Inlet—radiograph is taken with patient supine. Beam is directed caudally approximately 60 degrees but can be variable depending on an individual's pelvic tilt and body habitus.

   i. Helpful for demonstrating posterior displacement or (less commonly) anterior displacement of osseous structures.

   ii. Demonstrates internal or external rotation.

c. Outlet—radiograph is taken with patient supine with variable cranial tilt, often between 20 and 40 degrees, ideally superimposing the cranial aspect of the symphysis at the level of the second sacral segment.

   i. Reveals sacral morphology.

   ii. Highlights cranial or (less commonly) caudal displacement of osseous structures.

2. CT scan:

   a. Axial scan may demonstrate fine detail of posterior pelvic ring injuries and morphology.

   b. Soft tissue windows may reveal visceral injury, bleeding, occult open injuries, and core muscle anatomy.

   c. Three-dimensional reconstructions, while not generally necessary, can be useful for understating complex injury patterns.

3. Dynamic exam under anesthesia with fluoroscopy (EUAF):

   a. Patient is placed supine with fluoroscope brought in for inlet and outlet views.

   b. Examination is done with physician applying manual stress to cause deformity (▶ **Fig. 30.5**).

      i. Push-pull maneuver (push on one side and pull on the contralateral leg).

      ii. External rotation stress accomplished by frog-legging both extremities.

      iii. Internal rotation stress done by internally rotating one leg with or without a lateral force applied to the ipsilateral greater trochanter.

   c. Dynamic imaging may reveal occult instability that may not be evident on static pelvic radiographs (▶ **Fig. 30.6**).

E. Classification of pelvic ring fractures: Young and Burgess (▶ **Fig. 30.7**).

   1. Based on the force vector applied to the pelvis that leads to predictable patterns of deformity and instability.

   2. Predictive of associated injuries, mortality, and resuscitative requirements.

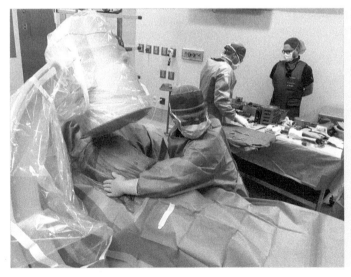

Fig. 30.5 Application of manual stress on a minimally displaced pelvic ring fracture to demonstrate instability. The fluoroscope is brought in on inlet tilt. The physician is examining the patient in ▶ **Fig. 30.6.**

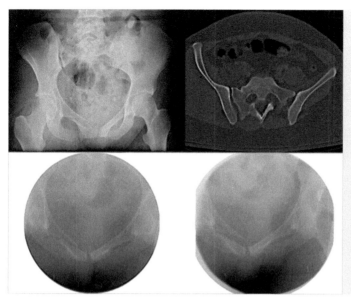

Fig. 30.6 A 23-year-old female sustains a minimally displaced pelvic ring injury as a result of a t-bone injury in a motor vehicle crash. Despite her minimally displaced fracture pattern, gross instability was demonstrated on lateral compression testing.

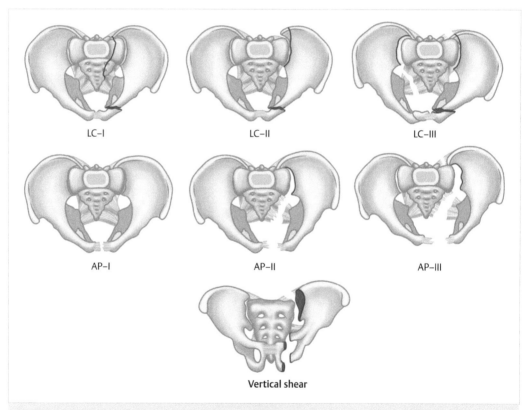

Fig. 30.7 The Young and Burgess classification system of pelvic ring injuries.

3. Fracture types:
   a. Lateral compression (LC):
      i. Laterally directed force causing variable anterior (typically horizontally oriented ramus fractures) and posterior injuries.

  ii. Likelihood of instability increases from LC-1 to LC-3.

  iii. LC-1—laterally directed force applied to the posterior pelvis resulting in a wide spectrum of sacral injury ranging from incomplete anterior sacral buckle fractures to complete fractures of the sacrum with or without displacement.

  iv. LC-2—laterally directed force applied to the anterior pelvis leading to rami fracture(s), internal rotation deformity, and posterior SI joint fracture dislocation (crescent fracture).

  v. LC-3—greater force leading to internal rotation of the pelvis on the side of impact and contralateral external rotation deformity ("windswept pelvis").

  vi. Mortality increases from LC-1 to LC-3 usually due to factors outside the pelvis (head, neck, and chest trauma).

 b. Anterior-posterior compression (APC):

  i. Anteriorly directed force resulting in opening of anterior pelvic ring usually at symphysis pubis or less commonly vertically oriented rami fractures with variable degrees of posterior SI joint injury.

  ii. Instability increases from APC-1 (stable) to APC-2 (rotationally unstable) to APC-3 (completely unstable).

  iii. APC-1—anterior ring injury without posterior element disruption typically manifested by pubic symphysis diastasis less than 2.5 cm.

  iv. APC-2—classically described as pubic symphysis diastasis > 2.5 cm (not absolute) and displacement of the anterior SI joint resulting in a rotationally unstable hemipelvis. The following ligaments are proposed to be injured to variable degrees leading to rotational instability: anterior SI ligament, sacrotuberous ligament, and sacrospinous ligament.

   • APC-3—pubic symphyseal displacement and SI joint dislocation described as rotationally and vertically unstable. The posterior SI ligamentous complex is completely disrupted.

  v. Mortality increases from APC-1 to APC-3 usually due to pelvic hemorrhage.

  vi. APC-3 has the highest resuscitative fluid requirements, blood product requirements, and risk of mortality of all pelvic ring fractures.

 c. Vertical shear (VS):

  i. Cranial displacement of unstable pelvic segment.

  ii. Similar mortality and resuscitation requirements of an APC-2 fracture.

 d. Combined mechanical injury (CMI): Fracture pattern that does not fit in to the other categories.

  i. No specific mechanism can be applied to the injury pattern.

  ii. AO/OTA/Pennal–Tile classification (▶ Fig. 30.8).

   • Alphanumeric system

   • Intended to predict stability.

   • Ideal for research cataloging—not generally used in daily communication.

II. Treatment

A. Initial management

 1. Advanced Trauma Life Support (ATLS) protocol (see Chapter 9, Polytrauma, for details) as the majority of patients with pelvic ring disruptions are multiply injured.

 2. Patients with hemodynamic instability and pelvic ring instability may benefit from circumferential pelvic antishock sheeting (CPAS) or pelvic binder application (▶ Fig. 30.9).

 3. Anterior external fixator may be indicated in certain fracture types as a resuscitative adjunct.

 a. It should be placed in the operating room under fluoroscopy.

 b. Patients with rotational instability with an incomplete posterior injury may realize the most benefit with this technique.

 c. It may be useful to apply external fixator prior to positioning patient in lithotomy position if needed to inspect and debride an open perineal wound.

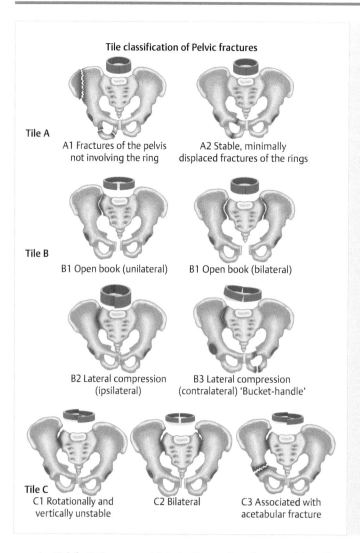

Tile classification of Pelvic fractures

Fig. 30.8 Pennal–Tile classification system of pelvic ring injuries.

Tile A

A1 Fractures of the pelvis not involving the ring

A2 Stable, minimally displaced fractures of the rings

Tile B

B1 Open book (unilateral)

B1 Open book (bilateral)

B2 Lateral compression (ipsilateral)

B3 Lateral compression (contralateral) 'Bucket-handle'

Tile C

C1 Rotationally and vertically unstable

C2 Bilateral

C3 Associated with acetabular fracture

4. Pelvic C-clamp was historically employed to provisionally secure posterior ring—may be used rarely and requires fluoroscopy to apply safely.

5. Hemodynamically unstable patients with arterial bleeding as demonstrated by contrast extravasation on CT scan may benefit from arterial embolization.

    a. Selective embolization is preferred to nonselective embolization.

    b. Embolization is only effective in select patients as 80 to 85% of pelvic hemorrhage is from cancellous bleeding or retroperitoneal veins.

6. Skeletal traction for select vertically unstable fractures to reduce injuries with cranial displacement or potential cranial displacement.

B. Nonoperative management

    1. Low-energy fractures with minimal displacement.

    2. Stable fracture patterns (those that do not deform under physiologic force): APC-1 and most LC-1.

        a. Dynamic stability is difficult to predict with static imaging studies.

        b. Stress view under anesthesia (EUAF) may be useful for assessing stability in patients with indeterminate stability by plain films and physical exam.

    3. Patients with medical comorbidities that would preclude safe operative management.

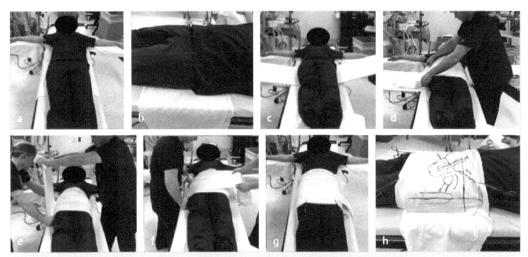

Fig. 30.9 The application of a circumferential antishock sheet (CPAS). The patient is placed supine and a smooth drawsheet is placed centered on the patient's greater trochanters (**a, b**). Two providers stand on either side of the patient to pull the drawsheet taut (**c**). One side of the sheet is passed to the opposite provider (**d**). The second provider tucks and holds tension while passing his/her sheet to the first provider (**e, f**). The sheet is held in place with self-retaining clamps (**g**). Knowledge of structures under the sheet can allow the provider to cut working portals in the sheet for external fixator placement, iliosacral screw insertion, and vascular cannulation (**h**).

C. Operative treatment:
1. Unstable fractures
    a. Rotationally unstable (classically): LC-2 and LC-3:
        i. There is considerable heterogeneity within the LC-1 classification. Select LC-1s with significant sacral fracture displacement may benefit from operative stabilization but this remains controversial.
        ii. Severe persistent pain and inability to mobilize are frequently cited as relative indications for surgery although data has not demonstrated that surgical stabilization leads to pain relief and improved mobility.
    b. Completely unstable (classically): APC-2, APC-3, VS, and CMI.
2. Instability noted on clinical examination or on examination under anesthesia (EUA).
3. Failure of nonoperative care.
4. Associated acetabular fracture.
5. Open fractures.
D. Timing of surgery
1. Surgery should be undertaken when the patient is physiologically optimized. Early fixation in physiologically stable patients is associated with shorter ICU and hospital stays as well as fewer complications including pneumonia and acute respiratory distress syndrome (ARDS).
2. Rarely, acute fixation may be performed as a life-saving resuscitative measure especially when percutaneous techniques are employed.
E. Surgical approaches:
1. Posterior pelvis and SI joint:
    a. Anterior exposure (iliac exposure):
        i. With the patient supine, dissection begins at the ASIS and proceeds posteriorly along the peripheral ilium.
        ii. The fascia between the external oblique and the tensor fascia lata is incised.
        iii. The iliopsoas is elevated in subperiosteal fashion to expose the posterior pelvic ring and SI joint.

b. Posterior exposure (▶Fig. 30.10):

    i. With the patient prone, an incision is created in a vertical paramedian or curvilinear fashion centered vertically on the posterior superior iliac spine (PSIS).
    ii. The skin incision is placed lateral to PSIS for posterior pelvic ring fractures and SI joint injuries.
    iii. The skin incision is placed medial to the PSIS or in the midline to expose a sacral fracture.
    iv. Elevate the gluteus muscle flap off the lumbodorsal fascia.
        • Allows for more secure coverage and closure than incising muscle.
        • Caudally, the gluteus maximus origin is at or very near to the sacral spinous processes.

2. Symphysis pubis and anterior pelvis (▶Fig. 30.11):

    a. Pfannenstiel incision 2 to 3 cm above pubis. The rectus is identified in the midline. Anterior dissection is carried peripherally just beyond the pubic tubercles to facilitate clamp application, assessment of reduction, and implant placement.

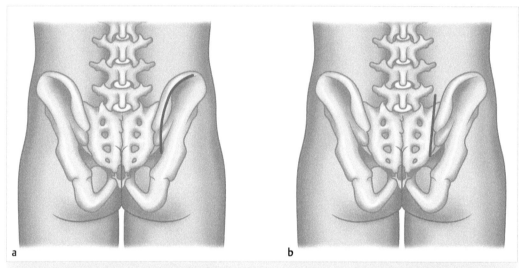

Fig. 30.10 Posterior exposure to the pelvic ring. **(a)** A curvilinear approach typically used for a posterior approach to the ilium. **(b)** A more vertical approach typically used for exposure of the sacrum and posterior sacroiliac joint.

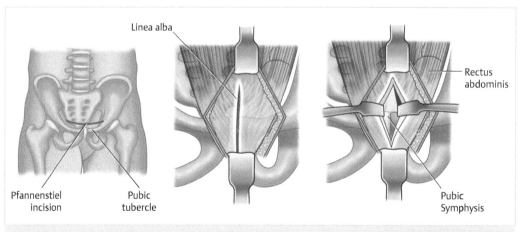

Fig. 30.11 Anterior exposure to the pelvic ring. The surgeon can access the symphysis pubis, the pubic rami, and the intrapelvic region.

b. Posterior osseous morphology of the parasymphyseal region is smooth—dissection of the area will help the surgeon to assess reduction.

3. Percutaneous fixation:

   a. Accomplished via osseous fixation pathways within the pelvic ring (▶ **Fig. 30.12**).

   b. Includes iliosacral screws, ramus screws, AIIS-PSIS (LC-2) screws, and posterior column screws.

   c. Successful screw fixation by percutaneous technique can be accomplished with a thorough understanding of osseous morphology and its radiographic correlates.

   d. Anterior osseous variation is not as well classified but incomplete understanding may lead to hazardous implant insertion when percutaneously instrumenting the anterior pelvic ring.

F. Fixation techniques

   1. Posterior pelvic ring:

      a. Iliosacral screws (▶ **Fig. 30.12**).

      b. Transiliac, transsacral screws (▶ **Fig. 30.13**).

         i. Improved purchase into the contralateral ilium.

         ii. May not be possible if the sacrum is dysmorphic.

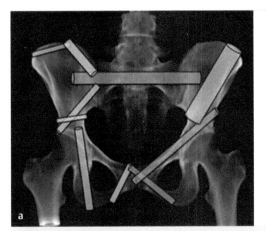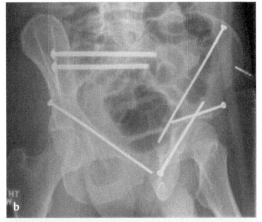

Fig. 30.12 **(a)** Potential osseous fixation pathways. **(b)** Clinical example of percutaneously inserted screws into some of the osseous fixation pathways.

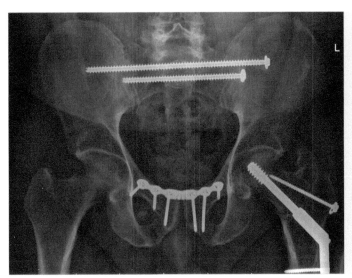

Fig. 30.13 Anteroposterior pelvis radiograph following fixation of a pelvic ring injury with an anterior pubic symphysis plate and posterior transiliac, transsacral screws.

    c. Posterior tension band plate.

    d. Lumbopelvic fixation—pedicle screws inserted into the PSIS (bypass the sacrum) and pedicle screws inserted into the lower lumbar spine pedicles are connected to by bars.

  2. Anterior pelvic ring:

    a. Pubic symphyseal plate (▶ **Fig. 30.13**; small fragment or large fragment).

    b. Ramus screws (▶ **Fig. 30.12**).

    c. Anterior external fixator—pins can be placed into the supra-acetabular region (under fluoroscopy) or into the iliac crest.

    d. Anterior (subcutaneous) internal fixator (infix)—pedicle screws inserted into the supra-acetabular region and connected by a 5 to 6 mm bar tunneled in the subcutaneous tissue of the lower abdomen, being careful to stay superficial to the fascia.

G. Complications

  1. Infection—rate of infection for posterior exposures has been reported to be as high as 25%.

  2. Hemorrhage:

    a. Injury

      i. Approximately 80 to 85% from cancellous bone or retroperitoneal veins.
      ii. Infrequently a result of arterial bleeding.

    b. Intra-/postoperative

      i. Intraoperative hemorrhage from arterial injury may exist.
      ii. Surgeon must be knowledgeable of anatomy.

  3. Death:

    a. Reported to be 6 to 20% risk of death historically in closed injuries.

    b. Up to 50% mortality (historically) in patients with open fractures.

  4. ARDS/multisystem organ failure:

    a. May occur in patients with incomplete resuscitation.

    b. May be a result of high-energy injury.

  5. Nonunion:

    a. Rare.

    b. May occur in neglected/undiagnosed unstable fractures.

  6. Malunion:

    a. Can occur in cases of neglected or undiagnosed instability.

    b. May result in limb-length inequality, sitting imbalance, dyspareunia, and chronic pain.

  7. Deep vein thrombosis (DVT):

    a. DVT risk is high (up to 40–50%) when no chemoprophylaxis is prescribed.

    b. No consensus for type of chemoprophylaxis.

    c. Sequential compression devices (SCDs) for mechanical prophylaxis have been demonstrated to be beneficial.

    d. Insertion of inferior vena cava (IVC) filter may be beneficial in high-risk patients with contraindications to chemoprophylaxis (e.g., intra/extracranial hemorrhage, spinal cord injury).

  8. Neurologic injury:

    a. May be a result of traction on lumbosacral plexus—thorough examination of patient's lower extremity function is paramount.

    b. May be a result of insertion of iliosacral screw into sacral canal—can be avoided with thorough understanding of anatomy, radiography, and operative steps (▶ **Fig. 30.14**).

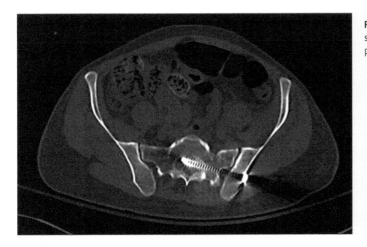

Fig. 30.14 A screw placed into the sacral canal may be a source of postoperative neurologic deficit.

H.   Rehabilitation

1.   Immediate mobilization.

2.   Weight-bearing restrictions usually dictated by the side of the posterior pelvic ring injury, typically 8 to 12 weeks nonweight-bearing on the side with an unstable posterior ring injury or bed to transfer only if bilateral posterior pelvic ring injury.

I.   Outcomes

1.   Some studies have demonstrated that degree of displacement may affect patient outcomes, especially with pure SI dislocations.

2.   Return to work outcomes vary between 40 and 100%.

3.   Associated injuries may be more important than the pelvic ring injury itself in determining patient outcomes.

a.   Most significant factor may be magnitude of the neurological injury.

b.   Neurological injury may be a source of substantial disability for patients.

III. Special Considerations for Pediatric Patients

A.   Very little literature exists regarding the effect of internal fixation on pelvic physes.

B.   In general, most pediatric patients have sufficient osseous volume to instrument with iliosacral screws if indicated by the injury pattern.

C.   Symphyseal disruptions may be secured with suture through bone tunnels to obviate the need for implant removal after injury has healed.

D.   Most pediatric pelvic ring injuries can be treated nonoperatively.

E.   Treatment parameters for adults can guide pediatric treatment.

Suggested Readings

Avilucea FR, Whiting PS, Mir H. Posterior fixation of APC-2 pelvic ring injuries decreases rates of anterior plate failure and malunion. J Bone Joint Surg Am 2016;98(11):944–951

Burgess AR, Eastridge BJ, Young JW, et al. Pelvic ring disruptions: effective classification system and treatment protocols. J Trauma 1990;30(7):848–856

Lybrand K, Bell A, Rodericks D, Templeman D, Tornetta P III. APC injuries with symphyseal fixation: what affects outcome? J Orthop Trauma 2017;31(1):27–30

Pennal GF, Tile M, Waddell JP, Garside H. Pelvic disruption: assessment and classification. Clin Orthop Relat Res 1980(151):12–21

Routt MLC Jr, Nork SE, Mills WJ. Percutaneous fixation of pelvic ring disruptions. Clin Orthop Relat Res 2000(375):15–29

Sagi HC, Coniglione FM, Stanford JH. Examination under anesthetic for occult pelvic ring instability. J Orthop Trauma 2011;25(9):529–536

31 Acetabular Fractures

Greg E. Gaski

Introduction

Acetabular fractures are complex injuries that require a thorough understanding of pelvic anatomy, underlying fracture pattern, and host factors. Radiographic classification aids in determining the optimal surgical approach, reduction tactics, and sequence of fixation. Percutaneous treatment methods and acute total hip arthroplasty (THA) are evolving as treatment options for specific types of acetabular fractures (▶Video 31.1).

I. Preoperative

A. History

1. Typically results from a high-energy mechanism of injury in young patients (motor vehicle accident, motorcycle accident, bicycle accident, pedestrian struck, fall from height).

2. Can result from low-energy mechanism in elderly patients (fall from standing).

3. Frequently occur in multiply-injured patients (head, neck, chest, abdomen, retroperitoneum, and associated extremity injuries).

B. Physical examination

1. Pain with rotation of the affected hip.

2. Hip and flank ecchymosis: Morel–Lavallée lesion.

   a. Closed, internal degloving injury due to severe trauma.

   b. Commonly associated with pelvis, acetabulum, and femur fractures.

   c. A potential space is created by separation of the skin and subcutaneous tissue from the underlying fascia. This space fills with blood and/or serous fluid.

   d. Typically debrided when treating the associated fracture operatively.

   e. In the setting of nonoperative fracture management, observation of the Morel–Lavallée lesion is warranted with consideration of surgical debridement if signs of infection develop.

3. Flexed, adducted, and internally rotated leg in the presence of an associated posterior hip dislocation.

4. Abducted, externally rotated leg in the presence of an associated anterior hip dislocation.

5. Nerve palsy:

   a. Sciatic nerve involvement in 10 to 15% of posteriorly displaced acetabular fractures, usually in conjunction with posterior hip dislocations.

   b. Absence of foot dorsiflexion and decreased dorsal foot sensation signifies injury to the peroneal division of the sciatic nerve.

   c. Absence of foot dorsiflexion and plantar flexion with diminished sensation on the dorsal and plantar surfaces of the foot signifies injury to both the peroneal and tibial divisions of the sciatic nerve (medial foot sensation intact from the saphenous nerve contribution).

C. Anatomy

1. Osteology (▶Fig. 31.1a, b):

   a. Judet and Letournel described the acetabulum as consisting of two columns of bone in an inverted Y.

   b. The anterior column consists of the superior pubic ramus, anterior wall, anterior pelvic brim, iliopectineal eminence, anterior iliac wing (including the anteroinferior iliac spine [AIIS] and anterosuperior iliac spine [ASIS]), and iliac crest.

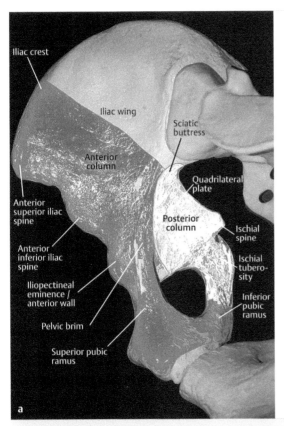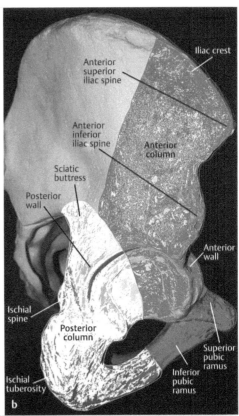

Fig. 31.1 Osteology of the acetabulum depicting the anterior and posterior columns as viewed **(a)** from inside the pelvis and **(b)** from outside the pelvis.

    c. The posterior column consists of the ischial tuberosity, ischial spine, majority of the quadrilateral plate, posterior wall, and inferior aspect of the sciatic buttress (adjacent to the greater sciatic notch).

2. Soft tissue: Labrum—ring of fibrocartilage around the acetabulum that contributes to stability of the hip by increasing the surface area and deepening the joint.

3. Vascular supply (▶ Fig. 31.2a, b):

    a. Anterior:

        i. External iliac artery and vein.

       ii. Obturator artery and vein.

     iii. Corona mortis—connection between the external iliac artery and obturator artery.

    b. Posterior:

        i. Superior gluteal and inferior gluteal arteries and veins are branches of the internal iliac system and exit the sciatic notch above and below the piriformis, respectively.

       ii. Ascending branch of the medial femoral circumflex artery within the quadratus femoris muscle—main blood supply to the femoral head.

D. Imaging

1. Radiographs—anteroposterior (AP) pelvis and Judet (45-degree oblique) radiographs:

    a. Obturator oblique—visualization of the anterior column and posterior wall.

    b. Iliac oblique—visualization of the posterior column and anterior wall.

2. Classic radiographic landmarks (▶ Fig. 31.3):

    a. Iliopectineal line—anterior column.

    b. Ilioischial line—posterior column.

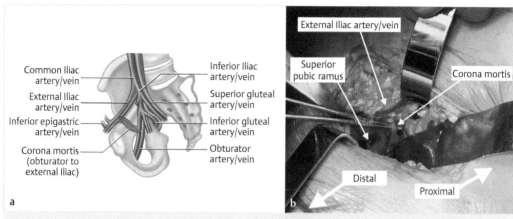

Fig. 31.2 (a) Illustration of the vascular anatomy inside the pelvis. (b) Clinical photograph of the "corona mortis."

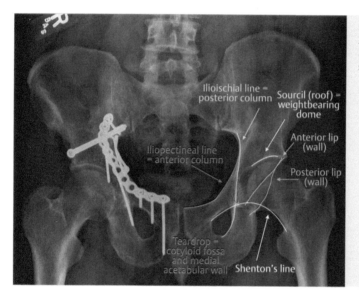

Fig. 31.3 Anteroposterior pelvis X-ray with radiographic landmarks and corresponding anatomic structures.

    c. Teardrop: bone between the cotyloid fossa and anterior quadrilateral plate (also considered the medial wall of the acetabulum).

    d. Roof (sourcil)—acetabular dome.

    e. Anterior lip—anterior wall.

    f. Posterior lip—posterior wall.

3. Roof arc measurements provide information regarding fracture stability:

    a. Vertical line drawn through the center of the acetabulum.

    b. Second line drawn from the center of the acetabulum to the point of fracture extension into the acetabulum.

    c. Roof arc angle measured at the intersection of the two lines.

    d. Medial roof arc angle is measured on the AP pelvis for evaluation of transverse fracture patterns. An angle less than 45 degrees is concerning for instability.

    e. Anterior roof arc angle is measured on the obturator oblique radiograph for evaluation of anterior column fractures. An angle less than 30 degrees potentially signifies instability.

    f. Posterior roof arc angle is measured on the iliac oblique radiograph for evaluation of posterior column fractures. An angle less than 70 degrees potentially signifies instability.

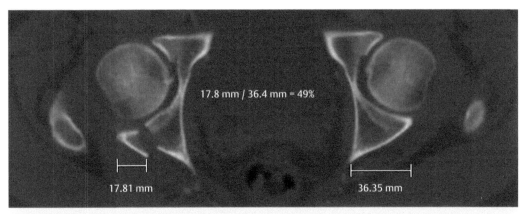

Fig. 31.4 Moed et al.'s technique for measurement of the amount (%) of posterior wall fracture involvement compared to the intact wall of the contralateral acetabulum.

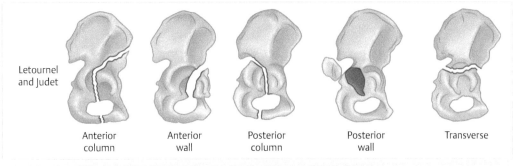

Fig. 31.5 Elementary acetabular fracture patterns according to Letournel and Judet.

    g.   CT scan subchondral arc as described by Olson and Matta—the superior 10 mm of the acetabular articular surface (dome) corresponds to the area encompassed by 45-degree roof arc measurements.

4.   CT scan with coronal and sagittal reconstructions:

    a.   Improved identification of fracture fragments with respective translational and rotational displacement.

    b.   Accurate measure of articular displacement (millimeters).

    c.   Assessment of marginal impaction of the articular surface.

    d.   Evaluation of intra-articular fracture fragments.

    e.   Posterior wall involvement to predict hip stability measured on axial cuts: Moed et al.'s technique—at the level of the largest posterior wall fracture involvement, measure the mediolateral width of the fracture. Divide that number by the width of the intact wall/acetabulum (►**Fig. 31.4**).

5.   Three-dimensional (3D) reconstructions provide an enhanced understanding of the complex anatomy of the pelvis and acetabulum. 3D imaging aids in delineation of fracture lines and preoperative planning.

E.   Classification of acetabular fractures according to letournel and judet

1.   Elementary patterns: single fracture plane (►**Fig. 31.5**):

    a.   Posterior wall:

       i.   Most common type of acetabular fracture (20–30%).

      ii.   Marginal impaction is common and best identified on CT.

     iii.   "Gull sign" signifies dome impaction.

  b. Posterior column—fracture disrupts the ilioischial line.

  c. Anterior wall:

   i. Rare.

   ii. Does not involve the iliopectineal line (pelvic brim).

  d. Anterior column:

   i. Fracture disrupts the iliopectineal line.

   ii. The superior point at which the fracture line exits the ilium influences treatment and may be described as exiting:

    • Low: AIIS or below.

    • Intermediate: between the AIIS and ASIS.

    • High: above the ASIS along the iliac crest.

  e. Transverse:

   i. The only elementary pattern that involves both columns.

   ii. Transtectal—fracture through the roof or dome of the acetabulum.

   iii. Juxtatectal—fracture through the superior extent of the cotyloid fossa with the majority of the dome intact.

   iv. Infratectal: fracture through the cotyloid fossa and involving the anterior and posterior walls without dome involvement.

2. Associated patterns (▶ **Fig. 31.6**):

  a. Posterior column/posterior wall.

  b. Transverse/posterior wall.

  c. T-shaped—transverse fracture with a vertical stem that travels inferiorly into the obturator foramen (most common), posteroinferior to divide the ischium, or anteroinferior to divide the pubis.

  d. Anterior column or wall/posterior hemitransverse:

   i. Anterior column fracture combined with a transverse fracture line exiting posterior from the primary anterior fracture, effectively dividing the posterior column into superior and inferior components.

   ii. Most common fracture pattern in elderly patients.

  e. Associated both columns:

   i. No portion of the articular surface is in continuity with the intact ilium.

   ii. "Spur sign" seen on the obturator oblique radiograph corresponds to the intact ilium and is pathognomonic for this fracture type.

   iii. "Secondary congruence" refers to the maintenance of femoral head congruity with the fractured acetabulum although dissociated from the innominate bone.

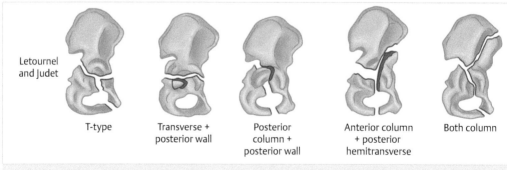

Letournel and Judet

T-type Transverse + posterior wall Posterior column + posterior wall Anterior column + posterior hemitransverse Both column

Fig. 31.6 Associated acetabular fracture patterns according to Letournel and Judet.

II. Treatment

A. Initial management

1. Advanced trauma life support (ATLS) protocol (see Chapter 9, Polytrauma, for details) as the majority of patients with acetabular fractures are multiply injured.

2. Hemodynamically unstable patients with or without associated chest and abdominal injuries may require angioembolization of arterial bleeding:

   a. Selective embolization is preferred to nonselective embolization.

   b. There is a 5 to 10 times increased risk of deep infection in patients undergoing open reduction and internal fixation (ORIF) of an acetabular fracture after angioembolization.

3. Urgent reduction of hip dislocations:

   a. Typically performed in the ED under conscious sedation.

   b. Temporary relaxation (paralysis) is necessary.

   c. Hip reduction in ED is contraindicated if a femoral neck fracture is present.

   d. For additional treatment details, refer to Chapter 32, Hip Dislocation.

4. Skeletal traction for select fractures to maintain hip reduction, aid in fracture reduction prior to definitive stabilization, and as a damage control measure (hemorrhage control and clot stabilization).

B. Nonoperative management

1. Fractures that do not involve the weight-bearing dome. The dome is typically defined by roof arc measurements below 45 degrees on X-ray and/or 1 cm on CT (does not apply to both columns or wall fractures).

2. Articular displacement less than 2 mm without hip instability.

3. Secondary congruence (defined above) of associated both column fractures.

4. Posterior wall fractures with less than 20% of wall involvement (wall measurement technique described by Moed et al defined above) in the absence of instability.

   a. Although uncommon, reports of instability with wall fractures less than 20% have been described.

   b. Fluoroscopic examination under anesthesia (EUA) remains the best determinant of hip stability.

   c. Fractures encompassing 20 to 40% of the wall with concentric reduction on injury CT are typically evaluated with a dynamic EUA. If stable, closed treatment is acceptable.

5. Geriatric patients with extensive comorbidities.

C. Operative treatment

1. Displaced fractures (≥ 2 mm) within the weight-bearing dome.

2. Instability noted on clinical examination or on EUA.

3. Hip incongruity.

4. Intra-articular fragment superior to the fovea.

5. Open fractures.

D. Timing of surgery

1. Classically, improved reductions were noted when ORIF is performed within 2 to 3 weeks.

2. Typically, surgery is undertaken when the patient is physiologically stable and the appropriate surgical team is assembled (rarely greater than 1 week from injury).

3. No increased blood loss noted when surgery is performed early (< 24 hours) compared to later (> 24 hours) for posterior wall fractures.

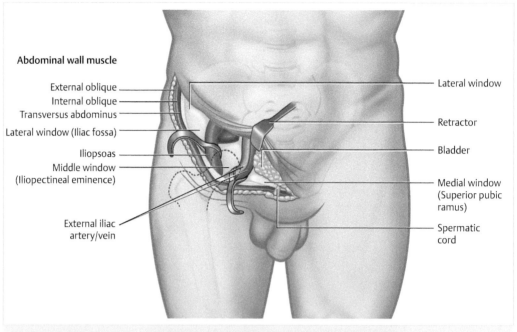

Fig. 31.7 Ilioinguinal approach illustrating the "three windows": lateral, middle, and medial.

4. Timing of fixation for anterior approaches is controversial. Some surgeons advocate waiting 2 to 3 days to allow the clot to stabilize in an effort to minimize blood loss although recent data suggest there is no difference when ORIF is performed before or after 48 hours postinjury.

E. Surgical approaches

1. Ilioinguinal (anterior; ▶ Fig. 31.7):

   a. Three windows—medial, middle, and lateral.

   b. Curvilinear incision from midline proximal to the symphysis toward the ASIS and posteriorly just lateral to the iliac crest.

   c. Lateral window—incise fascia between the external oblique and the tensor fascia lata from the ASIS posteriorly along the iliac crest. Continue the dissection along the inner table of the pelvis by working underneath the iliopsoas.

   d. Middle window—incise the roof of the inguinal ligament toward the superficial inguinal ring. Next, incise the iliopectineal fascia and work between the external iliac vessels medially and the iliopsoas laterally (femoral nerve).

   e. Medial window—identify and protect the spermatic cord or round ligament. The rectus muscle serves as the medial border. Dissection can continue between the two rectus heads (see anterior intrapelvic approach below).

2. Anterior intrapelvic (modified Stoppa; ▶ Fig. 31.8):

   a. With and without lateral window (see above).

   b. Pfannenstiel incision 2 to 3 cm above the pubis. Divide the rectus heads; partially or completely elevate the head of the rectus ipsilateral to the fracture.

   c. Work along the superior ramus, retract and protect the bladder, and identify and ligate the corona mortis (▶ Fig. 31.2).

   d. Continue the periosteal dissection posteriorly along the pelvic brim. Expose the quadrilateral plate inferiorly in the true pelvis and superiorly in the false pelvis onto the ilium.

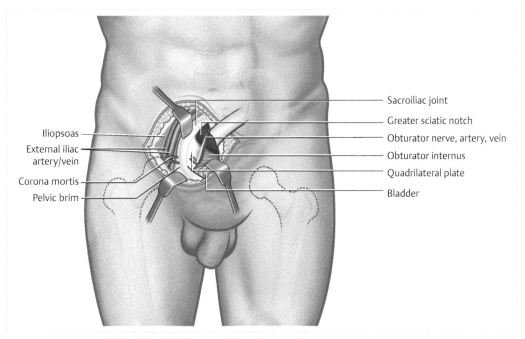

Fig. 31.8 Anterior intrapelvic approach ("Stoppa window").

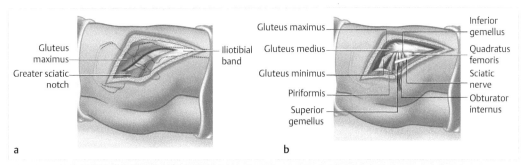

Fig. 31.9 Kocher–Langenbeck approach demonstrating the **(a)** superficial dissection and **(b)** deep dissection.

3. Kocher–Langenbeck (posterior; ▶ **Fig. 31.9 (a, b)**):
   a. Can be performed lateral or prone.
   b. Prone positioning facilitates reduction of transverse fractures and may reduce the risk of sciatic nerve palsy. Maintain hip extension and knee flexion to relax the sciatic nerve.
   c. Incision along the posterolateral border of the proximal femur toward the greater trochanter and curve toward the posterosuperior iliac spine (PSIS).
   d. Superficial dissection—incise the iliotibial band distally and the gluteus maximus in line with its fibers proximally.
   e. Deep dissection: retract the gluteus medius anteriorly, and identify and ligate the short external rotators near the femoral attachment.
      i. Piriformis can be traced back to the greater sciatic notch. The sciatic nerve lies anterior to piriformis in 85% of patients, divides the piriformis in 5 to 10% of patients, and rests posterior to the piriformis in 2 to 5% of patients.
      ii. Obturator internus tendon, superior gemellus, and inferior gemellus. These can be traced back to the lesser sciatic notch. Retraction of the internus tendon usually protects the sciatic nerve (the sciatic nerve lies posterior to the internus).

    4. Extended iliofemoral:

        a. Highest risk of infection and heterotopic ossification (HO; up to 50%).

        b. Rarely used.

        c. Consider this approach when fractures are older than 3 weeks.

    5. Combined anterior and posterior approaches.

    6. Percutaneous approaches:

        a. Minimally or nondisplaced fracture to prevent migration and/or promote early weight bearing.

        b. Elderly patients with extensive comorbidities that portend an increased risk of complications with an open approach. The goal of surgery is stabilization in a potentially nonanatomic position.

F. Reduction and fixation techniques

    1. Wall fractures:

        a. Marginal impaction reduced and allograft used to fill any voids.

        b. Small fragment lag screw and buttress plate fixation, usually with small fragment pelvic reconstruction plates.

        c. Peripheral wall fractures not amenable to lag screws are secured with spring plates (undercontoured one-third tubular plate) prior to buttress plate application (▶ **Fig. 31.10a, b**).

    2. One-column fractures: small fragment lag screw and "recon" buttress plate fixation.

    3. Fractures involving both columns:

        a. Direct reduction and small fragment fixation of one column/wall followed by indirect reduction and fixation of the other column.

        b. Exception: the anterior intrapelvic approach (modified Stoppa) allows direct access for reduction and fixation to the anterior column and select posterior column fractures.

        c. Cannulated screw fixation (4.0 to 7.3 mm).

        d. Precontoured implants have recently been developed to span both columns and buttress the quadrilateral plate (▶ **Fig. 31.3**).

G. Total Hip Arthroplasty

    1. Indications are controversial.

    2. Consider ORIF and acute THA in medically stable patients with fracture characteristics associated with an increased risk of post-traumatic arthritis:

        a. Comminution of the posterior wall.

        b. Marginal impaction.

        c. Posterior wall fracture in conjunction with hip dislocation and femoral head fracture.

        d. Underlying osteopenia with associated fracture comminution.

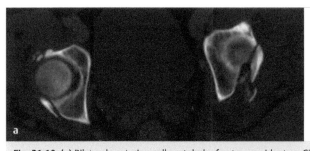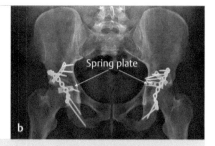

Fig. 31.10 (a) Bilateral posterior wall acetabular fractures evident on CT scan axial cut. **(b)** Anteroposterior pelvis radiograph following open reduction and internal fixation (ORIF) of bilateral posterior wall fractures with a buttress plate and 2 spring plates on each side.

3. Critical to obtain column stability through ORIF—traditional recon plates and/or cup cage.

4. Consider multiple cup screws to enhance stability.

H. Complications

1. Infection:

    a. Two to 15%.

    b. Risk factors:

        i. Multiply-injured patients.

        ii. Previous embolization (up to 60%).

        iii. Comorbidities including diabetes mellitus, kidney disease, liver disease.

        iv. Presence of Morel–Lavallée lesion.

        v. Smoking.

        vi. Morbid obesity.

2. Post-traumatic osteoarthritis (PTOA):

    a. Twenty percent require conversion to THA after ORIF for all patients.

    b. Thirty percent of elderly patients older than 65 years converted to THA after ORIF.

    c. Directly correlated with reduction quality (increased risk of PTOA with postoperative malreduction ≥2 mm).

    d. Risk factors—wall comminution, femoral head fracture/chondral injury, associated fracture pattern, age older than 40 years.

3. Nonunion: uncommon.

4. Anemia:

    a. Significant blood loss necessitating blood transfusion is common after acetabular surgery.

    b. Red blood cell salvage (cell saver) is more useful for anterior approaches than posterior approaches.

    c. Tranexamic acid (TXA) has been shown to decrease blood loss and transfusion rates after select acetabular ORIF.

5. Deep vein thrombosis:

    a. Up to 40 to 50% risk of deep vein thrombosis when no chemoprophylaxis is initially prescribed.

    b. Type of chemoprophylaxis controversial (low-molecular-weight heparin, aspirin, warfarin).

    c. Mechanoprophylaxis with sequential compression devices (SCDs) has been demonstrated to be beneficial.

    d. Consider inferior vena cava (IVC) filter in high-risk patients that cannot be prescribed chemoprophylaxis (e.g., intra-/extracranial hemorrhage, spinal cord injury).

6. Neurologic injury:

    a. Posterior approaches:

        i. Sciatic nerve at risk during posterior approaches (up to 10%).

        ii. Superior and inferior gluteal nerves at risk during posterior approaches (exit sciatic notch).

    b. Anterior approaches:

        i. Femoral nerve at risk during anterior (ilioinguinal) approach (usually attributed to traction).

        ii. Lateral femoral cutaneous nerve at risk during anterior approaches.

        iii. Obturator nerve at risk during anterior intrapelvic approach.

        iv. Pudendal nerve (traction injury).

7. Vascular injury:

    a. Posterior approaches:

        i. Superior and inferior gluteal vessels are at risk during a posterior approach.

        ii. Medial femoral circumflex artery is at risk during the caudal dissection of a posterior approach.

   b. Anterior approaches:
      i. External iliac vessels are at risk of laceration and thrombosis during an anterior approach.
      ii. Obturator vessels are at risk during an anterior intrapelvic approach.
      iii. Corona mortis is at risk during an anterior approach.
8. Avascular necrosis:
   a. Five percent risk.
   b. Greater risk with associated hip dislocation and femoral head fracture.
9. HO:
   a. Very common in extended iliofemoral approach.
   b. Common following posterior approaches: 15 to 60%.
   c. HO prophylaxis is controversial for posterior approaches or extended approaches:
      i. Radiation therapy (XRT) administered as a one-time dose within 72 hours has been shown to decrease HO.
      ii. Nonsteroidal anti-inflammatory drugs (NSAIDs) are an alternative to XRT. Indomethacin has been shown to increase the risk of acetabular nonunion and concomitant long bone nonunion without significantly reducing risk of symptomatic HO.

I. Rehabilitation
   1. Immediate mobilization.
   2. Restricted weight bearing for 8 to 12 weeks.
   3. Posterior hip precautions for patients with a history of posterior instability (controversial).

J. Outcomes
   1. Reduction quality has been shown in multiple studies to directly influence radiographic and functional outcomes.
   2. Goal of acetabular ORIF is less than 2 mm articular step-off.
   3. Seventy-five to 80% hip survivorship after 20 years in all patients treated with ORIF.
   4. Posterior wall fractures carry the worst prognosis. Risk factors for reoperation and PTOA include the following:
      a. Comminution.
      b. Advanced age (older than 60 years).
      c. Marginal impaction.
      d. Femoral head involvement.

III. Special Considerations for Pediatric Patients

A. Triradiate cartilage closes at the age of 12 years in girls and 14 years in boys.
B. Classification and treatment similar to adults.
C. Post-traumatic hip dysplasia may manifest as an uncommon late complication. It can result in a shallow, retroverted acetabulum.

Summary

Acetabular fractures are complex injuries and often associated with polytrauma. Careful neurologic examination may identify deficits, especially sciatic nerve dysfunction after posterior hip fracture-dislocations. Critical analysis of radiographs and CT scan with reconstructed images (including 3D) aids in management decisions, choice of surgial approach, and preoperative planning for reduction tactics and implant selection. Classic indications for operative treatment include: hip instability, articular displacement >2 mm in the weight-bearing dome, hip incongruity, and residual intra-articular fragment(s). Post-traumatic arthritis remains a common complication in up to 20-30% of patients sustaining acetabular fractures. The role of primary total hip arthroplasty has yet to be clearly defined, but is being increasingly performed in older patients with unfavorable fracture characteristics such as posterior wall impaction, posterior wall comminution, and femoral head involvement.

Suggested Readings

Cole JD, Bolhofner BR. Acetabular fracture fixation via a modified Stoppa limited intrapelvic approach. Description of operative technique and preliminary treatment results. Clin Orthop Relat Res 1994(305):112–123

Firoozabadi R, Swenson A, Kleweno C, Routt MC. Cell saver use in acetabular surgery: does approach matter? J Orthop Trauma 2015;29(8):349–353

Judet R, Judet J, Letournel E. Fractures of the acetabulum: classification and surgical approaches for open reduction. Preliminary report. J Bone Joint Surg Am 1964;46:1615–1646

Letournel E. Acetabulum fractures: classification and management. Clin Orthop Relat Res 1980(151):81–106

Manson TT, Perdue PW, Pollak AN, O'Toole RV. Embolization of pelvic arterial injury is a risk factor for deep infection after acetabular fracture surgery. J Orthop Trauma 2013;27(1):11–15

Matta JM, Merritt PO. Displaced acetabular fractures. Clin Orthop Relat Res 1988(230):83–97

Moed BR, Ajibade DA, Israel H. Computed tomography as a predictor of hip stability status in posterior wall fractures of the acetabulum. J Orthop Trauma 2009;23(1):7–15

O'Toole RV, Hui E, Chandra A, Nascone JW. How often does open reduction and internal fixation of geriatric acetabular fractures lead to hip arthroplasty? J Orthop Trauma 2014;28(3):148–153

Sagi HC, Jordan CJ, Barei DP, Serrano-Riera R, Steverson B. Indomethacin prophylaxis for heterotopic ossification after acetabular fracture surgery increases the risk for nonunion of the posterior wall. J Orthop Trauma 2014;28(7):377–383

Tannast M, Najibi S, Matta JM. Two to twenty-year survivorship of the hip in 810 patients with operatively treated acetabular fractures. J Bone Joint Surg Am 2012;94(17):1559–1567

Tornetta P III. Non-operative management of acetabular fractures. The use of dynamic stress views. J Bone Joint Surg Br 1999;81(1):67–70

32 Hip Dislocation

Elizabeth P. Davis and Joshua L. Gary

Introduction

A. Uncommon injury usually requiring high-energy mechanism.

   1. Ninety to 95% of patients have concomitant injuries.

B. Four types of dislocations—posterior, anterior, obturator, and medial.

   1. Ninety percent are posterior, 10% are anterior, and < 1% are obturator dislocations.

   2. Medial dislocations through the fossa acetabulum are seen with complex acetabular fractures or with severe rheumatoid arthritis.

C. Timely reduction is critical to limit the risk of avascular necrosis (AVN) and for preservation of hip function.

D. The primary goal in treatment is obtaining urgent concentric reduction and maintaining stability.

E. Dislocations of the hip are often associated with fractures of the femoral head, acetabulum, and femoral neck. Partial or full-thickness delamination of cartilage with or without femoral head impaction are expected with any injury (▶**Video 32.1**).

Keywords: hip dislocations, orthopaedic trauma, anatomy, imaging, preoperative evaluation, treatment

I. Preoperative

A. History and physical examination

   1. The alert patient will be in significant discomfort, will typically refuse to move the injured extremity, and may complain of numbness in the affected extremity.

   2. Patients can have "distracting injuries" and may be repeat offenders.

   3. Patients with a traumatic hip dislocation warrant a trauma surgery evaluation. Advanced Trauma Life Support (ATLS) protocol ensures a full and complete workup for these patients.

   4. Observe the position of the affected leg.

      a. Posterior dislocations—the hip will be held in flexion, internal rotation, and adduction. It may also be shorter than the other leg (▶**Fig. 32.1**, left hip).

      b. "Irreducible" posterior fracture-dislocations—the hip will be held in flexion, adduction, and neutral rotation.

      c. Obturator dislocations—the hip will be held in extension, external rotation, and significant abduction (▶**Fig. 32.1**, right hip). It is a variant of an anterior dislocation where the femoral head is inferior as opposed to superior in a pubic ramus dislocation.

      d. Anterior dislocations—the hip will be held in mild flexion, external rotation, and abduction (▶**Fig. 32.2**).

      e. Medial fracture dislocation (protrusion)—the limb will be shortened and with some abduction.

   5. The physical exam must include the entire affected lower extremity from the pelvis and hip joint to the foot.

   6. It is very important to document a detailed neurovascular exam, if possible, prior to any reduction attempt.

      a. The sciatic nerve is most commonly affected. Peroneal division is affected more often than the tibial division.

      b. Lower extremity nerve function should be documented pre and post reduction.

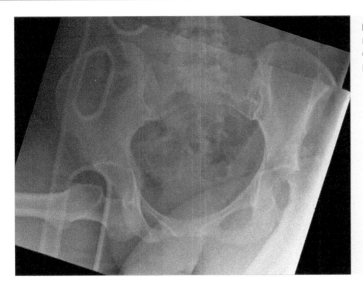

Fig. 32.1 Anteroposterior pelvis radiograph demonstrating a right obturator hip dislocation and a left posterior hip dislocation.

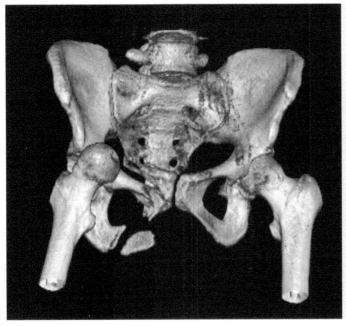

Fig. 32.2 Computed tomography 3D reconstruction of an anterior hip dislocation.

7. Ligamentous knee injuries, distal femur fractures, and patella fractures are associated with dashboard injuries and posterior hip dislocations.

B. Anatomy

1. The hip joint is made up of the pelvic acetabulum and the femoral head.

   a. The acetabulum is an articular surface formed by the convergence of the ilium, ischium, and pubis.

   b. The femoral head articulates with the acetabulum and is attached to the cotyloid fossa by the ligamentum teres.

2. The hip joint is inherently stable due to the depth of the bony acetabulum and labrum, diameter of the femoral head relative to the femoral neck, the capsule, and strong surrounding soft tissue. The capsule is thick and formed by a confluence of ligaments that extend from the pelvis to the femur including the iliofemoral, ischiofemoral, and pubofemoral ligaments (▶ **Fig. 32.3**).

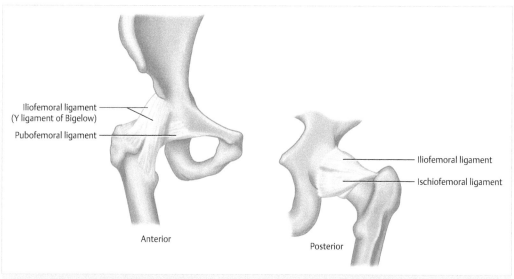

Fig. 32.3 Ligaments surrounding the hip joint.

3. Blood supply is predominantly derived from the ascending branch of the medial femoral circumflex artery. The lateral epiphyseal vessels enter in the cranial and posterior portion of the femoral neck. (See Chapter 33, Femoral Neck and Head Fractures, ▶ **Fig. 33.1**).

4. Approximately 50% of the femoral head is covered by the bony acetabulum and labrum.

   a. Femoral head anteversion averages 10 to 15 degrees relative to the femoral condyles.

   b. Decreased anteversion predisposes to posterior dislocation—acetabular dysplasia, femoral retroversion, crossover sign.

5. Soft tissues, including the piriformis tendon, iliopsoas tendon, or displaced fracture fragments may obstruct closed reduction.

C. Imaging

   1. Plain film analysis

      a. The anteroposterior pelvis is key for diagnosing dislocations and confirming reduction.

      b. Systematic evaluation is paramount every time—joint space and femoral heads should be symmetric, Shenton's line intact, and rotation assessed by the greater and lesser trochanters.

   2. Computed tomography (CT)

      a. Obtain the CT after successful reduction unless reduction cannot be achieved.

      b. 2-mm cuts through the pelvis allow for enhanced assessment of the bony anatomy.

      c. CT scans can identify intra-articular fragments, osteochondral lesions on the femoral head, fracture displacement, and details about an acetabular injury.

      d. Three-dimensional CT scans serve as a useful adjunct in preoperative planning for acetabular fracture-dislocations.

D. Classification

   1. Anatomic classification using the location of the distal segment relative to the acetabulum (See 'Introduction' of this chapter). Other previously described systems are not commonly used.

II. Treatment

A. Initial management

   1. Evaluation

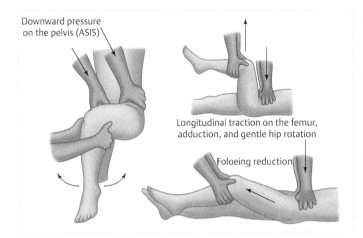

Downward pressure on the pelvis (ASIS)

Longitudinal traction on the femur, adduction, and gentle hip rotation

Foloeing reduction

Fig. 32.4 Allis reduction maneuver.

a. Life, limb, and then function.

b. Hip dislocations are an orthopaedic urgency and require prompt attention. Reduction within 6 hours decreases the risk of AVN of the femoral head.

   i. Timing is controversial but it is generally accepted that the sooner the hip can be safely reduced, the better.

   ii. Reduction will require deep conscious sedation in the emergency room versus paralysis in the operating room for most patients.

   iii. Placement of the extremity in skeletal traction may be necessary to prevent recurrent dislocation in the unstable hip, especially with posterior dislocations associated with acetabular fracture.

c. If closed reduction cannot be performed in the emergency department, the patient should be taken to the operating room for closed versus open reduction.

2. Reduction techniques:

a. Most dislocations regardless of the type can be reduced in a supine position. Like all reductions, reproduction of the deformity *followed by* maneuvers opposite the insult should result in successful reduction. Pre-reduction planning should be done based upon the direction of dislocation prior to sedation.

b. Described maneuvers for posterior dislocations:

   i. The Allis maneuver requires traction in line with the deformity, the pelvis stabilized by one or two assistants pressing downward force on each anterior superior iliac spine (ASIS) of the pelvis, and the hip is slowly flexed and adducted (▶ Fig. 32.4).

   ii. The lateral traction method utilizes a sheet wrapped around the inner thigh, proximally, to help pull the femoral head laterally to clear the acetabulum (▶ Fig. 32.5).

3. Post reduction:

a. Always obtain an anteroposterior pelvis demonstrating concentric reduction. A CT scan is usually obtained to rule out loose bodies (more sensitive than plain films). Note that a CT scan is generally not helpful prior to closed reduction.

b. Repeat neurovascular exam.

c. Stability examination is done after hip reduction while the patient is still sedated.

   i. Flex the hip to 90 degrees in neutral rotation and abduction/ adduction, apply a posterior force. If subluxation occurs, this patient will likely need surgical stabilization. This is subjective as the force applied is variable between clinicians and involvement of the most experienced member of the surgical team is ideal.

   ii. Unnecessary if clear surgical indications exist.

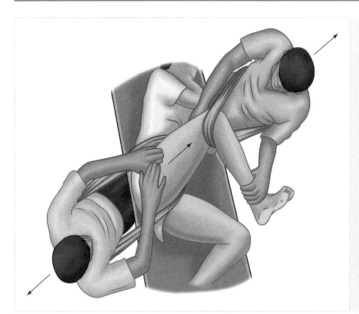

Fig. 32.5 Lateral traction hip reduction maneuver.

B. Definitive management

The goal of treatment is simple: Obtain a stable, concentric reduction of the hip. The treatment to obtain these goals may be simple or complex.

1. Pure dislocations:

a. Dislocation with successful closed reduction: A hip dislocation without associated fractures, concentric reduction, and with stable stress exam may be treated conservatively without operative intervention. The role for arthroscopic evaluation is controversial. Depending on institution preference, weight-bearing as tolerated immediately after or touchdown weight-bearing for 4 to 6 weeks with dislocation precautions is recommended.

b. Irreducible dislocation: A hip that is irreducible without associated fractures is likely to have soft tissue interposition that prevents reduction of the femoral head under the acetabulum.

    i. Urgent open reduction must be performed. A posterior approach is used for posterior dislocations and a Smith–Peterson approach is used for anterior or obturator dislocations.

    ii. Stability exam should be done after an open reduction.

2. Fracture-dislocations:

a. Fracture-dislocations require preoperative planning.

b. Acetabular or femoral head fracture dislocations may necessitate open reduction and internal fixation to restore congruity and stability.

c. Dislocations associated with a femoral neck fracture require open reduction and internal fixation of the femoral neck fracture before reduction of the hip joint. This is a rare time a posterior approach may be indicated for fixation of a femoral neck fracture. Patient factors may indicate the patient for total hip arthroplasty given significant rates of AVN.

d. Femoral neck fractures with an associated femoral head fracture have been reported to have up to a 100% incidence of AVN and total hip arthroplasty should be considered for elderly and low-demand patients.

e. Small debris within the acetabular fossa is acceptable in the non-weight-bearing portion of the dome.

C. Surgical approaches

1. Anterior (Chapter 33, Femoral Neck and Head Fractures, ▶Fig. 33.7)

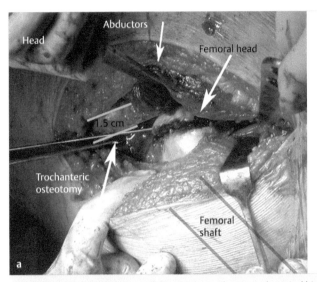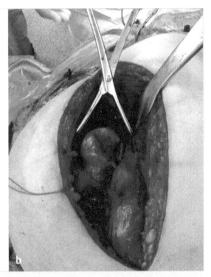

Fig. 32.6 Digastric osteotomy of the greater trochanter and surgical hip dislocation (a) with initial femoral head fracture reduction (b).

    a. Smith–Petersen: The patient is placed supine on a flat, radiolucent table.

      i. Incision is made starting along the iliac crest and curves inferiorly after the ASIS.

      ii. The superficial surgical interval is between the sartorius (femoral nerve) and tensor fascia latae (superior gluteal nerve). The deep interval lies between the gluteus medius (superior gluteal nerve) and rectus femoris (femoral nerve).

  2. Posterior (Chapter 31, Acetabular Fractures, ▶ Fig. 31.9):

    a. Kocher–Langenbeck: The patient is placed lateral or prone. Hip and extension and knee flexion intraoperatively decrease tension on the sciatic nerve.

      i. The gluteus maximus is split.

      ii. The sciatic nerve must be identified and protected. Some advocate for a neurolysis for patients with neuropraxia.

      iii. The blood supply to the femoral head runs anterior to the quadratus femoris, which must be left undisturbed.

    b. Digastric trochanteric osteotomy with anterior surgical dislocation is an extension of the posterior approach (▶ Fig. 32.6a, b).

      i. Lateral decubitus positioning opposed to prone.

      ii. Osteotomy of the greater trochanter is made approximately 1 cm thick along from the posterior border of the gluteus medius insertion and vastus lateralis origin, sparing and dissection of the muscle bellies.

      iii. Anterior dislocation of the femoral head allows for direct visualization.

D. Complications

  1. AVN:

    a. Varies from 1–2% to 15–17% incidence after traumatic dislocation of the hip.

    b. The risk of AVN increases the longer the hip is dislocated.

  2. Recurrent instability and dislocation:

    a. Results from failure to recreate a stable, concentric reduction.

    b. Decreased femoral anteversion.

    c. Acetabular retroversion.

    d. Posterior wall fractures (especially cranial and peripheral) with inadequate fixation.

3. Post-traumatic arthritis:

   a. Most common complication of hip dislocations. May be present immediately after dislocations with cartilage loss.

   b. Instability of the joint will lead to more rapid progression.

4. Infection:

   a. Longer surgical times and extensile exposures have a higher risk of infection.

   b. Open approaches should be treated with perioperative antibiotics.

5. Sciatic nerve palsy:

   a. Consider surgical exploration if there is a change in exam after a closed reduction.

   b. Consider neurolysis if present on initial evaluation and an open posterior approach is performed.

   c. Delayed sciatic nerve palsy due to scar formation, hematoma, heterotopic ossification.

   d. Most recover within 18 to 30 months of injury. Intense rehabilitation and use of braces to prevent equinus deformity is important.

6. Heterotopic ossification:

   a. More commonly seen with fracture dislocations.

   b. Single dose radiation is effective; there is a rare associated risk of delayed sarcoma. Anti-inflammatories are controversial and may not be effective in preventing symptomatic HO.

   c. Debridement of all nonviable muscle intraoperatively mandatory. Gluteus minimus below the superior gluteal bundle, and superior and inferior gemelli may be debrided as prophylactic measure without functional sequelae.

E. Rehabilitation

1. Hip precautions are utilized to prevent recurrent dislocations:

   a. Recurrent posterior dislocation at risk with hip flexion, adduction, and internal rotation. Posterior precautions—no hip flexion past 90 degrees, no internal rotation past 10 degrees, and no adduction.

   b. Recurrent anterior dislocation at risk with extension and external rotation. Anterior precautions—no hip hyperextension, no external rotation, no abduction beyond 30 degrees.

   c. Abduction pillows or braces and knee immobilizers can be used.

F. Outcomes

1. Those who do not develop AVN, post-traumatic arthritis, or infection generally do well.

2. Posterior hip dislocations carry up to a 20% risk of AVN and up to 25% risk of post-traumatic arthritis.

3. Obturator dislocations are frequently associated with cartilage loss or femoral head impaction to the weight-bearing portion and may have early functional limitations.

III. Special Considerations for Pediatric and Geriatric Patients

A. Pediatric patients

1. Pediatric hip dislocations are very rare, but when they occur they are usually pure dislocations without fractures of the hip. They are treated using the same principles as adult patients.

2. MRI is recommended postreduction to evaluate for posterior wall fractures. Skeletally immature patients have peripheral areas of the acetabulum that are not calcified and cannot be evaluated by plain radiographs or CT.

B.   Geriatric patients

   1.   Prosthetic hip dislocations:

      a.   These patients require reduction; however, the urgency is not as critical as in a native hip. Revision of the arthroplasty components may be required for recurrent prosthetic dislocation.

      b.   Assess implants, stability, presence of a constrained liner, and bone quality.

      c.   Reduce in the operating room if closed reduction cannot be obtained in the emergency room.

Summary

Traumatic hip dislocations are uncommon injuries, and the majority of them occur after high-energy mechanisms. Prompt reduction remains the mainstay of treatment of native hip dislocations to limit the risk of avascular necrosis. Inability to obtain a closed reduction with adequate sedation requires urgent open reduction. These patients have a high incidence of concomitant injuries and necessitate meticulous evaluation beginning with Advanced Trauma Life Support algorithms. Physical examination can alert the physician of a dislocation before a confirmatory anteroposterior pelvis radiograph is obtained. Advanced imaging should be reserved for postreduction evaluation of associated fractures and intra-articular osteochondral debris. Associated complications including avascular necrosis of the femoral head, recurrent instability, acetabular and labral pathology, heterotopic ossification, and post-traumatic arthritis should be openly discussed with patients early in their course of treatment.

Suggested Readings

Blanchard C, Kushare I, Boyles A, Mundy A, Beebe AC, Klingele KE. Traumatic, posterior pediatric hip dislocations with associated posterior labrum osteochondral avulsion: recognizing the acetabular "Fleck" sign. J Pediatr Orthop 2016;36(6):602–607

Foulk DM, Mullis BH. Hip dislocation: evaluation and management. J Am Acad Orthop Surg 2010;18(4):199–209

Kellam P, Ostrum RF. Systematic review and meta-analysis of avascular necrosis and post-traumatic arthritis after traumatic hip dislocation. J Orthop Trauma 2016;30(1):10–16

Mehta S, Routt ML Jr. Irreducible fracture-dislocations of the femoral head without posterior wall acetabular fractures. J Orthop Trauma 2008;22(10):686–692

Thompson VP, Epstein HC. Traumatic dislocation of the hip; a survey of two hundred and four cases covering a period of twenty-one years. J Bone Joint Surg Am 1951;33-A(3):746–778, passim

Upadhyay SS, Moulton A. The long-term results of traumatic posterior dislocation of the hip. J Bone Joint Surg Br 1981;63B(4):548–551

33 Femoral Neck and Head Fractures

Thuan V. Ly and Christopher B. Sugalski

Introduction

Femoral head fractures are often associated with posterior hip dislocation. Anatomic reduction and restoration of the concentric hip joint are paramount for a favorable outcome. Femoral neck fractures have a bimodal distribution. Open reduction and internal fixation is recommended for young adults with displaced femoral neck fracture. Displaced femoral neck fractures in elderly patients are best treated with hemi or total hip arthroplasty (▶**Video 33.1**).

Femoral Neck Fractures

I. Preoperative

A. History and physical examination

1. Bimodal age distribution.

   a. Young patient—usually high-energy injury.

   b. Older patient—usually low-energy injury, typically ground-level fall.

2. Preoperative functional activity level, especially important when considering fractures in the elderly.

3. Preexisting hip pain can correlate with pathologic fracture or longstanding hip arthritis, necessitating biopsy or total hip arthroplasty.

4. A complete history and physical examination should be coordinated with the appropriate medical team, especially in the case of an elderly patient with preexisting medical comorbidities.

5. High-energy injuries have a high suspicion for associated femoral head and neck trauma, chest and abdominal injuries, and coexisting extremity injuries.

6. Frail elderly patients may sustain coexisting injuries such as cervical and rib fractures that could adversely affect the treatment outcomes.

7. The affected extremity will be shortened and externally rotated in displaced fractures.

8. A complete neurovascular examination of all extremities is imperative, as well as palpation and range of motion for all joints.

B. Anatomy

1. Femoral neck-shaft angle is approximately 130 degrees with 10 degrees of anteversion.

2. Typical femoral head diameter is between 40 to 60 mm with a 3 to 4 mm hyaline cartilage cap.

3. Femoral head and neck blood supply (▶**Fig. 33.1**) is predominantly from the branches of the medial femoral circumflex artery, with secondary supply from the lateral femoral circumflex and the artery of the ligamentum teres. Retinacular arteries arise from terminal branches of the medial femoral circumflex artery and provide critical blood supply to the weight-bearing portions of the femoral head.

4. The calcar femorale is a strong bony buttress along the posteromedial aspect of the neck.

5. The greater trochanter serves as an attachment for the hip abductors (gluteus medius and minimus).

6. The iliopsoas inserts at the lesser trochanter.

7. A thick capsule encases the femoral neck and head consisting of the iliofemoral, ischiofemoral, and pubofemoral ligaments (see Chapter 32, Hip Dislocation, ▶**Fig. 32.3**).

8. Congruency of the femoroacetabular joint is increased by the presence of circular fibrocartilaginous labrum.

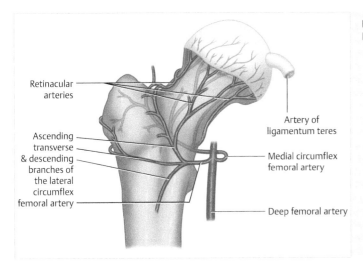

Fig. 33.1 Femoral head and neck blood supply.

Retinacular arteries

Artery of ligamentum teres

Ascending transverse & descending branches of the lateral circumflex femoral artery

Medial circumflex femoral artery

Deep femoral artery

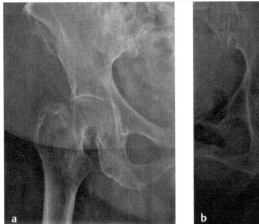
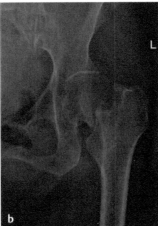
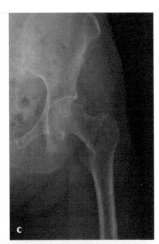

Fig. 33.2 (a) Subcapital femoral neck fracture; (b) transcervical femoral neck fracture; (c) basicervical femoral neck fracture.

C. Imaging

1. Plain radiographic imaging (XR) should include views of anteroposterior (AP) pelvis, AP hip, and lateral hip to adequately visualize the fracture morphology.

2. If difficult to differentiate an intertrochanteric fracture from a femoral neck fracture, therefore additional imaging may be required—AP traction view in internal rotation or computerized tomography (CT) scan can be obtained to further categorize the fracture pattern.

3. Full-length femur films (AP, lateral) should be obtained to evaluate for any preexisting deformity, hardware/prosthesis, or excessive anterior bowing which could affect treatment.

4. With a suspected occult femoral neck fracture, MRI is the study of choice as it demonstrates higher sensitivity than CT for detection of nondisplaced fractures.

D. Classification

1. Subcapital—fracture abutting femoral head (▶ **Fig. 33.2a**).

2. Transcervical—fracture along midneck (▶ **Fig. 33.2b**).

3. Basicervical—fracture along base of femoral neck (▶ **Fig. 33.2c**).

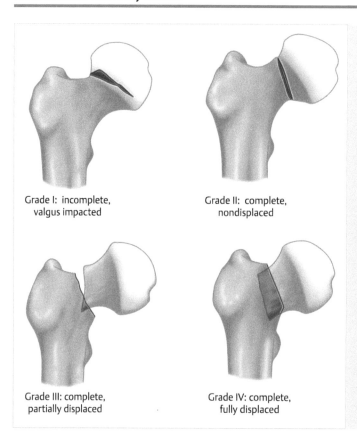

Fig. 33.3 Garden classification for femoral neck fractures.

Grade I: incomplete, valgus impacted

Grade II: complete, nondisplaced

Grade III: complete, partially displaced

Grade IV: complete, fully displaced

4. Garden classification (**Fig. 33.3**)—based on displacement and risk of avascular necrosis (AVN), which increases with increasing grade.
   a. Grade I—incomplete, valgus impacted.
   b. Grade II—complete, nondisplaced.
   c. Grade III—complete, partially displaced.
   d. Grade IV—complete, fully displaced.
   e. More accurately defined as nondisplaced Garden I/II and displaced Garden III/IV.
5. Pauwels classification (▶ **Fig. 33.4**) is based on fracture inclination and with reference to the horizontal plane which determines classification. Increased verticality is associated with increased instability due to shear forces transferred during weight bearing.
   a. Type I: < 30 degrees.
   b. Type II: 30 to 50 degrees.
   c. Type III: > 50 degrees.
6. Femoral neck stress fractures—fatigue fracture that occurs when bone is subjected to repetitive abnormal forces which overcome innate reparative biology.
   a. High-risk patients
      i. Military recruits, runners, and females.
      ii. Young recreational athletes with rapid increase in activity duration, frequency, or intensity.
      iii. Female athlete triad—eating disorder, amenorrhea, and osteoporosis.

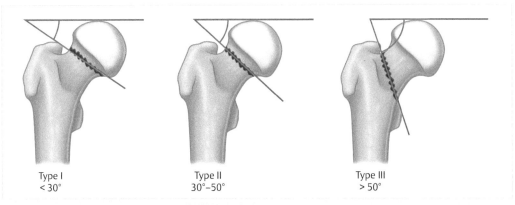

| Type I | Type II | Type III |
| <30° | 30°–50° | >50° |

Fig. 33.4 Pauwels classification for femoral neck fractures.

   b. Workup
      i. History
         • Menstrual irregularities.
         • Assess calcium and vitamin D levels and supplement accordingly.
      ii. XR—initially nondiagnostic, but may show endosteal/periosteal changes or a thin black line as the fatigue fracture progresses.
      iii. Magnetic resonance imaging (MRI)—gold standard imaging modality.
      iv. Bone scan—sensitive but nonspecific.
   c. Types
      i. Compression—fracture initiating on inferior aspect of the femoral neck.
         • Conservative treatment with nonweight bearing until asymptomatic, followed by gradual return to activities.
         • If fatigue line > 50% neck diameter, treat with percutaneous pinning (as described in operative management section).
      ii. Tension—fracture initiating on superior aspect of the femoral neck– treat with percutaneous pinning.
      iii. Displaced—open reduction and internal fixation.

II. Treatment

A. Initial management
   1. Management in the emergency department begins with a complete history and physical examination, and assessment of associated injuries and medical comorbidities.
   2. More than half (50–70%) of nonelderly patients sustaining high-energy injuries with femoral neck fractures will have significant coexisting injuries.
   3. Excessive manipulation of the hip should be avoided to decrease unnecessary discomfort and risk of further fracture displacement.
   4. A foley catheter should be placed for patient comfort; transferring to a bedpan can be difficult and painful.
   5. Judicious use of pain medication is advised, especially among elderly patients who are prone to excessive sedation.

B. Definitive management

   1. Nonoperative treatment:

      a. An option for stable, nondisplaced, valgus-impacted fractures.

         i. Around 6 to 12 weeks of touchdown weight-bearing with a walker should be allowed for sufficient healing.

         ii. Associated with an increased risk of future displacement resulting in nonunion, AVN, and a poor functional outcome.

      b. Elderly patients with extensive medical comorbidities at high risk of perioperative cardiopulmonary complications.

         i. Renders mobilization more difficult.

         ii. Consider supplemental pain management via regional anesthesia (nerve blocks and catheters).

         iii. This route of management should be discussed with the patient and family, emphasizing the high risk of associated medical complications associated with prolonged immobility.

         iv. The consideration of transfer to end of life/comfort care is a real discussion for these patients.

   2. Operative management and fixation:

      a. Standard of care.

      b. A stabilized fracture allows more rapid mobilization and decreases morbidity and mortality, which often occurs with prolonged bed rest, and improves patient function.

      c. Improved outcomes are associated with surgical fixation within 24 to 48 hours of presentation.

C. Surgical approaches and fixation techniques (▶ **Fig. 33.5**)

   1. Open reduction internal fixation—ideal for a young patient with displaced femoral neck fracture.

      a. Anterolateral approach (Watson-Jones) (▶ **Fig. 33.6**).

         i. Lateral incision centered over the greater trochanter, extending 6 to 8 cm distally along the femoral shaft and 6 to 10 cm proximally curving slightly anterior (incision remains 3 cm posterior to the anterior superior iliac spine [ASIS]).

         ii. Superficial dissection: Incise the iliotibial band at the distal extent of the incision and proceed toward the anterior half of the greater trochanter. Proximally, incise fascia along the posterior border of the tensor fascia lata.

         iii. Deep dissection: Retract tensor fascia lata (superior gluteal nerve) anteriorly and gluteus medius (superior gluteal nerve) posteriorly. Mobilize the reflected head of the rectus femoris (femoral nerve) medially, as needed, to expose the anterior hip capsule.

         iv. Externally rotate the femur and perform a capsulotomy to expose the femoral neck.

         v. To improve visualization of the base of the femoral neck, incise the anterior 1 to 2 cm of the gluteus medius insertion and vastus lateralis origin. This also facilitates placement of a lateral side plate (for sliding hip screw fixation) or insertion of cancellous screws.

         vi. Be aware that this approach provides only limited visualization of subcapital femoral neck fractures.

      b. Anterior approach (Smith-Petersen) (▶ **Fig. 33.7**).

         i. Anterior incision from the iliac crest 2 to 3 cm proximal to the ASIS, extending toward the ASIS and then 10 cm distal toward the lateral border of the patella.

         ii. Superficial dissection: Identify and the develop the interval between the sartorius (femoral nerve) medially and tensor fascia lata (superior gluteal nerve) laterally.

         iii. Avoid injury to the lateral femoral cutaneous nerve that pierces the fascia near the ASIS and lies superficial to the sartorius.

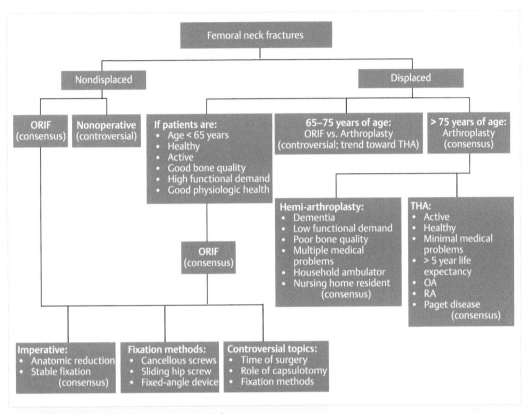

Fig. 33.5 Treatment algorithm for femoral neck fractures.

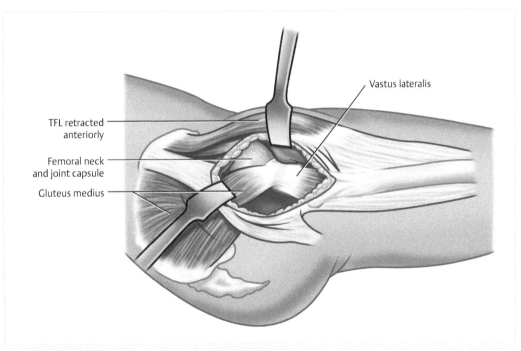

Fig. 33.6 Anterolateral approach (Watson-Jones) to the hip.

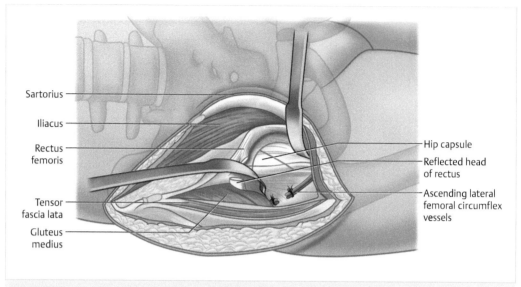

Sartorius

Iliacus

Rectus
femoris

Hip capsule

Reflected head
of rectus

Ascending lateral
femoral circumflex
vessels

Tensor
fascia lata

Gluteus
medius

Fig. 33.7 Anterior approach (Smith-Petersen) to the hip.

    iv. Ligate ascending branches of the lateral femoral circumflex artery as needed.

    v. Deep dissection: Retract the gluteus medius (superior gluteal nerve) laterally and the two heads of the rectus femoris (femoral nerve) medially off the hip capsule.

      • The direct (straight) head arises from the AIIS and should be mobilized medially.

      • The indirect (reflected) head originates on the superior acetabulum and may need to be detached to expose subcapital femoral neck fractues and femoral head fractures.

    vi. Adduct and externally rotate the femur to place the hip capsule on stretch.

    vii. Perform a capsulotomy to expose the femoral neck.

    viii. This approach provides excellent exposure for most femoral neck fractures and facilitates fracture reduction; however, a separate lateral incision is typically required for implant fixation.

2. Percutaneous screw fixation (▶ **Fig. 33.8**):

    a. Placement of multiple cancellous (typically cannulated) screws via a limited lateral incision provides stable fixation in anatomically-reduced or valgus-impacted fractures.

    b. If further reduction of the fracture is required, extension of the incision to an anterolateral approach (Watson-Jones) or a separate anterior approach (Smith-Petersen) to the hip is required for access to the femoral neck.

    c. Patient is positioned supine on a fracture table and the contralateral leg is either scissored or placed in the lithotomy position, allowing appropriate fluoroscopic imaging access (▶ **Fig. 33.9a**).

    d. C-arm is brought in from the nonoperative side at approximately 45 degrees to obtain adequate AP and lateral images of the affected hip (▶ **Fig. 33.9b**).

    e. Appropriate placement of the incision and guide pin entry can be marked by the intersection of the lines created by laying a guide pin on the skin in line with the central femoral head and neck in the both the AP and lateral projections (▶ **Fig. 33.9c, d**).

    f. A straight lateral incision is made through skin and through the fascia lata for placement of the guide pins which are later replaced by cannulated screws.

    g. The first screw is placed in a central inferior location within 3 mm of the stronger cortical bone followed by 2 parallel superior screws (anterosuperior and posterosuperior) in an inverted triangle position.

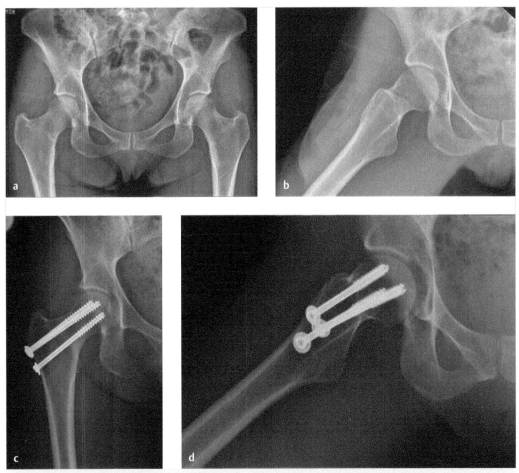

Fig. 33.8 **(a)** A 36-year-old female with nondisplaced femoral neck fracture. Anteroposterior (AP) pelvis; **(b)** right hip lateral; **(c)** X-rays showing the femoral neck fracture. Postoperative right hip; **(d)** lateral X-rays showing the percutaneous 7.3 mm partially threaded cancellous screws.

    h. Pin length is then measured with the appropriate depth gauge, and the appropriate size cancellous screws (6.5–8.0 mm) are then chosen.

        i. Partially threaded screws allow adequate compression of the fracture.

    i. Washers can be placed along the lateral cortex to increase the purchase of the screw head or adjust for excessive screw length.

    j. Fully threaded screws can subsequently be placed for length stability, if needed.

3. Sliding hip screw (▶ **Fig. 33.10**)

    a. Patient positioned supine on the fracture table.

    b. A straight lateral incision is made along the proximal lateral thigh, deep to fascia. A slightly large incision is required compared to the technique described for percutaneous screws.

    c. Using the device appropriate aiming guide (based on the neck-shaft angle), a guide pin is placed in a central position on both the AP and lateral projections to within 5 mm of subchondral bone.

    d. Consider inserting an antirotation screw to prevent rotary displacement of the fracture.

    e. The pin is overdrilled with care to keep the tip of the pin engaged in the subchondral bone.

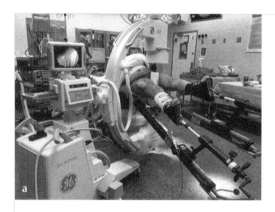
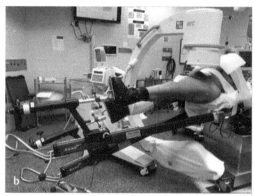
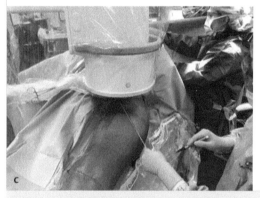
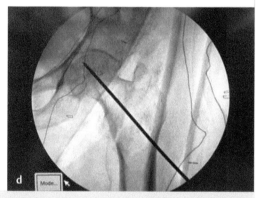

Fig. 33.9 **(a)** Patient in a scissored position. **(b)** C-arm advanced from nonoperative side. **(c, d)** Method utilized for marking of the incision and guide pin entry.

    f.   The screw path is then tapped.

    g.   The appropriate length compression screw is then placed followed by placement of the slide plate which is secured by two or more screws.

    h.   This technique may provide more stable fixation for vertical fracture patterns and basicervical fractures.

4. Arthroplasty (▶ **Fig. 33.11**):

    a.   Displaced femoral neck fractures in physiologically older patients may be treated definitively with prosthetic replacement.

    b.   Hemiarthroplasty is generally reserved for elderly patients with low demands and without preexisting hip arthritis.

    c.   Total hip arthroplasty (THA) should be considered for the more active patient.

       i.   Better pain relief.

      ii.   Improved functional outcomes compared to hemiarthroplasty.

     iii.   Decreased risk of requiring revision surgery as osteoarthritis progresses on the acetabulum.

    d.   There are a variety of surgical approaches (anterior, anterolateral, direct lateral, and posterior), each with distinct advantages and disadvantages. The anterior and anterolateral approaches are described above; the posterior approach is described in detail in the acetabular chapter).

    e.   Posterolateral approach:

       i.   Split iliotibial fascia and gluteus maximus. Requires take down of the short external rotators.

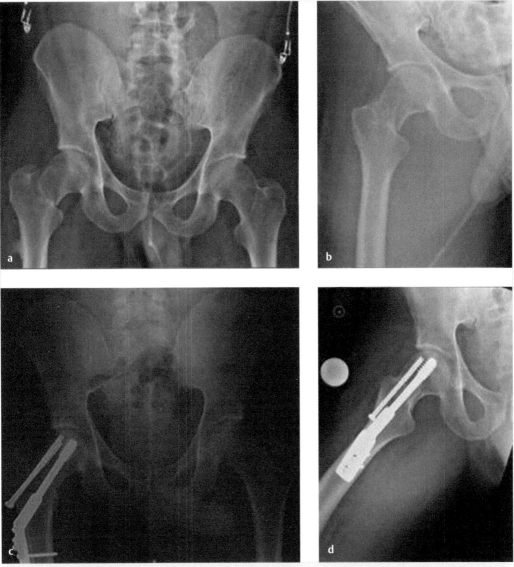

Fig. 33.10 A 35-year-old healthy male with a displaced femoral neck fracture. Anteroposterior (AP) pelvis **(a)** and lateral hip X-rays **(b)** showing the displaced femoral neck fracture. Three months postoperative right hip AP **(c)** and lateral **(d)** X-rays showing a sliding hip screw and two cannulated 7.3 mm screws.

    ii.   Familiar to most surgeons.

    iii.   Requires secure posterior capsule and short external rotator repair to minimize dislocation risk.

  f.   Anterior approach:

    i.   Interval between sartorius (femoral nerve) and tensor fascia lata (superior gluteal nerve).

    ii.   Improved early mobilization in some studies.

    iii.   More difficult femoral exposure and increased risk of intraoperative femur fracture.

    iv.   Steep learning curve.

  g.   Anterolateral approach:

    i.   Interval between tensor fascia lata and gluteus medius.

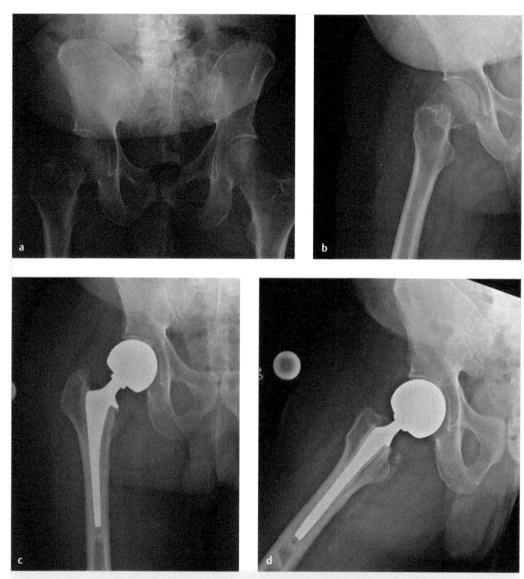

Fig. 33.11 A 69-year-old male with a displaced femoral neck fracture. Anteroposterior (AP) pelvis (**a**) and right lateral hip (**b**) X-rays showing the displaced femoral neck fracture. Three months postoperative right hip AP (**c**) and lateral hip (**d**) X-rays of hemiarthroplasty.

        ii. Decreased dislocation risk.

       iii. Violates abductors and may lead to postoperative limp.

    h. Direct lateral approach:

        i. Splits gluteus medius and vastus lateralis.

        ii. Decreased risk of dislocation.

       iii. Violates abductors and may lead to postoperative limp and higher rates of heterotopic ossification.

D. Complications

    1. Avascular necrosis:

       a. 10 to 30%.

b. Intracapsular femoral neck fractures disrupt the blood supply to the femoral head to varying degrees.

c. Increased risk with increasing displacement and subcapital fracture.

d. Decreased risk with timely anatomic reduction.

2. Fixation failure:

a. 10 to 20%.

b. Increased risk with posterior comminution, initial displacement, age, and osteoporosis.

3. Nonunion:

a. 10 to 20%.

b. Same risk factors as fixation failure.

4. Dislocation:

a. 1 to 10%.

b. Higher dislocation rates of THA for fracture compared to elective THA for arthritis.

i. Lack of preoperative stiffness associated with arthritis.
ii. Baseline cognitive dysfunction (i.e., dementia and alcoholism).

c. Higher dislocation rates of THA compared to hemiarthroplasty—larger femoral heads utilized in hemiarthroplasty have increased jump distance.

5. Acetabular erosion (hemiarthroplasty):

a. 10 to 40%.

b. Less of an issue if hemiarthroplasty is selected for lower demand patients.

6. Prosthesis failure (component wear and loosening)—2 to 8%.

7. Infection:

a. 1 to 5%.

b. Increased risk with arthroplasty.

8. Mortality—30% at one year for the elderly patient.

E. Rehabilitation

1. Optimal treatment of femoral neck fractures allows early mobilization with immediate weight-bearing in an effort to decrease medical complications associated with recumbency.

2. Typically, elderly patients are weight-bearing as tolerated immediately following surgery, as they are unable to comply with more limited restrictions.

3. Younger patients sustain higher energy and comminuted fractures and are typically prescribed a period of touchdown weight-bearing for 6 to 12 weeks.

4. Weight-bearing as tolerated is recommended following arthroplasty. Range of motion precautions are dependent upon the surgical approach chosen.

5. Most physiologically older patients require a prolonged stay in a rehabilitation facility. Half of these patients will require permanent gait aids and experience some decrease in overall mobility and function.

F. Outcomes

1. Debate exists in the literature regarding optimal treatment of femoral neck fractures:

a. Fixation with cancellous (cannulated) screws versus sliding hip screw in young adults (< 50 years old).

b. Fixation versus arthroplasty for middle-aged adults (50–65 years old).

c. Type of arthroplasty in elderly patients.

2. In general, anatomic restoration of the native femoral head and neck will produce optimal results; however, as age increases and the quality of bone decreases, results of fixation are not as reliable due to potential loss of fixation, nonunion, and AVN.

3. In a physiologically older patient, prosthetic replacement with THA will produce satisfactory results and decrease the need for future surgery if fixation were to fail.

4. In the low demand, elderly patient, treatment with hemiarthroplasty may suffice, and is associated with a lower risk of dislocation when compared to THA

Femoral Head Fractures

I. Preoperative

A. History and physical examination

1. Femoral head fractures generally result from high-energy trauma such as motor vehicle accidents (dashboard injury), pedestrians versus motor vehicle, and fall from height. These trauma patients should be evaluated in accordance with appropriate advanced trauma life support (ATLS) protocols.

2. With the exception of penetrating trauma, these injuries are caused by shear of the femoral head against the acetabulum.

3. Typically, there is an associated posterior hip dislocation at the time of injury. However, anterior hip dislocation or central dislocation and impaction against acetabular fragments can also lead to fracture of the femoral head.

4. With a posterior hip dislocation, the limb will be shortened and internally rotated. This may not be the case if there is an associated femoral shaft fracture.

5. A thorough examination of the affected extremity, including neurovascular status, is imperative as the sciatic nerve can be stretched by the persistent or prior displacement of the proximal femur.

B. Anatomy: See Anatomy section on femoral neck fractures.

C. Imaging

1. AP pelvis XR—if hip dislocation is identified, closed reduction of the hip should take priority over further imaging.

2. Lateral hip XR and full length femur XR.

3. Judet views of acetabulum to evaluate associated acetabular fractures, including commonly associated posterior wall fragments.

4. Inlet and outlet views of pelvis if associated with pelvic ring injury.

5. Postreduction pelvis CT:

   a. Further evaluate fracture characteristics and concentric reduction.

   b. Check for intraarticular fragments and associated acetabular and femoral neck fracture.

   c. Will ultimately determine operative planning.

D. Classification

1. Pipkin (▶Fig. 33.12):

   a. Type I—fracture line inferior to ligamentum teres.

   b. Type II—fracture line superior to ligamentum teres.

   c. Type III—associated femoral neck fracture.

   d. Type IV—associated acetabular fracture.

II. Treatment

A. Initial management

1. Trauma patients should be evaluated utilizing ATLS protocols.

2. Care should be taken to not overlook associated injuries such as ipsilateral femoral shaft fractures, knee injuries, and femoral neck fractures which may displace further during attempted reduction.

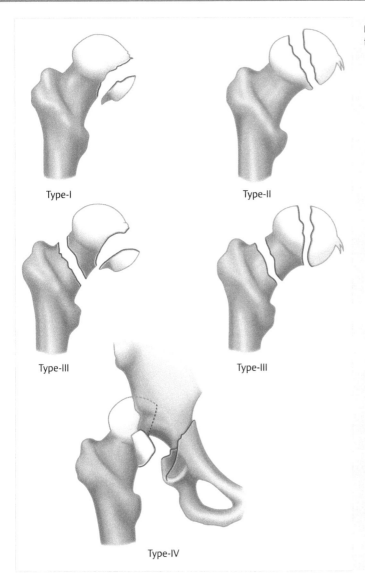

Type-I

Type-II

Type-III

Type-III

Type-IV

Fig. 33.12 Pipkin classification for femoral head fracture.

3. Hip dislocation should be urgently reduced, either under deep conscious sedation in the emergency department or in the operating room.

4. The limb should be placed in skeletal traction in the case of intraarticular fragments or irreducible dislocations.

B. Definitive management

1. Nonoperative treatment:

a. Most Pipkin type I fractures that meet the following criteria:

i. Weight-bearing portion of the femoral head is concentrically reduced.

ii. Hip is stable.

iii. No loose bodies superior to the fovea.

b. Pipkin type II fractures with < 1 to 2 mm displacement and the same criteria stated above.

c. Touchdown weight-bearing for 8 to 12 weeks with serial radiographs.

2. Operative treatment:

    a. Displaced Pipkin type II fractures ≥ 1 to 2 mm.

    b. Most Pipkin type III suprafoveal fractures with consideration of operative indications listed above.

    c. Most Pipkin type IV suprafoveal or any type IV with associated operative acetabular fracture.

3. Fragment excision is indicated for intraarticular fragments and small areas of comminution not in the weight-bearing portion of the femoral head—can be performed arthroscopically.

4. Arthroplasty should be considered in Pipkin type III fractures in the physiologically older patient or as a salvage procedure following attempted open reduction and internal fixation (ORIF).

C. Surgical approaches

1. Anterior approach (Smith-Petersen) (▶ **Fig. 33.7**).

    a. See description of this approach in the preceding section on femoral neck fractures.

    b. Reduction can be aided by 5 mm Schanz pin placed in the proximal femur and Kirschner wires (joysticks) in the femoral head.

    c. The anterior approach generally offers the best exposure of the typical anterior and medial fracture fragments, but does not allow simultaneous treatment of associated posterior wall fractures.

2. Posterior approach (Kocher-Langenbeck).

    a. Lateral position.

    b. See a full description of the approach with illustrations in the acetabulum chapter.

    c. Capsulotomy permits limited access to the femoral head, but often the fracture pattern will dictate a separate anterior approach or surgical hip dislocation for adequate visualization and fracture fixation.

3. Posterior approach with surgical hip dislocation (see Chapter 32, Hip Dislocation ▶ **Fig. 32.6a, b**)

    a. Superficial approach identical to the above (Kocher-Langenbeck).

    b. Short external rotators are preserved.

    c. Greater trochanter osteotomy and periacetabular capsulotomy are performed to allow anterior dislocation of the hip and visualization of the acetabulum and femoral head (see suggested reading 5 for further description).

D. Fixation techniques (▶ **Fig. 33.13**).

1. Anatomic reduction and interfragmentary compression provide stable reduction and allow for early hip range of motion.

2. Typical small fragments implants (2.7–3.5 mm) are used and should either be headless or countersunk to avoid future articular damage with joint motion. Minifragment fixation can also be used for small osteochondral fractures (2.0–2.7 mm).

E. Complications

1. Traumatic osteoarthritis:

    a. 20 to 50%.

    b. Treat with arthroplasty versus hip arthrodesis.

2. AVN:

    a. 0 to 23%.

    b. Increased with delay in hip reduction.

3. Heterotopic ossification (HO):

    a. 6 to 64%.

    b. Increases risk with anterior approach; decreases risk by limited stripping of musculature from ilium.

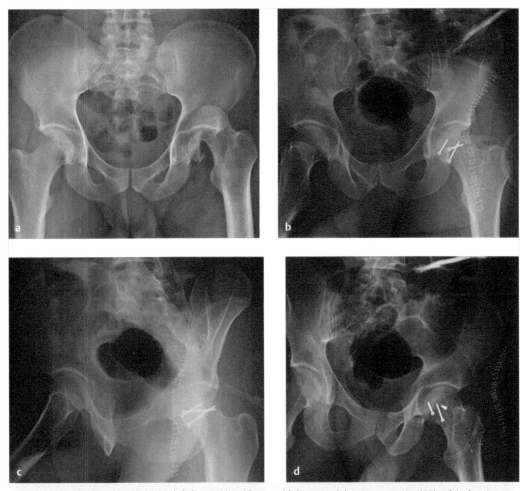

Fig. 33.13 A 27-year-old male with a left femoral head fracture/dislocation, **(a)** Anteroposterior (AP) pelvis showing the femoral head fracture and dislocation. Postoperative AP pelvis **(b)** and Judet views **(c, d)** showing femoral head fixation with 2.7 mm counter sunk screws.

    c.   Risk may be mitigated by prophylactic nonsteroidal anti-inflammatory drugs (NSAIDs) or radiation.

  4. Sciatic nerve palsy: 10%.

F. Rehabilitation

  1. Touchdown weight-bearing 8 to 12 weeks.

  2. Avoid hip flexion beyond 70 degrees for 8 to 12 weeks to avoid shear forces along the healing fracture.

  3. Long-term follow-up for 2 years to rule out AVN.

G. Outcomes

  1. Limited conclusions can be made regarding the treatment of femoral head fractures due to the rarity of the injury and lack of long-term follow-up data.

  2. Approximately half of patients with anatomic reduction of femoral head fractures and associated injuries can expect good to excellent results in the intermediate term.

  3. As noted above, post-traumatic arthritis, AVN, and HO may require additional surgical procedures and eventual hip arthroplasty.

Conclusion

The goals of treatment for Femoral Neck and Head Fractures are anatomic reduction with stable fixation, and a concentric hip joint. Treatment options depend on the fracture pattern, physiologic age, and medical comorbidities of the patient. Open reduction and internal fixation is ideal in the young adult. Arthroplasty (hemi or total hip) is the recommended treatment for elderly patients with displaced fracture patterns and significant medical comorbidities.

Suggested Readings

Asghar FA, Karunakar MA. Femoral head fractures: diagnosis, management, and complications. Orthop Clin North Am 2004; 35(4):463–472

Baker RP, Squires B, Gargan MF, Bannister GC. Total hip arthroplasty and hemiarthroplasty in mobile, independent patients with a displaced intracapsular fracture of the femoral neck. A randomized, controlled trial. J Bone Joint Surg Am 2006;88(12):2583–2589

Bhandari M, Devereaux PJ, Swiontkowski MF, et al. Internal fixation compared with arthroplasty for displaced fractures of the femoral neck. A meta-analysis. J Bone Joint Surg Am 2003;85(9):1673–1681

Fixation using Alternative Implants for the Treatment of Hip fractures (FAITH) Investigators. Fracture fixation in the operative management of hip fractures (FAITH): an international, multicentre, randomised controlled trial. Lancet 2017;389:1519–1527

Gardner MJ, Suk M, Pearle A, Buly RL, Helfet DL, Lorich DG. Surgical dislocation of the hip for fractures of the femoral head. J Orthop Trauma 2005;19(5):334–342

Ly TV, Swiontkowski MF. Treatment of femoral neck fractures in young adults. J Bone Joint Surg Am 2008;90(10):2254–2266

Swiontkowski MF. Intracapsular fractures of the hip. J Bone Joint Surg Am 1994;76(1):129–138

34 Intertrochanteric, Pertrochanteric, and Subtrochanteric Femur Fractures

Thomas A. Russell

Introduction

The incidence of hip fractures in the United States is over 250,000 hospitalizations per year with approximately half the cases in the pertrochanteric/subtrochanteric group, and femoral neck and head fractures accounting for the remainder.

Ninety-five percent of hip fractures occur in people older than 65 years. Lifetime incidence of hip fracture is 20% for women and 10% for men. Males have three times higher risk of death compared to females.

Keywords: intertrochanteric fracture, pertrochanteric fracture, subtrochanteric fracture, hip fracture, hip fracture fixation, hip fracture devices, geriatric fractures, hip fracture surgery

I. Preoperative

A. History and physical examination

1. The presenting complaint is pain about the groin or hip with possible radiation to the knee and inability to ambulate or bear weight on the affected leg.

2. Mechanism of injury—ground level fall (elderly patients) or high-energy trauma (typically younger patients).

3. Past history may include an osteoporosis diagnosis, previous contralateral hip or other fragility fracture, and prior bisphosphonate therapy.

4. Physical findings may consist of lower extremity deformity with external rotation and shortening, bruising of the lateral proximal thigh or buttocks, and the inability to lift the affected leg off the stretcher with pain.

5. Auscultation test is a helpful screening tool. Percuss both patellae with the stethoscope bell overlying the symphysis pubis. A difference in sound or pitch between extremities implies a fracture defect between femur and pelvis resulting in impedance of percussive conduction.

6. Do not manipulate the extremity until after evaluation of radiographic examination if the extremity is deformed or auscultation test is positive.

B. Anatomy

1. The pertrochanteric–subtrochanteric hip originates from the extracapsular femoral neck extending to the proximal one-third of the femoral diaphysis (~5 cm below the lesser trochanter).

2. Components of the hip fracture include the following:

   a. Pertrochanteric metaphyseal primary fracture line.

   b. Femoral head and intracapsular neck fragment.

   c. Greater trochanter and lateral wall.

   d. Lesser trochanter.

   e. Subtrochanteric diaphysis (origin of the intramedullary canal).

3. The proximal femur is NOT SOLID. It is composed of a cortical shell adjacent to and covering an internal trabecular cancellous bone network extending from the head through the femoral neck and terminating in the thickened cortical tubular diaphysis below the lesser trochanter (▶ **Fig. 34.1a, b**). The two primary trabecular arcade patterns are dense cancellous bone

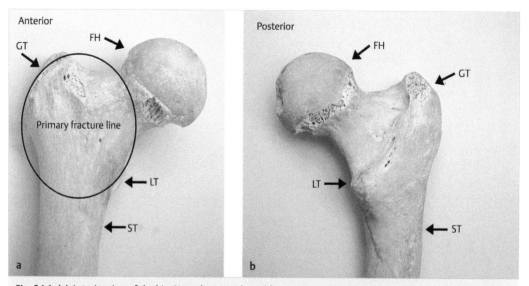

Fig. 34.1 **(a)** Anterior view of the hip. Note the metaphyseal fracture zone and components greater trochanter (GT), lesser trochanter (LT), femoral head and neck (FH), subtrochanteric (ST) shaft. **(b)** Posterior view of the hip. Vascular foramina enter the posterior neck from the 1 to 9 o'clock positions as branches of the medial circumflex femoral artery.

columns that are formed in response to load transfer from standing and sitting. Loss of these arcades predisposes to weakening of the hip structure and propensity to fracture (▶ **Fig. 34.2**).

    a. Posteromedial corticocancellous trabecular column (calcar).

    b. Anterolateral corticocancellous trabecular column.

  4. The femoral neck shaft angle averages 128 to 132 degrees on the anteroposterior (AP) view and the femoral head and neck are oriented in 0 to 30 degrees of anteversion (average 15 degrees) in relation to the coronal plane of the femur in most adults. Appreciation of these orientations is important in reduction and fixation tactics.

  5. Neurologic and vascular structures are rarely at risk from these fractures.

  6. Local preexisting disease, from osseous deformity, soft-tissue contractures, arthropathy, and microarchitecture pathology (osteomalacia and osteoporosis), may affect the surgical tactics and prognosis.

C. Diagnostic imaging

  1. Plain film radiographs are the mainstay of diagnosis.

    a. AP pelvis including hips (compare to normal side).

    b. AP hip and cross-table lateral hip views.

    c. Traction internal rotation AP view may be helpful in understanding fracture pattern, especially if shortened or excessively rotated on presentation.

  2. CT scans may be useful for multiplanar fractures from high-energy trauma.

  3. MRI scan most useful for diagnosis of occult fractures of the hip.

D. Classification of hip fractures

  1. AP and lateral view radiographic images are used to classify the fracture to give insight into fixation tactics and implant selection. They also relate to complexity of the reduction and the loads imparted to the implant.

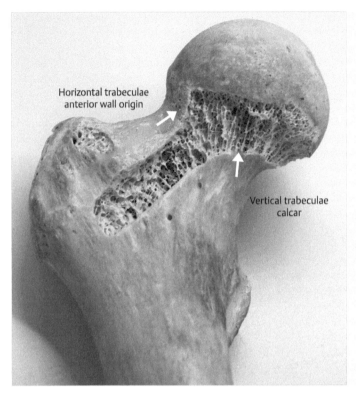

Fig. 34.2 Anteroposterior view of the hip. Note the cut-away of thin (2–4 mm) cortical wall and trabecular internal structures. Vertical trabecular column corresponding to the calcar and the horizontal trabecular column arising from the anterior wall to the neck and femoral head as described by Hammer.

Horizontal trabeculae anterior wall origin

Vertical trabeculae calcar

Table 34.1 Common classifications for pertrochanteric and subtrochanteric hip fractures

Name	Year	Class	Note
Boyd and Griffin	1934	1. Stable two-part 2. Unstable posteromedial comminution 3. Subtrochanteric extension laterally and reverse obliquity 4. Subtrochanteric/intertrochanteric multiplanar	Correlated implant failure rate increases from classes 1 to 4 with plate fixation
OTA/AO 31A	2018	A1: Simple pertrochanteric fracture with intact lateral wall A2: Incompetent lateral wall A3: Reverse obliquity or transverse pattern	AP radiograph only
Russell and Taylor	1988	1A: GT intact: LT intact 1B: GT intact: LT unstable 2A: GT unstable: LT intact 2B: GT unstable: LT unstable	Subtrochanteric classification relates optimal stability from interlocking nail vs. CMN vs. plate/screw

Abbreviations: AP, anteroposterior; CMN, cephalomedullary nail; GT, greater trochanteric region including lateral wall; LT, lesser trochanter and adjacent wall.

2. Common classifications for pertrochanteric and subtrochanteric hip fractures (▶ Table 34.1).

3. AO/OTA Fracture and Dislocation Classification Compendium-2018 is an alphanumeric classification most commonly used for pertrochanteric fractures. Proximal metaphyseal fractures of the hip are grouped into the 31A category (▶ Fig. 34.3a–c).

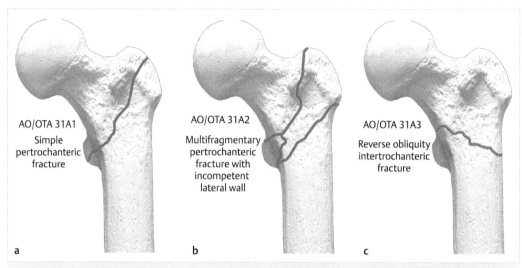

Fig. 34.3 AO/OTA classification 2018 of intertrochanteric femur fractures. **(a)** 31A1: Simple pertrochanteric femur fracture with intact lateral wall. **(b)** 31A2: Multifragmentary pertrochanteric femur fracture with incompetent lateral wall. **(c)** 31A3: Reverse obliquity intertrochanteric femur fracture. (Adapted from Meinberg E, Agel J, Roberts C. Fracture and dislocation classification compendium 2018. J Orthop Trauma 2018;32(1): 1–170.)

  a. 31A1 fractures are intertrochanteric fractures with an intact lateral wall (wall thickness > 20.5 mm). A stable reduction should be obtainable. Sliding hip screw (SHS) plates and cephalomedullary nails (CMNs) are equally effective.

  b. 31A2 fractures are multifragmentary intertrochanteric fractures with an incompetent lateral wall (wall thickness of ≤ 20.5 mm). These fractures are unstable and typically treated with a CMN. Alternative implants include SHS with a trochanteric buttress plate, blade plate, and locking plate.

  c. 31A3 intertrochanteric fractures are unstable with standard SHS plating due to reverse obliquity patterns and subtrochanteric extension in this group. CMNs are commonly recommended.

4. The Russell–Taylor Classification for subtrochanteric fractures (1988) relates the consideration of implant selection based on involvement of the greater and lesser trochanteric components in proximal femur fractures (▶Fig. 34.4).

  a. Fractures below the lesser trochanter and not involving the greater trochanter and lateral wall (type IA) can be treated with conventional static interlocking nails (**Fig. 34.4a**).

  b. For fractures of the lesser trochanter and the medial column, but intact greater trochanteric region (type IB), the implant requires increased structural design strength such as a CMN (▶Fig. 34.4b).

  c. Type II fractures relate to greater trochanteric region and piriformis fossa involvement.

  d. If the greater trochanteric fragment is stable and there is no lesser trochanteric fracture comminution (type IIA), a trochanteric portal CMN is commonly used (▶Fig. 34.4c).

  e. In type IIB fractures, the greater trochanteric lateral wall complex is unstable and there is medial comminution of the lesser trochanteric region (▶Fig. 34.4d).

    i. This is the most unstable type of fracture and open reduction with the use of trochanteric buttress type lateral plates with ancillary fixation may be required.

    ii. Alternatively, CMNs are commonly used for this fracture pattern; however, several challenges exist: nails can be difficult to use in this class of fracture, as the split in

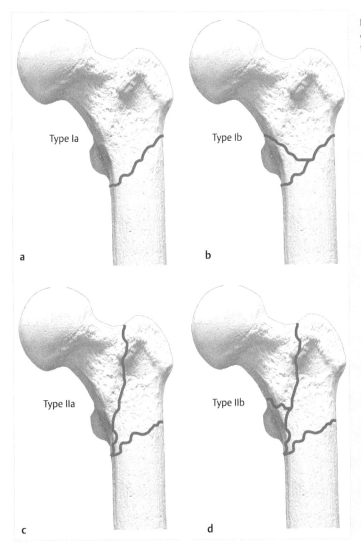

Fig. 34.4 (a–d) Russell–Taylor classification for subtrochanteric fractures.

Type Ia

Type Ib

a

b

Type IIa

Type IIb

c

d

the proximal fracture does not permit stable containment of the nail in the proximal femur.

5. Intraoperative change in classification may occur resulting in a tactical change:

   a. Lateral wall failure during plate application occurs up to 74% intraoperatively and may necessitate change to trochanteric buttress addition or CMN.

   b. Subtrochanteric extension below the lesser trochanter during surgery necessitates change to trochanteric extension and longer plates or conversion to longer nail if short nail was the original plan.

II. Treatment in Adults

A. The focus of treatment is the optimal conditioning of the patient for anesthesia and surgery within a 24- to 48-hour window after injury with anatomic reduction of the anteromedial wall and stable definitive fixation sufficient to permit early pain-free weight-bearing rehabilitation with the goal of restoration of prefracture functional independence.

B. Initial management optimizes the medical health of the patient for surgery.

1. After diagnosis, the extremity is placed in gentle alignment without traction; a pillow under the injured hip may help. A medical survey and physical examination are continued to rule out other injuries and preexisting diseases. Chest radiograph, electrocardiogram, and laboratory studies for blood electrolytes and blood typing and urinalysis are standard. IV access is achieved and dehydration and electrolyte replacement are initiated.

2. Consultation with geriatric service in conjunction with orthopaedic care in a team approach is optimal to maximize patient safety and optimize hospital efficiency.

   a. Frequent associated traumatic injuries include head (intracranial lesions and lacerations), neck (fractures and spondylosis), and upper extremity (proximal humerus and distal radius fractures) injuries in low-energy falls.

   b. Many patients in the geriatric population have medical comorbidities complicating urgent surgery. The most common to rule out are the following:

      i. Anticoagulation or coagulopathies.
      ii. Unstable arrhythmias.
      iii. Renal dysfunction.
      iv. Liver dysfunction.
      v. Dehydration/electrolyte imbalances, especially hypokalemia.
      vi. Systemic bacterial infection.

C. Definitive management

1. Nonoperative treatment is rarely indicated but might be appropriate in long-term nonambulatory patients or patients unlikely to survive surgery.

   a. Nonoperative care involves high-intensity nursing care with immobilization of the limb in an extended position with pillow support only.

   b. There is high risk for decubiti ulcers, malnutrition, and renal and thromboembolic complications; however, most patients have minimal pain after the first 3 weeks.

   c. Varus deformity and limb shortening are common after nonoperative treatment, but nonunion is rare.

2. Operative care—surgical management with operative open reduction and stable fixation minimizes pain and permits next-day mobility into chair or assisted ambulation. It is the current recommendation for all patients without medical contraindications with ambulatory capability prior to injury.

   a. Surgical approaches:

      i. Universally either the straight lateral approach or Watson-Jones approach (Chapter 33, Femoral Neck and Head Fractures, ▶ Fig. 33.6) is used for pertrochanteric fracture repair.
      ii. Approaches may be performed in the supine or lateral position with a fluoroscopic tabletop with or without a traction table attachment.
      iii. The clock model for hip incisions (▶ Fig. 34.5) conceptually places the tip of greater trochanter in line with the center of the femoral head and is represented as the center of the clock hands (0) with the femoral shaft aligned with the 6 o'clock position and proximally the 12 o'clock position is the extension of the clock face to the pelvic iliac brim.

         • Hip approaches for pertrochanteric fracture plating and intramedullary nailing are aligned in the 12–0–6 or the 1–0–6 lines, if more extensile exposure of the anteromedial femoral neck is required.
         • The subcutaneous interval is through the iliotibial tract in the 0–6 region for SHS plates and between the tensor fascia lata (TFL) and gluteus medius for the 1–0–6 interval.
         • For cephalomedullary nailing, two shorter incisions are used along the 12–0–6 interval with the proximal incision 2 cm proximal to the tip of the greater trochanter (0) approximately 2-cm long and the 2-cm second incision is in the 0 to 6 segment juxtaposed from the lesser trochanteric region on c-arm fluoroscopy.

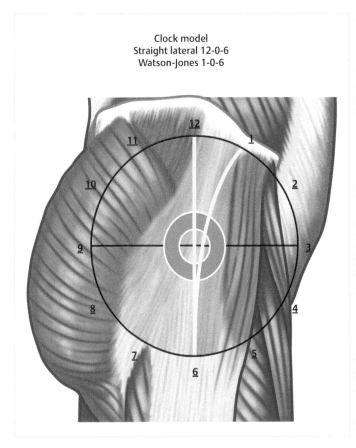

Clock model
Straight lateral 12-0-6
Watson-Jones 1-0-6

Fig. 34.5 Clock diagram for surgical approach to hip for fracture fixation based on a lateral view of the hip. The center of the clock face is 0 representing the tip of the greater trochanter aligned with the center of the femoral head. The 12 o'clock position is at the iliac brim and the 6 o'clock position overlies the femoral shaft axis.

b. Surgical reduction maneuver:
   i. Distraction—pull axial traction on the leg to regain length; excessive traction in geriatric patients may disrupt soft-tissue capsular attachments; monitor femoral head distraction from the acetabulum with C-arm fluoroscopy to avoid overdistraction.
   ii. Angulation—align the limb to the head/neck component using manual manipulation of the extremity or with clamps and/or joysticks in hip and/or shaft; avoid varus.
   iii. Translation—lift the shaft anteriorly to align with head and neck component and confirm with adequate lateral C-arm fluoroscopy.
   iv. Rotation—rotate the shaft and/or head/neck component to reduce the anteromedial wall of the hip of lower extremity to complete anteromedial neck anatomic reduction. If uncertain, directly palpate or visualize the anteromedial neck that is just proximal to the anterolateral origin of the vastus lateralis muscle. An anatomic anteromedial reduction of the femoral neck and anterior greater trochanteric ridge guarantees correct length, angulation, translation, and rotation of the intertrochanteric fracture.

D. Fixation techniques

Devices for fixation include plate and screw combinations and CMN and screw combinations. They may be grouped according to their insertion techniques and relative mechanical stability.

1. Plate and screw devices (▶ **Fig. 34.6**) typically include a specialized plate component that attaches to the lateral femur and specialized blades or screws for fixation into the femoral head and shaft. Russell et al have proposed a mechanical classification based on failure modes and rotational stability for plate and nail devices.

2. Plate and sliding screw designs are economical implants for stable fractures in low-demand patients.

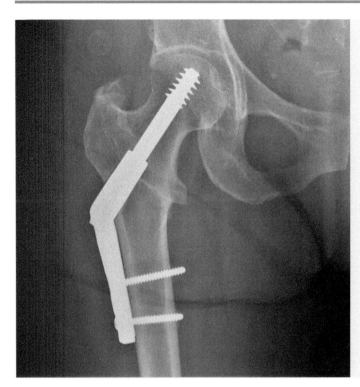

Fig. 34.6 Anteroposterior hip radiograph demonstrating fixation of an intertrochanteric femur fracture with a sliding hip screw.

3. CMN (▶**Fig. 34.7**) and screw designs behave differently biomechanically and are indicated in the following situations:
   a. Lateral wall incompetence.
   b. Reverse obliquity intertrochanteric fractures.
   c. Subtrochanteric fractures.
4. A "tip–apex distance" from the tip of the lag screw (for an SHS device with side plate or a CMN) should be less than 25 mm. Tip–apex distances is defined as the sum of the distance from the tip of the lag screw to the apex of the femoral head on AP and lateral radiographs.

E. Complications
   1. Mortality rate of 12 to 37% at 1-year postinjury, higher with increasing age.
   2. Postoperative medical complications occur in 19% of cases, primarily cardiovascular, pulmonary, and thromboembolic in nature.
   3. Nonunion rate of 1 to 5%.
   4. Malunion rates are underreported, but exceed 50%:
      a. Secondary to malreduction.
      b. Secondary to loss of fixation due to progressive fracture collapse causing shortening and varus.
      c. The addition of orthobiologics to internal fixation for osteopenic hip fractures is evolving and may be an important addition to surgical treatment to minimize malunion.
   5. Implant failure of screw breakage, pullout, or plate failure is 5%.
   6. Deep infections are reported in 1 to 2% of cases and superficial infection 1%.
   7. Delirium, dementia and/or depression occur in 35 to 65% of hip fracture patients.

F. Postoperative rehabilitation with weight bearing assistive devices
   1. With stable fixation, patients are aggressively mobilized to minimize complications. Up in chair and ambulation with walker/crutches and assistance is begun twice a day the first postoperative day and continued until the patient is independent.

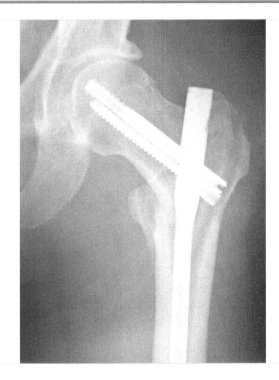

Fig. 34.7 Anteroposterior hip radiograph demonstrating fixation of an intertrochanteric femur fracture with a cephalomedullary nail.

2. Patients are allowed full weight bearing as tolerated and they will self-regulate their weight bearing based on their pain and stability of the fracture fixation. If patients complain of excessive pain with assisted weight bearing or at rest, reevaluate the stability of the fixation.

3. Most patients older than 65 years will require hospitalization in acute care for 3 days before transfer to an orthogeriatric rehabilitation center for 2 to 4 weeks depending on their general health and preinjury ambulatory activities of daily living capabilities.

G. Outcomes—general comments

1. Fracture healing occurs in 95% of patients in 8 to 16 weeks depending on the general health and nutrition of the patient and the extent of comminution of the fracture.

2. Adequate protein nutrition and vitamin D therapy are critical to healing and participation in rehabilitation.

3. Bone metabolism abnormalities including osteoporosis must be diagnosed and treated to prevent future fractures.

4. Socioeconomic morbidity:

   a. Fifty percent of patients are unable to live independently after injury.

   b. Fifty percent of patients require cane/walker assistance permanently.

   c. Average direct cost of medical care for a hip fracture is $40,000 for the first year.

III. Special Considerations: Pediatric Hip Fractures

A. Hip fractures in children are rare (< 1% of fractures in children).

B. The physeal growth plates are still open and these plates affect the fracture patterns and treatment.

C. The Delbet classification system (1928) is widely used with type IV fractures, most closely resembling adult pertrochanteric fractures.

D. These fractures are usually treated in pediatric orthopaedic centers with child-sized hip screw (SHS) implants. Minimize depth of femoral neck fixation to avoid screw intrusion into the capital physis. Spica casts are used in addition for small children and noncompliant patients.

E. Osteonecrosis and coxa vara are the most serious complications after pediatric hip fractures.

Summary

Hip fractures are the most frequent cause of emergent orthopaedic hospitalization. They are the most frequently surgically treated long bone fractures and have the highest postoperative mortality. After 100 years of surgical treatment and advances, most patients do not recover their preinjury function. Treatment is almost universally surgical in adults and as the majority are older than 65 years of age, medical comorbidities are common. Surgery includes reduction and stabilization with either extramedullary or intramedullary devices specifically designed for the unique hip anatomy. The goal of treatment is functional recovery to the preinjury status without residual deformity; however, postoperative loss of reduction and implant failure are still relatively high in the osteopenic elderly patient. Advances in optimized morphological and biomechanical implant design are beginning to show improved results in implant survival and fixation stability. The accurate reduction of the anteromedial wall and the preservation of the lateral wall extension of the greater trochanteric component are critical to success. Restoration of the anteromedial wall restores the femoral neck shaft angulation and rotation. The implant is optimally effective only when the reduction is correct. Malunion is more common than nonunion and may be progressive postoperatively. The development of the orthogeriatric team approach to these patients is improving efficiency and decreasing complications postoperatively. Rehabilitation to regain the patient's confidence in the extremity is critical to functional recovery. Future advances in augmentation orthobiologics may improve the fracture fixation interface and accelerate fracture healing.

Suggested Readings

Ahrengart L, Törnkvist H, Fornander P, et al. A randomized study of the compression hip screw and Gamma nail in 426 fractures. Clin Orthop Relat Res 2002(401):209–222

Baumgaertner MR, Curtin SL, Lindskog DM, Keggi JM. The value of the tip-apex distance in predicting failure of fixation of peritrochanteric fractures of the hip. J Bone Joint Surg Am 1995;77(7):1058–1064

Hammer A. The structure of the femoral neck: a physical dissection with emphasis on the internal trabecular system. Ann Anat 2010;192(3):168–177

Palm H, Jacobsen S, Sonne-Holm S, Gebuhr P; Hip Fracture Study Group. Integrity of the lateral femoral wall in intertrochanteric hip fractures: an important predictor of a reoperation. J Bone Joint Surg Am 2007;89(3):470–475

Reindl R, Harvey EJ, Berry GK, Rahme E; Canadian Orthopaedic Trauma Society (COTS). Intramedullary versus extramedullary fixation for unstable intertrochanteric fractures: a prospective randomized controlled trial. J Bone Joint Surg Am 2015;97(23):1905–1912

Russell TA, Mir HR, Stoneback J, Cohen J, Downs B. Avoidance of malreduction of proximal femoral shaft fractures with the use of a minimally invasive nail insertion technique (MINIT). J Orthop Trauma 2008;22(6):391–398

Sadowski C, Lübbeke A, Saudan M, Riand N, Stern R, Hoffmeyer P. Treatment of reverse oblique and transverse intertrochanteric fractures with use of an intramedullary nail or a 95 degrees screw-plate: a prospective, randomized study. J Bone Joint Surg Am 2002;84(3): 372–381– Recent articles

Sanders D, Bryant D, Tieszer C, et al. A multicenter randomized control trial comparing a novel intramedullary device (InterTAN) versus conventional treatment (sliding hip screw) of geriatric hip fractures. J Orthop Trauma 2017;31(1):1–8

35 Femoral Shaft Fractures

Marcus F. Sciadini and Christopher Lee

Introduction

Major injuries are commonly the result of high-energy mechanisms. They are often associated with life-threatening conditions. Reported incidence of femoral shaft fractures is 37.1 per 100,000 person-years. The mortality rate was upward of 80% during the early part of the First World War. Treatment progressed with the introduction of the Thomas splint (▶ **Fig. 35.1**). Subsequently, femoral shaft fractures were treated with traction typically for weeks or months. Intramedullary fixation was first introduced by Gerhard Kuntscher in 1939.

Keywords: femoral shaft fracture, treatment

I. Preoperative

A. History and physical examination

1. Age and medical comorbidities:

    a. Older patients with osteoporosis may have excessive bow (smaller radius of curvature) to the femur.

    b. Comorbidities including morbid obesity may influence patient positioning and choice of nailing technique.

2. Mechanism of injury:

    a. High-energy mechanisms in younger populations are frequently a result of high-speed motor vehicle accidents.

    b. Low-energy mechanism is more common in the elderly population as a result of a ground level fall; also rule out metastatic lesion in the elderly populations, especially if there are prodromal symptoms.

3. Other pertinent information from history:

    a. Time elapse from injury to presentation.

    b. Need for prolonged extrication.

4. Physical examination:

    a. Advanced trauma life support protocols are followed in initial evaluation.

    b. Examination should include visual inspection and palpation of all extremities, the pelvis, and the spine. Circumferential inspection of the extremity is done to look for associated open wounds, degloving injuries, bruising, and abrasions.

    c. Pain and swelling at the thigh with obvious deformity is common. Blood loss ranges from 1,000 to 1,500 mL for closed injuries.

    d. Focused examination of the knee ligaments and associated soft tissues is necessary, though often optimally performed at the conclusion of surgical stabilization.

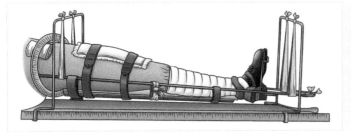

Fig. 35.1 An example of the Thomas splint used to treat femoral shaft fractures in the late 1800s and early 1900s.

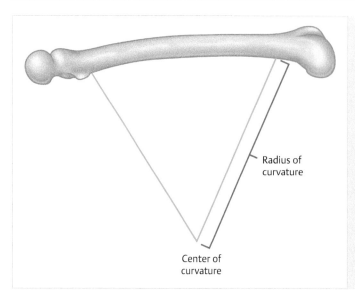

Fig. 35.2 A lateral image of a femur indicating the radius of curvature.

Radius of curvature

Center of curvature

5. Associated orthopaedic injuries:
    a. Ipsilateral femoral neck fractures:
        i. Incidence of 2 to 6%; missed up to 31% of the time.
        ii. Often vertical and basicervical.
    b. Ipsilateral knee injuries:
        i. Ligamentous laxity reported as high as 50%.
        ii. Approximately 25% risk of lateral or medial meniscus injury.

B. Anatomy
    1. The femoral shaft is the longest and strongest bone in the body.
    2. The femoral diaphysis extends from 5 cm distal to the lesser trochanter to 5 cm proximal to the adductor tubercle.
    3. The anterior bow is 12 to 15 degrees with a radius of curvature of approximately 120 cm. The radius of curvature decreases with age and the diameter of the intramedullary canal increases with age (▶ **Fig. 35.2**).
    4. The thickened posterior cortex coalesces into a ridge known as the linea aspera.
    5. The lateral cortex is under tension and the medial cortex is under compression.
    6. Compartments (▶ **Fig. 35.3**):
        a. Anterior:
            i. Sartorius, quadriceps.
            ii. Most commonly involved in compartment syndrome of the thigh.
        b. Posterior—biceps femoris, semitendinosus, semimembranosus.
        c. Medial—gracilis, adductor longus, adductor brevis, adductor magnus.
    7. Major muscle-deforming forces:
        a. Proximally—iliopsoas on the lesser trochanter (flexion, external rotation), the gluteus medius/minimus on the greater trochanter, and the gluteus maximus on the linea aspera.
        b. Distally—adductors on the linea aspera and pectineal line, and gastrocnemius on the posterior aspect of the lateral and medial femoral condyles.
    8. Vascular:
        a. External iliac artery becomes the femoral artery as it passes underneath the inguinal ligament and enters the anterior compartment through the femoral triangle.

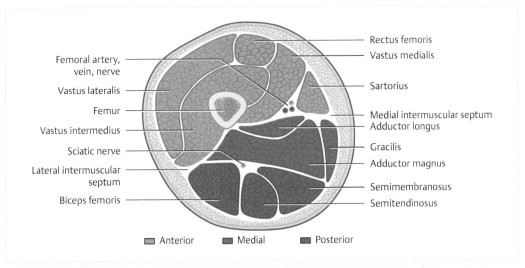

Fig. 35.3 Cross-section of the mid-thigh depicting the three compartments and respective muscles.

b. Profundus gives off numerous perforating branches along the length of the femur.

c. Main blood supply to the femur comes from the profunda and nutrient vessel, which enters posteriorly and proximally near the linea aspera.

d. Femoral artery is closest to the medial aspect of the femur 4 cm distal to the lesser trochanter. AP interlocks placed in retrograde nails are at risk of injuring the artery when the proximal nail ends below the lesser trochanter.

C. Imaging

1. Initial workup:

a. Anteroposterior (AP) and lateral views of the entire femur including the hip and knee.

b. AP and lateral views of the hip.

c. AP and lateral views of the knee.

2. Additional imaging—fine-cut (2-mm) CT scan advocated as screening tool to evaluate for femoral neck fracture.

3. Special considerations—intraoperative fluoroscopic view of the femoral neck with the leg internally rotated 15 degrees and intraoperative AP view of the pelvis and AP and lateral views of the femur following surgical fixation to evaluate for femoral neck fracture (▶Fig. 35.4a–d).

D. Classification

1. AO/OTA: the femur is designated as zone "3" and the shaft is designated as zone "2."

a. 32A: simple:

i. A1: spiral.
ii. A2: oblique, angle ≥ 30 degrees.
iii. A3: transverse, angle less than 30 degrees.

b. 32B: wedge:

i. B2: intact wedge.
ii. B3: fragmentary wedge.

c. 32C: multifragmentary:

i. C2: intact segmental.
ii. C3: fragmentary segmental.

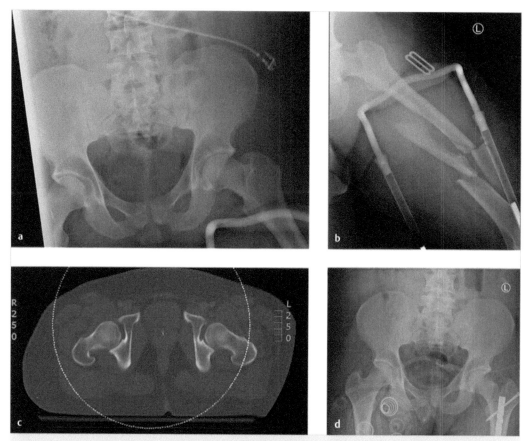

Fig. 35.4 Anteroposterior (AP) views of **(a)** the pelvis and **(b)** the left femur in a patient with a left femur fracture without evidence of a femoral neck fracture. **(c)** Axial CT view of the pelvis showing no evidence of a femoral neck fracture. **(d)** Intraoperative AP pelvis clearly showing a left femoral neck fracture.

II. Treatment

A. Initial management

This includes emergency room (ER) management:

1. Long leg splint or knee immobilizer for pain control and soft-tissue stabilization for distal fractures.

2. Traction:

a. Noninvasive traction is typically placed by Emergency medical technician (EMT) (danger, if left in place may quickly lead to pressure ulcer).

b. Skeletal traction is placed in the distal femur or proximal tibia to provide length and pain relief:

i. Safe placement is from medial to lateral at the distal femur and lateral to medial at the proximal tibia (contraindicated in suspected knee ligamentous injury).

ii. Typically 10% of one's body weight is applied.

B. Definitive management

1. Nonoperative management is rarely indicated:

a. Includes traction, long leg casting, and cast bracing.

b. Possible for nondisplaced or unicortical fractures (such as gunshot wounds) but even high-risk patients with limited life expectancy would typically be offered surgery for pain control.

2. Operative management:

    a. Absolute indications—all displaced fractures.

    b. Relative indications—nondisplaced fractures.

C. Surgical Approaches and Fixation Techniques

  1. External fixation:

    a. Quick means of bone stabilization.

    b. Indications:

      i. Severe soft-tissue injuries.

      ii. Extensive contamination at fracture site.

      iii. Associated vascular injury requiring repair.

      iv. Polytrauma patients initially treated with damage control measures.

    c. Pin size and number—typically 5 mm in diameter, with a minimum of two pins per segment.

    d. Pin location:

      i. Anterior—placed through the extensor mechanism and can limit knee motion.

      ii. Anterolateral.

      iii. Lateral—placed through the iliotibial (IT) band and can limit knee motion.

    e. Pin tract infection:

      i. Can be treated with oral antibiotics.

      ii. May lead to osteomyelitis.

    f. Conversion to intramedullary nailing:

      i. Optimally within 2 weeks.

      ii. Greater than 2 weeks increases the rate of pin site infections and definitive hardware infections.

    g. Most stable construct—near–far pin placement with rods applied as close to the skin as possible.

  2. Antegrade intramedullary nailing:

    a. Patient positioning:

      i. Supine fracture table:

        • Pros: consistent traction, allows unencumbered access to the patient, allows for multiple procedures simultaneously, and ease of fluoroscopic landmarks.

        • Cons: difficult starting point, can introduce internal rotation deformity to femur, and compartment syndrome can develop in well-leg due to positioning.

      ii. Supine radiolucent table:

        • Pros: Rrequires traction pin versus surgical assistance for traction and well-leg without compromising positioning.

        • Cons: Difficult starting point and more difficult imaging.

      iii. Lateral fracture table (▶ **Fig. 35.5**):

        • Pros: Easier access to starting point and consistent traction.

        • Cons: Rotational assessment can be challenging, more difficult imaging, and may not be possible in polytrauma patients.

      iv. Lateral radiolucent table (▶ **Fig. 35.6**):

        • Pros: Easier access to starting point.

        • Cons: Requires manual traction by surgical assistant, imaging can be difficult, may not be possible in polytrauma patients with thoracic or pulmonary issues, and similarly can be challenging to judge rotation.

    b. Approach:

      i. 2- to 3-cm incision proximal to the greater trochanter in line with the femoral canal.

      ii. The incision may need to be extended proximally and distally in obese patients.

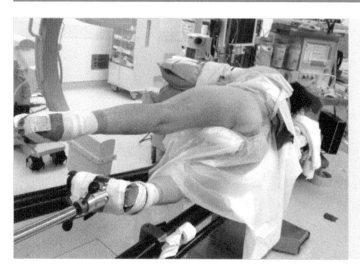

Fig. 35.5 Lateral positioning of a patient on a fracture table.

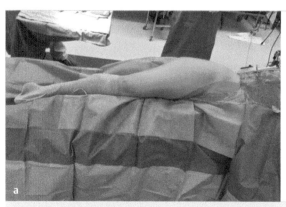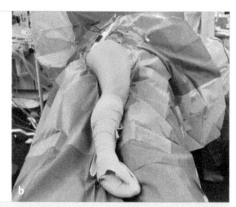

Fig. 35.6 (a, b) Lateral positioning of a patient with a beanbag on a radiolucent table.

    c. Technique:
       i. Starting point—piriformis entry (▶**Fig. 35.7**):
         • Pros: In line with the axis of the femoral canal.
         • Cons: More difficult start point, especially in obese patients, increased abductor muscle damage, associated with iatrogenic femoral neck fractures, and avoid in pediatric patients as it may cause avascular necrosis (AVN).
      ii. Starting point—trochanteric entry:
         • Pros: Easier start point, less abductor muscle damage, and less fluoroscopic time.
         • Cons: Can lead to varus or valgus malalignment of the fracture.
         • Adduction and limited hip flexion increase risk to the superior gluteal nerve and gluteus medius during antegrade nailing.
      iii. Typical fracture deformity:
         • Proximal segment typically externally rotated, flexed, and abducted.
         • Distal segment typically extended and adducted.
      iv. Reduction tools:
         • Schanz pins.
         • Femoral distractor.

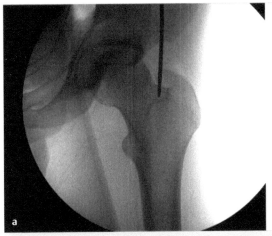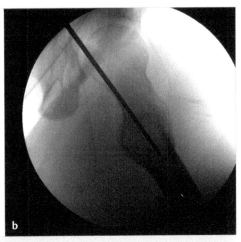

Fig. 35.7 (a, b) Anteroposterior and lateral intraoperative fluoroscopic images showing a proper piriformis start point.

- F-tool.
- Curved ball-tip guide.
- Unicortical plates.
- Finger reduction tool.

3. Retrograde intramedullary nailing:
   a. Indications:
      i. Ipsilateral femoral neck fractures.
      ii. Bilateral femoral shaft fractures.
      iii. Distal third femoral shaft fractures and some distal femur fractures with simple intra-articular extension.
      iv. Ipsilateral tibial shaft fractures.
      v. Pregnant patients (to reduce radiation to fetus).
      vi. Polytrauma patient requiring surgery to multiple extremities.
   b. Contraindications:
      i. Minimal knee range of motion.
      ii. Patella baja.
   c. Patient positioning—supine on radiolucent table with knee flexed 30 to 50 degrees.
   d. Approach:
      i. 2-cm incision starting at the distal pole of the patella.
      ii. Medial parapatellar versus patellar split.
   e. Technique:
      i. Starting point:
         - Anterior to the posterior cruciate ligament and slightly medial to the intercondylar sulcus in line with canal.
         - Radiographically at the apex of Blumensaat's line (▶ **Fig. 35.8**).
      ii. Reduction maneuver:
         - Bump placed beneath the distal segment of the femur can counteract a hyperextension deformity at the fracture site.
         - Adjunctive tools including Schanz pins (▶ **Fig. 35.9**), femoral distractor, periarticular reduction clamps, blocking screws, finger reduction tool, and manual manipulation employed.

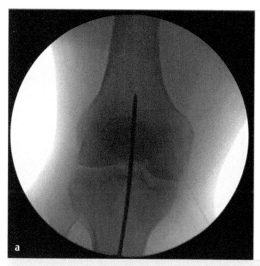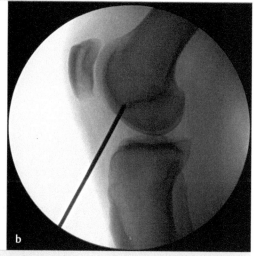

Fig. 35.8 Intraoperative fluoroscopic images demonstrating the appropriate starting point for a retrograde nail on **(a)** anteroposterior knee, **(b)** lateral knee at the anterior tip of Blumensaat's line.

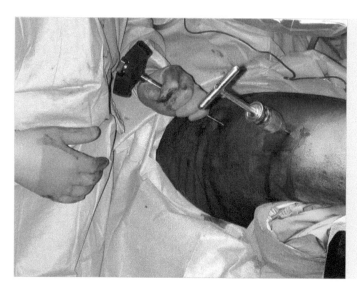

Fig. 35.9 Intraoperative photograph of a femoral shaft fracture reduction obtained with use of Schanz pins.

4. Plate fixation:

    a. Indications:

        i. Previous malunion.

        ii. Obliteration of canal due to infection or prior fracture.

        iii. Periprosthetic or peri-implant fractures.

        iv. Skeletal immaturity.

    b. Patient positioning:

        i. Supine—optimal for polytrauma patients, but can increase difficulty of exposure.

        ii. Lateral—increases ease of exposure, but can be contraindicated in polytrauma patients.

    c. Approach:

        i. Subvastus approach (▶ **Fig. 35.10**).

        ii. Lateral approach—incise the IT band, elevate vastus lateralis from linea aspera with care to cauterize and/or ligate perforators.

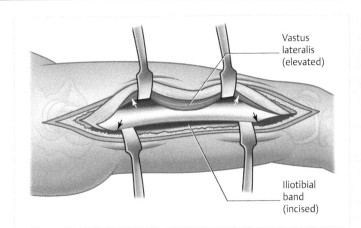

Vastus
lateralis
(elevated)

Iliotibial
band
(incised)

Fig. 35.10 The lateral subvastus approach to the femur. The iliotibial band is incised and the vastus lateralis is elevated anteriorly to expose the femur.

    d. Technique:
        i. Minimum of a 10-hole 4.5-mm plate should be employed.
       ii. Eight cortices are recommended proximal and distal to the fracture. Lag screw through the plate increases construct rigidity.

D. Complications
   1. Nerve injury:
      a. Pudendal nerve palsy: associated with use of the perineal post on the fracture table and longer surgical times.
      b. Sciatic and peroneal nerve palsy: associated with overdistraction and longer surgical times.
   2. Muscle weakness and entry site injury:
      a. Increased hip pain with antegrade nailing.
      b. Increased knee pain with retrograde nailing.
      c. Knee stiffness:
         i. Usually improves in the first 6 to 12 weeks.
        ii. Persistent knee stiffness at 3 to 6 months may warrant knee manipulation and/or surgical release.
   3. Angular malalignment: more common in proximal and distal fractures treated with nailing.
   4. Rotational deformity:
      a. Typically defined as 15 degrees or more (external rotation clinically tolerated better than internal rotation).
      b. Ranges from 9 to 28%.
      c. CT scanogram is the gold standard of measuring rotational difference.
      d. Prevention: image the hip and knee of the contralateral, uninjured limb. Compare the lesser trochanter profiles and the femoral neck profile on the AP view.
   5. Heterotopic ossification (HO):
      a. Incidence of 9 to 60% after antegrade nailing.
      b. Clinically significant HO present in only 5 to 10% of patients
      c. Most common location is near the greater trochanter.
   6. Delayed union and nonunion: nonunion rates of 8% in unreamed nails and 2% in reamed nails.
   7. Infection:
      a. Less than 1% in closed fractures.
      b. Ranges from 2 to 5% in open fractures.
   8. Compartment syndrome: infrequent, though estimated to be from 1 to 2%.

E. Rehabilitation
1. Immediate weight bearing and unrestricted active and passive range of motion of the hip and knee can be instituted after intramedullary fixation.
F. Outcomes
1. Reamed, static intramedullary fixation of the femoral shaft fractures has a 98% union rate.
2. Radiographic union at approximately 4 to 6 months with no significant difference between antegrade and retrograde approaches.

III. Special Considerations

A. Pediatric Patients

Treatment varies according to age.
1. 0 to 6 months—Pavlik harness.
2. 6 months to 5 years—closed reduction and spica casting.
3. 5 to 10 years—flexible nailing versus submuscular plate.
4. Older than 10 years—submuscular plating versus antegrade nailing. For this age group, avoid piriformis entry nails in adolescents due to increased risk of AVN.

B. Geriatric Patients
1. Mismatch in radius of curvature of the nail versus femoral shaft can lead to anterior perforation of the distal femur:
    a. Atypical bisphosphonate fractures (see Chapter 10, Osteoporosis, for additional information) have prolonged healing times.

Summary

This chapter provided an overview of the initial presentation and treatment options for femoral shaft fractures. Pertinent imaging and anatomy were reviewed, in addition to various surgical options with associated complications. Special treatment considerations for pediatric and geriatric patients were discussed at the conclusion of the chapter.

Suggested Readings

Bone LB, Johnson KD, Weigelt J, Scheinberg R. Early versus delayed stabilization of femoral fractures. A prospective randomized study. J Bone Joint Surg Am 1989;71(3):336–340

Brumback RJ, Uwagie-Ero S, Lakatos RP, Poka A, Bathon GH, Burgess AR. Intramedullary nailing of femoral shaft fractures. Part II: fracture-healing with static interlocking fixation. J Bone Joint Surg Am 1988;70(10):1453–1462

O'Toole RV, Dancy L, Dietz AR, Pollak AN, Johnson AJ, Osgood G, Nascone JW, Sciadini MF, Castillo RC. Diagnosis of femoral neck fracture associated with femoral shaft fracture: blinded comparison of computed tomography and plain radiography. J Orthop Trauma 2013;27(6):325–330

Ostrum RF, Agarwal A, Lakatos R, Poka A. Prospective comparison of retrograde and antegrade femoral intramedullary nailing. Orthop Trauma 2000;14(7):496–501

Stannard JP, Bankston L, Futch LA, McGwin G, Volgas DA. Functional outcome following intramedullary nailing of the femur: a prospective randomized comparison of piriformis fossa and greater trochanteric entry portals. J Bone Joint Surg Am 2011;93(15):1385–1391

Winquist RA, Hansen ST Jr, Clawson DK. Closed intramedullary nailing of femoral fractures. A report of five hundred and twenty cases. J Bone Joint Surg Am 1984;66(4):529–539

36 Distal Femur Fractures

Aaron Johnson and Gerard P. Slobogean

Introduction

Distal femur fractures comprise various injury patterns ranging from high-energy trauma to low-energy fragility fractures. High-energy injuries may occur in either young or old patients, while low-energy fractures tend to occur in the elderly population, or patients who have previously sustained spinal cord injuries. Furthermore, with increasing incidence of arthroplasty being performed, these fractures may be periprosthetic above a total knee arthroplasty (TKA), below a total hip arthroplasty (THA), or interprosthetic between a THA and TKA.

Keywords: Distal femur fracture, distal femur locking plates, retrograde distal femoral nail, nonunion, malunion, periprosthetic fractures

I. Preoperative

A. History and physical examination
    A detailed history and physical examination can offer key insights that can help guide the treating physician when deciding on an appropriate treatment strategy. Specific areas to focus on include the following:

    1. Patient age and medical comorbidities.

    2. Mechanism of injury.

    3. Previous surgical procedures (especially around the hip or knee).

    4. Preinjury ambulatory status.

    5. Any history of spinal cord injury.

    6. Associated injuries.

    7. Assessing neurologic function distally (motor and sensory).

    8. Assessing skin for any signs of open injury or traumatic arthrotomy.

B. Anatomy
    It is important to understand the normal anatomy of the distal articular block, as well as deformities of the articular block in relation to the shaft. Preoperative imaging of the contralateral femur taken with fluoroscopy can help establish normal articular morphology, coronal alignment, femoral length, and rotational alignment of the femur.

    1. Articular anatomy:

        a. The articular block of the distal femur is trapezoidal (the posterior width of the distal femur is wider than the anterior width; see ▶ **Fig. 36.1c**).

        b. This must be taken into account when restoring the articular anatomy and placing lateral plate fixation.

    2. Coronal deformity alignment (varus–valgus alignment; ▶ **Fig. 36.1a**):

        a. Normal femoral shaft is oriented 7 to 11 degrees of valgus in relation to the articular surface. It is designated as the anatomic lateral distal femoral angle (aLDFA) = 79 to 83 degrees.

        b. The fracture deformity is related to the location of the fracture with respect to the adductor tubercle.

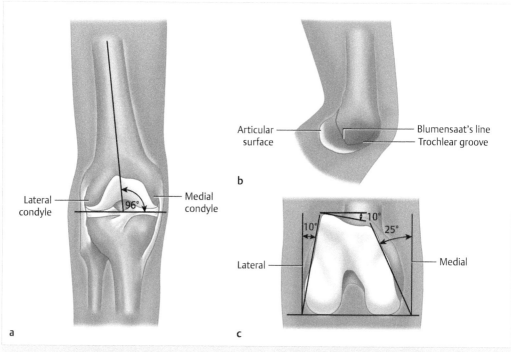

Fig. 36.1 (a–c) Illustration of the trapezoidal shape of the articular surface of the distal femur.

3. Sagittal alignment (▶Fig. 36.1b):

   a. Normal posterior distal femoral angle (PDFA) is 79 to 87 degrees. This is represented by the angle formed by a line drawn along the axis of the femoral shaft and a line drawn between the anterior and posterior points where the femoral condyle meets the metaphysis.

   b. There is typically an extension (apex posterior) deformity through the fracture site.

   c. Deformity is due to the pull of the gastrocnemius muscle.

4. Length and rotation:

   a. Both can be assessed in comparison to the contralateral side.

   b. Length can be measured with a radiolucent ruler overlaid on the opposite femur.

   c. Rotation can be matched with the lesser trochanter profile views of the opposite femur, ensuring similar rotational profile of the knee.

5. Mechanical axis of the femur and extremity:

   a. The native femur has a lateral distal femoral mechanical axis of typically 88 degrees. It is important to keep this relationship in mind during preoperative planning and intraoperatively.

   b. Matching the mechanical axis to the contralateral limb is often beneficial for comminuted fracture patterns.

C. Imaging

   1. Conventional radiology:

      a. Anteroposterior and lateral radiographs of the knee.

      b. Full-length orthogonal imaging of the femur.

   2. Computed tomography—two-dimensional imaging with reconstruction views is useful for identifying the following:

      a. Coronal plane articular fragments.

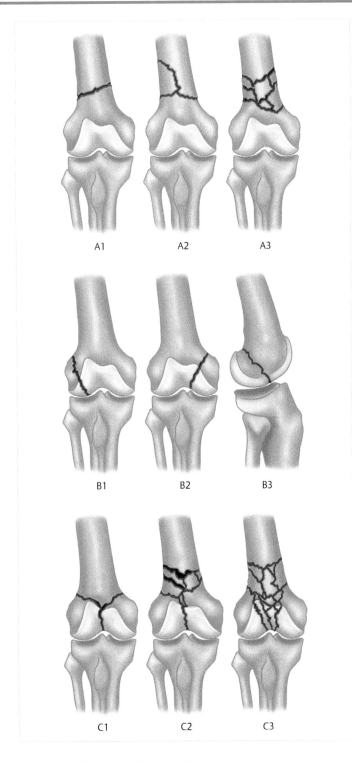

Fig. 36.2 Schematic depictions of the AO/OTA classification.

A1 A2 A3

B1 B2 B3

C1 C2 C3

    b.   Intra-articular extension.

    c.   Intercondylar comminution.

D.   Classification

    The AO/OTA fracture classification is the most useful for guiding treatment (see ▸ Fig. 36.2).

1. Type A—extra-articular fractures (supracondylar).
2. Type B—partial articular fractures are typically unicondylar, and can be either medial or lateral condyle fractures:
   a. Type B1—lateral condyle.
   b. Type B2—medial condyle.
   c. Type B3—isolated coronal fracture ("Hoffa's" fragment).
3. Type C—complete intercondylar (Note: Any type C pattern may also be associated with a coronal plane articular fracture).
   a. Type C1—simple intercondylar fracture line with no metaphyseal comminution.
   b. Type C2—simple intercondylar fracture line with metaphyseal comminution.
   c. Type C3—comminuted intercondylar fracture with metaphyseal comminution.

II. Treatment

A. Initial management
   1. Initial management should consist of gross realignment of the limb and application of a stabilizing device:
      a. Well-padded long leg splint.
      b. Knee immobilizer.
      c. Hinged knee brace if the definitive treatment will be nonoperative.
   2. The purpose of immobilization is to facilitate patient care, mobilization, and pain control.
   3. There is rarely a role for skeletal traction, as this usually exacerbates the deforming forces.
B. Definitive management
   1. Operative versus nonoperative management:
      a. Distal femur fractures are typically treated surgically.
      b. There may be occasions when medical comorbidities preclude surgical treatment:
         i. Medically ill patients where the risks of anesthesia and blood loss outweigh benefit.
         ii. Severely debilitated, nonambulatory patients.
         iii. Paraplegic or spinal cord injured patients.
      c. Nonoperative management should consist of a well-padded brace or knee immobilizer.
      d. Evaluate neuropathic or spinal cord injury patients on a weekly or biweekly basis to ensure there is no skin or soft-tissue compromise. Impending open fractures or threatened skin should be considered indications for surgical intervention in these patients.
C. Surgical approaches and fixation techniques—Preoperative imaging should be scrutinized and the preoperative plan should be determined prior to the OR. Patient positioning and implants will depend on the type of fixation strategy that is planned. Furthermore, based on whether or not articular reduction will be required may affect the ultimate surgical approach chosen.
   1. Extra-articular fractures (AO/OTA type A):
      a. Extra-articular fractures may be treated with either plate fixation or intramedullary nail.
      b. Intramedullary nails:
         i. If there is space distally for multiple points of fixation in the intramedullary nail (▶Fig. 36.3).
         ii. Multiplanar interlocking screws distally may improve stability.
      c. The same reduction techniques as outlined later may be used in order to position the fragments appropriately for nail fixation. Blocking screws may also be used during and after nail placement to prevent later displacement of the fracture fragments. The surgical approach for this procedure is the same as for a retrograde femoral nail.

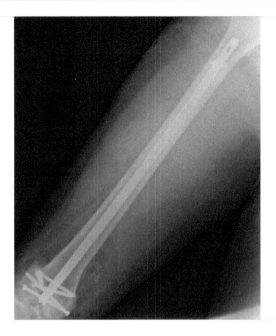

Fig. 36.3 Postoperative radiograph demonstrating anatomic alignment of a distal supracondylar fracture treated with a retrograde intramedullary nail.

  d. Lateral plate fixation:

    i. Reduction techniques can be either direct or indirect.

    ii. Simple fracture patterns may be fixed with lag screws and a lateral neutralization plate.

    iii. Supracondylar fractures with metaphyseal comminution may best be treated with a bridge plating technique (Refer Chapter 4, Biomechanics of Internal Fracture Fixation).

    iv. A lateral approach is typically sufficient for reduction and fixation.

2. Partial articular fractures (AO/OTA type B):

  a. Type B1 bridge lateral condyle fracture—lateral buttress plate fixation.

    i. If a lateral approach is used, then the reduction is assessed using radiographic assessment of the articular surface and alignment.

    ii. If the anterolateral approach is used, then the joint surface is directly visualized and reduced anatomically

  b. Type B2 bridge medial condyle fracture—medial buttress plate fixation.

    i. This is typically the only fracture pattern that requires a medial approach to the distal femur.

    ii. A standard anteromedial approach to the femur is used, elevating the vastus medialis muscle.

  c. Type B3 bridge articular fracture in the coronal plane (Hoffa's fracture).

    i. Anteromedial or anterolateral approach to assess the joint surface.

    ii. The fragment may be provisionally reduced with a variety of pointed reduction clamps and Kirschner's wires (K-wires).

    iii. Fixation with headless compression screws or mini/small fragment screws countersunk beneath the articular surface. Two to three screws are typically used, and should be placed in a divergent orientation for maximal stability.

3. Complete articular fractures (AO/OTA type C):

  a. The first priority in fixation of type C fractures is restoration of the articular congruity.

  b. Reduction and provisional fixation can be achieved with smooth K-wires, bone clamps, large periarticular clamps, or Steinmann's pins (often used as joysticks in the femoral condyles).

  c. Fragment-specific fixation should be performed with threaded K-wires or interfragmentary screws (either mini fragment, or small fragment fixation).

  d. Think about the ultimate fixation construct, to ensure that the interfragmentary screws are not in the path of the primary fixation construct.

  e. Following reduction of the articular surface, fixation proceeds in a similar fashion to type A fractures.

  f. The implant of choice is typically a fixed-angle device. Examples include the following:
   i. Blade plates.
   ii. Condylar sliding-barrel plates.
   iii. Distal femur locking plates.
   iv. Intramedullary nail for select simple articular fracture patterns.

  g. When reducing the articular surface to the shaft, the following parameters should be considered (imaging of the contralateral femur can provide the surgeon with a template):
   i. Overall length of the femur.
   ii. Alignment of the mechanical axis of the limb (e.g., varus/valgus alignment).
   iii. Flexion/extension of the distal femur.
   iv. Rotation of the articular block with respect to the shaft.

4. Surgical approach:

  a. Regardless of specific surgical approach used, the patient is typically positioned supine. The lateral decubitus position may be used to facilitate proximal exposure; however, distal joint work and alignment are more difficult in the lateral position.

  b. Supine bridge a bump under the hip may or may not be used.
   i. If a bump is used, it is more difficult to obtain intraoperative imaging to compare length and rotation with the contralateral side.
   ii. The use of a bump, however, facilitates proximal exposure if a long plate is required that extends toward the vastus ridge.

  c. The entire hindquarter is prepped into the sterile field.

  d. If a tourniquet is used, a sterile tourniquet is preferred.

  e. Lateral approach:
   i. Preferred for type A and simple type C fractures that do not require direct visualization of the articular cartilage.
   ii. As illustrated in ▶ Fig. 36.4 (posterior line), the incision is centered laterally over the distal femur.
   iii. Split the iliotibial band in line with its fibers.

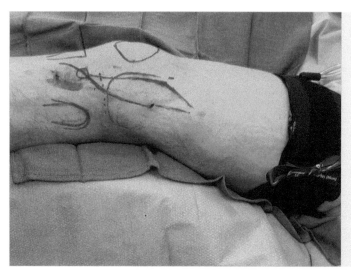

Fig. 36.4 Standard incisions for direct lateral and anterolateral approaches to the distal femur.

    iv. Reflect the vastus lateralis muscle anteriorly to expose the distal femur.

    v. Care should be taken to leave a cuff of muscle attached to the posterior intermuscular septum in order to prevent profunda perforator vessels from retracting into the posterior compartment during the approach.

  f. Anterolateral approach:

    i. Facilitates direct visualization of the joint surface.

    ii. Useful for complex intra-articular fractures (OTA C2, C3, and select displaced C1).

    iii. As depicted in ▶ Fig. 36.4 (anterior line), the incision is curvilinear from lateral toward midline.

    iv. Perform a lateral parapatellar arthrotomy to directly visualize the articular cartilage of the distal femur and patellofemoral joint.

  g. Either incision may be extended proximally as far as desired. Many plate fixation systems have percutaneous targeting jigs that allow for minimally invasive proximal fixation through cannulas that minimize soft-tissue dissection proximally.

  h. Modification when the primary implant is an intramedullary nail:

    i. Use the anterolateral approach as necessary for joint reduction and fixation.

    ii. Alternatively, an anterior knee incision can be performed with a medial or lateral arthrotomy to access the joint.

    iii. Continue the parapatellar arthrotomy distally to gain access for the starting point of a retrograde femoral nail.

5. Reduction, hardware construct, and fixation strategy:

  a. The first step is obtaining an anatomic reduction of the articular block through direct or indirect visualization.

  b. Simple (minimally displaced or nondisplaced) articular fractures:

    i. Reduction may be assessed on fluoroscopic imaging without a full anterolateral approach and arthrotomy.

    ii. Large bone clamps may be placed through percutaneous stab incisions.

    iii. Reduction can be temporarily held with K-wires until interfragmentary lag screws are placed orthogonal to the fracture line (▶ Fig. 36.5).

  c. Complex intra-articular fractures:

    i. Coronal fractures should be reduced first:

- Anterior to posterior directed interfragmentary (countersunk) lag screws.
- Typically 2.0-, 2.7-, or 3.5-mm diameter screws.
- Divergent on lateral fluoroscopy.

    ii. Intercondylar fragments should then be reduced and provisionally held with K-wires and/or large bone clamps.

    iii. Interfragmentary screws should be placed from a lateral to medial orientation, and should be placed in the periphery of the condyle in order to avoid later placement of lateral plate construct.

  d. The implant of choice is typically a distal femoral locking plate.

    i. Additional options are listed above.

    ii. There are numerous options by multiple manufacturers, all of which can be applied using the same fundamental concepts.

    iii. Following articular reduction (or if there is no intra-articular extension), the articular block must then be reduced to the shaft.

    iv. Simple fracture patterns in patients with adequate bone stock:

- Femur is exposed, fracture reduced, clamped, and absolute stability may be obtained with multiple small fragment or large fragment lag screws orthogonal to the fracture line.
- The lateral plate subsequently functions as a neutralization plate for the construct (▶ Fig. 36.6).

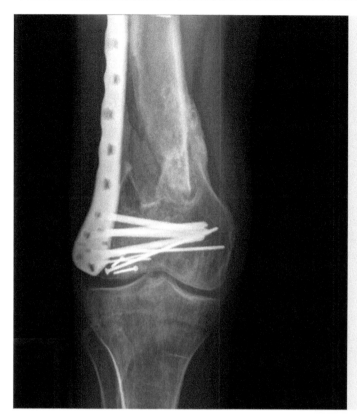

Fig. 36.5 Anteroposterior knee radiograph 6 months postoperatively that demonstrates multiple mini- and small-fragment interfragmentary screws used to reduce the components of the articular block in a 20-year-old male patient. The metaphyseal comminution above the distal segment was bridged with the lateral locking plate, and notable medial callus is seen.

    v.   Metaphyseal comminution or poor bone quality:
- Bridge the metaphyseal region with the lateral plate construct.
- The working length of the particular fracture characteristics must be taken into consideration, and screw placement must be modulated to minimize the risk of creating too stiff of a construct.

    vi.   Plate length. Comminuted fractures are often treated by a bridge plating technique with longer plates, fewer screws proximally, and more screws in the articular segment.

    vii.   Plate placement:
- Most plating systems offer an optional targeting arm. Affix the jig to the plate and slide the plate underneath the vastus lateralis muscle to position it on the lateral aspect of the femur.
- Plate position is confirmed via fluoroscopy.
- Most plates are designed to sit on the anterior aspect of the distal femoral condyle. Due to the trapezoidal nature of the distal femur, care should be taken to avoid placement of the plate too posterior on the lateral condyle, as doing so may increase the risk of medialization, or "golf club deformity" of the distal segment.
- Most plates contain a distal screw hole designed to restore the anatomic axis of the femur. When inserted, this screw should be approximately parallel to the joint line. This should be placed first, and sets the coronal alignment.

    viii.   Pin the most proximal hole in the plate to the shaft:
- The sagittal deformity (typically extension through the fracture site) should be corrected during this step.
- Towel bumps or percutaneous Schanz pins (placed in the distal and proximal segment placed orthogonal to one another) allow for control of the extension deformity.

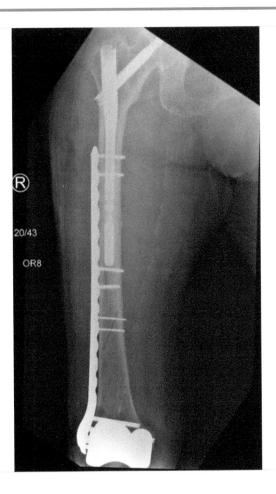

Fig. 36.6 Postoperative anteroposterior radiograph of a type B extra-articular fracture above a total knee arthroplasty with a long spiral component into the shaft that was treated with lag screws and lateral plate neutralization.

ix. The distal shaft segment is then reduced to the plate with a cortical screw:
   - If the plate is a straight, then it should sit on the anterolateral cortex of the femur.
   - Some plates have a built-in 11-degree twist, which allows the plate to sit on the direct lateral surface of the femur when the fracture is correctly reduced.
   - Cortical screws can be used for fixation to the femoral shaft if the precontoured plate matches the reduced femur.
   - However, if the plate is not in contact with the lateral cortex of the femur when the reduction otherwise matches the contralateral limb, consider insertion of locking screws in the shaft segment (▶ **Fig. 36.7**). This strategy prevents drawing the femoral shaft toward the plate and creation of a medial translational ("golf club") deformity of the articular block.

x. An electrocautery cord may be stretched from the center of the femoral head to the center of the ankle to provide a gross assessment of overall limb alignment (▶ **Fig. 36.8**). Comparison to the contralateral limb provides a template for the patient's native alignment.

xi. Once the alignment is acceptable, the distal segment of the plate is filled with locking screws. Oblique views of the medial condyle can be taken to assess screw length.
   - Long screws in this position may be symptomatic postoperatively.

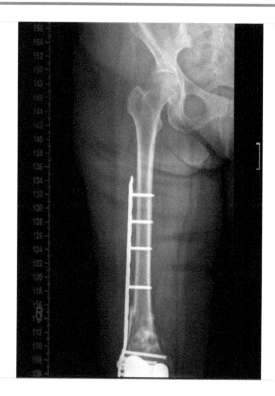

Fig. 36.7 One-year postoperative images in a patient who has no pain, knee range of motion of 0 to 120 degrees, and is full weight bearing who had plate fixation locked off the bone laterally to prevent medial displacement of the distal articular block.

D. Complications

1. Nonunion is the most common complication, with reports ranging in the literature from 3 to 24%.

   a. There are few prospective studies describing nonunion rates, but the existing literature suggests that nonunion risk is dependent on the following:

   i. Fracture type.

   ii. Type of implant used.

   iii. Screw configuration (generally recommended to skip one to two holes proximal to fracture between screws).

   iv. Obesity.

   v. Open fracture:

   • Nonunion treatment—typically repaired with a plate or nail fixation. Distal femoral replacement is a less commonly used treatment option.

   b. Malunion occurs in up to one-third of patients, and may be due to rotational deformity, angular deformity, or a medialization of the distal articular block.

   c. Knee stiffness—physical therapy may be of benefit to regain motion faster and prevent contracture.

   d. Infection rates are low in closed injury, but are as high as 7% in open fractures.

   e. Post-traumatic arthritis is uncommon.

E. Rehabilitation

1. Postoperative bracing (knee immobilizer or hinged knee brace) is optional. There is no evidence that bracing improves clinical outcomes.

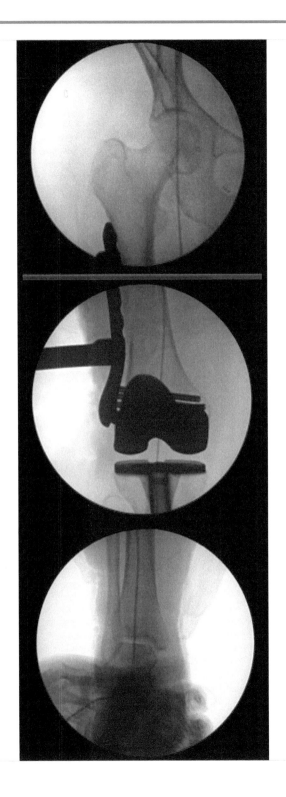

Fig. 36.8 Intraoperative fluoroscopic views of the hip, knee, and ankle demonstrating a neutral mechanical axis.

2. Non-weight-bearing (touchdown weight bearing) for 6 to 12 weeks for most young adults with intra-articular fractures.

3. Weight bearing in geriatric patients is controversial. Recent reports have shown improved outcomes with immediate weight-bearing protocols in patients with extra-articular or periprosthetic fractures in patients older than 65 years.

4. Early active range of motion as tolerated.

F. Outcomes

1. Functional and radiographic outcomes demonstrate 85 to 90% excellent results.

2. Outcomes are poor when complicated by nonunion, stiffness, or infection.

3. Patients require second procedures at reported rates from 16 to 25%.

4. The majority of evidence reports similar outcomes between locking plates and intramedullary nails.

III. Special Considerations

A. Open fractures

1. Increased risk of infection and nonunion.

2. Controversy exists over the extent to which devitalized bone should be debrided. Aggressive debridement of devitalized bone has been shown to increase nonunion rates, whereas less aggressive debridement has been associated with higher union rates with a potential increase in infection rates.

B. Periprosthetic fractures

1. Fractures above a TKA should be carefully examined to determine if the implant is loose.

   a. Loosening of a knee prosthesis following supracondylar femur fracture is rare.

   b. Loose implants may show condylar widening on anteroposterior radiograph, or fracture lines that extend distal to the flange on computed tomography.

   c. Loose components should be treated with revision TKA or distal femoral replacement.

2. Well-fixed components should be fixed as described above.

3. The majority of TKA implants are amenable to fixation with retrograde intramedullary nails if desired.

   a. The prosthesis must have an open box design.

   b. Due to the location of the box, the starting point may be more posterior than the ideal starting point.

   c. Diligence should be paid to avoid an extension deformity at the fracture site during reaming and nail passage.

C. Geriatric or severely osteopenic

1. In patients who have poor bone quality, metaphyseal comminution, and extreme distal extent of the fracture, a distal femoral replacement may be considered.

2. Outcomes of distal femoral replacement are inferior to primary TKA; however, they do allow immediate weight bearing postoperatively.

Summary

It is important to understand the unique shape of the distal femur, the anatomic axis of the femur, and the mechanical axis of the limb when treating these injuries. Although they are treated surgically, the indications for nonoperative management are detailed. For fractures treated operatively, reduction strategies and fixation techniques are provided for various different fracture patterns and clinical scenarios. Surgical technique varies depending on if the fracture is extra-articular, partial articular, or intra-articular. Furthermore, host factors must be taken into account, as distal femur fractures occur in a bimodal distribution, affecting both young healthy patients and older patients who may have poor bone quality. Fractures can be treated with intramedullary fixation, lag screw and neutralization plating, or bridge plating for relative stability. Open fractures pose a particular dilemma; more extensive debridement has lower infection rates but higher nonunion rates. Conversely, less extensive debridement results in higher rates of infection but lower nonunion rates. The treating surgeon must therefore weigh the risks of infection versus nonunion. Overall outcomes of distal femur fractures are good in 85 to 90% of patients. Although there is no difference in reported outcomes between the different treatment types (e.g., intramedullary nail vs. distal femoral locking plates), outcomes are worse when malreduction and nonunion are present, and the overall reoperation rate for this injury ranges from 16 to 25%.

Suggested Readings

Collinge CA, Gardner MJ, Crist BD. Pitfalls in the application of distal femur plates for fractures. J Orthop Trauma 2011;25(11):695–706

Nork SE, Segina DN, Aflatoon K, et al. The association between supracondylar-intercondylar distal femoral fractures and coronal plane fractures. J Bone Joint Surg Am 2005;87(3):564–569

Ricci WM, Collinge C, Streubel PN, McAndrew CM, Gardner MJ. A comparison of more and less aggressive bone debridement protocols for the treatment of open supracondylar femur fractures. J Orthop Trauma 2013;27(12):722–725

Ricci WM, Streubel PN, Morshed S, Collinge CA, Nork SE, Gardner MJ. Risk factors for failure of locked plate fixation of distal femur fractures: an analysis of 335 cases. J Orthop Trauma 2014;28(2):83–89

Southeast Fracture C; Southeast Fracture Consortium. LCP versus LISS in the treatment of open and closed distal femur fractures: does it make a difference? J Orthop Trauma 2016;30(6):e212–e216

Starr AJ, Jones AL, Reinert CM. The "swashbuckler": a modified anterior approach for fractures of the distal femur. J Orthop Trauma 1999;13(2):138–140

37 Knee Dislocation

Michael G. Baraga, Hayley E. Ennis, and Dylan N. Greif

Introduction

A knee dislocation is the disruption of the tibiofemoral articulation. An acute knee dislocation is an orthopaedic emergency that can result in severe consequences if untreated. Importantly, knee dislocations do not always present with obvious deformity, making it crucial that the evaluating physician remain clinically suspicious when evaluating patients with knee pain and be aware of proper treatment algorithms (▶Video 37.1).

Keywords: knee, dislocation, subluxation, trauma, multiligament injury

I. Preoperative

A. History and physical examination
1. Mechanism—high versus low energy:
    a. High energy—motor vehicle accident, pedestrian hit by car, crush.
    b. Low energy—athletic injury, misstep (usually with twisting fall), morbidly obese patient.
2. Appearance:
    a. Obvious deformity:
        i. Do not delay reduction for formal X-rays (XRs) if obvious deformity is present—reduce immediately.
        ii. If irreducible via closed means, there may be interposition of medial tissue from the medial femoral condyle buttonholing through the medial capsule (▶Fig. 37.1). This may require open reduction in the operating room.
    b. No obvious deformity. Note that only subtle signs of trauma (swelling, bruising, abrasions) may present since roughly 50% of knee dislocations spontaneously reduce. One must have a high index of suspicion and perform a ligamentous examination for knee stability.
3. Vascular examination (▶Fig. 37.2)—a good vascular exam is crucial as up to 40 to 50% of knee dislocations can be associated with vascular injury. There is approximately an 85% amputation rate with greater than 8 hour interrupted blood flow.

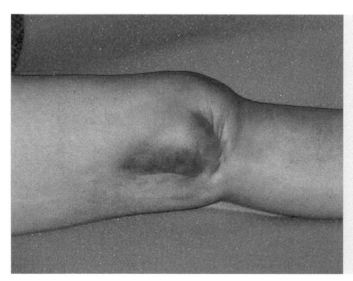

Fig. 37.1 Knee "dimple" usually seen in lateral dislocations may indicate irreducible dislocation via closed means. (Adapted from Harb A, Lincoln D, Michaelson J. The MR dimple sign in irreducible posterolateral knee dislocations. Skeletal Radiology 2009;38(11):1111–1114.)

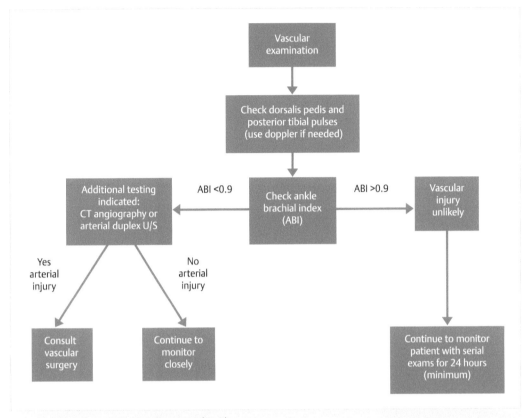

Fig. 37.2 Vascular examination diagnostic algorithm.

a. Palpable pulse:
   i. Dorsalis pedis and posterior tibial pulses should be checked immediately and compared to the uninjured limb.
   ii. Pulses should be checked serially—pulse may be present initially in 5 to 15% of those with vascular injury (collateral circulation may initially mask injury) and then may decrease or become nonpalpable with time.
   iii. Pulses should be documented before and after the reduction along with subsequent serial examination.
   iv. If the pulse is not palpable, or unequal to the contralateral (uninjured) limb, use Doppler.
b. Ankle-brachial index (ABI):
   i. ABI should be measured even if pulse is palpable.
   ii. When ABI is greater than 0.9, vascular injury is unlikely (99–100% negative predictive value), continue to monitor with serial examinations.
   iii. When ABI is less than 0.9, further testing is needed, like CT angiography or arterial duplex ultrasound (if patient cannot be given contrast). Consult vascular surgery if arterial injury is diagnosed.

4. Neurologic examination:
   a. Neurologic examination is important for detecting nerve deficits and detecting vascular injury as nerve injury is significantly associated with vascular disruption.
   b. The common peroneal nerve (CPN) is most commonly injured due to its superficial anatomical location traversing around the proximal fibula near the knee joint.

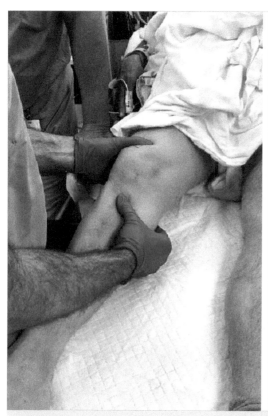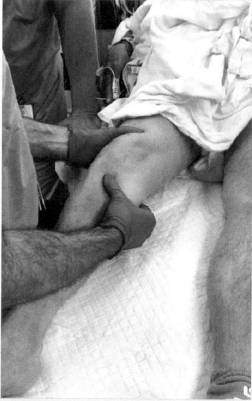

Fig. 37.3 Anterior drawer and Lachman's tests for anterior cruciate ligament.

   i. Injury occurs in up to 40% of knee dislocations.

   ii. Sensory (numbness on dorsum of foot and/or dorsum of the first web space) and/or motor deficits (foot drop).

   iii. Highly associated with injury to the posterolateral corner (PLC).

  c. Tibial nerve is less likely to be injured due to its protected location and more consistent blood supply.

 5. Examination of knee stability:

  a. Cruciate ligaments:

   i. Anterior cruciate ligament (ACL):

    • Test: Lachman's test, anterior drawer test (▶ **Fig. 37.3**).

   ii. Posterior cruciate ligament (PCL):

    • Test: posterior sag sign, posterior drawer test (▶ **Fig. 37.4**).

    • Dial test at 90 degrees (combined with PLC injury).

  b. Collateral ligaments:

   i. Medial collateral ligament (MCL):

    • Test—valgus stress at 30-degree flexion to isolate MCL (▶ **Fig. 37.5**).

    • Note—laxity to valgus stress at 0 degrees indicates likely presence of cruciate ligament injury in addition to MCL/posteromedial corner injury.

   ii. Lateral collateral ligament (LCL):

    • Test—varus stress at 30-degree flexion isolates LCL (▶ **Fig. 37.6**).

    • Note—laxity to varus stress at 0 degrees indicates likely presence of cruciate ligament injury in addition to LCL/PLC injury.

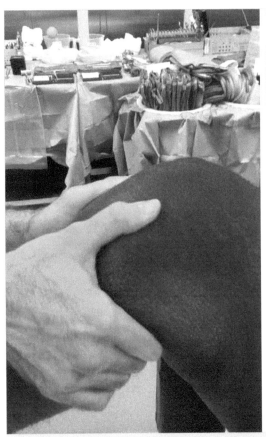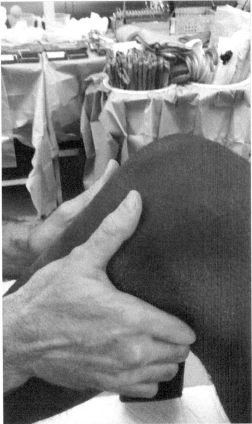

Fig. 37.4 Posterior drawer test for posterior cruciate ligament (start and end of stress test).

    c. PLC:

        i. Composed of LCL, popliteus tendon, popliteofibular ligament, lateral capsule, biceps femoris, iliotibial band, and lateral head of gastrocnemius.

        ii. Test—dial test:

- Greater than 10 degrees increased external rotation of foot (when compared to contralateral uninjured limb) with knee in 30-degree flexion ONLY = PLC injury; PCL likely intact.
- Greater than 10 degrees increased external rotation of foot with knee in 30- AND 90-degree flexion = PLC and PCL injury.

B. Anatomy (▶ **Fig. 37.7**):

    1. Disruption of the tibiofemoral articulation in any direction—involves damage to at least two ligaments of the knee, often more.

    2. ACL—origin: lateral femoral condyle; insertion: anterior between intercondylar eminences of tibia.

    3. PCL—origin: lateral edge of medial femoral condyle; insertion: tibial sulcus.

    4. MCL—origin: proximal and posterior to medial epicondyle of femur; insertion: proximal: 1.2 cm distal to joint line; distal: medial surface of tibia 6 cm distal to joint line.

    5. PLC:

        a. LCL—origin: lateral epicondyle of femur; insertion: anterolateral fibular head.

        b. Popliteus—origin: muscle originates posteromedial proximal tibia; insertion: tendon inserts lateral femoral condyle 18.5 mm distal and anterior to LCL femoral origin.

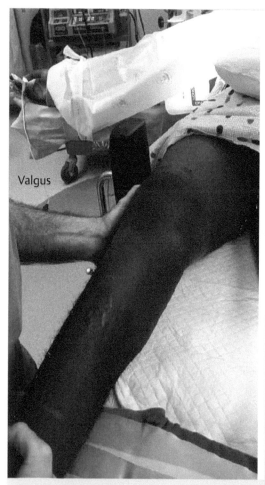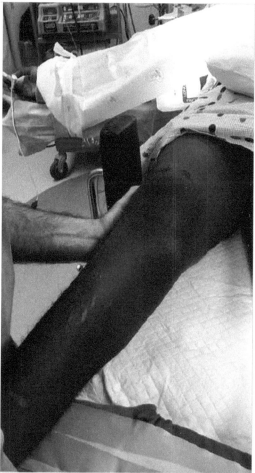

Valgus

Fig. 37.5 Valgus examination for medial collateral ligament (start and end of stress test).

    c. Popliteofibular ligament—origin: musculotendinous junction popliteus tendon; insertion: fibular head.

    d. Arcuate ligament—origin: posterior portion of head of fibula; insertion: popliteus muscle and lateral epicondyle of femur.

    e. Lateral capsule.

C. Imaging

  1. Radiographs:

    a. Gross deformity on XR is obvious—immediate reduction should not be postponed for initial XRs.

    b. Since approximately half of knee dislocations will present reduced, subtle signs of knee dislocation on XR should be noted:

      i. Avulsion fractures:

        • Segond fracture (▶ **Fig. 37.8**)—avulsion of the proximal, lateral tibia near joint line, which occurs due to avulsion of the anterolateral ligament off of the tibia. Considered a pathognomonic sign for ACL tear.

        • Arcuate fracture—avulsion fracture of the proximal fibula, which is significant for a PLC injury.

        • Rim fracture of the tibia.

      ii. Osteochondral defects.

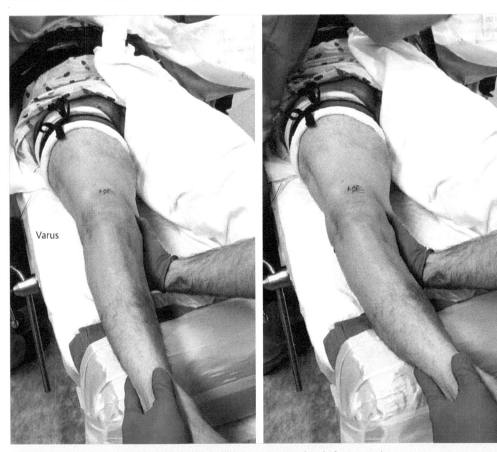

Fig. 37.6 Varus examinations for lateral collateral ligament (start and end of stress test).

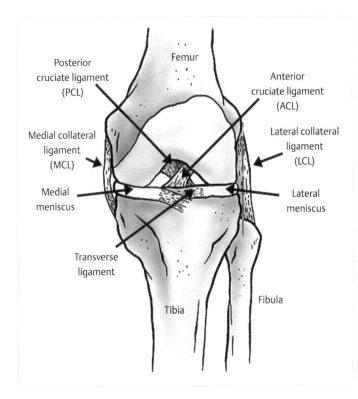

Posterior
cruciate ligament
(PCL)

Femur

Anterior
cruciate ligament
(ACL)

Medial collateral
ligament
(MCL)

Lateral collateral
ligament
(LCL)

Medial
meniscus

Lateral
meniscus

Transverse
ligament

Fibula

Tibia

Fig. 37.7 Anatomy of the knee joint: anterior view. (Adapted from Makris EA, Hadidi P, Athanasiou KA. The knee meniscus: structure–function, pathophysiology, current repair techniques, and prospects for regeneration. Biomaterials 2011;32(30):7411–7431.)

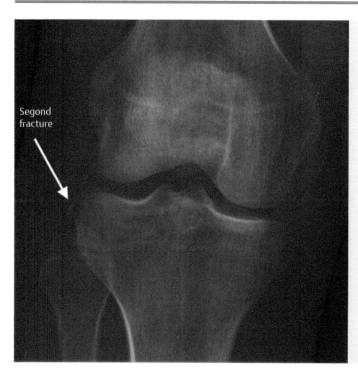

Fig. 37.8 Avulsion fracture in a right knee showing a Segond fracture (*arrow*).

Segond fracture

Table 37.1 Schenck's classification

Type	Description
KD I	Single cruciate (ACL or PCL) + 1 collateral
KD II	Dual cruciate (ACL + PCL)
KD III-M	ACL, PCL, and MCL injury
KD III-L	ACL, PCL, and LCL + PCL injury
KD IV	ACL, PCL, MCL, and LCL +PLC injury
KD V	Dislocation + fracture
	C = arterial injury; N = nerve injury

Abbreviations: ACL, anterior cruciate ligament; KD, knee dislocation; LCL, lateral collateral ligament; MCL, medial collateral ligament; PCL, posterior cruciate ligament; PLC, posterolateral corner.

2. MRI:

   a. Not necessary for acute evaluation.

   b. Should be obtained after the patient is stabilized in order to fully evaluate ligamentous and meniscal injury and plan for future reconstruction.

D. Classification

   1. Three classification schemes:

      a. Kennedy's (anatomic) classification—based on the direction of tibial displacement but does not provide information on ligaments involved.

         i. Anterior (most common).

         ii. Posterior.

         iii. Lateral.

         iv. Medial.

         v. Rotational.

         vi. Anterior/posterior: 40 to 50% associated with vascular injury.

      b. Schenck's classification (▶Table 37.1)—based on ligamentous injury (grade III injuries) and allows description of neurologic or vascular injuries.

II. Treatment

A. Initial management

   1. Immobilization—radiolucent knee immobilizer or long leg plaster splint.

      a. Acceptable if the knee is stable after reduction and vascular examination is within normal limits.

      b. An XR of the knee well reduced in the knee immobilizer is necessary.

      c. Avoid range of motion (ROM) as hinges will obscure proper radiographic evaluation.

      d. Serial radiographs to monitor if patient is in an ICU setting.

   2. Knee spanning external fixation—infrequently necessary. Indications include the following:

      a. Vascular repair.

      b. Extensive soft-tissue injury.

      c. Knee is unstable after reduction in knee immobilizer or splint.

      d. Morbid obesity precludes splinting/immobilization.

B. Definitive management

   1. Nonsurgical management:

      a. Surgical management has better outcomes than nonsurgical management.

      b. Nonsurgical management is only appropriate for poor operative candidates who are sedentary and/or have severe comorbidities.

         i. Patient should be immobilized for 6 weeks and receive frequent XRs to confirm maintained knee reduction.

         ii. ROM is gradually progressed in a knee brace.

   2. Surgical management:

      a. Timing:

         i. No consensus on definition of early or late (3 or 6 weeks):

            • Early surgical management is preferred for settings of bony avulsions or associated fractures.

            • Caution with use of arthroscopy within 10 to 14 days of injury as extravasation of fluid may cause compartment syndrome.

            • Early intervention is associated with loss of ROM in some studies, but improved functional outcomes.

            • Late/chronic reconstructions result in less joint stiffness; however, patients have higher rates of chondral injury and lower functional scores.

         ii. Staged surgical treatment:

            • Involves early repair/augmentations/reconstruction of collateral injury with delayed cruciate reconstruction.

            • May be less favorable than surgical management of all injured ligaments simultaneously due to studies showing higher failure rates associated with staged surgical treatment.

      b. Multiligamentous reconstruction versus repair—ligamentous reconstruction/augmentation (i.e., use of allograft or autograft) has more favorable outcomes with regard to lower failure rate and higher return to activity when compared to ligamentous repair.

   3. Rehabilitation:

      a. Specifics are dependent upon which ligaments are reconstructed and what type of tissue is used (allograft vs. autograft).

      b. Rehabilitation guidelines are surgeon/technique specific regarding ROM and weight bearing.

      c. Important to maintain communication between treatment team (surgeon/physical therapists) regarding specific restrictions.

      d. Return to sport likely in 9 to 12 months.

4. Outcomes:

    a. Functional outcomes in terms of knee function and return to work/activity/sports have been shown in some studies to be superior for those who are treated operatively with ligamentous reconstruction in the early time frame.

    b. However, all patients who suffer a knee dislocation are at risk for post-traumatic osteoarthritis and decreased knee ROM regardless of management specifics.

III. Special Considerations for Pediatric Patients

A. No dedicated reports exist on the predictive ability of ABI in skeletally immature patients. Currently, the same treatment algorithm applied to adults is used in the pediatric population, with consideration of open physes in the reconstruction plan.

Summary

Knee dislocations are orthopaedic emergencies due to potential vascular injury and compartment syndrome, which carry a poor prognosis if not promptly recognized and treated. Knee dislocations may not always present with an obvious deformity and approximately half of knee dislocations spontaneously reduce prior to formal evaluation. Therefore, the evaluating physician must remain clinically suspicious when evaluating patients with knee pain, examine knee stability, and perform a thorough vascular and neurologic examination. Treatment algorithms consisting of ligament repair and/or reconstruction are individualized based on specific patient and injury characteristics.

Suggested Readings

Boyce RH, Singh K, Obremskey WT. Acute management of traumatic knee dislocations for the generalist. J Am Acad Orthop Surg 2015;23(12):761–768

Halvorson JJ, Anz A, Langfitt M, et al. Vascular injury associated with extremity trauma: initial diagnosis and management. J Am Acad Orthop Surg 2011;19(8):495–504

Levy BA, Fanelli GC, Whelan DB, et al; Knee Dislocation Study Group. Controversies in the treatment of knee dislocations and multiligament reconstruction. J Am Acad Orthop Surg 2009;17(4):197–206

Mayer S, Albright JC, Stoneback JW. Pediatric knee dislocations and physeal fractures about the knee. J Am Acad Orthop Surg 2015;23(9):571–580

Mook WR, Ligh CA, Moorman CT III, Leversedge FJ. Nerve injury complicating multiligament knee injury: current concepts and treatment algorithm. J Am Acad Orthop Surg 2013;21(6):343–354

Rihn JA, Groff YJ, Harner CD, Cha PS. The acutely dislocated knee: evaluation and management. J Am Acad Orthop Surg 2004;12(5):334–346

38 Patella Fractures

Benjamin M. Wheatley and Jean-Claude G. D'Alleyrand

Introduction

The patella serves a critical role in the function of the extensor mechanism by increasing its moment arm. Functioning as a sliding lever, it translates the quadriceps and patellar tendons anterior to the trochlea and the knee's axis of rotation, which generates compressive forces across the patellofemoral joint. These forces can exceed three times the body weight while climbing stairs and as much as seven times the body weight while squatting. Patellar fracture is the most common cause of disruption of the extensor mechanism and is approximately six times as common as either quadriceps or patellar tendon rupture. These fractures account for 0.5 to 1.5% of skeletal injuries, with the majority resulting either from falls from heights or from traffic accidents.

Keywords: patella, fracture, tension band, extensor mechanism, complications of treatment

I. Preoperative

A. History and physical examination

1. The majority of these fractures occur in patients 20 to 50 years of age, with a 2:1 male-to-female ratio. They may occur either as a result of direct or indirect forces or as a combination of the two.

2. Examination may reveal a large, tense hemarthrosis. Widely displaced fractures in which the retinacula have been disrupted may result in a less tense effusion as the capsule is disrupted.

3. Failure to perform a straight leg raise or to actively extend the knee. Nondisplaced or minimally displaced fractures may spare the retinacula, preserving the patient's ability to perform a straight leg raise.

4. Palpable defect.

5. Open fractures occur in 6 to 30% of patellar fractures. The majority of open fractures (up to 75%) are Gustilo–Anderson type II.

B. Anatomy

1. Osteology:

   a. The patella is the largest sesamoid bone in the body. Its articular surface is divided longitudinally by a central ridge that separates the medial and lateral facets (▶ **Fig. 38.1**). The odd facet is a third, smaller facet, and is located more medially.

   b. The proximal three-quarters of the patella is covered by cartilage, which can be up to 1-cm thick. The distal quarter of the patella is nonarticular and devoid of cartilage.

   c. Bipartite patella results from failure of fusion of the accessory patellar ossification center and occurs in approximately 2 to 8% of the population and are bilateral in 50% of cases. The most common location is superolateral. Unlike a fracture, a bipartite fragment will appear well corticated on radiographs and lack edema on MRI (▶ **Fig. 38.2**).

2. Neurovascular anatomy:

   a. The blood supply is formed by an anastomotic ring surrounding the patella (▶ **Fig. 38.3**). This is formed by the confluence of six arteries: the supreme genicular artery, medial and lateral superior genicular arteries, medial and lateral inferior genicular arteries, and the anterior tibia recurrent artery.

   b. The supreme genicular artery, also known as the descending genicular artery, arises from the superficial femoral artery. The anterior tibial artery gives rise to the anterior tibial

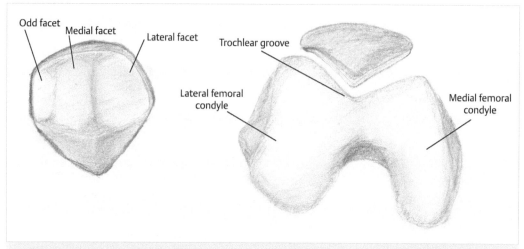

Fig. 38.1 The normal anatomy of the patella. The dorsal surface contains a large medial and lateral facets that are covered in a thick articular cartilage as well as a third, more medial facet, named the odd facet, which is devoid of cartilage. The shape of the femoral sulcus provides some bony stability during flexion.

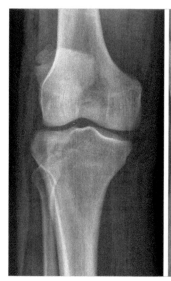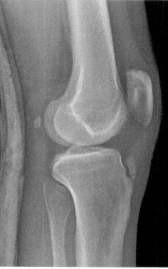

Fig. 38.2 A bipartite patella is the result of a failure of fusion of an accessory ossification center and most commonly occurs in the superolateral portion of the patella, as in this radiograph.

recurrent artery. The remaining four vessels arise from the popliteal artery. The inferior portion of the ring is formed by the transverse infrapatellar branch, which runs within the infrapatellar fat pad, deep to the patellar tendon.

c. The intraosseous blood supply comes from mid-patellar vessels, which enter on the anterior surface in the middle third of the bone to supply the proximal two-thirds and from polar vessels, which come from the transverse infrapatellar branch to the inferior third of the patella.

d. The dominant blood supply enters retrograde through the inferior pole. As a result of this retrograde blood flow, displaced transverse fractures may place proximal fragments at risk of avascular necrosis (AVN).

e. The infrapatellar branch of the saphenous nerve provides sensation to the anterior knee and anterolateral leg. It branches from the saphenous nerve distal to the adductor canal and courses from superomedial to inferolateral crossing the patellar tendon approximately 3 cm inferior to the patella.

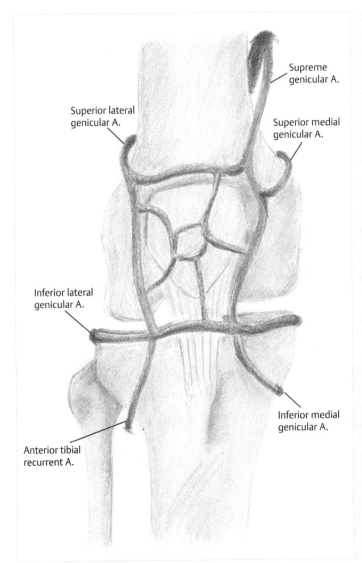

Fig. 38.3 The vascular supply of the patella is provided by a circumferential plexus. The plexus is supplied by six arteries: the supreme genicular artery, lateral superior genicular artery, medial superior genicular artery, lateral inferior genicular artery, medial inferior genicular artery, and the anterior tibial recurrent artery.

Supreme genicular A.

Superior lateral genicular A.

Superior medial genicular A.

Inferior lateral genicular A.

Inferior medial genicular A.

Anterior tibial recurrent A.

3. Ligamentous and tendinous insertions:
   a. Medial patellofemoral ligament (MPFL): It originates on the adductor tubercle and inserts on the superomedial portion of the patella. It resists lateral displacement of the patella (►Fig. 38.4).
   b. Lateral patellofemoral ligament (LPFL): It originates on the proximal lateral epicondyle and inserts on the superolateral portion of the patella. It resists medial displacement of the patella (►Fig. 38.4).
   c. The vastus intermedius originates on the anterior surface of the femur and inserts directly on the superior pole of the patella and forms the deep layer of the aponeurosis.
   d. The remainder of the quadriceps (rectus femoris, vastus lateralis, vastus medialis, vastus medialis obliquus (VMO), and the vastus lateralis obliquus) terminate in an aponeurosis that merges into the anterior third of the joint capsule and is superficial to the vastus intermedius.
   e. The aponeurosis courses over and is adherent to the ventral surface of the patella. It continues to course distally and is contiguous with the superficial portion of the patellar tendon.

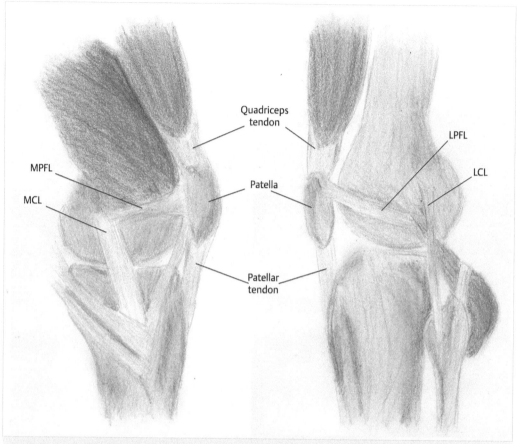

Fig. 38.4 The medial and lateral ligamentous structures of the knee. LCL, lateral collateral ligament; LPFL, lateral patellofemoral ligament; MCL, medial collateral ligament; MPFL, medial patellofemoral ligament.

    f.   The VMO is a dynamic stabilizer and prevents lateral subluxation of the patella.

    g.   The patellar tendon extends from the inferior pole of the patella to the tibial tubercle.

C. Imaging

    1.   Plain radiographs:

       a.   Anteroposterior, lateral, and skyline or merchant views (▶**Fig. 38.5**).

       b.   Plain radiographs underestimate the degree of comminution and articular incongruity.

    2.   Advanced imaging:

       a.   CT scan can be used to further delineate the extent of comminution. The addition of a CT scan has been shown to lead to changes in management plans in nearly 50% of cases.

       b.   MRI is not routinely used but may be beneficial for occult or osteochondral fractures.

D. Classification

    1.   Descriptive classification:

       a.   Nondisplaced, transverse, vertical, stellate, distal pole, and osteochondral (▶**Fig. 38.6**).

       b.   Sixty-five percent of fractures are nondisplaced.

       c.   Transverse fractures account for 50 to 80% of patellar fractures. The majority of these are in the middle to lower third of the patella.

       d.   Vertical fractures account for up to 20% of patellar fractures. Vertical fractures are typically not displaced and do not compromise the extensor mechanism.

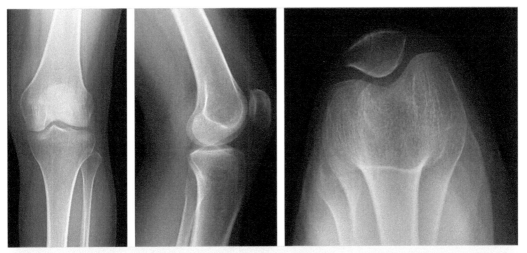

Fig. 38.5 Standard radiographic analysis of the patella includes an anteroposterior, lateral, and skyline or merchant view of the patella.

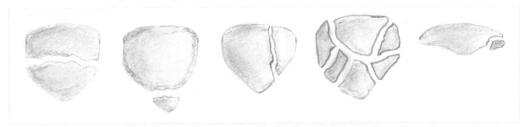

Fig. 38.6 The descriptive classification is the most commonly used system for patellar fractures. The most common types include transverse, inferior pole, vertical, stellate, and osteochondral fractures.

      e.   Stellate pattern fractures may be seen in 30 to 35% of cases.

      f.   Osteochondral fractures occur as the result of a patellar dislocation.

      g.   Frontal plane fractures have been reported but are exceedingly rare.

  2. AO/OTA classification:

      a.   The patella is labeled 34.

      b.   Fracture types include the following: A, extra-articular; B, partial articular (vertical); and C, complete articular (nonvertical).

      c.   Fractures are then further subclassified based on location (medial vs. lateral and proximal vs. distal) and the degree of comminution.

      d.   This classification is not commonly used in practice and is primarily reserved for research.

II. Treatment

A. Initial management

  1. Patellar fractures commonly occur due to falls from height or motor vehicle accidents.

  2. A thorough primary survey should be conducted to evaluate for other injuries.

  3. If the fracture is an open injury, it should be treated as such, to include removal of gross contamination, administration of appropriate antibiotics, and tetanus vaccine if indicated.

  4. A knee immobilizer should be applied while awaiting further treatment.

B. Definitive management
   1. Nonoperative management:
      a. Indications: General guidelines, up to 3 mm of displacement and/or up to 2 mm of articular incongruity, closed, and an intact extensor mechanism.
      b. Initially weight bearing as tolerated in extension with a knee immobilizer or range-of-motion (ROM) brace that is locked in extension.
      c. May begin passive ROM or closed chain exercises (heel slides) after 2 to 3 weeks with weekly increases in motion. Some surgeons will prescribe a more conservative approach and wait until 6 weeks to initiate knee ROM.
      d. Nonoperative management of displaced fractures may also be reasonable in cases of knee joint ankylosis, nonambulatory patients, or patients who are not suitably fit for surgery.
   2. Operative management:
      a. Indications: General guidelines, greater than 3 mm of displacement or 2 mm of articular incongruity, open fracture, or failure of the extensor mechanism.
      b. Goals of treatment are to restore the extensor mechanism and articular congruity.
      c. The articular reduction can be assessed by palpation through the retinacular tears that typically accompany displaced fractures. Alternatively, in the cases where the retinacula are intact, arthroscopic-assisted fixation has been described, which utilizes an arthroscope to view the quality of reduction.
C. Surgical approaches
   1. Anterior approach to the knee:
      a. Longitudinal midline incision.
      b. Develop medial and lateral skin flaps.
      c. The patella lies relatively superficial.
      d. Identify medial and lateral retinacular tears if present.
D. Fixation techniques
   1. Modified anterior tension band:
      a. This is the preferred technique for simple transverse fractures, as patellar fractures are subjected to tensile deforming forces.
      b. A tension band construct converts tensile forces into compressive forces (▶Fig. 38.7a, b), which are ideal for stability and fracture healing.
      c. By placing a wire or suture anterior to the fracture, the tensile forces are neutralized, which allows for compressive forces to be exhibited across the entire fracture.
      d. The modified anterior tension band (MATB) construct consists of two Kirschner's wires placed perpendicular to the fracture and left slightly prominent at both the proximal and distal aspects.
      e. A stainless steel wire is then passed posterior to the ends of the Kirschner wires in a figure-of-eight over the anterior surface of the patella.
      f. Cannulated screws can be used instead of Kirschner's wires, with the steel wire passed through the screws and crossed anteriorly. A cannulated screw tension band construct has been shown to have a higher load to failure than either MATB or screws alone.
   2. Lag screw fixation is most appropriate in vertical fractures or as an adjuvant to another fixation method. Lag screws can be used in comminuted fractures to create two larger fragments, which can then be repaired with a tension band construct.
   3. Plating:
      a. Mini-fragment (2.0–2.7 mm) locking plates.
      b. Recent studies have advocated using patella-specific fixed-angle plates (mesh plates) for comminuted fractures.

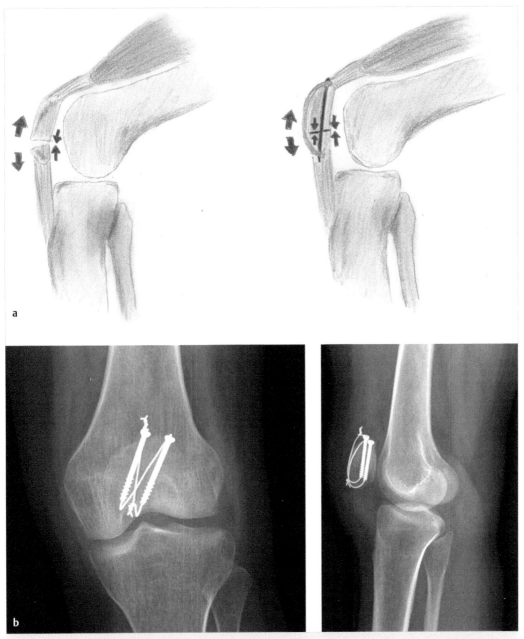

Fig. 38.7 When a three-point bending moment is applied, it will create compressive forces on one side and tensile forces on the other. **(a)** The tension band principle is utilized to convert the tensile forces on one side of the fracture into compressive forces such that there will be equal compression across the entire fractured surface. The tensile forces remain but are transferred to the band that spans the opposite side from the load. **(b)** A radiographic image of a modified tension band technique utilizing cannulated screws for the treatment of an oblique patellar fracture.

4. Partial patellectomy:
   a. Commonly performed for severely comminuted inferior and superior pole fractures—consider inferior pole patellectomy and tendon repair for simple inferior pole fractures involving the distal third (see Chapter 39, Quadriceps and Patellar Tendon Ruptures, for patellar tendon repair technique).

  b. Good to excellent results have been reported in 80 to 90% of patients with a mean quadriceps strength of 85% at final follow-up.

  c. Removal of greater than 40% of the patella has been shown to result in poor outcomes.

 5. Total patellectomy

  a. Used only as a salvage procedure.

  b. On average, patellectomy results in a 50% reduction in quadriceps strength, which may result in difficulty with daily activities such as rising from a seated position or climbing stairs.

  c. Total patellectomy may also result in knee instability.

E. Complications

 1. Stiffness is a common complication following either operative or nonoperative treatment.

  a. It is usually limited to the terminal extent of motion and does not interfere with function.

  b. Length of immobilization has not been shown to be a significant factor.

 2. Implant-related complications are very common due to the subcutaneous position of the patella.

  a. Hardware removal secondary to symptomatic implants has been reported to be as high as 70% in some series, but is more typically reported at 20 to 50%.

  b. It is more common in patients younger than 60 years of age.

  c. More common with Kirschner's wire fixation than with cannulated screws.

  d. Other implant-related complications include wire breakage or migration.

 3. Anterior knee pain is seen in the majority of patients.

 4. Patellofemoral arthritis is a common complication, in as many as 50% of patients, and may be the result of the initial injury, iatrogenic damage to the articular surface, or secondary to inadequate articular reduction.

 5. Nonunion has been reported in up to 12.5% of cases.

  a. Often results in an asymptomatic fibrous nonunion and typically does not require additional surgery.

  b. A higher incidence has been reported with open fractures.

 6. Loss of reduction may occur in 20 to 45% of fractures treated operatively.

  a. Most commonly due to improper fixation technique, unrecognized comminution, and patient noncompliance.

  b. Additional reasons for loss of reduction include inappropriate rehabilitation protocol and morbid obesity.

 7. Infection is reported in 3 to 10% of cases and delayed wound healing may be as high as 12%. It is more common in open fractures and with increasing severity of soft-tissue injury.

F. Rehabilitation

 1. Postoperative rehabilitation should be based on intraoperative findings to include fracture pattern and stability of the fixation.

 2. Immediate weight bearing in extension is acceptable in nearly all cases.

 3. After a period of immobilization, patients may begin a regimen of active flexion and passive extension. This will provide the benefits of motion while reducing tensile forces on the implants.

  a. Initial ROM restrictions depend on several host factors including age, bone quality, comorbidities, and potential for compliance.

  b. A typical postoperative protocol may allow immediate ROM of 0 to 30 degrees with full weight bearing in a brace locked in extension. The permitted ROM is then increased 30 degrees every 2 weeks, with an ROM goal of 0 to 90 degrees at 6 weeks after surgery.

  c. In patients with osteopenia, substantial fracture comminution, questionable fixation, or a tenuous wound closure, a brief period of immobilization and a slower advance of motion may be warranted, although this may compromise the patient's final ROM.

 4. Resistance exercises should be delayed until adequate healing, approximately 12 weeks.

G. Outcomes

 1. Clinical improvement can continue over the first 6 months after surgery.

 2. Functional impairment including strength, power, and endurance can persist for 12 months.

 3. The majority of patients regain near-normal ROM and comparable strength following rehabilitation.

III. Special Considerations for Pediatric and/or Geriatric Patients

 1. Patellar sleeve fracture:

  a. Most commonly seen in patients aged 8 to 12 years.

  b. An avulsion-type injury due to an eccentric load of the extensor mechanism (▶Fig. 38.8a, b).

  c. Typically results in a sleeve of cartilage being avulsed from the remainder of the patella.

  d. Radiographs may reveal patella baja or alta and an ossified fragment may or may not accompany the avulsion.

   i. The Insall–Salvati index is a ratio of the patellar tendon length divided by the length of the patella. It is measured at 30 degrees of knee flexion. Patella baja (low patella) is less than 0.8, while a measurement of greater than 1.2 indicates patella alta (high patella).

  e. Patients will report pain and exhibit an inability to bear weight or perform a straight leg raise.

  f. Nondisplaced fractures with an intact extensor mechanism may be treated nonoperatively, while displaced fractures will require fixation.

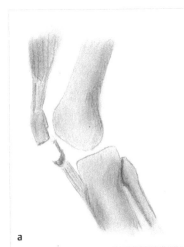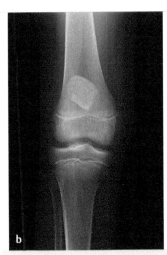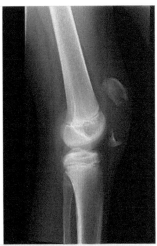

Fig. 38.8 Patellar sleeve fractures are typically seen in patients 8 to 12 years of age. **(a)** They are the result of a severe eccentric load placed on the extensor mechanism. A portion of the articular cartilage will be avulsed from the remainder of the patella. **(b)** In some cases, a large portion of the ossified inferior pole may be avulsed with the articular cartilage making them readily apparent on radiographs.

Summary

Patellar fractures, while rare, can be devastating injuries. The patella is a crucial component of the extensor mechanism of the knee. It functions to redirect the force generated by the quadriceps muscle and to magnify its effect by increasing the moment arm of the muscle. Fractures of the patella frequently disrupt the extensor mechanism, which can potentially make ambulation difficult without appropriate management.

Suggested Readings

Benjamin J, Bried J, Dohm M, McMurtry M. Biomechanical evaluation of various forms of fixation of transverse patellar fractures. J Orthop Trauma 1987;1(3):219–222

Bryant TL, Anderson CL, Stevens CG, Conrad BP, Vincent HK, Sadasivan KK. Comparison of cannulated screws with FiberWire or stainless steel wire for patella fracture fixation: a pilot study. J Orthop 2014;12(2):92–96

Hoshino CM, Tran W, Tiberi JV, et al. Complications following tension-band fixation of patellar fractures with cannulated screws compared with Kirschner wires. J Bone Joint Surg Am 2013;95(7):653–659

Hung LK, Chan KM, Chow YN, Leung PC. Fractured patella: operative treatment using the tension band principle. Injury 1985;16(5):343–347

LeBrun CT, Langford JR, Sagi HC. Functional outcomes after operatively treated patella fractures. J Orthop Trauma 2012;26(7):422–426

Sutton FS Jr, Thompson CH, Lipke J, Kettelkamp DB. The effect of patellectomy on knee function. J Bone Joint Surg Am 1976;58(4):537–540

39 Quadriceps and Patellar Tendon Ruptures

Kyle J. Jeray and Michael D. Hunter

Introduction

Quadriceps and patellar tendon ruptures are relatively uncommon injuries, but proper management is essential given the importance of maintaining knee extensor mechanism function. Quadriceps tendon ruptures are more common than patellar tendon ruptures and occur at an older age, typically greater than 40. The risk factors for rupture are similar between both entities and consist of chronic steroid use, diabetes, renal disease, lupus, gout, hyperparathyroidism, and rheumatoid arthritis. Generally, the mechanism of injury is described as eccentric loading of the tendon against a flexed knee. With increasing flexion angle at the time of injury, more stress is put on the patellar tendon and likely to lead to patellar tendon rupture instead of quadriceps tendon rupture. Early diagnosis and surgical management is of paramount importance to achieve excellent results in complete ruptures (▶ **Video 39.1**).

Keywords: patellar tendon rupture, quadriceps tendon rupture, extensor mechanism rupture, quadriceps tendon repair, patellar tendon repair

I. Preoperative

A. History

   1. Past medical history (lupus, rheumatoid, diabetes, gout, hyperparathyroidism).

   2. Medications (chronic steroid use, local steroid injection).

   3. Mechanism of injury (i.e., flexed knee, jumping).

   4. Activities (sports, history of overuse, previous tendinitis).

   5. High index of suspicion (reports of 10–50% missed diagnosis rates).

B. Physical examination

   1. Quadriceps tendon rupture:

     a. Palpable defect near proximal pole of patella.

     b. Knee effusion/hemarthrosis.

     c. Tenderness to palpation over quadriceps tendon.

     d. Weakness/pain with resisted knee extension.

     e. Inability to perform straight leg raise with complete rupture.

     f. Patella baja or normal patellar height.

   2. Patellar tendon rupture:

     a. Palpable defect near inferior pole of patella.

     b. Patella alta.

     c. Pain over patellar tendon.

     d. Knee effusion/hemarthrosis.

     e. Weak knee extension (partial tear).

     f. Inability to perform straight leg raise with complete tear.

C. Anatomy

   1. Quadriceps tendon:

     a. Coalescence of rectus femoris, vastus lateralis, vastus intermedius, and vastus medialis.

     b. Forms a tendon 3 cm proximal to the superior pole of the patella.

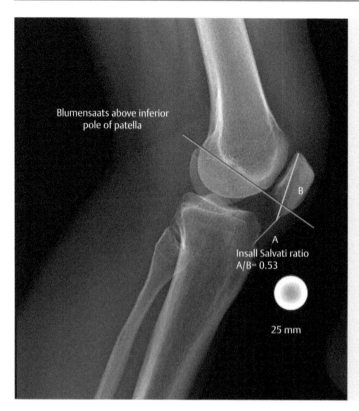

Fig. 39.1 Lateral knee X-ray showing patella baja and quadriceps tendon rupture.

Blumensaats above inferior pole of patella

B

A

Insall Salvati ratio
A/B= 0.53

25 mm

   c. Distinct layers:

      i. Superficial—rectus femoris fibers.

      ii. Middle—vastus lateralis and vastus medialis fibers.

      iii. Deep—vastus intermedius fibers in continuity with synovium.

2. Patellar tendon:

   a. Continuation of the quadriceps tendon as it envelopes the patella (the largest sesamoid bone) and attaches to the tibial tubercle.

   b. Average thickness of the tendon is 4 mm and increases to 5 to 6 mm at the tibial tubercle.

   c. Tightly invested with the medial and lateral retinacula, so frequently these are torn as well.

D. Imaging

1. Quadriceps and patella tendon rupture.

   a. Anteroposterior and lateral X-ray of the knee.

      i. Can show obliteration of quadriceps/patellar tendon shadow.

      ii. Patella baja or normal in quadriceps tendon ruptures (▶ Fig. 39.1).

      iii. Patella alta in patellar tendon ruptures (▶ Fig. 39.2).

2. Arthrography:

   a. Mostly historical with the increased access to MRI.

   b. Injection of contrast material can show extravasation.

3. Ultrasound:

   a. Very sensitive and noninvasive.

   b. Can distinguish complete from partial tears.

   c. Downside is that reliability is operator dependent and does not evaluate associated injuries.

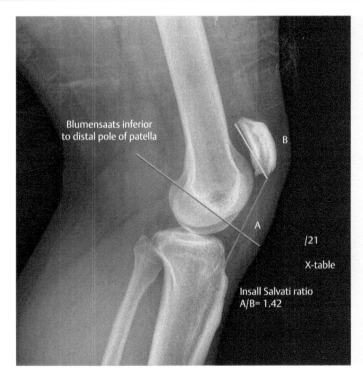

Fig. 39.2 Lateral knee X-ray showing patella alta and patella tendon rupture.

Blumensaats inferior to distal pole of patella

B

A

/21

X-table

Insall Salvati ratio
A/B= 1.42

4. MRI:

    a. High sensitivity, used if suspicion for partial tearing.

    b. Useful to determine tear location for surgical planning or diagnosis of concomitant injuries.

    c. High cost, not necessary for most cases.

II. Treatment

A. Initial and definitive management

    1. Quadriceps tendon tear:

        a. Partial tendon tear with no functional deficit:

            i. Can be treated closed, or nonoperatively.

            ii. Immobilize in full extension with brace for 6 weeks, followed by physical therapy.

            iii. Aggressively treat effusion due to quadriceps deactivation by using ice, compression, anti-inflammatories, ± aspiration.

            iv. Discontinue brace once quadriceps strength has been regained.

        b. Complete tear or partial with functional deficit:

            i. Immediately immobilize in extension.

            ii. Ice, compression, and aspiration may help pain and quadriceps deactivation; however, there is no proven benefit from aspiration.

            iii. Poor results with nonsurgical management.

            iv. Outcomes are better with surgical fixation within 2 to 3 weeks.

            v. Delayed surgical repair results in increased complications and less satisfactory results.

            vi. Many surgical methods have been described with no clear benefit of one or the other and is dependent on location of tear.

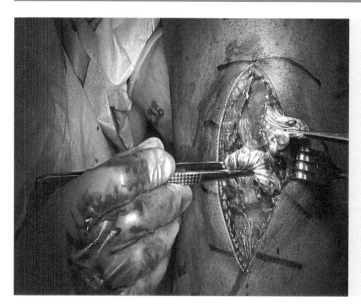

Fig. 39.3 Midline incision centered over patella with full-thickness skin flaps and patellar tendon.

2. Patellar tendon rupture:
   a. Partial tendon tear with intact extensor mechanism:
      i. Can be treated closed, or nonoperatively.
      ii. Immobilize in full extension 2 to 4 weeks followed by range-of-motion (ROM) exercises at 4 to 6 weeks.
      iii. Rest, ice, elevation, compression, and aspiration can improve early pain and ROM; however, these controversies remained unresolved.
   b. Complete tear or partial tear with functional deficits:
      i. Immobilize in full extension immediately.
      ii. Aspiration, ice, and compression remain controversial with regard to benefit.
      iii. Early surgical planning is important as these cannot be managed nonoperatively.
      iv. These injuries require timely surgical repair to avoid retraction or complications associated with delayed treatment.
      v. Several techniques have been described based on location of tear, including use of patellar drill holes and suture anchors.

B. Surgical approaches
   1. Quadriceps tendon rupture—midline incision centered over the quadriceps tendon.
      a. Create full thickness flaps to expose entire tendon.
      b. Evacuate hematoma and debride free edges of the tendon.
   2. Patellar tendon rupture—midline incision based from mid-patella to the tibial tubercle.
      a. Create full-thickness flaps to expose tendon and likely ruptured retinaculum (▶Fig. 39.3).
      b. Evacuate hematoma and clean free edges of tendon (▶Fig. 39.4).
      c. If avulsion of distal pole of patella, clean free bone edge.

C. Fixation techniques
   1. Quadriceps tendon rupture:
      a. Midsubstance tearing—primary end-to-end repair with nonabsorbable sutures.
      b. Osteotendinous junction tearing of the quadriceps tendon.
         i. Two nonabsorbable sutures passed in a Krackow fashion leaving four free strands in the distal stump (▶Fig. 39.5a).
         ii. Roughen the superior pole of the patella to promote bone–tendon healing.

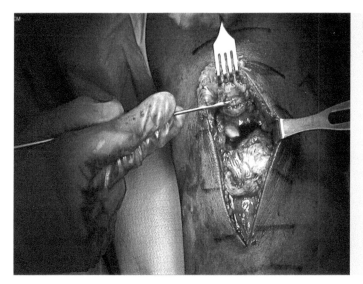

Fig. 39.4 Debridement of free patellar tendon edges and osteotendinous junction.

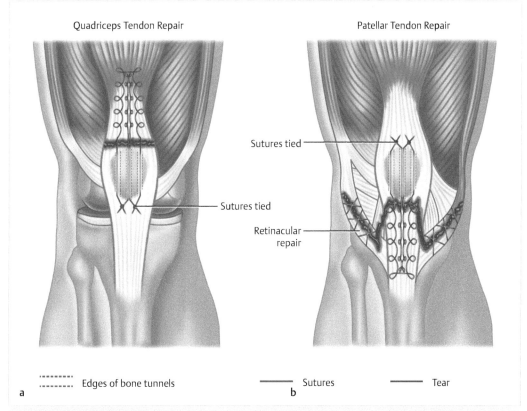

Quadriceps Tendon Repair

Patellar Tendon Repair

Sutures tied

Sutures tied

Retinacular repair

·········· Edges of bone tunnels ———— Sutures ———— Tear

a

b

Fig. 39.5 **(a)** Quadriceps tendon repair technique using three patellar bone tunnels with Krackow stitch pattern. **(b)** Patellar tendon repair technique using three patellar bone tunnels with Krackow stitch pattern and simple retinacular closure.

iii. Drill three parallel 2-mm paths in the longitudinal axis of the patella and pass the lateral and medial strands through the lateral and medial drill holes.

iv. The two central strands are passed through the middle drill hole and each side is tied on the inferior pole.

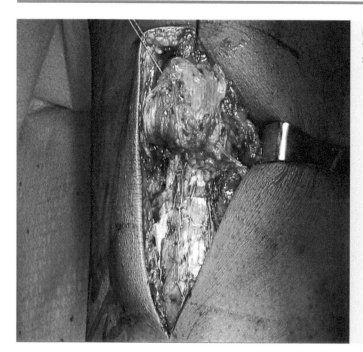

Fig. 39.6 Krackow sutures passed through patella and tied over superior pole closure.

   v. Close the retinaculum and take the knee through ROM to ensure appropriate patellar tracking.

   vi. Newer techniques involve the use of suture anchors due to simplicity and shorter operative time.

   vii. Scuderi quadriceps turndown of fascia lata graft used for augmentation if repair is tenuous.

2. Patellar tendon rupture:

  a. Midsubstance tearing.

    i. Two nonabsorbable sutures passed in a Bunnell or a Krackow fashion.

    ii. Tension can be approximated intraoperatively with use of a lateral knee X-ray and comparison of patellar height to the contralateral side.

    iii. Once the correct tension is obtained, the tear can be oversewn with nonabsorbable suture in a simple fashion.

  b. Osteotendinous junction tear at the patella:

    i. Two nonabsorbable sutures passed in a Krackow fashion.

    ii. These are passed through three vertical bone tunnels in the patella in similar fashion as described above (▶Fig. 39.5b).

    iii. Sutures are tied on the superior pole of the patella (▶Fig. 39.6).

    iv. Tension can be compared by taking a lateral knee X-ray and matching patellar height to contralateral limb X-ray.

    v. Once correct tension is obtained, the tear can be oversewn with nonabsorbable suture in a simple fashion (▶Fig. 39.7).

    vi. Augmentation with Mersilene Tape (Ethicon, United States) or number 5 Mersilene suture using medial to lateral drill holes near the tubercle and through the patella or quadriceps tendon insertion to relieve tension off the repair is becoming more historical.

    vii. Use of suture anchors has been shown to be stronger in cadaveric studies, but reports of higher rerupture rates clinically have called this into question.

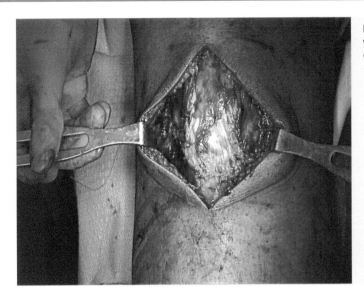

Fig. 39.7 Patellar tendon over sewn with medial and lateral retinacula closure.

D. Complications

    1. Quadriceps tendon repair:

        a. Loss of ROM is the most common complication.

        b. Patella fracture from osseous tunnels.

        c. Rerupture of quadriceps tendon.

    2. Patellar tendon repair:

        a. Recurrent hemarthrosis requiring drainage.

        b. Wound complications and infections.

        c. Tendon rerupture.

        d. Patella baja with decreased ROM from overtensioning.

        e. Patella fracture from osseous tunnels.

E. Rehabilitation

    1. Quadriceps tendon repair:

        a. Postoperatively, the knee is placed into a locked knee brace and allowed to weight-bear in full extension.

        b. ROM typically begins around 4 to 6 weeks post-op.

        c. Therapy focuses on ROM and quadriceps strengthening.

        d. Brace is typically removed around 12 weeks when good quadriceps function is regained and the patient is able to perform a straight leg raise.

    2. Patellar tendon repair:

        a. Touchdown weight bearing in extension with crutches postoperatively—Many surgeons may allow immediate weight bearing with the knee locked in extension.

        b. Isometric hamstring exercises begin day 1.

        c. Active flexion and passive extension 0 to 45 degrees begin at week 2.

        d. Active knee extension begins at 3 weeks.

        e. Full weight bearing in extension begins at week 6 if it was previously restricted.

        f. Recent studies reported higher complications and failure rates of both quadriceps and patellar tendon repairs with prolonged immobilization.

F. Outcomes
    1. Quadriceps tendon repair outcomes:

        a. Early surgical repair results in more satisfactory outcomes in ROM and strength. Multicenter studies have reported successful outcomes between 83 and 100% with good to excellent results and return to activity.

        b. Delay of surgical repair of 2 weeks post injury yielded good results, but 4-, 12-, and 14-week delays had unsatisfactory results.

        c. Up to 85% of patients are able to return to previous occupation, but may lose up to 12% of quadriceps strength, and up to 10 degrees of motion.

    2. Patellar tendon repair outcomes:

        a. Repair within 7 days has shown 80% excellent and 16% good results.

        b. Delayed repair is associated with longer quadriceps atrophy.

Summary

Quadriceps and patellar tendon ruptures are uncommon injuries and may be difficult to diagnose. Identifying medical risk factors such as diabetes and chronic steroid use can decrease missed diagnosis rates. Proper physical examination of the knee extensor mechanism can be helpful in determining partial versus complete tears and whether functional deficits are present. Radiographs aid in diagnosis and MRI is sometimes indicated if a partial tear is suspected. Partial quadriceps and patellar tendon tears with no functional deficits are treated with immobilization in full extension followed by physical therapy initiation at 4 to 6 weeks. For complete tears of the quadriceps tendon or partial tear with functional deficit, early surgery is key. Surgery consists of nonabsorbable suture woven through the tendon and passed through drill holes in the patella or suture anchors. For complete patellar tendon tears, nonabsorbable suture is used with subsequent closure of the retinaculum. Rehabilitation for quadriceps tendon repair includes locked extension bracing with weight bearing as tolerated for 6 weeks followed by range of motion and strengthening exercises. Patellar tendon rehabilitation consists of gradual return to active knee extension starting as early as 3 weeks. Complications of surgery include stiffness, rerupture, and increased risk of patella fracture. Overall, with proper diagnosis and management patients can achieve excellent results and get back to their previous activity level.

Suggested Readings

Ciriello V, Gudipati S, Tosounidis T, Soucacos PN, Giannoudis PV. Clinical outcomes after repair of quadriceps tendon rupture: a systematic review. Injury 2012;43(11):1931–1938

Gilmore JH, Clayton-Smith ZJ, Aguilar M, Pneumaticos SG, Giannoudis PV. Reconstruction techniques and clinical results of patellar tendon ruptures: evidence today. Knee 2015;22(3):148–155

Ilan DI, Tejwani N, Keschner M, Leibman M. Quadriceps tendon rupture. J Am Acad Orthop Surg 2003;11(3):192–200

Konrath GA, Chen D, Lock T, et al. Outcomes following repair of quadriceps tendon ruptures. J Orthop Trauma 1998;12(4):273–279

Matava MJ. Patellar tendon ruptures. J Am Acad Orthop Surg 1996;4(6):287–296

Rauh M, Parker R. Patellar and quadriceps tendinopathies and ruptures. In: DeLee JC, ed. DeLee and Drez's Orthopaedic Sports Medicine. Philadelphia, PA: Sanders; 2009:1513–1577

40 Tibial Plateau Fractures

Camden Burns and Stephen Oleszkiewicz

Introduction

Tibial plateau fractures account for approximately 1% of all fractures with a frequency similar to the calcaneus and humeral shaft. Serial neurovascular monitoring of tibial plateau fractures is important as high-energy fractures are at risk of compartment syndrome. Goals of surgical management include restoration of the articular surface, alignment, and joint stability. Emphasis is placed on soft-tissue management with the use of staged surgeries, dual incisions, and minimally invasive surgical techniques (**Video 40.1**).

I. Preoperative

A. History and physical examination

1. Mechanism of injury:

   a. Low energy—twisting, slip, and fall from standing height injuries:

      i. Varus and valgus forces can drive the femoral condyle into the underlying corresponding tibial plateau.

      ii. These injuries commonly occur in the elderly population with osteoporotic bone.

   b. High energy—falls from height, skiing/sport injuries, motor vehicle accidents:

      i. Axial load to the knee that can cause bicondylar tibial plateau fractures.

      ii. Usually occurs in younger patients with more dense bone.

2. Weight-bearing status:

   The patient is typically unable to bear weight.

3. Patient comorbidities:

   a. Smoking status.

   b. Medical history.

4. Patient employment and activity level.

5. Inspection:

   a. View the soft tissues circumferentially (including posterior aspect of knee) to ensure there are no open wounds or lacerations.

   b. Usually a significant joint effusion indicative of lipohemarthrosis (fat and blood contents from the exposed underlying bone marrow) is present.

   c. Significant soft-tissue swelling and bruising may be present.

6. Palpation:

   a. Significant tenderness to palpation about the proximal tibia.

   b. May palpate crepitus from subcutaneous fracture fragments.

7. Range of motion:

   a. Usually deferred in more severe fractures due to pain and instability from the fracture.

   b. In minimally displaced or nondisplaced fractures, patients may have a painful arc of motion that is limited.

8. Neurovascular examination:

   a. The importance of a thorough neurovascular examination cannot be overstated.

   b. Neurological:

      i. Motor: Ankle dorsiflexion (deep peroneal nerve), extensor hallucis longus (deep peroneal nerve), gastrocnemius (tibial nerve), flexor hallucis longus (tibial nerve), and peroneals (superficial peroneal nerve) should be documented.

     ii. Sensation: Gross sensation in sural, saphenous, deep peroneal, superficial peroneal, and tibial nerves should be documented.

  c. Vascular:

     i. The dorsalis pedis and posterior tibial arterial pulses should be palpated. The quality of the pulse should be compared to the contralateral extremity and documented.

     ii. If the pulses are unable to be palpated, a Doppler ultrasound should be used to document the presence or absence of pulses.

     iii. If there is any mismatch in pulses compared to the contralateral extremity, an ankle brachial index (ABI) should be obtained.

     iv. ABIs less than 0.9 warrant further vascular workup (angiography) and consultation.

9. Stability testing:

  a. In high-energy fractures with severe comminution, this step can be skipped initially due to patient discomfort.

  b. In minimally displaced or borderline operative fractures, the stability of the knee should be tested by applying a varus and valgus force with the knee in full extension.

  c. This maneuver may be too uncomfortable due to fracture pain and a large joint effusion. In order to obtain a reliable examination, the hemarthrosis can be aspirated with a large bore needle (18–21 gauge) and the knee injected with approximately 10 to 20 mL of local anesthetic (1% lidocaine with or without epinephrine, 0.5% Marcaine with or without epinephrine).

  d. Any increase in joint laxity to varus or valgus stress examination greater than 10 degrees compared to the contralateral side is deemed unstable.

10. Compartment syndrome monitoring:

  a. Reported incidence up to 20% in high-energy bicondylar tibial plateau fractures.

  b. Requires vigilant monitoring and expeditious diagnosis with subsequent surgical fascial release.

B. Anatomy

1. Definition:

  a. According to the AO/OTA classification, tibial plateau fractures encompass fractures of the proximal tibial articular surface and a portion of the tibial metaphysis equal to the width of the joint at its widest point (▶ **Fig. 40.1**).

2. Skeletal:

  a. The skeletal anatomy includes the medial condylar articular surface, lateral condylar articular surface, and medial/lateral intercondylar eminences (also called tibial spines; ▶ **Fig. 40.2a, b**).

     i. The medial condyle of the tibial plateau is larger than the lateral condyle, concave, has stronger subchondral bone, and sits lower on a lateral radiograph.

     ii. The lateral condyle is smaller, convex, has weaker subchondral bone, and sits higher on a lateral radiograph compared to the medial condyle.

     iii. The intercondylar eminence has anterior and posterior areas that serve as attachment points for the anterior cruciate ligament (ACL) and posterior cruciate ligament (PCL), respectively.

3. Alignment (▶ **Fig. 40.3**):

  a. The proximal tibia articular surface is in 3-degree anatomic varus, meaning the lateral condyle is slightly higher than the medial condyle when viewing an anteroposterior (AP) radiograph (average medial proximal tibia angle = 87 degrees).

  b. The proximal tibia articular surface has approximately 5 to 10 degrees of posterior slope (average posterior proximal tibia angle = 81 degrees).

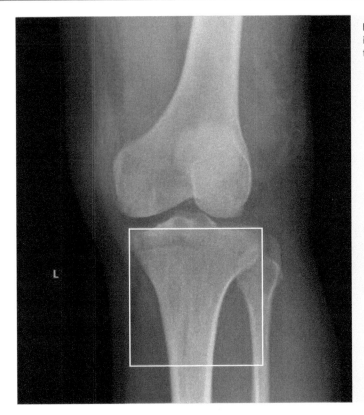

Fig. 40.1 The square outline identifies AO/OTA 41 or proximal tibia periarticular fractures.

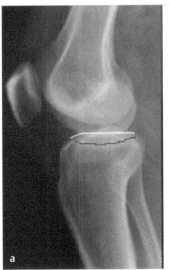
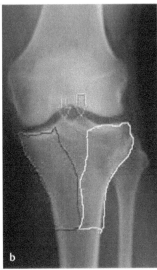

Fig. 40.2 (a) A lateral plain film and (b) an anteroposterior film showing the medial condyle outlined in red, lateral condyle outlined in yellow, green arrow showing the medial tibial spine and blue arrow showing the lateral tibial spine.

4. Soft tissue (▶ Fig. 40.4):
   a. Meniscus:
      i. The medial and lateral menisci are fibrocartilaginous rings of tissue that are located on top of the medial and lateral condyles.
      ii. Function:
         • Cushion the knee joint to allow for smooth articulation between the distal femur and proximal tibia.

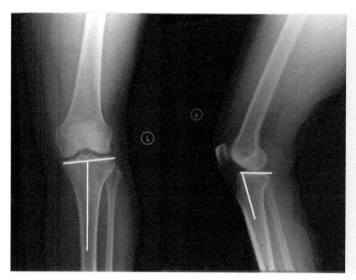

Fig. 40.3 Anteroposterior and lateral knee films with yellow lines showing the medial proximal tibia angle and and posterior proximal tibia angle.

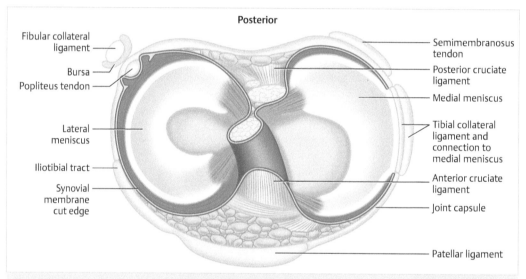

Posterior

Fibular collateral ligament

Bursa

Popliteus tendon

Lateral meniscus

Iliotibial tract

Synovial membrane cut edge

Semimembranosus tendon

Posterior cruciate ligament

Medial meniscus

Tibial collateral ligament and connection to medial meniscus

Anterior cruciate ligament

Joint capsule

Patellar ligament

Fig. 40.4 Soft tissue structures of the tibial plateau. These structures may also be injured in tibial plateau fractures.

- Stress distribution.
- Load transmission.

iii. These structures are frequently torn in association with tibial plateau fractures (typically reported incidence of 40% but has been described in up to 80%), most commonly tearing off its peripheral attachment to the capsule of the knee joint (meniscocapsular avulsions).

b. Ligaments:

i. There are four main ligaments surrounding the knee joint. These structures can be injured at their proximal or distal bony insertions while remaining attached to the bone (avulsion fracture) or can be torn in the middle of the ligament (intrasubstance tear).

- ACL—resists excessive anterior translation of the tibia in relation to the femur.
- PCL—resists excessive posterior translation of the tibia in relation to the femur.
- Medial collateral ligament (MCL):
  - Function—resists excessive valgus force to the knee joint.
  - Clinical significance—may be injured in lateral condyle tibial plateau fractures.

- Lateral collateral ligament (LCL):
  - Function—resists excessive varus force to the knee joint.
  - Clinical significance—may be injured in medial condyle tibial plateau fractures.
  c. Tendons:
    i. Patellar tendon—inserts into the anterior aspect of the proximal tibia at the tibial tubercle.
       - Function—knee extension.
    ii. Iliotibial band—inserts into anterolateral aspect of proximal tibia at "Gerdy's tubercle."
       - Function—part of the "posterolateral corner," a group of tendons, ligaments, and the knee capsule that stabilize the knee in extension/slight flexion.
    iii. Hamstring tendons—group of three hamstring tendons (gracilis, semitendinosus, sartorius), referred to as the pes anserine, insert into anteromedial aspect of proximal tibia.
       - Function—knee flexion.
5. Neurovascular structures:
   a. Common peroneal nerve—winds around the fibular neck (upper aspect of fibula) and is the most common nerve injury in tibial plateau fractures.
      i. The nerve most commonly is stretched due to a varus injury to the knee.
      ii. The resulting nerve injury usually resolves with observation.
      iii. Function:
         - Deep peroneal nerve controls ankle dorsiflexion and provides sensation between the first and second web space dorsally on the foot.
         - Superficial peroneal nerve controls ankle eversion and provides sensation to the majority of the dorsum of the foot.
   b. Tibial nerve and popliteal artery:
      i. Course along the posterior aspect of the knee immediately behind the knee capsule.
      ii. Can suffer stretch injuries due to the mechanism of injury, displaced bony fragments, or knee dislocations in association with fracture.
      iii. Rarely, the popliteal artery can be transected.

C. Imaging assessment
   1. Radiographs:
      a. High-quality AP and lateral radiographs of the knee and tibia—Visualize the joint above and below the fracture.
      b. Tibial plateau view:
         i. X-ray beam angled similarly as an AP radiograph of the knee but with 10 degrees of caudal tilt. This is due to the approximately 10-degree slope of the proximal tibia articular surface.
   2. CT scan:
      a. Usually obtained for operative fractures to measure displacement and/or precisely define fracture fragments for preoperative planning.
      b. Aids the surgeon in identifying occult fractures that would otherwise be missed on plain radiographs:
         i. Lipohemarthrosis visualized on CT scan is a clue that an occult fracture is present.
         ii. Especially helpful in identifying posteromedial shear fractures that could require an additional incision and surgical fixation in the operating room (▶ **Fig. 40.5**).
      c. If there is significant soft-tissue injury or fracture displacement and external fixator placement is planned, the CT scan should be obtained after placement of the external fixator to aid in fracture pattern recognition (see 'External Fixation' section later in this chapter).
   3. MRI:
      a. The role of MRI in tibial plateau fractures is controversial.

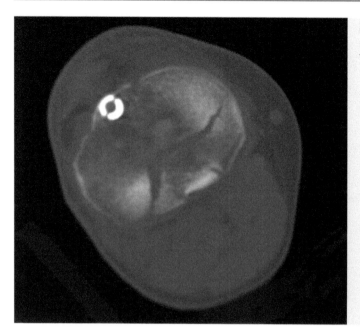

Fig. 40.5 CT scan showing posteromedial tibial plateau fracture fragment.

    b. Identifies soft-tissue injuries that are not visible on X-ray or CT (meniscus and ligament tears).

    c. Oftentimes, the lateral meniscus is routinely visualized during surgery (see "Open reduction internal fixation"). However, during the posteromedial approach, the medial meniscus is not routinely visualized.

D. Classification

  1. OTA-AO classification:

    a. The fracture can be subdivided into either type A, B, or C.

      i. Extra-articular (type A)—the articular surface is not fractured, but there is a fracture of the proximal tibia metaphysis that is a distance equal to or less than the width of the joint at its widest point.

      ii. Partial articular (type B)—there is a fracture of the articular surface of the tibia, but a portion of the articular surface remains in continuity with the metaphysis/diaphysis.

      iii. Complete articular (type C)—there is a fracture of the articular surface, and no portion of the articular surface remains attached to the underlying metaphysis/diaphysis.

  2. Schatzker's classification (▶ **Fig. 40.6**):

    a. This classification is the most commonly used to describe the general characteristics of a tibial plateau fracture.

    b. The classification is intended to describe increasing severity of fractures with each number.

      i. Schatzker I—isolated split fracture of the lateral tibia plateau; often occurs in young patients with strong subchondral bone.

      ii. Schatzker II (▶ **Fig. 40.7**)—split fracture of the lateral tibia plateau with associated depression of the articular surface; most common tibial plateau fracture.

      iii. Schatzker III—pure depression fracture of the lateral tibial plateau:

        • Relatively uncommon fracture pattern.

        • Usually occurs in the elderly population and/or those with osteoporotic bone.

        • Be aware of the difference between a lateral tibial plateau split fracture with displacement versus a lateral tibial plateau fracture with depression as they can be easily confused radiographically.

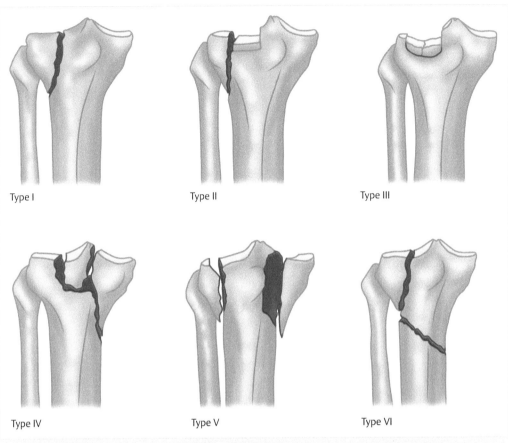

Fig. 40.6 Schatzker classification (I–VI) of tibial plateau fractures; I: Lateral split fracture, II: Lateral split + depression fractures, III: lateral depression fracture, IV: medial plateau fracture; V: fracture of medial and lateral condyles, VI: bicondylar fracture with complete metadiaphyseal discontinuity.

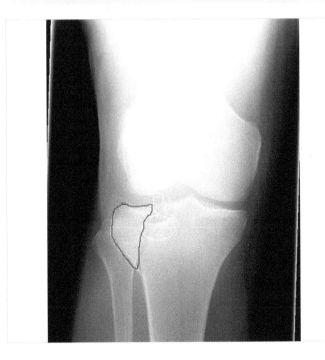

Fig. 40.7 Schatzker 2 fracture with red outline showing split fragment and yellow outline showing depressed segment.

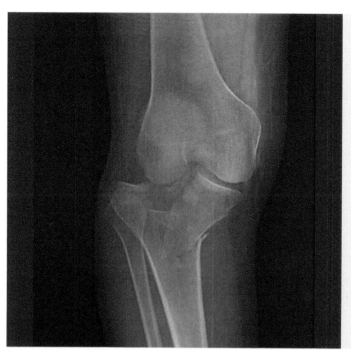

Fig. 40.8 Schatzker IV medial tibia plateau fracture.

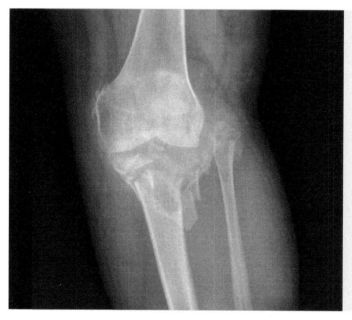

Fig. 40.9 Schatzker VI bicondylar tibia plateau fracture.

iv. Schatzker IV (▶**Fig. 40.8**)—split fracture of the medial condyle often with extension into the intercondylar eminence:

- These fractures tend to be highly unstable as they can be associated with a fracture dislocation.
- Have the highest rate of associated neurovascular and ligamentous injuries.
- Require a high level of vigilance to avoid devastating complications.

v. Schatzker V—fracture of the medial and lateral condyles of the tibial plateau ("bicondylar fracture") typically with the tibial spines remaining in continuity with the diaphysis. This pattern is relatively uncommon.

vi. Schatzker VI (▶**Fig. 40.9**)—fracture of the medial and lateral condyles of the tibial plateau ("bicondylar fracture") with no remaining attachment of the articular surface to the diaphysis:

- Usually associated with significant soft-tissue injury.
- Medial and bicondylar tibial plateau fractures (Schatzker IV–VI) have the highest rates of compartment syndrome.

II. Treatment

A. Initial management

1. The knee should be immobilized in order to help decrease patient discomfort with either a knee immobilizer or long leg plaster splint with the knee in slight flexion.

2. Serial examination in patients at risk of developing compartment syndrome.

B. Nonoperative treatment

1. Indications:

a. Nondisplaced or minimally displaced lateral plateau fracture stable to stress examination.

i. Long-term studies have demonstrated that an unstable joint significantly contributes to the development of post-traumatic osteoarthritis.

ii. The exact amount of condylar widening and joint depression that is acceptable to treat without surgery is not known. However, any joint depression or condylar widening that produces joint instability is an indication for surgery. Generally accepted guidelines for fracture displacement include the following:

- Joint depression: 5 to 10 mm.
- Condylar widening: greater than 5 mm.

b. Avulsion fractures of the tibial plateau that do not involve a significant amount of the articular surface (typically minimally displaced tibia spine fractures).

C. Operative treatment

1. Indications:

a. Absolute:

i. Open tibial plateau fracture.

ii. Concomitant compartment syndrome or arterial injury.

b. Relative:

i. Bicondylar plateau fractures.

ii. Nondisplaced or displaced medial plateau fractures. Nondisplaced medial plateau fractures are prone to late secondary displacement with nonoperative management.

iii. Lateral plateau fractures with associated joint instability.

iv. "Floating knee" injury (tibial plateau fracture associated with a femur fracture).

v. Tibial plateau fracture in a multiply injured patient to facilitate mobilization.

2. Treatment options:

a. External fixation:

i. Indications:

- High-energy fractures with significant soft-tissue swelling, length unstable patterns (fractures with significant shortening), or fractures with associated joint dislocations or subluxation. Usually Schatzker's fractures IV to VI.

ii. Purpose:

- Allows soft tissues to rest before definitive fixation.
- Indirectly reduces the fracture via fracture fragment soft-tissue attachments (ligamentotaxis).
- Restores length and alignment of the fracture, which aids in preoperative planning when obtaining a CT scan.

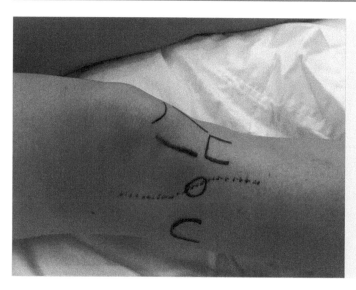

Fig. 40.10 Anterolateral incision to the tibial plateau.

iii. Technique:
- Two Schanz pins placed in the femur from an anterior or anterolateral position and two Schanz pins placed in anterior tibia just medial to tibial crest.
- Pins are typically placed outside of the anticipated location of definitive fixation.

b. Open reduction internal fixation (ORIF):

i. Approaches:
- Anterolateral (▶**Fig. 40.10**): Lazy "S" or "hockey stick" incision that begins at the lateral aspect of the tibial crest at the level of the tibial tubercle, crosses obliquely over Gerdy's tubercle, and either continues up the lateral aspect of the femur or turns posteriorly at the joint line.
- Incision is sharply continued down to level of fascia.
- The anterior compartment fascia and iliotibial band are incised in line with the skin incision.
- The anterior compartment musculature is elevated off the proximal tibia exposing the underlying anterolateral tibial plateau.
- A submeniscal arthrotomy may be performed at this point in time to gain access to the joint and directly visualize the joint surface. The lateral meniscus can be visualized and inspected for tears.

ii. Posteromedial (▶**Fig. 40.11**):
- Straight incision 2 cm posterior to the posteromedial border of the tibia to the adductor tubercle of the medial femoral condyle.
  Alternatively, the incision can be curved 90 degrees posteriorly at the joint line.
- Sharp dissection through subcutaneous tissue down to fascia and pes anserine tendons. Be aware of the saphenous nerve and vein that course in the subcutaneous tissue.
- The pes anserine tendons need to be dissected to increase their mobility in order to work in the interval between the pes anserine tendons and the medial head of the gastrocnemius. Alternatively, some surgeons will elect to transect the tendons and repair them at the end of the case to enhance visualization.
- The gastrocnemius fascia is sharply incised along the posteromedial aspect of the tibia, exposing the underlying tibial plateau bone and fracture.
- The joint surface is not routinely visualized from the medial approach with intraoperative fluoroscopy used to determine reduction or arthroscopically assisted.

iii. Direct posterior: May be indicated for rare posterior fracture patterns.

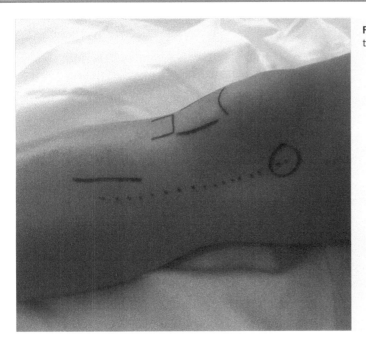

Fig. 40.11 Posteromedial incision to the tibial plateau.

    iv. Reduction techniques:

- Depressed portions of the tibial plateau are elevated back to their original position. This can be achieved with use of bone tamps and a lamina spreader.
- Access to the depressed portion requires opening a fractured piece of tibial plateau ("opening the book") or creating a window using a drill bit and/or osteotomes ("cortical window").
- The articular piece is held in place provisionally or definitively with K-wires:
  - Small fragment screws placed close to the articular surface (subchondral screws) are used to hold the articular piece in place ("rafter" screws) to prevent recurrence of depression.
  - More small fragment screws are better at supporting a depressed articular surface than fewer large screws (6.5 mm).
- After the depressed articular piece is anatomically reduced, the void left behind in the metaphyseal bone can be filled with different substances.
  - Autograft obtained from the patient's distal femur or iliac crest (done historically, but rarely done today).
  - Biological bone graft substitute: cancellous chips (typically used as an intraoperative tool to help with depressed segments).
  - Synthetic bone graft substitutes: calcium phosphate, calcium sulfate. Studies have shown that synthetic bone graft substitutes, specifically calcium phosphate, have greater compressive strength and lead to less articular subsidence than autogenous iliac crest bone graft.

3. Definitive fixation options:
   a. Nonlocked buttress plating:
      i. Indications are partial articular fractures (AO/OTA type B); posteromedial shear fractures (either in isolation or as part of a bicondylar fracture pattern); these fractures are oriented coronally on CT scan; young, healthy dense bone:
         - Techniques are commercially available precontoured small fragment and large fragment periarticular plates. Small fragment are most commonly used but large fragment plates are used in select circumstances.

b. Locked plating:

    i. Indications are osteoporotic bone, comminuted fractures with poor screw purchase. Precontoured lateral locked plates may not be necessary when dual nonlocking plate fixation strategies are undertaken in bicondylar fracture patterns.

    ii. Technique: There are conflicting reports comparing the ability of a single lateral locked plate to maintain alignment as well as dual-plate fixation in bicondylar fractures.

c. Circular frames ("thin-wire" fixation)/hybrid fixation:

    i. Indications:

- Similar indications as ORIF but especially useful for injuries associated with severe soft-tissue compromise (fasciotomy wounds, severe open tibial plateau fractures, or closed high-energy bicondylar tibia plateau fractures with extensive soft-tissue injury).
- A prospective, randomized controlled trial demonstrated equivalent long-term outcomes as ORIF but with less frequent rates of deep infection and wound complications.

    ii. Contraindications—partial articular fractures.

    iii. Technique:

- Requires preoperative CT scan for meticulous preoperative planning.
- Limited incisions are used to place percutaneous clamps and screws.
- Thin wires are used to aid in reduction of large fragments:
  - Thin wires should be placed greater than 14 mm from joint surface to avoid intracapsular placement.
  - If wires are placed intracapsular, a subsequent pin tract infection could develop into septic arthritis.
- Schanz pins are used to attach the articular segment to the diaphysis via circular rings.

D. Postoperative rehabilitation

1. Range of motion:

a. Early range of motion is encouraged since articular cartilage receives its nutrition through passive diffusion due to motion.

b. The exact timing of range of motion depends on the stability of the fracture and soft-tissue integrity.

c. Some surgeons will start immediate range of motion, while others may immobilize the patient in a splint for 7 to 10 days until the incisions are healed.

d. Consider a knee brace if there is associated ligamentous injury; some surgeons use a brace routinely for pain control and to "protect" the repair.

2. Weight-bearing status

a. The topic of weight bearing is controversial as it depends on the personality of the fracture and stability of fixation.

b. In general, most surgeons will initiate a period of nonweight bearing for at least 6 weeks. Some surgeons may start partial weight bearing at 6 weeks, while others may keep patients nonweight bearing until 12 weeks.

c. In general, the goal is to have the patient weight bearing as tolerated by 12 weeks.

E. Complications

1. Arthrofibrosis (Knee stiffness):

a. Significant knee stiffness is defined as less than 90 degrees of knee flexion.

b. More common in higher-energy fractures or if early range of motion is not instituted in the immediate postoperative period.

c. May require a return trip to the operating room for knee manipulation performed under anesthesia.

    d. The patient should be encouraged to maintain full knee extension when resting in bed in the early postoperative period to avoid losing knee extension. Loss of 5 to 10 degrees of knee extension results in an abnormal gait.

2. Post-traumatic osteoarthritis:

    a. Thirty-one percent secondary degenerative changes in a long-term cohort study, although two-thirds of patients did not have associated symptoms.

    b. Patients with malalignment of more than 5 degrees may develop more severe arthritis.

    c. Studies have not shown differences in outcomes with articular displacements ≤ 4 mm compared to anatomic reduction.

3. Infection:

    a. Varies based on severity of fracture pattern, integrity of soft tissues, open fractures, or dysvascular limbs:

        i. Reported rates of deep infection are 5 to 10%.
        ii. Up to 30 to 40% risk of infection when an associated compartment syndrome is present.

    b. Delayed surgical repair with the aid of external fixator application for soft-tissue rest has shown to decrease deep wound infection rates in high-energy bicondylar tibial plateau fractures.

    c. Can present as septic arthritis requiring emergent surgical irrigation and debridement.

    d. Nonunion:

        i. Typically occurs at junction between metaphysis and diaphysis in higher-energy fractures.
        ii. Reported rate of approximately 5% in the literature in high-energy fractures.

F. Prognosis:

1. Unicondylar fractures, as expected, have better outcomes than bicondylar fractures.

2. Mean knee range of motion in one cohort was 130 degrees at 1-year follow-up (range 10–145 degrees).

3. At 1-year follow-up, up to 90% of patients can be expected to return to working activities.

Suggested Readings

Barei DP, Nork SE, Mills WJ, Henley MB, Benirschke SK. Complications associated with internal fixation of high-energy bicondylar tibial plateau fractures utilizing a two-incision technique. J Orthop Trauma 2004;18(10):649–657

Canadian Orthopaedic Trauma Society. Open reduction and internal fixation compared with circular fixator application for bicondylar tibial plateau fractures. Results of a multicenter, prospective, randomized clinical trial. J Bone Joint Surg Am 2006;88(12):2613–2623

Lansinger O, Bergman B, Körner L, Andersson GB. Tibial condylar fractures. A twenty-year follow-up. J Bone Joint Surg Am 1986;68(1):13–19

Rademakers MV, Kerkhoffs GM, Sierevelt IN, Raaymakers EL, Marti RK. Operative treatment of 109 tibial plateau fractures: five- to 27-year follow-up results. J Orthop Trauma 2007;21(1):5–10

Russell TA, Leighton RK; Alpha-BSM Tibial Plateau Fracture Study Group. Comparison of autogenous bone graft and endothermic calcium phosphate cement for defect augmentation in tibial plateau fractures. A multicenter, prospective, randomized study. J Bone Joint Surg Am 2008;90(10):2057–2061

Schatzker J, McBroom R, Bruce D. The tibial plateau fracture. The Toronto experience 1968–1975. Clin Orthop Relat Res 1979(138):94–104

Shepherd L, Abdollahi K, Lee J, Vangsness CT Jr. The prevalence of soft tissue injuries in nonoperative tibial plateau fractures as determined by magnetic resonance imaging. J Orthop Trauma 2002;16(9):628–631

41 Tibia and Fibula Shaft Fractures

Jonah Hebert-Davies and Conor P. Kleweno

Introduction

The tibia is the most commonly fractured long bone. Tibial fractures can result either from direct, high-energy impact mechanism or from low-energy twisting or fall mechanisms. The relatively subcutaneous location makes it particularly at risk for open fractures. Thorough initial management, adequate preoperative imaging and planning, as well as good surgical techniques are necessary to ensure optimal outcomes.

Keywords: tibia, tibia fracture, intramedullary nailing, compartment syndrome

I. Preoperative Evaluation and Assessment

A. History and physical examination

    1. Commonly associated with high-energy mechanism.

    2. Full orthopaedic workup including careful examination for associated fractures.

    3. Skin integrity must be evaluated to look for open fractures.

    4. Detailed initial neurovascular and compartment examination should be documented. Repeat (and document) neurovascular examination after reduction and splinting.

    5. Patients are at risk for compartment syndrome and should be re-examined frequently with corresponding documentation. Disproportionate pain or pain with passive flexion/extension should alert the surgeon to the high probability of compartment syndrome (see section "**III, Complications**" in this chapter).

B. Imaging and anatomy

    1. Adequate quality orthogonal X-ray views of the tibia.

    2. X-rays of knee and ankle are also recommended because articular extension at both the knee and at the ankle is common (▶ **Fig. 41.1a**).

       a. Distal third fractures—high rate of associated posterior malleolus fracture.

       b. If this is suspected and not seen on X-ray, a CT scan should be obtained. The axial views are most helpful to plan potential fixation of the posterior malleolus fragment (▶ **Fig. 41.1b**).

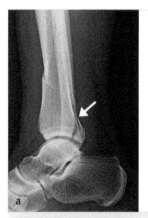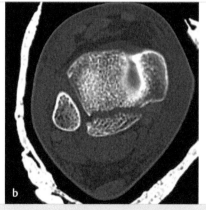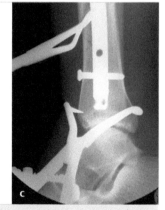

Fig. 41.1 Distal third tibia shaft fracture with (**a**) lateral X-ray revealing associated posterior malleolar fracture (*arrow*). (**b**) CT scan axial cut at tibial plafond showing associated posterior malleolar fracture that can guide trajectory of clamp and screw. (**c**) Lateral X-ray after placement of clamps, reducing the fracture.

3. Plain radiographs can help identify many specific details about the fracture.

    a. Suspected open fractures, high-energy mechanisms (segmental, comminuted) with severe soft-tissue injury can be identified on X-rays.

    b. Fibula fractures seen on X-ray can also give clues to the energy of the fracture mechanism. Fibula fractures at the same level as the tibia fracture tend to be higher energy than at distant (either proximal or distal) sites.

C. Classification

    1. The AO/OTA classification is useful to describe tibia shaft fractures.

        a. Type A—simple patterns, progressing from spiral (A1) to transverse (A3).

        b. Type B—wedge fractures increasing in complexity from B1 to B3.

        c. Type C—complex fractures with increasing comminution from C1 to C3.

    2. Open fractures are typically classified according to the Gustilo–Anderson classification (for further reference, please see Chapter 2, Open Fractures).

II. Treatment

A. Initial management

    1. Reduction in the emergency department and placement into a padded long leg splint as soon as possible.

    2. Open wounds should have sterile dressings applied. Any gross contamination should be removed, but formal debridement should be reserved for the operating room.

    3. Appropriate antibiotics (typically a first-generation cephalosporin) and tetanus update are administered.

B. Definitive management

    1. Historical data suggest that many tibia fractures can be treated nonoperatively with reduction and casting.

    2. However, most displaced tibia fractures are currently treated surgically.

    3. Operative management has the following advantages: improved alignment, earlier ankle and knee range of motion, immediate weight bearing, and improved functional outcomes.

    4. Rarely fractures treated nonoperatively should meet the following criteria:

        a. Closed, isolated, simple, nondisplaced, or minimally displaced tibial shaft fractures in patients willing to comply with non–weight bearing.

        b. Able to tolerate multiple cast changes and frequent X-ray follow-ups.

        c. Medically moribund patients are also candidates for cast treatment.

    5. Open fractures should undergo urgent surgical debridement:

        a. Types I, II, and IIIA can generally be treated definitively immediately following debridement assuming there is not gross contamination present.

        b. Types IIIB and IIIC typically undergo staged management with an external fixator prior to definitive fixation depending on the amount of contamination and severity of soft-tissue injury.

        c. Traumatic wounds are extended proximally and distally to expose the entire zone of injury and facilitate adequate debridement.

        d. Consider soft-tissue friendly counter incisions for debridement in select locations. For example, small to medium traumatic anterior medial wounds can be accessed through an anterolateral approach.

    6. The vast majority of extra-articular fractures are treated with intramedullary nails (IMN).

7. Proximal third and distal third fractures (with or without simple articular fracture involvement) can be treated with open reduction and internal fixation (ORIF) with plates and screws or IMN. Recent data suggest no clinically significant difference in malalignment rates and infectious/wound complications between ORIF with plates and IMN.

8. Modern nail designs incorporate far proximal and far distal multiplanar interlocking screw options to allow for treatment of proximal and distal fractures (i.e., "extreme nailing").

9. Compartment syndrome (Refer to Chapter 13, Compartment Syndrome, for detailed discussion of pathophysiology, diagnosis, and treatment).

   a. Tibia fracture is the most common cause of compartment syndrome.

      i. High risk in crush injuries even with minimally displaced fractures.
      ii. Common in tibia fractures associated with sports (football and soccer).
      iii. Dysvascular limbs following revascularization.

   b. Primarily a clinical diagnosis. Intracompartmental pressure monitor can assist in diagnosis when the clinical examination is equivocal and in obtunded patients.

   c. Treatment is emergent fasciotomy.

C. Surgical approaches

   1. Most common approaches for tibial nailing are the following:

      a. Infrapatellar (or transpatellar).

      b. Suprapatellar ("retropatellar").

      c. Lateral parapatellar (retinacular release).

   2. Advantages of infrapatellar:

      a. Avoiding articular involvement.

      b. No need for specific instrumentation.

   3. Advantages of suprapatellar approach:

      a. Semi-extended leg position: minimizes knee range of motion throughout nailing (▶ Fig. 41.2).

         i. Easier to maintain starting point.
         ii. Facilitates achieving and maintaining fracture reduction.
         iii. Improved quality of fluoroscopic imaging.

      b. Patellar mobility should be evaluated prior to committing to suprapatellar nailing.

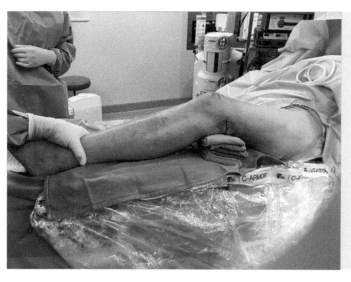

Fig. 41.2 Intraoperative image showing semiextended leg position used for suprapatellar and lateral parapatellar retinacular release approaches.

4. Advantages of lateral parapatellar retinacular release include the following:

    a. All advantages of semi-extended position.

    b. Remain extra-articular.

5. If plate fixation is planned:

    a. Typically, laterally based plate is used for proximal to mid-shaft fractures.

    b. Standard anterolateral approach is used, centered on Gerdy's tubercle.

    c. Anterior compartment fascia is opened and plate can be slid distally in minimally invasive, submuscular fashion.

    d. Distal third fractures can also be treated with either direct medial or anterolateral plate used in a minimally invasive technique.

D. Reduction techniques

1. Indirect reduction—standard closed/indirect methods include traction, manual manipulation, universal distractor, and external fixator.

2. Percutaneously placed clamps are placed through small (<1 cm) incisions (▶ **Fig. 41.3a, b**).

3. Unicortical plates can be placed in open or closed fractures either temporarily (diaphyseal) or permanently (metaphyseal) to effect and maintain a reduction (▶ **Fig. 41.4**).

4. Open reduction remains an appropriate option with good soft-tissue handling (typically lateral or posterior medial approaches; avoid anterior medial incisions).

5. Supra- or infraisthmic fractures must be reduced prior to reaming and nailing—nail insertion will *not* fix malreduction and often will only accentuate it.

E. Fixation techniques

1. Tibia shaft fractures are typically treated with reamed, statically locked nails with at least one, and preferably two, interlocking bolt above and below the fracture.

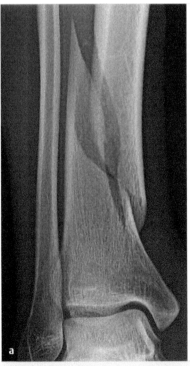
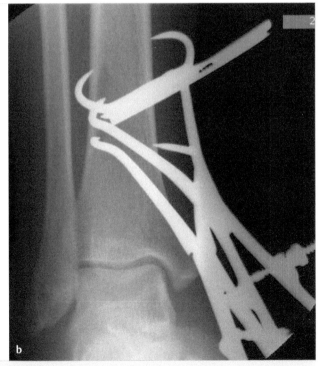

Fig. 41.3 Distal third tibia spiral shaft fracture. **(a)** Initial anteroposterior view and **(b)** after placement of multiple percutaneous clamps. Care should be take when placing these to respect soft tissue.

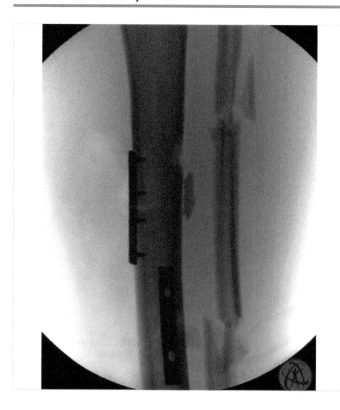

Fig. 41.4 Intraoperative fluoroscopic anteroposterior image of type 3b open, segmental tibia shaft fracture. Multiple 2.7-mm plates with unicortical screws were utilized to temporarily maintain reduction during nailing.

2. Starting point for tibial nail insertion:
   a. Medial to the lateral tibial eminence on the anteroposterior (AP) view.
   b. Anterior to the articular margin and at or posterior to the apex of the tibia on the lateral view.
   c. Guidewire should be inserted in line with the medullary canal.
   d. The starting point ultimately determines nail position and is especially critical for IMN of proximal third and distal third fractures.

3. Important to obtain accurate AP and lateral fluoroscopic views as inadequate views can result in as much as 1 cm of displacement of the starting point.

4. Proximal tibial fractures:
   a. High propensity for malreduction into valgus, procurvatum (apex anterior) and posterior translation of the distal segment.
   b. Techniques to help avoid malalignment include the following:
      i. Correct starting point (▶ **Fig. 41.5a**).
      ii. Semi-extended positioning.
      iii. Large universal distractor.
      iv. Provisional unicortical plate.
      v. Blocking (Poller) screws (▶ **Fig. 41.5a, b**).
      vi. Percutaneous clamps.
   c. Insert multiple (three if possible) multiplanar interlocking screws proximally.

5. Distal tibia fractures:
   a. Most common direction of malalignment is valgus, followed by recurvatum and varus.

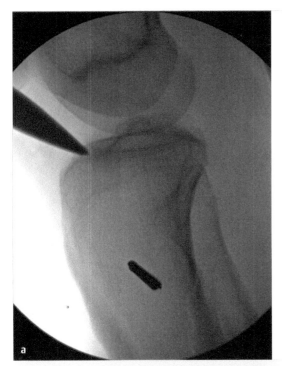 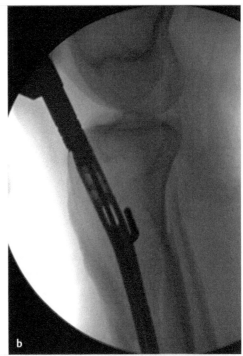

Fig. 41.5 (a, b) Demonstrates the use of a blocking drill bit to avoid malpositioning of the nail and to prevent and/or correct a procurvatum deformity in this proximal tibia fracture.

    b. Techniques to avoid malalignment:
        i. Precise positioning of the distal aspect of the nail:
            • Center or slightly lateral to the center of the tibia/talus on the AP view.
            • Center on the lateral fluoroscopic views.
        ii. Blocking screws.
        iii. Percutaneous clamps.
        iv. Semi-extended positioning.
        v. Fibula fixation may help improve alignment if there is difficulty obtaining a reduction:
            • Conflicting results on whether ORIF fibula increases the risk of tibia nonunion.
            • ORIF fibula may prevent late malunion, although this was found with previous generation nails with fewer interlocking options.
    c. Insert multiple (three if possible) multiplanar interlocking screws distally.
6. Associated posterior malleolus fractures:
    a. Common in distal third tibial fractures (▶ **Fig. 41.1a–c**).
    b. Minimally displaced and small fractures can be clamped anterior to posterior (▶ **Fig. 41.1c**) and fixed prior to beginning reaming or can be fixed after the nail has been inserted.
    c. Fixation: independent AP screws and possibly AP interlocking screw.
    d. Large fractures should be reduced and fixed prior to nail insertion; a separate formal posterior approach to ankle should be considered.
7. Bone loss:
    a. Antibiotic cement spacer can be placed into the bone defect for induced membrane formation and secondary bone grafting (Masquelet's technique).
    b. Bone transport through use of ring fixator.

III. Complications

A. Sequela of missed compartment syndrome

    1. Misdiagnosis, late diagnosis, and/or inadequate treatment lead to severe morbidity, including possible amputation.

    2. Common cause of litigation.

B. Nonunion

    1. Five to 10% risk (higher in open fractures, especially with bone loss).

    2. Reaming improves union rate for closed fractures.

    3. In general, the tibia heals slowly. Six- to 9-month follow-up may be necessary to determine failure to progress to union.

    4. Options for treatment include exchange nailing, autograft, and ring fixator (must exclude infection as cause).

C. Knee/kneeling pain

    1. Unknown etiology but common issue.

    2. Reported incidence highly variable (11–69% in literature).

    3. Important to counsel patients preoperatively.

IV. Rehabilitation

A. Weight bearing/range of motion

    1. Weight bearing as tolerated is standard with IMN.

    2. Some surgeons recommend a 1- to 2-week period of soft-tissue rest with splint depending on the severity of soft-tissue injury. Splint foot in neutral flexion to avoid equinus contracture.

    3. Early range of motion of the ankle and knee is encouraged.

    4. Delayed weight bearing if plate fixation or casting technique is used.

B. Therapy regimen

    1. Therapy for strengthening, stretching (particularly to treat equinus contracture), and proprioception can be prescribed, although not necessary in many patients.

V. Outcomes

A. Functional outcomes

    1. Knee pain (see above).

    2. Goal is full recovery, but many patients can have limitations in activity. At 1 year, up to three-fourths of patients have difficulty performing routine daily activities: kneeling, running, stair climbing, or walking prolonged distances.

VI. Special Considerations for Pediatric and/or Geriatric Patients

A. Pediatric patients

    1. Nonoperative treatment with closed reduction and casting is common.

    2. If closed reduction is unacceptable, flexible tibial nailing or ORIF with rigid plating may be used.

    3. IMN is reserved for patients whose physeal closure is nearly complete.

B. Geriatric patients

    1. Focus on rapid return to weight bearing. Non–weight bearing is poorly tolerated and patients are at higher risk of complications including thromboembolism.

Summary

Tibial shaft fractures are the most common long bone fracture. The subcutaneous nature of the bone makes it at high risk for open fractures. There is also an increased risk for compartment syndrome. Most of these fractures are treated with reamed intrameduallry nails, but sometimes require staged management, open reduction with plate fixation or even non-operative treatment. Early weightbearing and range of motion should be a focus of rehabilitation. Excellent union rates can be expected for most fractures and outcomes are generally good with regards to function in well healed fractures.

Suggested Readings

Bhandari M, Guyatt G, Tornetta P III, et al; Study to Prospectively Evaluate Reamed Intramedullary Nails in Patients with Tibial Fractures Investigators. Randomized trial of reamed and unreamed intramedullary nailing of tibial shaft fractures. J Bone Joint Surg Am 2008;90(12):2567–2578

Bone LB, Sucato D, Stegemann PM, Rohrbacher BJ. Displaced isolated fractures of the tibial shaft treated with either a cast or intramedullary nailing. An outcome analysis of matched pairs of patients. J Bone Joint Surg Am 1997;79(9):1336–1341

Chan DS, Serrano-Riera R, Griffing R, et al. Suprapatellar versus infrapatellar tibial nail insertion: a prospective randomized control pilot study. J Orthop Trauma 2016;30(3):130–134

Obremskey W, Agel J, Archer K, To P, Tornetta P III; SPRINT Investigators. Character, incidence, and predictors of knee pain and activity after infrapatellar intramedullary nailing of an isolated tibia fracture. J Orthop Trauma 2016;30(3):135–141

Sarmiento A, Gersten LM, Sobol PA, Shankwiler JA, Vangsness CT. Tibial shaft fractures treated with functional braces. Experience with 780 fractures. J Bone Joint Surg Br 1989;71(4):602–609

42 Pilon Fractures

Jonah Hebert-Davies and Reza Firoozabadi

Introduction

Pilon fractures are routinely due to high-energy mechanisms secondary to axial loading of the talus into the tibial plafond. They had been associated with unacceptably high rates of complications prior to the implementation of staged management. Although this has changed, these fractures remain challenging and rigorous application of treatment principles is imperative to ensure optimal outcomes.

Keywords: pilon, plafond, distal tibia, staged fixation

I. Preoperative

A. History and physical examination

1. Due to the high-energy mechanism of these injuries, patients should be evaluated according to standard advanced trauma life support (ATLS) protocol.

2. Fall from height mechanism is often associated with calcaneal and thoracolumbar spine fractures.

3. Vascular and neurological injuries are commonly associated with pilon fractures and a thorough examination should be documented.

4. Dysvascular limbs that do not recover following initial reduction should be investigated with vascular surgery according to local protocols.

B. Anatomy

1. Axial compression with foot in dorsiflexion leads to comminution of the anterior aspect of the plafond.

2. Axial loading with the foot in plantar flexion causes injury to the posterior aspect of the plafond.

3. Injury to lateral and medial aspects of plafond are associated with the hindfoot being abducted and adducted, respectively. The foot being in a neutral position results in injury to the anterior and posterior regions.

4. Pilon fractures occur in a typical fracture pattern. Although variations exist, most fractures are comprised of an anterolateral fragment (Chaput's), a posterolateral fragment (Volkmann's), a medial malleolus fragment, and a central die-punch region (▶ **Fig. 42.1**).

C. Imaging

1. High-quality orthogonal X-rays of the ankle should be obtained.

2. As these are generally high-energy fractures, foot- and full-length tibia X-rays should also be obtained.

3. Postreduction X-rays to determine quality of reduction.

4. CT scans are generally obtained following external fixation; they can be obtained prior in certain situations (where partial or acute definitive fixation is considered).

5. CT scan should be used to evaluate articular fragments, location of fracture lines, degree of impaction, associated injures (tendon sheath avulsions, kissing lesions on talus, other associated fractured bones), and fibular fracture.

6. Axial cuts are most useful for surgical planning and fragment evaluation. Special attention should be given to assessing for entrapped posteromedial structures within fractures, such as posterior tibial tendon or the posterior tibial neurovascular bundle.

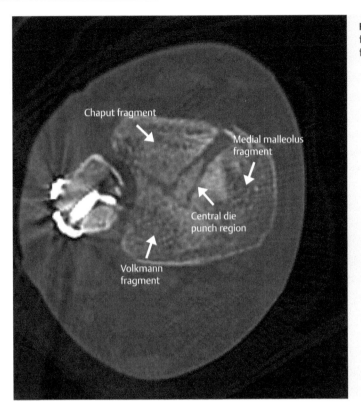

Fig. 42.1 Axial CT scan of pilon fracture showing typical fracture fragments.

7. Coronal and sagittal reformats should be analyzed to aid in preoperative planning and assess for areas of impaction.

8. If the fibula was fixed during initial stage of management, length can be assessed on coronal CT.

D. Classification

1. AO/OTA classification is most useful for pilon fracture nomenclature: A type is extra-articular, B type is partial articular, and C type is complete articular.

   Degree of comminution will dictate severity of injury (i.e., 43C1 vs. 43C3).

II. Treatment

A. Initial management

1. Fractures should be reduced in the emergency department and placed into a bulky splint.

2. Soft-tissue swelling can be surprisingly severe. Blisters can be covered with nonadherent dressings.

3. Most pilon fractures will undergo staged management with external fixation initially, followed by definitive fixation when soft-tissue swelling improves. Recent evidence has shown equivalent results with acute (< 24 hours) definitive fixation of pilon fractures; however, results have not been widely replicated.

4. Low-energy pilon fractures or variants (geriatric/osteoporotic) may be amenable to primary fixation.

5. External fixation of pilon fractures should focus on restoring length, alignment, and rotation.

6. Ligamentotaxis, strategically placed Schanz pins, and appropriate distraction vectors will help achieve reduction.

     7.   Associated fibula fractures can undergo ORIF in this initial setting if soft tissues permit. Fibula fixation should not take place during the initial surgery under the following circumstances:

        a.   Complex fractures when malreduction can occur.

        b.   The definitive fixation will be performed by a different surgeon.

B.   Definitive management

     1.   Nonoperative management of pilon fractures is uncommon except for nondisplaced fractures (< 2 mm displacement with normal length and alignment) and in patients with prohibitive medical comorbidities or nonambulating patients.

     2.   Historically, definitive management should be delayed until soft-tissue swelling has subsided (positive wrinkle sign) and fracture blisters have sufficiently re-epithelialized; however, some studies have shown early definitive fixation may yield equivalent outcomes for select patients.

     3.   Because pilon fractures involve the articular surface, open reduction and internal fixation (ORIF) is the mainstay of treatment.

     4.   ORIF of pilon fractures consists of four major points:

        a.   Anatomic reduction of the articular surface.

        b.   Solid fixation of the articular segment to the diaphysis.

        c.   Fixation of the fibular fracture.

        d.   Potential grafting or filling with bone substitutes of metaphyseal bone defects/loss.

     5.   Most fractures are treated with plate and screw fixation; however, some type A and C1 (simple articular) fractures may be amenable to intramedullary fixation.

     6.   There is continued controversy regarding definitive management with external fixation and limited ORIF versus formal ORIF with direct visualization of the articular surface and key fracture elements. The following apply to external fixation and limited ORIF:

        a.   Typically can be done earlier than formal ORIF.

        b.   The fibula is typically not fixed as this has been shown to have a higher complication rate with no clinical benefit.

        c.   Both joint spanning frames and ring fixators (without spanning the joint) can be used. If a ring fixator is used, many times a temporary "foot plate" will be added initially and then removed 4 to 6 weeks post-op to allow early ankle range of motion.

        d.   External fixation and limited ORIF may be a better option for grossly contaminated open injuries or injuries with significant soft-tissue loss.

C.   Surgical approaches

     1.   Several approaches are described to treat pilon fractures. Often a combination of these approaches is needed to adequately address these fractures (▶Fig. 42.2).

     2.   Anteromedial:

        a.   Medial to the tibialis anterior and lateral to the tribal crest proximal to the ankle joint.

        b.   The incision is curved at the joint toward the tip of the medial malleolus.

        c.   Allows good visualization of the joint and medial gutter (▶Fig. 42.3).

     3.   Anterolateral:

        a.   Lateral to the peroneus tertius/extensor digitorum communis and medial to the peroneal muscles in line with the fourth ray of the foot.

        b.   Offers great visualization of the lateral fragments.

     4.   Posteromedial:

        a.   Between the tibialis posterior tendon and flexor digitorum communis or between the flexor hallucis longus and the flexor digitorum communis.

        b.   Permits good visualization and direct fixation of the medial posterior malleolus.

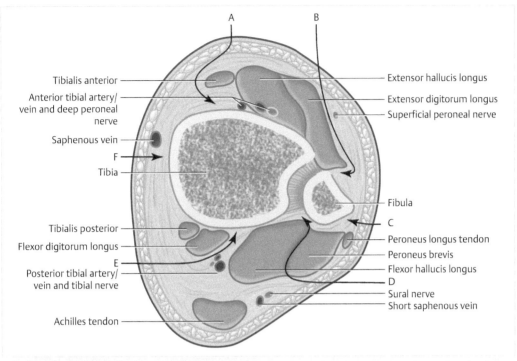

A, Tibialis anterior
Anterior tibial artery/ vein and deep peroneal nerve
Saphenous vein
F
Tibia
Tibialis posterior
Flexor digitorum longus
E
Posterior tibial artery/ vein and tibial nerve
Achilles tendon

Extensor hallucis longus
Extensor digitorum longus
Superficial peroneal nerve
Fibula
C
Peroneus longus tendon
Peroneus brevis
Flexor hallucis longus
D
Sural nerve
Short saphenous vein

Fig. 42.2 Cross-sectional schematic displaying the intervals for commonly utilized approached to pilon fractures. A, anteromedial; B, anterolateral; C, posterolateral fibula; D, posterolateral tibia, E, posteromedial tibia; F, medial tibia. (Adapted from Howard JK, Agel J, Barei DP, Benirschke SK, Nork SE. A prospective study evaluating incision placement and wound healing for tibial plafond fractures. J Orthop Trauma 2008;22:299–305.)

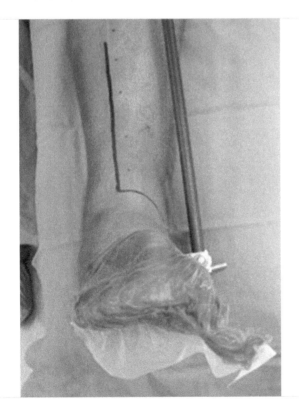

Fig. 42.3 This image depicts the markings for making an incision for anteromedial approach. Note the external fixator was left in place due to significant anterior joint comminution in this case.

5. Posterolateral:

    a. Uses the interval between the peroneal tendons and the flexor hallucis longus.

    b. Facilitates exposure of the fibula and the posterior malleolus for buttress plate application.

6. Direct medial:

    a. Between the tibialis anterior and posterior tendons along the medial face of the tibia.

    b. Less commonly used due to soft-tissue concerns.

    c. It can be used for minimally invasive plating of extra-articular fractures.

D. Fixation techniques

1. Several strategies can be used to achieve this; however, two principles are frequently used for C-type fractures:

    a. Convert a C-type to a B-type fracture:

        i. This involves fixation of a specific fragment (medial malleolus, Chaput's, or Volkmann's) to the intact diaphysis.

        ii. Build back to the intact segment.

        iii. Most useful for fractures with little or no metaphyseal comminution.

    b. Convert a C-type to an A-type fracture:

        i. Anatomically reduce all joint fragments together before fixing them.

        ii. This strategy can be employed when there is significant metaphyseal comminution with or without articular comminution.

        iii. Most common fixation constructs include an anterolateral plate with a component of medial fixation (screws or plate fixation; ▶ Fig. 42.4a, b).

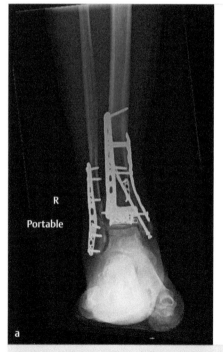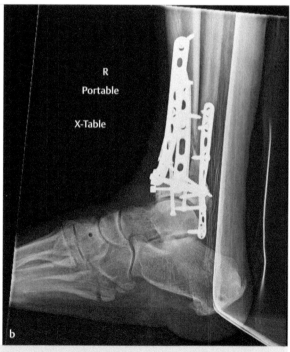

Fig. 42.4 (a, b) Fixation strategy for C-type pilon including an anterolateral plate, a minifragment rim plate, medial plate + screw fixation, and plating of the fibula.

2. External fixators can be kept on for 6 weeks following fixation to neutralize deforming forces, help maintain length, and protect the articular reduction in the following circumstances:

    a. Severely comminuted fractures.

    b. Severe soft-tissue injury.

    c. Patients with osteopenia.

3. Definitive external fixation with a ring fixator, with or without limited internal fixation, might be considered for open pilon fractures, compartment syndrome, or patients with poor healing potential due to high risk of soft-tissue complications.

E. Complications

1. Infection rate is approximately 5 to 15% for closed fractures.

2. Wound complication/dehiscence is relatively common and seen in up to 30% of patients. Often these can be treated with simple dressing changes but occasionally require return to the operating room for debridement.

3. Post-traumatic arthritis is common, but patients may not require further surgery for several years.

    a. Conservative treatment options include bracing, nonsteroidal anti-inflammatory medication, acetaminophen, and cortisone injection.

    b. Reconstructive options for symptomatic post-traumatic arthritis that has failed conservative measures include fusion (most common), arthroplasty (rarely performed), and amputation in severe cases.

F. Rehabilitation

1. Patients are placed in a splint for 2 to 3 weeks for soft-tissue rest. Sutures are removed at this time.

2. Patients are kept non–weight bearing for 8 to 12 weeks and then progressed to full weight bearing.

3. Gentle range of motion exercises of the ankle can be started once the wound has healed.

G. Outcomes

1. Open fractures lead to higher complication rates and worse outcomes.

2. Staged management of most pilon fractures with meticulous soft-tissue management is vital in improving outcomes.

3. Nonoperative management with displaced intra-articular fractures lead to poor outcomes

4. Quality of reduction and ankle range of motion correlate with quality of life (QOL) and Olerud–Molander ankle score.

III. Special Considerations for Pediatric Patients

A. Pediatric pilon fractures are rare. They need to be distinguished from triplane fractures.

B. The requirement of greater than 5 mm of displacement distinguishes pediatric pilon fractures from undisplaced triplane fractures.

C. Growth plate disturbances should be anticipated.

D. ORIF is advocated in the adolescent population.

IV. Special Considerations for Elderly Patients

A. Can occur due to low energy.

B. Be cognizant of the level of impaction that can occur in this patient population and the need for allograft augmentation.

C. Consider leaving external fixation in place for 4 to 6 weeks postfixation if the patient has significant comminution and/or injury to the anterior aspect of the plafond that is causing subluxation of the talus anteriorly on the sagittal view.

Summary

Pilon fractures are complex fractures associated with significant high-energy soft tissue injuries. Optimal management requires thoughtful preoperative planning and careful management of soft tissues. Despite this, there is still a high risk for complications. Even with optimal care, outcomes can be poor with regards to function and pain.

Suggested Readings

Cole PA, Mehrle RK, Bhandari M, Zlowodzki M. The pilon map: fracture lines and comminution zones in OTA/AO type 43C3 pilon fractures. J Orthop Trauma 2013;27(7):e152–e156

De-Las-Heras-Romero J, Lledo-Alvarez AM, Lizaur-Utrilla A, Lopez-Prats FA. Quality of life and prognostic factors after intra-articular tibial pilon fracture. Injury 2017;48(6):1258–1263

Duckworth AD, Jefferies JG, Clement ND, White TO. Type C tibial pilon fractures: short- and long-term outcome following operative intervention. Bone Joint J 2016;98-B(8):1106–1111

Eastman JG, Firoozabadi R, Benirschke SK, Barei DP, Dunbar RP. Entrapped posteromedial structures in pilon fractures. J Orthop Trauma 2014;28(9):528–533

Gardner MJ, Mehta S, Barei DP, Nork SE. Treatment protocol for open AO/OTA type C3 pilon fractures with segmental bone loss. J Orthop Trauma 2008;22(7):451–457

Rüedi TP, Allogower M. Fractures of the lower end of the tibia into the ankle joint. Injury 1969;1(2):92–99

Sirkin M, Sanders R, DiPasquale T, Herscovici D Jr. A staged protocol for soft tissue management in the treatment of complex pilon fractures. J Orthop Trauma 1999;13(2):78–84

White TO, Guy P, Cooke CJ, et al. The results of early primary open reduction and internal fixation for treatment of OTA 43.C-type tibial pilon fractures: a cohort study. J Orthop Trauma 2010;24(12):757–763

43 Ankle Fractures and Dislocations

Michael T. Archdeacon and Adam P. Schumaier

Introduction

Ankle fractures and fracture dislocations are the most frequent intra-articular fracture of the weight-bearing joints. Approximately 70% of ankle fractures are unimalleolar, 20% bimalleolar, and 10% trimalleolar (▶ **Video 43.1**).

Keywords: ankle, plafond, mortise, syndesmosis, malleolus, tibia, fibula, dislocation, fracture

I. Preoperative

A. History and physical examination

1. Mechanism of injury (typically rotational or abduction/adduction), ability to bear weight following injury, location(s) of pain, and prior injuries to ankle.

2. Comorbid conditions are particularly relevant including diabetes mellitus, peripheral vascular disease, and preoperative ambulatory status.

3. Inspection—look for swelling, blistering, and abrasions. The soft-tissue envelope around the ankle can be tenuous, so definitive fixation may be delayed to allow soft-tissue recovery.

4. Palpation: entire length of the tibia, fibula, and foot should be palpated for tenderness. Pain over the proximal fibula may suggest Maisonneuve's fracture, a proximal third fibular fracture with an associated syndesmotic injury, and medial malleolus fracture or deep deltoid ligament rupture.

5. Vascular examination: posterior tibial artery (posterior to the medial malleolus) and dorsalis pedis artery (lateral to the extensor hallucis longus tendon).

6. Neurologic examination:

    a. Typically evaluate dorsal foot (superficial peroneal), plantar foot (tibial), and first web space (deep peroneal) sensation.

    b. Motor function is difficult to evaluate in a fracture situation, but assessing toe flexion and extension is usually possible.

B. Anatomy (▶ **Fig. 43.1**)

1. Osteology:

    a. Fibula—slightly posterior to the tibia at the ankle; forms the lateral malleolus.

    b. Tibia—forms the medial and posterior malleoli:

        i. Medial malleolus has an anterior and posterior colliculus with an intercollicular groove, where the deltoid ligament attaches.

        ii. Incisura: notch in distal tibia where the fibula rests. The notch is formed by anterior (Chaput's) and posterior (Volkmann's) tubercles, which serve as attachment sites for the anterior and posterior inferior tibiofibular ligaments.

        iii. Plafond—distal articular surface of tibia. Plafond and malleoli form the ankle mortise with the talus.

    c. Talus—wider anteriorly than posteriorly. The dome is mostly covered with articular cartilage and is housed in the ankle mortise. It is composed of dense bone, which is generally not injured in ankle fractures.

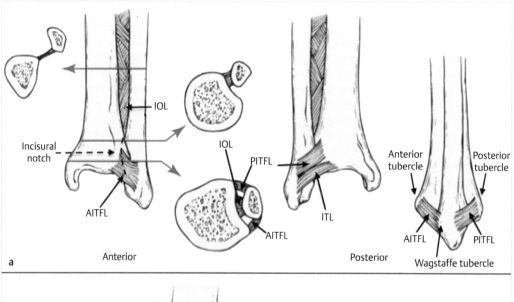

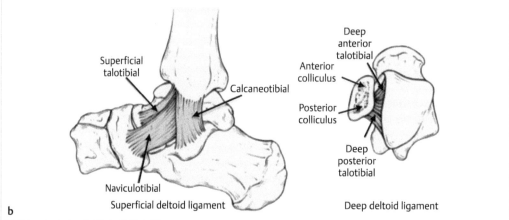

Fig. 43.1 Multiple views illustrating the **(a)** syndesmotic and **(b)** deltoid ligaments of the ankle joint. (Adapted from Browner BD, Jupiter JB, Levine AM, et al. Skeletal Trauma. 4th ed. Philadelphia, PA: Saunders; 2009:2516–2517).

2. Ligaments (▶ **Fig. 43.1**):

    a. Syndesmosis—composed of four ligaments between the distal tibia and fibula, which allow small amounts of motion. Syndesmotic injury is known as a "high ankle sprain":

        i. Anteroinferior tibiofibular ligament (AITFL):

- Attaches to the anterior (Chaput's) tubercle on the anterolateral tibia and Wagstaffe's tubercle on the anterior fibula.
- Weaker than the posteroinferior tibiofibular ligament (PITFL) and ruptures more frequently than avulses.

        ii. PITFL:

- Attaches to posterior (Volkmann's) tubercle on posterolateral tibia.
- Stronger than the AITFL and avulses more frequently than ruptures.

        iii. Transverse tibiofibular ligament/inferior transverse ligament (TTFL/ITL). Just inferior to PITFL.

        iv. Interosseous ligament (IOL). Located between AITFL and PITFL, continuous with the interosseous membrane proximally.

    b. Medial collateral ligament (MCL or deltoid ligament)—important restraint to external rotation:

        i. The superficial component connects the anterior colliculus of the medial malleolus with the navicular, talus, and calcaneus.

        ii. The deep component is mostly transverse and practically intra-articular, and connects the posterior colliculus of the medial malleolus to the talus. It is the strongest component and primary stabilizer, and can avulse the medial malleolus before tearing.

    c. Lateral collateral ligament—all the components attach to the lateral malleolus:

        i. Anterior talofibular ligament (ATFL):

- Primary inversion restraint during plantar flexion.
- Most commonly injured ligament in low ankle sprains.

        ii. Posterior talofibular ligament (PTFL).

        iii. Calcaneofibular ligament—primary inversion restraint during dorsiflexion.

C. Imaging

  1. Indications to obtain plain radiographs—history of frank dislocation, inability to bear weight following the injury, palpable tenderness of either malleolus.

    a. Anteroposterior (AP), lateral, and mortise views are required:

        i. Mortise view—acquired by internally rotating the leg and foot 15 to 20 degrees until malleoli are equidistant from the image detector; it improves visualization of the joint space.

        ii. External rotation and gravity stress views assess integrity of the deltoid ligament.

- External rotation stress view—the mortise view taken while the foot is manually rotated externally (▶ Fig. 43.2).
- Gravity stress view—this is an AP view taken with the patient in the lateral decubitus position, with the medial malleolus pointing upward, and without ankle support.

    b. Normal measurements—medial clear space (< 5 mm), lateral clear space (< 5 mm), tibiotalar clear space (< 5 mm), and tibiofibular overlap (> 10 mm; ▶ Fig. 43.3).

  2. CT may be used for evaluating syndesmotic injuries, loose bodies, and for preoperative planning of complex injury patterns such as trimalleolar and severe fracture dislocations.

  3. MRI may be useful for soft-tissue evaluation if the stress examination is equivocal.

D. Classification

  1. Ankle fractures are typically described based on number of malleoli involved (unimalleolar, bimalleolar, trimalleolar).

  2. Classifications commonly encountered in the literature: Lauge–Hansen and Danis–Weber.

    a. Lauge–Hansen: describes a pattern of injury progression based on which structures are under tension (▶ Fig. 43.4). Supination initially places lateral structures under tension, and pronation initially places medial structures under tension. There are two terms for each pattern.

        i. First term—position of ankle during injury.

        ii. Second term—direction of force applied to ankle:

- Supination-external rotation (SER): ATFL disruption [1] → oblique fibula fracture [2] → PTFL rupture or posterior malleolus avulsion [3] → medial malleolus transverse fracture or deltoid disruption [4].
- Supination-adduction (SA)—talofibular sprain or distal fibula avulsion [1] → vertical medial malleolus fracture [2].
- Pronation-abduction (PA): medial malleolus avulsion fracture or deltoid disruption [1] → ATFL disruption [2] → transverse or comminuted fibula fracture [3].
- Pronation-external rotation (PER)—medial malleolus transverse fracture or deltoid disruption [1] → ATFL disruption [2] → high oblique fibula fracture [3] → PTFL rupture or posterior malleolus avulsion [4].

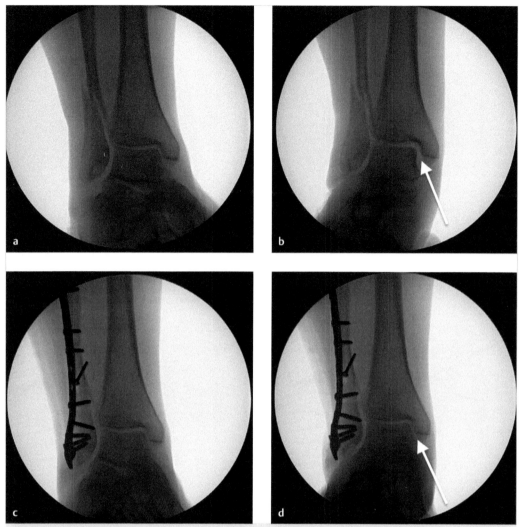

Fig. 43.2 Four fluoroscopic images that demonstrate the utilization of external rotation stress views for assessing ankle stability. **(a)** Fluoroscopic mortise view demonstrating an oblique fibular fracture with normal medial clear space. **(b)** External rotation stress view demonstrates subtle medial clear space widening, suggesting an unstable ankle or a "bimalleolar equivalent." **(c)** Fluoroscopic mortise view following stabilization of the fibular fracture with plate and screws. **(d)** External rotation stress view demonstrating resolution of the clear space widening.

    b. Danis–Weber—based on the level of fibula fracture (▶Fig. **43.4**):

        i. Type A occurs distal to the plafond, and the syndesmosis is usually stable.

       ii. Type B occurs at the plafond, and syndesmotic stability cannot be predicted.

      iii. Type C occurs proximal to the plafond, and the syndesmosis is usually unstable.

II. Treatment

A. Initial management (Chapter 3, Closed Fracture Management/Casting)

    1. Fracture dislocations should be reduced and splinted.

       a. Reduction is eased by applying distraction and reversing the mechanism of injury, focusing on talar reduction within the mortise.

       b. The following technique is useful for most fracture dislocations:

          i. Suspend the leg by holding the first and second toes, allowing gravity to reduce the fracture.

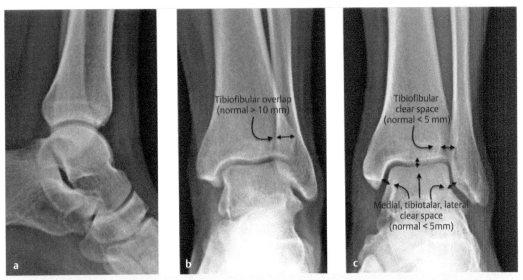

Fig. 43.3 (a–c) Lateral anteroposterior, and mortise views of a normal ankle. Black arrows illustrate the normal values for tibiofibular overlap and clear spaces.

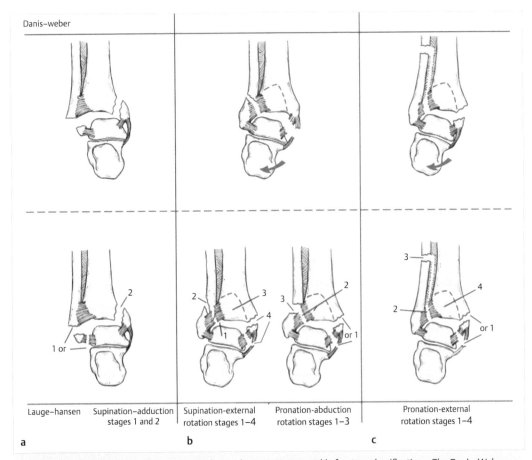

Fig. 43.4 (a–c) Comparison of the Danis–Weber and Lauge–Hansen ankle fracture classifications. The Danis–Weber system is based on the level of the fibular fracture, while the Lauge–Hansen system is based on injury sequences. (Adapted from Browner BD, Jupiter JB, Levine AM, et al. Skeletal Trauma. 4th ed. Philadelphia, PA: Saunders; 2009:2532).

      ii. Slightly flex knee to relax gastrocnemius.

      iii. Place the patient's foot against your chest with ankle in neutral, allowing the peroneal tendons and soft tissues to reduce fibula and talus; a lateral to medial force on the distal fibula may facilitate reduction of a laterally subluxed talus.

      iv. With the patient's foot against your chest, ankle in neutral, and knee in slight flexion, mold a short leg splint with extra padding on bony prominences.

  2. Open fractures require tetanus prophylaxis, antibiotics, and debridement.

B. Definitive management

  1. Nonoperative injuries:

    a. Minimally displaced (<3 mm) unimalleolar fractures can be treated with a short leg walking cast or boot. Long leg casts can be used if concerned about rotational stability.

      i. Stability should be assessed by measuring the medial clear space (stable < 4 mm, indeterminate 4–5 mm, and unstable > 5 mm). External rotation and gravity stress views can assess deltoid ligament integrity (▶ **Fig. 43.2**).

  2. Operative injuries:

    a. Unimalleolar fractures with greater than 3 mm displacement.

    b. Bimalleolar fractures, bimalleolar fracture equivalents, and trimalleolar fractures.

      i. Bimalleolar fractures and lateral malleolar fractures with disruption of the deltoid are considered equivalent. Medial tenderness or medial clear space widening greater than 5 mm suggest deltoid disruption; stress views can assess integrity of deltoid ligament.

    c. Posterior malleolar fractures:

      i. Primarily PITFL avulsions that frequently reduce following fixation of the lateral malleolus.

      ii. Fixation is recommended when there is greater than 25% involvement of the articular surface.

      iii. Some advocate for posterior malleolar fixation regardless of size if the syndesmosis is unstable.

    d. Syndesmotic injuries:

      i. Usually reduces following reduction of medial and/or lateral malleolus.

      ii. Signs of syndesmotic disruption and indications for fixation:

        • Irreparable medial structures.

        • Persistent medial or lateral clear space widening greater than 5 mm (▶ **Fig. 43.5**).

        • Intraoperative gross instability demonstrated via fibular traction (Cotton's test) or gravity stress view after fibular fixation (described above). Abnormal tibiofibular clear space is more than 5 mm and abnormal tibiofibular overlap is less than 10 mm.

C. Surgical approaches (▶ **Fig. 43.6a–d**)

  1. Anterior (▶ **Fig. 43.6a**) incision directly over anterior distal tibia, used for fixing posterior malleolar fractures with an anterior to posterior screw. Superficial peroneal nerve and dorsalis pedis artery: anterior to distal tibia.

  2. Lateral (▶ **Fig. 43.6b**) incision directly over lateral malleolus and extended proximally just posterior to the fibula. Dissect the peroneal fascia and retract the peroneal tendons and muscles posteriorly. Superficial peroneal nerve: position varies but is commonly found just anterior to the distal fibula approximately 7 cm proximal to tip of the distal fibula.

  3. Anteromedial (▶ **Fig. 43.6c**)—anterior and slightly curved incision around the medial malleolus:

    a. Saphenous vein and nerve—anterior to the medial malleolus.

    b. Posterior tibial tendon—first structure posterior to the medial malleolus.

  4. Posterolateral (▶ **Fig. 43.6d**) incision slightly lateral to Achilles tendon, used for direct access to posterior malleolar fractures.

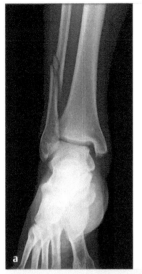
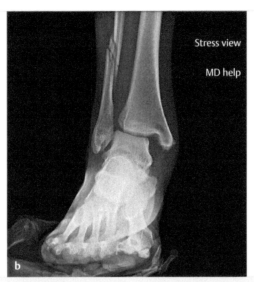
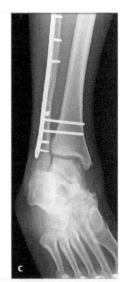

Fig. 43.5 Three X-rays illustrating a typical Weber C fibular fracture with syndesmotic and deltoid disruption. **(a)** Comminuted oblique fibular fracture. **(b)** External rotation stress view demonstrates significant tibiofibular and medial clear space widening. **(c)** Postoperative image demonstrating fixation with a lateral plate and two trans-syndesmotic screws with fixation across four cortices.

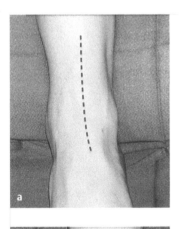
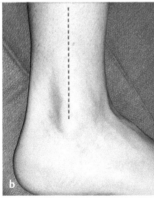
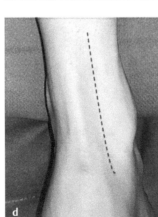

Fig. 43.6 Examples of surgical incisions for the **(a)** anterior, **(b)** lateral, **(c)** medial, and **(d)** posterolateral approaches to the ankle.

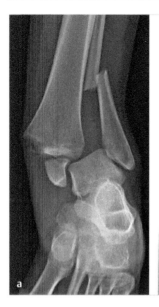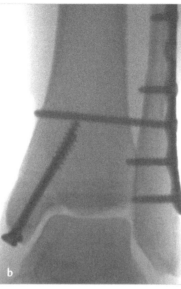

Fig. 43.7 Ankle fracture dislocation (a) with postoperative fluoroscopy (b). The medial malleolus was reduced with two lag screws perpendicular to the fracture, and the fibula was reduced with a one-third tubular plate. A trans-syndesmotic screw was placed through the fibular plate and bicortically through the fibula and the tibia.

D. Fixation techniques

1. Lateral malleolus should be fixed first in order to restore lateral length.

    a. Options for fixation:

        i. Lag screw perpendicular to the fracture and lateral neutralization (one-third tubular) plate.

        ii. Lateral buttress plate with or without a lag screw (▶ **Fig. 43.7**).

        iii. Posterior antiglide plate.

    b. If fibula fracture does not reduce, the medial malleolar fragment or deltoid ligament is likely blocking reduction and the medial joint should be explored.

2. Medial malleolus—usually repaired using one or two lag screws perpendicular to the fracture; however, tension band wiring or buttress plating may be useful for comminuted fractures (▶ **Fig. 43.7**). Disrupted deltoid ligaments do not need to be repaired because casting or bracing provides sufficient stability for healing.

3. Posterior malleolus—usually reduced with a lag screw placed either AP or posteroanterior; buttress plates may be used via posterolateral approach for large fracture fragments.

4. Syndesmosis—one or two screws (not in lag mode) should be placed through the fibula and tibia a few centimeters proximal to the plafond, directed 15 to 30 degrees anteriorly to remain perpendicular to the joint line.

5. Diabetic neuropathic patients—consider the "comb" technique with multiple screws across four cortices due to high failure rate with the standard technique (▶ **Fig. 43.8**).

E. Complications

1. Decreased range of motion, particularly dorsiflexion: 10% of patients have more than 10-degree loss.

2. Post-traumatic arthritis—evidence in up to 14% of patients; more common in women.

3. Painful hardware (up to 30%) and symptomatic peroneal tendonitis (~5%).

4. Malunion and nonunion are rare, but the following are risk factors: diabetes, peripheral vascular disease, elderly, and localized skin disease (venous ulcers).

5. Diabetic complications:

    a. Peripheral neuropathy and hemoglobin A1C ≥ 8% are independently associated with surgical site infection.

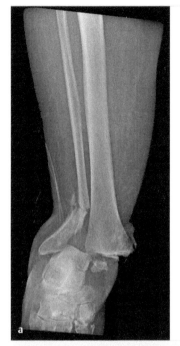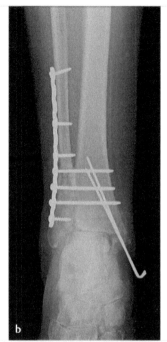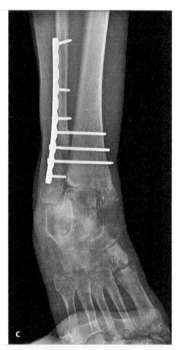

Fig. 43.8 Three ankle X-rays of a diabetic, neuropathic patient who sustained a fracture-dislocation.
(a) Comminuted fibular and medial malleolar fractures with syndesmotic disruption and tibiotalar dislocation.
(b) Postoperative X-ray demonstrates the "comb" technique, where multiple trans-syndesmotic screws are placed across four cortices. **(c)** The medial malleolar fracture was treated with percutaneous wires, which were removed at 6 weeks.

    b. Complicated diabetics (neuropathy, peripheral arterial disease, renal disease):
       i. Greater than seven times increased risk of infection compared with nondiabetic, nonneuropathic patients.
      ii. Greater than threefold risk of noninfectious complications (malunion, nonunion, Charcot's arthropathy) and five times more likely to require revision or arthrodesis.

F. Rehabilitation

1. Typically a posterior/sugar tong splint is applied in the OR transitioning to a removable boot once wounds have healed.

2. Nonoperative distal fibula fractures can be allowed to bear weight immediately in most circumstances.

3. Full weight bearing can begin immediately in uncomplicated, simple unimalleolar fractures with stable internal fixation.

4. Weight bearing was historically restricted for 4 to 6 weeks in patients with bimalleolar fractures; however, patients with bimalleolar fractures without syndesmotic injury may be allowed to fully bear weight as early as 2 weeks from injury.

5. Trimalleolar fractures, associated ankle dislocations, and syndesmosis injuries may require prolonged non–weight bearing up to 4 to 8 weeks. Highly comminuted fractures, complex medical patients (diabetes, peripheral neuropathy, etc.), and fractures with tenuous fixation may require more prolonged weight-bearing restrictions. It is not uncommon for diabetic patients to remain non–weight bearing for 16 weeks.

6. Rehabilitation with range of motion and gentle strengthening exercises can begin once wounds have healed and may last for several months before return to preinjury activities.

G. Outcomes

1. Excellent functional outcome for most patients with eventual full return to normal activity.

2. Poor prognostic signs include osteochondral injury, significant articular injury, residual talar displacement, late syndesmotic instability, and trimalleolar involvement.

III. Special Considerations for the Elderly

Elderly patients are more likely to suffer low-energy injuries, are usually lower demand, and may not be ideal surgical candidates due to poor skin quality, osteoporotic bone, or comorbid medical conditions. Close contact casting may be an acceptable alternative for some patients, but external fixation remains a viable option to reduce the risks of a formal surgical reconstruction.

Summary

Ankle fracture dislocations frequently require operative treatment. Initial assessment involves a history and physical to assess stability of the joint. Broadly, ankle stability depends on the integrity of 1) medial structures, 2) lateral structures, and 3) syndesmotic ligaments. Injury to more than one of these structures typically requires surgery. Surgical techniques usually involve a combination of plates and screws utilizing soft-tissue friendly approaches. Rehabilitation protocols vary based on the patient, but weight-bearing begins within 2–10 weeks depending on patient and injury specific factors. Functional gains can occur for more than a year post injury. The goal is to restore pre-injury levels of function, but post-traumatic changes can occur, particularly if articular congruency or ankle stability are not restored.

Suggested Readings

Alton TB, Harnden E, Hagen J, Firoozabadi R. Single provider reduction and splinting of displaced ankle fractures: a modification of Quigley's classic technique. J Orthop Trauma 2015;29(4):e166–e171

Brown OL, Dirschl DR, Obremskey WT. Incidence of hardware-related pain and its effect on functional outcomes after open reduction and internal fixation of ankle fractures. J Orthop Trauma 2001;15(4):271–274

Lauge-Hansen N. Fractures of the ankle. II. Combined experimental-surgical and experimental-roentgenologic investigations. Arch Surg 1950;60(5):957–985

Michelson JD. Fractures about the ankle. J Bone Joint Surg Am 1995;77(1):142–152

Smeeing DP, Houwert RM, Briet JP, et al. Weight-bearing and mobilization in the postoperative care of ankle fractures: a systematic review and meta-analysis of randomized controlled trials and cohort studies. PLoS One 2015;10(2):e0118320

Willett K, Keene DJ, Mistry D, et al. Ankle Injury Management (AIM) Trial Collaborators. Close contact casting vs surgery for initial treatment of unstable ankle fractures in older adults: a randomized clinical trial. JAMA 2016;316(14):1455–1463

44 Achilles Tendon Rupture

Jannat M. Khan, D. Landry Jarvis, Alejandro Marquez-Lara, and Eben A. Carroll

Introduction

Achilles tendon ruptures represent a spectrum of acute and chronic injuries. While acute injuries are more often associated with sports activity, chronic ruptures occur in the setting of chronic tendinopathy. Although the cause of Achilles tendinopathy is likely multifactorial, it has been associated with repetitive stress, such as running, and chronic metabolic conditions affecting the extracellular matrix of the Achilles tendon. Understanding the differences between these two conditions is essential to develop an appropriate treatment strategy and optimize patient outcomes (▶ **Video 44.1**).

Keywords: Achilles tendon rupture, diagnostic imaging, open repair, minimally invasive repair, rehabilitation

I. Preoperative

A. History and physical examination

1. Peak incidence in the third to fifth decade of life.

2. Higher incidence among males (5:1) with positive correlation of Achilles tendon pathology among obese, and elderly population (> 60 years old).

3. Common among nonathletes participating in intermittent high-performance activity ("Weekend Warrior").

4. At the time of injury, the patient may feel a snap sensation, hear an audible pop, and have instant pain that gradually dissipates.

5. Visible limp with difficulty with plantar flexion and weight bearing.

6. Etiology not clear but can be divided into degenerative theory or traumatic mechanical theory.

7. Risk of degenerative injury—recent oral or intrasubstance fluoroquinolones and corticosteroids, long-standing paratendinitis, or recent Achilles surgery.

   a. Degeneration postulated to occur due to impaired blood flow to the tendon, which may lead to hypoxia and altered metabolism.

   b. Rupture can occur without application of excessive loads.

8. Injury may be due to direct or indirect acute trauma:

   a. Direct—blow, laceration, or crush injury.

   b. Indirect—obliquely loaded at a short initial length with maximum muscle contraction when pushing off weight-bearing foot with knee in extension (most common), that is, lunging for a ball with a giving way sensation.

      i. Sharp unexpected dorsiflexion, that is, fall in hole.
      ii. Strong dorsiflexion force on a plantar-flexed ankle, that is, falling from a height.

9. Ecchymosis and edema.

10. Excessive dorsiflexion at rest.

11. Unable to stand on toes.

12. The American Academy of Orthopaedic Surgeons (AAOS) Clinical Practice Guidelines states that diagnosis made with two or more positive findings following examinations:

    a. Thompson's test (when compression of calf in prone position does not elicit passive plantar flexion): 96% sensitive (▶ **Fig. 44.1**).

    b. Decreased plantar flexion strength.

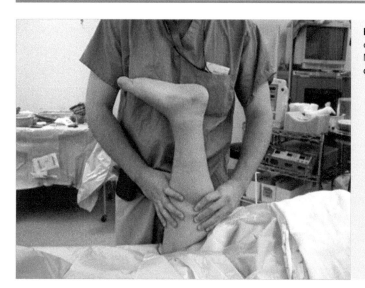

Fig. 44.1 Clinical picture demonstrating the Thompson test. Note the absence of dorsiflexion with compression of the calf muscle.

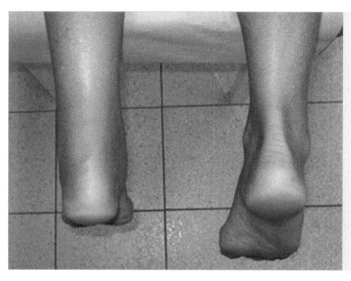

Fig. 44.2 Clinical photograph demonstrating Matles' positive for right leg. (Adapted from Wikimedia commons, public domain.)

    c.   Positive sulcus sign (palpable defect distal to insertion site).

    d.   Matles' test (increased passive ankle dorsiflexion at rest): 88% sensitive (▶ **Fig. 44.2**).

B.   Anatomy

    1.   Achilles tendon is the strongest and largest tendon in the human body.

    2.   Gastrocnemius–soleus complex (GSC):

        a.   Formed by conjoined tendon of the gastrocnemius and soleus muscles.

        b.   Integral in knee flexion, foot plantar flexion, and hindfoot inversion.

        c.   Tendon spans three different joints including the knee, tibiotalar, and subtalar joints.

        d.   Gastrocnemius arises from posterior femoral condyles: acts as an effective plantar flexor with knee in extension.

        e.   Soleus arises from the posterior aspect of the tibia, fibula, and interosseous membrane only traversing the ankle joint: acts as an effective plantar flexor with knee in flexion.

        f.   GSC inserts over the broad posterosuperior aspect of the calcaneal tuberosity.

3. Seventy-five percent of ruptures occur 2 to 6 cm proximal to the calcaneus.

    a. Tenuous vascular supply in this watershed area.

        i. Proximal—intramuscular arterial branches of posterior tibial artery.

        ii. Distal—interosseous arteriole branches from peroneal artery.

    b. High-peak stresses (70 MPa) experienced in this area. Most tendons experience stress below 30 MPa.

4. Extracellular matrix:

    a. Matrix metalloproteinase (MMP 1–3)—increase in MMP1 is associated with degradation of type I collagen and matrix remodeling.

    b. Transglutaminase (TG):

        i. Implicated in organogenesis, tissue repair, and tissue stabilization.

        ii. Decrease in TG associated with reparative tendon's capabilities.

C. Imaging

  1. X-ray:

    a. Helps assess Kager's triangle, which is the space between Achilles tendon, posterior tibia, and superior calcaneus (▶ Fig. 44.3). Irregular configuration in chronic ruptures.

  2. Ultrasound:

    a. Help differentiate partial and complete tears.

    b. Hypoechoic signal proximal to insertion of Achilles tendon.

    c. Greater than 5 mm gap noted between tendon edges indicates surgical intervention.

    d. Not recommended if suspicion of partial tendon tear (only 50% sensitive).

  3. MRI:

    a. Discontinuous Achilles tendon due to tear denoted by hypointense signal proximal to insertion in T1, hyperintense signal in T2 MRI.

    b. Disruption of signal in tendon substance on T1.

    c. Generalized high signal on T2 (▶ Fig. 44.4a, b).

    d. Recommended to reserve use for the following patient populations:

        i. Inconclusive clinical examination findings.

        ii. Subacute or chronic tears occurring more than 4 weeks prior to presentation.

        iii. Prior tears with concern for scar tissue in order to develop an appropriate surgical plan.

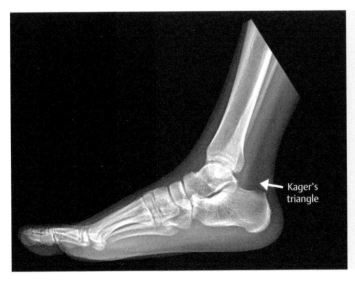

Fig. 44.3 Lateral plain film radiograph demonstrating normal-appearing space between the Achilles tendon, posterior tibia, and superior calcaneus (Kager's triangle).

Kager's triangle

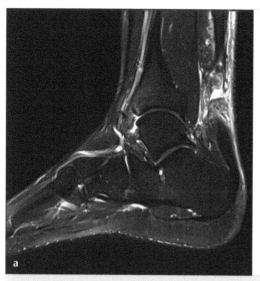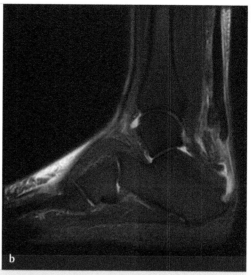

Fig. 44.4 (a) Sagittal cut of T2 MRI demonstrating acute achilles tendon rupture at the watershed area. **(b)** Sagittal cut T2 MRI demonstrating acute achilles tendon rupture at the calcaneus insertion.

Table 44.1 Kuwada's classification of Achilles tendon ruptures

Type	Injury	Treatment
I	Partial tear (< 50%)	Nonoperative treatment
II	Complete rupture with <3 cm tendinous gap	End-to-end anastomosis
III	Complete rupture with 3–6 cm tendinous gap	Tendon (flexor hallucis longus) flap with or without synthetic graft augmentation, V-Y advancement, a Bosworth turndown, tendon transfer
IV	Complete rupture with >6 cm tendinous gap	Gastrocnemius recession with tendon or synthetic graft

D. Classification
  1. Kawada classification (▶ **Table 44.1**):
    a. Derived from direct visualization of Achilles tendon; unclear if correlates with MRI.
    b. Developed to help guide treatment based on the completeness of the tear and the amount of gapping.

II. Treatment

A. Initial management
  1. The patient should be placed in a plantar-flexed splint or cast.
  2. Nonweight bearing (NWB).
B. Definitive management
  1. Nonoperative—acceptable functional results and lower complication rates than operative treatment; should be considered in patients with increased surgical risk factors and moderate to low physical activity demands.
    a. Functional rehabilitation:
      i. Conversion to functional bracing at 2 weeks.
      ii. Increased weight bearing and strengthening exercises.
      iii. Similar rerupture rate compared to operative results.

b. Strict immobilization—immobilization for up to 8 weeks, then conversion to heel lifts with slow advancement of weight bearing is associated with loss of power, strength endurance, and higher rerupture rate (reserved for elderly, less active).

2. Operative:

a. Multiple meta-analyses demonstrate similar outcomes as nonoperative management with functional rehabilitation such as early range-of-motion protocols. However, the rerupture rate after surgical treatment (4%) may be lower compared to nonoperative treatment (10%).

b. Recent studies support possible improved functional outcomes, specifically early and reliable restoration of calf muscle strength, and earlier return to activity compared to nonoperative treatment. This may be beneficial for high-activity professionals such as athletes.

c. No decreased functional outcome with delay up to 30 days; important to delay until swelling improves.

d. No significant difference between open and percutaneous technique regarding plantar flexion strength and return to sports.

C. Surgical approach/fixation technique

1. Open repair:

a. Incision:

i. Midline longitudinal incision—increased pressure due to repaired tendon.

ii. Medial longitudinal incision—avoids sural nerve and lesser saphenous plexus.

b. Dissection (▶ **Fig. 44.5**):

i. Layered dissection through skin, crural fascia, and paratenon.

ii. Protect sural nerve.

iii. Locate and debride ruptured tendon ends.

iv. Avoid significant retraction to prevent skin complications.

c. Repair:

i. Direct—for gaps less than 3 cm after debridement:

• Nonabsorbable suture.

• Various acceptable stitch patterns: Krackow (▶ **Fig. 44.6**), modified Bunnel, modified Kessler, triple bundle.

• Approximate tendon ends with tension similar to contralateral side.

ii. Augmented repair/reconstruction:

• Types of augments—flexor hallucis longus (FHL), flexor digitorum longus (FDL), and peroneus brevis (PB).

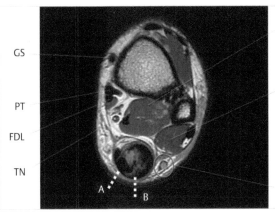

Fig. 44.5 Axial cut of T2 MRI depicting Achilles tendon tear. Surgical incision marked with dotted lines, posteromedial (A) and direct posterior (B) approaches. Note sural nerve (*red circle*) is lateral to Achilles tendon. (GS, greater saphenous vein; PT, posterior tibial tendon; FDL, flexor digitorum longus; TN, tibial nerve; FHL, flexor hallucis longus; PB, peroneus brevis; SN, sural nerve; LS, lesser saphenous.)

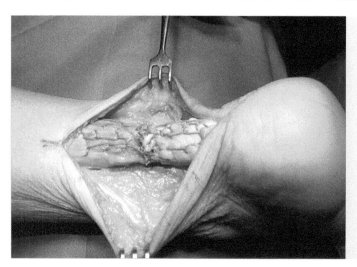

Fig. 44.6 Clinical photograph demonstrating Krackow's suture repair of an Achilles tendon rupture.

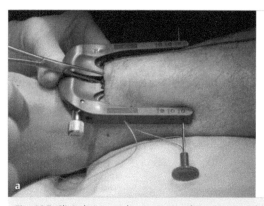
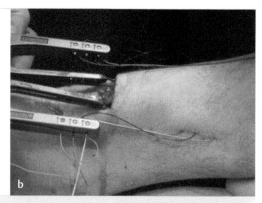

Fig. 44.7 Clinical pictures demonstrating the miniopen Achilles tendon repair utilizing the Achillon jig. (Reproduce with permission of Integra Lifesciences Corporation, USA.) **(a)** The jig is inserted with the central two branches beneath the paratenon and facilitates passing suture percutaneously. **(b)** The jig is then withdrawn leaving the sutures within the paratenon and traversing the midportion of the tendon. (Adapted from Carmont MR, Rossi R, Scheffler S, Mei-Dan O, Beaufils P. Percutaneous & Mini Invasive Achilles tendon repair. Sports Med Arthrosc Rehabil Ther Technol 2011;3:28.)

- FHL augmentation released from insertion through a medial arch incision. It is passed through a bone tunnel in the calcaneus near the tubercle and woven proximally through the achilles tendon.
- Sliding VY advancement of GSC.
- Medial and lateral fascial turndown flaps or plantaris weave.
- Acellular human dermal tissue matrix.
- Achilles tendon allograft for defects greater than 10 cm (case reports).

  d. Closure—layered closure to prevent adhesions.

2. Minimally invasive techniques:

  a. Significantly less wound complications and slight increase in sural nerve injuries.

  b. For ruptures between 2 and 8 cm proximal to the insertion.

  c. Cannot be used for chronic ruptures:

   i. Mini-open technique (▶ **Fig. 44.7a, b**):

   - Three-centimeter horizontal incision at the level of the tendon rupture.
   - Dissection to and debridement of the tendon ends.
   - Use of a percutaneous suture passing guide to tether and repair tendon ends.

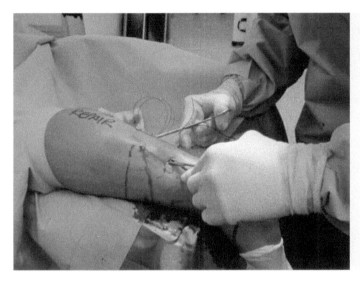

Fig. 44.8 Clinical picture demonstrating percutaneous Achilles tendon repair. (Adapted from Carmont MR, Rossi R, Scheffler S, Mei-Dan O, Beaufils P. Percutaneous & Mini Invasive Achilles tendon repair. Sports Med Arthrosc Rehabil Ther Technol 2011;3:28.)

    ii. Percutaneous technique (▸**Fig. 44.8**):
- No visualization of the tendon.
- Posteromedial and posterolateral stab incision.
- Percutaneous passage of suture.

D. Complications
1. Soft-tissue complications:
   a. Skin necrosis (up to 5% in open repair).
   b. Superficial infection: much greater in open repair.
   c. Deep infection (1–2%).
   d. Tendinous adhesions.
2. Rerupture (3%): compared to 9.8% with conservative management.
3. Sural nerve injury (3–9%).
4. Deep venous thrombosis (<1%).

E. Rehabilitation
1. Many different rehabilitation protocols with a recent shift toward accelerated programs with nonoperative treatment.
2. In general, most rehab protocols are as follows:
   a. Zero to 2 weeks—plantar-flexed immobilization and NWB—May be modified after operative fixation to full weight bearing (FWB).
   b. Two to 6 weeks—weight bearing as tolerated (WBAT) in heel lift with encouraged ankle range of motion (ROM) with no dorsiflexion past neutral—Early ankle mobilization with free plantar flexion encouraged after operative management.
   c. Six to 12 weeks—FWB in shoe with progressive dorsiflexion.
   d. Three months—begin jogging.
   e. Three to 6 months—return to sports.

F. Outcomes
1. Common outcome measures:
   a. Objective measures:
      i. Single heel rise test or heel-rise endurance test: measure ability to lift heel 2 cm off the ground or the number of repetitions until failure, respectively.
      ii. Ankle ROM.

b. Subjective measures:

    i. Clinician based: American Orthopaedic Foot and Ankle Society (AOFAS) Ankle-Hindfoot score.

    ii. Patient reported: Achilles Tendon Total Rupture Score.

- Validated 10-item questionnaire.
- A score of 0 suggests major limitations and symptoms.
- A score of 10 suggests no limitations or symptoms.

2. Expected outcomes:

a. Almost all patients will return to preinjury activity regardless of treatment option.

b. Return to sport:

    i. Around 80% will return to the same level of sport regardless of treatment.

    ii. Higher functioning athletes may benefit from surgery due to faster return to sport and lower rerupture rate compared to conservative management.

III. Special Considerations for Pediatric or Geriatric Patients

A. Pediatric patients

1. Commonly a tendon avulsion injury, not a defect within the tendon.

2. Optimal management has not been well established.

3. Nonoperative management generally favored with early rehabilitation to return patient to baseline activity.

4. Consider early operative repair in high-level adolescent athletes.

B. Geriatric patients

1. Management depends on clinical assessment of patient baseline physical activity, but further study is required to determine benefit of operative versus nonoperative management.

2. Generally managed nonoperatively with early rehabilitation protocol.

Summary

Achilles tendon ruptures are common injuries affecting active individuals that can result in significant disability. This increase may be related to a higher rate of sports activity in the general population and higher level of awareness for this type of injury. A prompt diagnosis is critical to determine appropriate management. This chapter describes pertinent physical examination findings validated to help diagnose these types of injuries as well as appropriate diagnostic imaging studies. Historically, Achilles tendon ruptures have been treated conservatively with nonoperative management. However select patients may benefit from operative management.

Suggested Readings

Claessen FM, de Vos RJ, Reijman M, Meuffels DE. Predictors of primary Achilles tendon ruptures. Sports Med 2014;44(9):1241–1259

Kuwada GT. Classification of tendo Achillis rupture with consideration of surgical repair techniques. J Foot Surg 1990;29(4):361–365

Lantto I, Heikkinen J, Flinkkila T, et al. A prospective randomized trial comparing surgical and nonsurgical treatments of acute Achilles tendon ruptures. Am J Sports Med 2016;44(9):2406–2414

Maffulli N, Via AG, Oliva F. Chronic Achilles tendon disorders: tendinopathy and chronic rupture. Clin Sports Med 2015;34(4):607–624

Maffulli N, Oliva F, Costa V, Del Buono A. The management of chronic rupture of the Achilles tendon: minimally invasive peroneus brevis tendon transfer. Bone Joint J 2015;97-B(3):353–357

Soroceanu A, Sidhwa F, Aarabi S, Kaufman A, Glazebrook M. Surgical versus nonsurgical treatment of acute Achilles tendon rupture: a meta-analysis of randomized trials. J Bone Joint Surg Am 2012;94(23):2136–2143

Uquillas CA, Guss MS, Ryan DJ, Jazrawi LM, Strauss EJ. Everything Achilles: knowledge update and current concepts in management: AAOS exhibit selection. J Bone Joint Surg Am 2015;97(14):1187–1195

45 Calcaneus Fractures

Christiaan N. Mamczak and Kevin C. Anderson

Keywords: calcaneus, displaced Intra-articular calcaneal fracture (DIACF), Essex-Lopresti fracture, Sander's Classification, Bohler's angle, Broden's view, axial Harris view, extensile lateral approach (ELA), sinus tarsi (ST) approach, subtalar fusion

I. Preoperative

A. History and physical examination

   1. Pain:

      a. Moderate to severe hindfoot pain is common.

      b. Rule out associated ankle injuries (i.e., peroneal tendon subluxation, fractures).

      c. Head-to-toe clinical examination is necessary to diagnosis other associated injuries.

   2. Swelling:

      a. Fracture swelling is expected and greatest within the first 72 hours.

         i. Acute foot compartment syndrome can occur (10%) with missed diagnosis resulting in lesser toe clawing; fasciotomies are controversial (refer to Chapter 13, Compartment Syndrome, for additional information).

      b. Resolution of swelling can dictate timing and surgical approach.

   3. Ecchymosis:

      a. Typically localized at the heel and into the midfoot arch.

   4. Skin at risk:

      a. Fracture blisters (▶ **Fig. 45.1**):

         i. Occur within 24 to 72 hours; blood-filled (vs. serous) blisters indicate deeper intradermal injury.

      b. Skin tenting:

         i. Most concerning in posterior tuberosity avulsion or certain tongue-type fractures. Emergent surgical reduction with fixation is critical to prevent the difficult sequelae of full-thickness heel skin necrosis.

         ii. Lateral wall blowout can result in inside-out skin pressure; may require external fixation.

      c. Open traumatic wounds—typically on the medial side with transverse/oblique orientation.

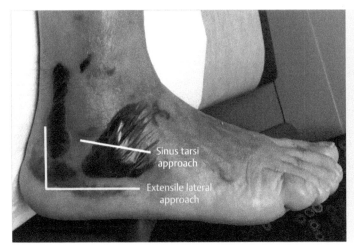

Fig. 45.1 Clinical example of blood-filled fracture blisters and ecchymosis. Surgical approach via the extensile lateral or sinus tarsi methods should be delayed in this patient due to the inherent risks of infection and wound complications.

5. Neurovascular injury:

    a. Sural nerve paresthesias occur secondary to lateral wall blowout.

    b. Medial more often than lateral plantar nerve paresthesias result from compartment syndrome, open medial wounds, or entrapment within the fracture.

    c. Vascular arterial transection or injury is rare.

6. Associated injuries:
Complete head-to-toe physical examination is warranted with high-energy injuries.

    a. Spine injuries are common with falls from a height (X-rays ± CT).

    b. Ipsilateral lower extremity or other appendicular injuries do occur.

B. Epidemiology and fracture anatomy

    1. The os calcis is the most commonly fractured tarsal bone.

        a. Extra-/intra-articular patterns depend upon the mechanism of injury and energy.

        b. Open fractures occur in up to 17% of patients, often with transverse or oblique medial wounds.

        c. Bilateral calcaneal fractures occur in 5 to 10% of patients.

        d. Associated injuries are common: axial spine (~10%) and lower extremities (~26%).

    2. Mechanism of injury and fracture lines:

        a. Axial loading injury:

            i. Falls from a height often lead to displaced intra-articular calcaneal fractures (DIACFs) as the lateral talar process is driven into the calcaneus to create primary and secondary fracture lines.

                • Have a high clinical suspicion for associated injuries (spine and lower extremities).

                • Thorough patient secondary survey examination is warranted.

                • **Primary fracture line** divides the posterior facet due to oblique shear forces from anterolateral (critical angle) to posteromedial (▶ **Fig. 45.2**).

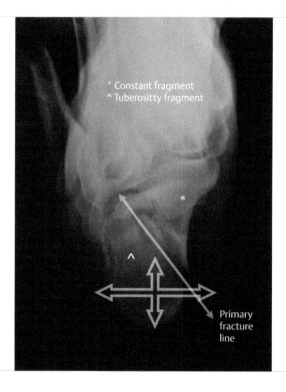

Fig. 45.2 Axial Harris radiograph demonstrates the oblique primary fracture line separating the anteromedial sustentacular fragment (*) from the posterior tuberosity (^) leading to the customary shortening and widening of the heel.

- Constant fragment (anteromedial)—includes the sustentaculum tali and typically remains anatomic ("constant") due to ligamentotaxis; may include the middle and anterior facets in less comminuted patterns.
- Posterolateral fragment—includes a variable portion of the posterior facet and the posterior tuberosity, comminution includes lateral wall.
- **Secondary fracture lines**—variable and occur with increasing energy.
  - Tongue-type—sagittal transverse line ± intra-articular involvement (▶Fig. 45.3).
  - Joint depression—variable size/number of posterior facet fragments.
  - Lateral wall blowout—occurs with increasing posterior facet depression and creates subfibular impingement due to increased heel width.

ii. Motor vehicle accidents result from pedal or floorboard impaction into the plantar foot surface with variable fracture patterns (as described earlier).

b. Rotational injury:

i. Usually a variety of extra-articular fracture patterns affecting the anterior process and calcaneocuboid joint or the sustentaculum.

c. Posterior tuberosity avulsion injury/tongue-type variants:

i. Result of a strong eccentric contraction of the triceps surae with an avulsion fracture of the Achilles tendon insertion at the posterior tuberosity with varying size.

ii. Urgent surgical fixation is warranted to prevent full skin necrosis.

C. Bony anatomy

The os calcis is an asymmetrically shaped bone with four important but irregular articulations to the talus and cuboid. Fracture patterns may disrupt the normal hindfoot function (▶Fig. 45.4).

1. The subtalar joint:

a. Posterior facet—largest and primary weight-bearing surface with mildly convex shape.

b. Anterior and middle facets may be confluent.

2. The calcaneocuboid joint:

a. Contributes to hindfoot–midfoot inversion and eversion.

b. Subluxation often reduces via ligamentotaxis following restoration of calcaneal height and length but may warrant open reduction and fracture-specific fixation.

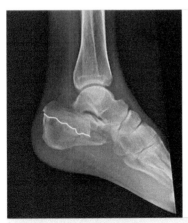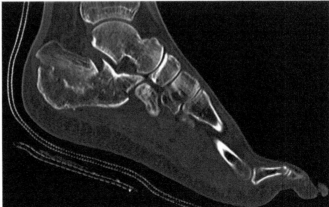

Fig. 45.3 Lateral radiograph and CT images depict a tongue-type secondary fracture line with intra-articular involvement and posterior facet joint depression.

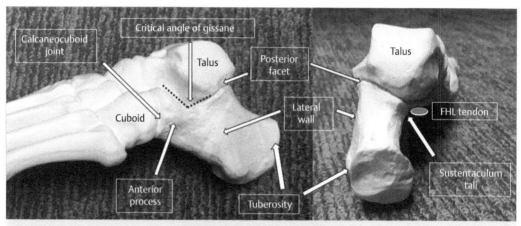

Fig. 45.4 Saw bone lateral and axial views depicting the relevant calcaneal anatomy.

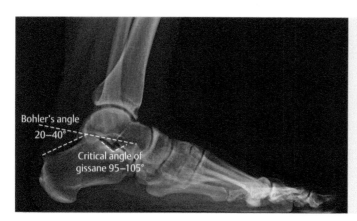

Fig. 45.5 Lateral radiograph demonstrates an intact calcaneus with normal Bohler's angle and normal critical angle of Gissane.

3. Sustentaculum tali:
    a. Dense cortical bone contained within the medial "constant" fragment.
    b. Flexor hallucis longus (FHL) runs directly below—at risk for injury with excessive screw length.
    c. Deltoid and talocalcaneal ligament attachments.
4. Posterior tuberosity:
    a. Provides calcaneal height, length, and width (often disrupted in fractures).
    b. Supports the posterior facet.
5. Anterior process:
    a. Supports anterior and middle facets, articulates with calcaneocuboid joint.
6. Lateral wall:
    a. Irregularly flat' cortical surface with peroneal tendon tubercle at risk for lateral displacement and resulting subfibular impingement pain.
D. Imaging
    1. Plain radiographs:
        a. Foot and ankle anteroposterior/lateral/oblique views to access adjacent joints:
            i. **Bohler's angle** (normal 20–40 degrees)—lateral radiographic angle between tangent line from superior aspect anterior process to crest of posterior facet and line from posterior facet to top of posterior tuberosity (▶ **Fig. 45.5**). Lower angles associated with

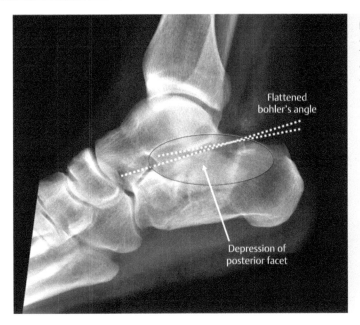

Fig. 45.6 Lateral radiograph depicts a displaced intra-articular calcaneal fracture with loss of Bohler's angle and depression of the posterior facet articular surface.

Flattened bohler's angle

Depression of posterior facet

greater intra-articular depression, increased fracture complexity, poorer functional scores, and increased risks for subtalar arthritis (▶**Fig. 45.6**).

ii. **Critical angle of gissane** (normal 95–105 degrees)—lateral radiographic angle denoting dense cortical bone supporting the lateral talar process (▶**Fig. 45.5**). Disruption associated with greater fracture comminution dividing the anterior, middle, and posterior facets.

b. Axial (Harris) view (▶**Fig. 45.2**):

i. Foot maximally dorsiflexed and beam directed 45 degrees cranial.

ii. Visualizes heel axial alignment (normal 10-degree valgus).

iii. Useful to assess: varus, tuberosity shortening/widening, medial comminution, and lateral wall blowout.

c. Broden's views: intraoperative adjunct (▶**Fig. 45.7d**):

i. Ankle in neutral dorsiflexion with 30-degree internal rotation and X-rays taken at various degrees of cranial inclination (10–40 degrees).

ii. Allows for visualization of the posterior facet reduction and safe fixation.

d. Typical DIACF X-ray findings include decreased Bohler's angle, increased angle of Gissane, calcaneal shortening (length and height), heel widening (hindfoot varus), and various degrees of comminution at the constant fragment and lateral wall.

2. CT scan:

a. Gold standard adjunct for fracture classification and preoperative planning.

b. Indicated for all DIACFs; basis for Sanders' classification (described later).

E. Classification

1. Extra-articular fractures (25%):

a. Anterior process fractures visible on lateral X-ray; present like lateral ankle sprain.

b. Calcaneal tuberosity (Achilles avulsion) fracture—visible on lateral X-ray; urgent fixation.

c. Sustentacular fractures—visible on axial X-ray; present like medial ankle sprain.

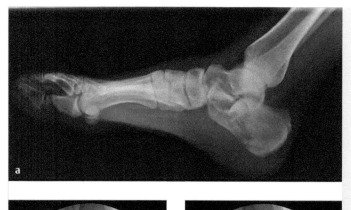

Fig. 45.7 (a) Essex-Lopresti tongue-type fracture. (b) Reduction is achieved through percutaneous Schanz pin techniques. (c–e) Intraoperative lateral, Broden, and axial views confirm anatomic reduction and safe hardware placement.

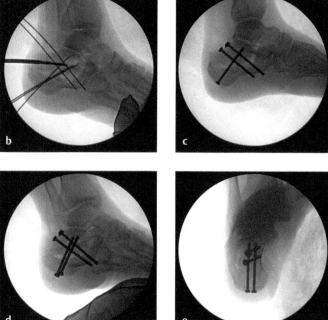

2. Intra-articular fractures (75%):
   a. Essex–Lopresti classification—based upon secondary fracture line on lateral X-ray:
      i. Joint depression—posterior tuberosity is not attached to the posterior facet.
      ii. Tongue type—posterior tuberosity is attached to the posterior facet (▸Fig. 45.7a–e).
   b. Sanders' classification—based on the number/location of posterior facet fragments seen on coronal CT image denoting the widest portion of the inferior talar facet. Three potential fracture lines (A, B, and C) with four possible fragments (lateral, middle, medial, sustentacular; ▸Fig. 45.8):
      i. Type I—nondisplaced fractures (rare); nonoperative.
      ii. Type II—two fracture fragments; consider open reduction and internal fixation (ORIF) in appropriate patient.
      iii. Type III—three fracture fragments; consider ORIF in appropriate patient.
      iv. Type IV—highly comminuted; consider ORIF ± primary ST fusion in ideal patient.

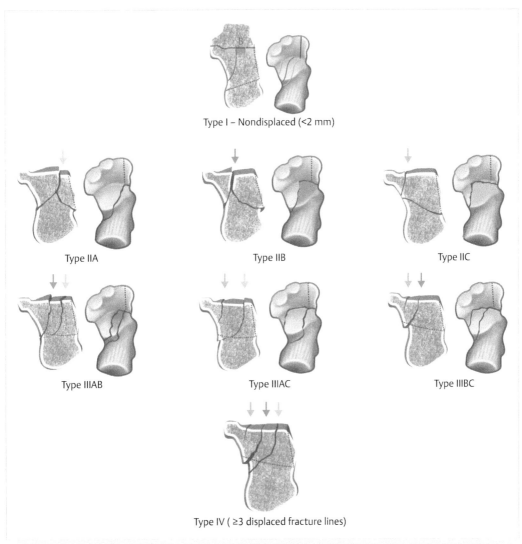

Type I – Nondisplaced (<2 mm)

Type IIA

Type IIB

Type IIC

Type IIIAB

Type IIIAC

Type IIIBC

Type IV (≥3 displaced fracture lines)

Fig. 45.8 Rendition of the Sanders CT classification for displaced intra-articular calcaneal fractures with coronal and axial views. Secondary intra-articular fracture lines as displayed based on their location within the posterior facet and the extent of fracture pattern.

II. Treatment

A. Initial management

1. Advanced trauma life support protocol.

   a. High-energy mechanisms of injury (i.e., falls, motor vehicle accidents [MVA]).

2. Well-padded bulky jones splint to protect soft tissues (neutral dorsiflexion).

3. Elevation and non–weight bearing.

   a. Elevation and non–weight bearing (NWB) are critical for soft-tissue management.

4. External fixation:

   a. External fixation is warranted for complex associated injuries and impending skin compromise.

5. Open fractures:

    a. Early intravenous (IV) antibiotics (preferably within 1 hour of injury).

    b. Thorough irrigation and debridement ± external fixation or provisional pinning.

    c. Primary closure versus negative pressure wound therapy.

B. Definitive management

  1. Nonoperative treatment

    a. Indications:
Nondisplaced fractures, minimally displaced extra-articular fractures, low-demand patients with osteopenia, comorbidities where risks outweigh the benefits (i.e., diabetes, nicotine dependence, peripheral vascular disease, and skin compromise).

    b. Brief splint immobilization with early ROM to prevent stiffness.

    c. Advance to weight bearing as tolerated at 8 to 12 weeks postoperatively.

    d. Late sequelae:
Post-traumatic arthritis, widened heel associated with poor shoe wearing, varus heel may lead to lateral ankle pain, painful exostoses.

  2. Operative treatment

    a. ORIF

      i. Indications: Displaced but reconstructable fracture patterns in younger patients with a good soft-tissue envelope.

    b. Primary ORIF with subtalar fusion (▶Fig. 45.9):

      i. Controversial versus ORIF without fusion.

      ii. Consideration in Sanders IV to prevent additional delayed ST fusion procedure (i.e., laborers who cannot "afford" a second surgery for recovery with time off work).

      iii. Surgical goal is to restore the height, length, and valgus with ORIF + subtalar joint debridement and fusion using large cannulated screws.

C. Surgical approach:

  1. Closed reduction percutaneous fixation:

    a. Tongue-type fractures via Essex-Lopresti technique.

    b. Extra-articular fractures (i.e., posterior tuberosity avulsion).

  2. ORIF via extensile lateral approach (ELA):

    a. Vertical limb 1 cm anterior to Achilles tendon.

    b. Horizontal limb along transition of plantar skin (glabrous border).

    c. No skin undermining; full-thickness flap developed by subperiosteal dissection to include peroneal tendons and sural nerve with K-wires to hold ('no touch'; ▶Fig. 45.10).

    d. Direct visualization of the lateral wall fragment, which is (often) removed to visualize impacted and displaced posterior facet.

    e. Begin rebuilding anterior and middle facets at the critical angle.

    f. Disimpact the primary fracture line to restore tuberosity height, length, and heel valgus with tuberosity Schanz pin and K-wires into the sustentaculum/anterior process.

    g. Posterior facet reduced under direct visualization; consider independent lag screws.

    h. Lateral wall replaced with definitive fixation plate and screws applied.

    i. Deep wound closure in layers and over a drain to prevent postoperative hematoma with tension-free skin Allgower–Donati suture technique.

  3. ORIF via ST approach:

    a. Less invasive—oblique incision from fibular tip distally over ST.

    b. Mobilize underneath and protect peroneal tendons and sural nerve.

    c. Reduction as described earlier, except for retention of lateral wall.

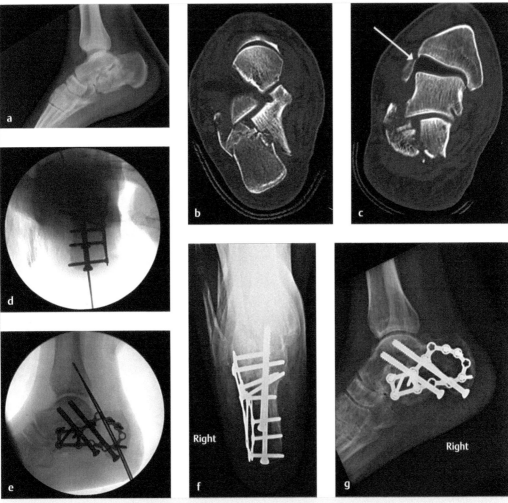

Fig. 45.9 **(a)** Displaced intra-articular calcaneal fracture after motor vehicle accident with significant impaction of the subtalar joint. **(b)** CT scan denotes marked lateral comminution of the posterior facet. **(c)** Associated ankle subluxation was present. **(d, e)** Extensile lateral approach was used for open reduction and internal fixation + primary subtalar fusion with percutaneous pinning of the ankle joint. **(f, g)** Radiographs demonstrate successful fusion with restoration of calcaneal height, length, and valgus.

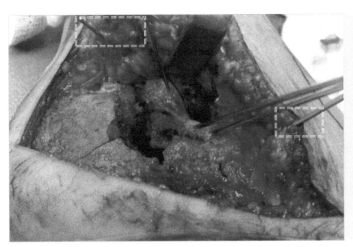

Fig. 45.10 Intraoperative image depicts the use of stout K-wires (*yellow highlight*) to retract the ELA flap. This "no-touch" technique helps prevent constant tension from retractors to allow visualization and reduction. (Reproduced with permission from Yoo BJ, Meeker JE. Calcaneus. In: Mamczak CN, ed. Illustrated Tips and Tricks for Intraoperative Imaging in Fracture Surgery. Philadelphia, PA: Wolters Kluwer Health; 2018:297–308.)

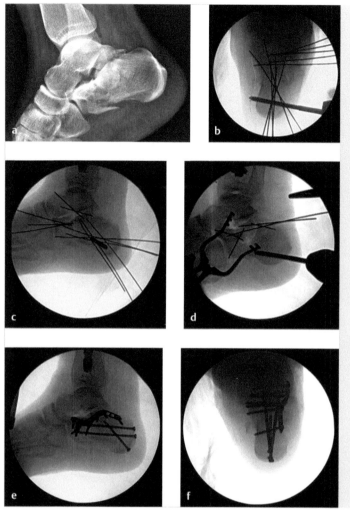

Fig. 45.11 (a) Radiograph demonstrating a displaced intra-articular calcaneal fracture (Sanders type 2) with posterior facet depression. (b–d) Intraoperative axial, lateral, and Broden views show restoration of calcaneal height, length, width, and valgus with joint reduction. (e, f) Final views highlight the use of a low-profile, sinus tarsi–specific plating construct with percutaneous cannulated screws supporting the reduction of the longitudinal axis and posterior facet.

    d. Specifically designed implants available with adjunctive percutaneous cannulated screws supporting fixation of the longitudinal axis and tuberosity height (▶Fig. 45.11).

    e. Less wound healing complications and OR time without sacrificed reduction when compared to ELA.

    f. Time to surgery typically performed earlier than ELA, but still predicated on soft-tissue envelope; reduction may be increasingly difficult for certain fracture patterns at a greater length of time from injury.

4. Medial approach:

    a. Oblique incision posterior to neurovascular bundle with limited access to address fixation of the sustentaculum and medial posterior tuberosity.

5. Percutaneous techniques/intramedullary implants (▶Fig. 45.12):

    a. Decreases incidence of skin flap necrosis and allows earlier operative intervention.

       i. Indirect fluoroscopic or mini-open reduction with percutaneous distractor restores heel height and reduces heel varus.

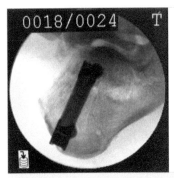 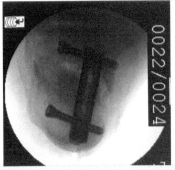 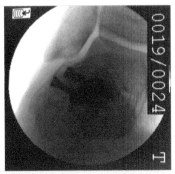

Fig. 45.12 Intraoperative fluoroscopic images demonstrate the percutaneous use of a Calcanail® to restore Bohler's angle, hindfoot valgus, and the articular reduction of the posterior facet.

      ii.   Plantar heel incision with less concern for skin necrosis out of injury zone.

     iii.   Guide pin along longitudinal axis of calcaneus with reamer allowing for reduction awls and posterior facet reduction "inside-out."

     iv.   Intramedullary implant supports the posterior facet with two interlocks with maintenance of reduction and limited wound complications.

D. Complications

  1. Subtalar arthritis:

    a. Correlates with severity of comminution and anatomic reduction.

    b. Treatment—nonsteroidal anti-inflammatory drugs, orthotics, or delayed subtalar arthrodesis.

  2. Wound drainage/dehiscence:

    a. Most common with ELA; less common with ST and percutaneous approaches.

    b. Early oral antibiotics with wound care; may require formal irrigation and debridement or flap.

  3. Subfibular impingement:

    a. Due to lateral wall displacement.

    b. Treat with delayed exostectomy.

  4. Increased heel width:

    a. Secondary to malunion.

    b. Difficulty with shoe fitting.

    c. Consider calcaneus slide osteotomy.

  5. Painful retained hardware:

    a. More common with larger ELA plates, screw over penetration of medial cortex (i.e., FHL).

  6. Osteomyelitis:

    a. Most common with open fractures and ELA flap necrosis.

    b. Aggressive surgical debridement with a prolonged course of IV antibiotics.

    c. Flap necrosis may require skin grafting or flap coverage.

    d. Transtibial amputation for failed salvage.

  7. Chronic pain:

    a. Spectrum—complex regional pain syndrome, post-traumatic arthritis, retained hardware, and stiff hindfoot with restricted function during stance.

E. Postoperative management and rehabilitation

1. Bulky plaster splint with elevation and pain control (regional anesthesia ± narcotics).
2. Drain for ELA.
3. Suture removal at 2 to 3 weeks and transition to walking boot with early ankle/foot range of motion (ROM).
4. NWB for 8 to 12 weeks then progressive ambulation with orthotic consideration.

F. Outcomes

1. Patient selection:
Patient selection is critically important to assess risks and benefits of treatment pathways.
   a. Thorough discussion of potential outcomes, expectations and common complications:
      i. Chronic pain, post-traumatic arthritis, hardware irritation, and wound-related complications are unfortunately common despite anatomic restoration.
   b. Operative versus nonoperative treatment remains controversial in certain patients.

2. Analysis of predictors for poor outcome:
   a. Workman's compensation.
   b. Initial Bohler's angle less than 0 degrees.
   c. Comminution (i.e., Sanders IV).
   d. Employed as a laborer.
   e. Nicotine dependence.
   f. Peripheral vascular disease.
   g. Uncontrolled diabetes.
   h. Male greater than female.

3. Variables predicting late subtalar fusion:
   a. Bohler's angle less than 0 degrees, Sanders IV, Workman's compensation, non-op, male laborers.

Summary

Fractures of the os calcis inherently represent complex anatomy with associated risks for challenging post-traumatic and surgical sequelae. The soft-tissue envelope, fracture pattern, and patient characteristics are critical aspects in deciding between operative and nonoperative treatment pathways. Proper patient selection, a keen understanding of restoring the calcaneal anatomy, and surgeon experience can optimize surgical outcomes. Regardless, patients should be counseled that post-traumatic arthritis and changes in the normal function of the hindfoot are common. Recent studies have attempted to identify which patient and fracture characteristics may benefit from surgical fixation. Debate still exists over which patients should have surgery and the use of primary subtalar fusion in the acute setting. Individualizing the risks and benefits of conservative nonoperative versus early or late operative treatment algorithms should be clearly reviewed to promote realistic expectations for both patients and surgeons. Displaced intra-articular calcaneal fractures occur in 75% of cases and denote the most complex injuries. Surgical goals entail restoring anatomic congruency of the subtalar joint surfaces, positive Bohler's angle, decreasing heel width, and recreating a nonvarus hindfoot. Modern advances in operative techniques have expanded the options for surgical approach, fixation constructs, and the timing of fixation with an effort to limit historic complications of these injuries. Postsurgical sequelae most commonly involve the risks of wound dehiscence, post-traumatic arthritis, and chronic hindfoot pain due to retained implants, abnormal heel width, and stiffness. A single method of treating these fractures, operative or not, may be inadequate and ultimately limit the potential for positive clinical outcomes.

Suggested Readings

Buckley R, Leighton R, Sanders D, et al. Open reduction and internal fixation compared with ORIF and primary subtalar arthrodesis for treatment of Sanders type IV calcaneal fractures: a randomized multicenter trial. J Orthop Trauma 2014;28(10):577–583

Csizy M, Buckley R, Tough S, et al. Displaced intra-articular calcaneal fractures: variables predicting late subtalar fusion. J Orthop Trauma 2003;17(2):106–112

Howard JL, Buckley R, McCormack R, et al. Complications following management of displaced intra-articular calcaneal fractures: a prospective randomized trial comparing open reduction internal fixation with nonoperative management. J Orthop Trauma 2003;17(4):241–249

Loucks C, Buckley R. Bohler's angle: correlation with outcome in displaced intra-articular calcaneal fractures. J Orthop Trauma 1999;13(8):554–558

Schepers T, Backes M, Dingemans SA, de Jong VM, Luitse JSK. Similar anatomical reduction and lower complication rates with the sinus tarsi approach compared with the extended lateral approach in displaced intra-articular calcaneal fractures. J Orthop Trauma 2017;31(6):293–298

Sanders R, Fortin P, DiPasquale T, Walling A. Operative treatment in 120 displaced intraarticular calcaneal fractures. Results using a prognostic computed tomography scan classification. Clin Orthop Relat Res 1993(290):87–95

Tufescu TV, Buckley R. Age, gender, work capability, and worker's compensation in patients with displaced intraarticular calcaneal fractures. J Orthop Trauma 2001;15(4):275–279

Zhang W, Lin F, Chen E, et al. Operative versus nonoperative treatment of displaced intra-articular calcaneal fractures: a meta-analysis of randomized controlled trials. J Orthop Trauma 2016;30:e75–e81

46 Talus Fractures

Laura S. Phieffer and Shan Lansing

Introduction

This chapter provides an overview of fractures that occur in the talus with an approach to examine patients with talus fractures, the anatomy of the talus and its blood supply. Treatment options including surgical approaches and fixation techniques are provided.

Keywords: talus fracture, ankle injury, talus surgery, talar neck fractures, talar body fractures.

I. Preoperative

A. History and physical examination

Talar neck fractures:

1. Fractures of the talar neck make up 45 to 50% of all talus fractures.

2. Talar neck fractures are produced by decelerating forces with axial impaction. This has also been described as a hyperdorsiflexion injury.

   a. Due to dorsiflexion, the posterior capsular ligaments of the subtalar joint are ruptured and the superior aspect of the talar neck is forced against the distal end of the tibia. As the force continues, the posterior ankle capsule, posterior talofibular ligaments, and the deltoid ligament give out and the talar neck sustains a fracture as it impacts the anterior lip of the distal tibia.

   b. Historically, fractures to the talar neck have been called "aviator's astragalus" because they were seen in pilots after crash landings of airplanes during World War I.

3. Patients present with swelling and hematoma over the ankle joint, especially near the proximal dorsal foot. Pain and swelling may mask a dislocation or fracture displacement.

4. Range of motion (ROM) at the talocrural and subtalar joints will likely be limited. Patients will have pain and be unable to bear weight on the injured side.

5. The foot and ankle should be evaluated for soft-tissue injuries and neurovascular deficits; blood supply can be evaluated through palpation or Doppler ultrasound.

6. Ecchymosis, abrasions, fracture blisters, and deformity should be noted.

7. Integrity of the medial malleolus and calcaneus should be evaluated:

   a. Twenty-eight percent of talar neck fractures present with concurrent fractures of the medial malleolus.

   b. Ten percent present with concurrent calcaneus fractures.

Talus body fractures:

1. Talar body fractures make up approximately 40% of talus fractures.

2. Often they involve the articular surface of the trochlea and the posterior facet of the subtalar joint.

3. Lateral process fractures will present as lateral ankle pain, which can be misdiagnosed as a sprained ankle.

Talar head fractures:

1. Fractures of the talar head make up 5 to 10% of all talus fractures.

2. Talar head fractures generally result from plantar flexion combined with axial compression.

3. Patients will present on examination with tenderness and swelling of the talonavicular joint.

B. Anatomy

Talar neck fractures:

1. Blood supply to the talus (▶ **Fig. 46.1**).

   a. The blood supply to the talus comes from the posterior tibial artery, anterior tibial (dorsalis pedis) artery, and peroneal artery, which connect to form an anastomosis.

   b. Medially the posterior tibial artery provides the following:

      i. Artery of the tarsal canal—entering along the inferior talar neck.

      ii. Deltoid branch—enters the talar body medially; often is the single source of blood supply to the talar body following talus fracture.

   c. Laterally the anterior tibial artery (becomes the dorsalis pedis artery as it crosses the ankle joint) and peroneal artery provide the following:

      i. Artery of the tarsal sinus—distal branch of the dorsalis pedis artery; supplies blood to the talar head.

2. The talus is one of the few bones in the foot that has no muscular attachments. It is held in place by surrounding bones and attached ligaments.

3. Osteology (▶ **Fig. 46.2a–c**):

   a. The talus neck is short and broad with relatively weak cortex.

Talus body fractures:

1. For blood supply to the talar body, see above section on talar neck fractures: anatomy, blood supply.

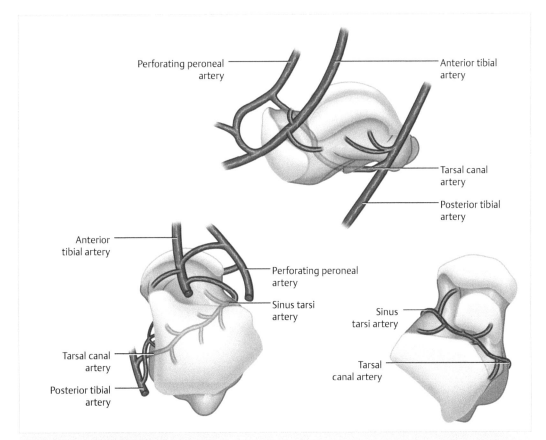

Fig. 46.1 Vascular supply to the talus.

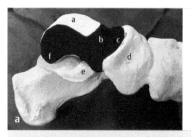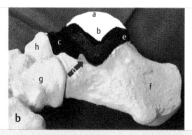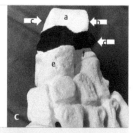

Fig. 46.2 **(a)** Medial view of a saw bone talus (a, body with articular surface for tibia; b, Neck; c, head of the talus articulating with navicular; d, navicular; e, sustentaculum tali of the calcaneus; f, medial process of the talus). **(b)** Lateral view of a saw bone talus (a, body with articular surface for tibia; b, articular surface for lateral malleolus; c, neck of the talus; d, lateral process of the talus, arrow pointing to the tarsal sinus; e, posterior process of the talus; f, calcaneus; g, cuboid; h, navicular). **(c)** Anterior view of a saw bone talus (a, body with articular surface for tibia; b, arrow indicating articular surface for lateral malleolus; c, arrow indicating articular surface for the medial malleolus; d, arrow indicating lateral talar process; e, navicular; g, calcaneus).

2. Talar body fractures primarily affect the articular surface and posterior facet of the subtalar joint, but include the lateral and posterior process as well:

   a. The lateral process articulates with the distal fibula superiorly and the calcaneus inferiorly:

      i. The lateral process fractures are often called "snowboarder's fractures."

   b. The posterior process has two tubercles (medial and lateral) through which the flexor hallucis longus runs.

Talar head fractures:

1. For blood supply of the talar head, see above section on talar neck fractures: anatomy, blood supply.

2. Bone density is highest in the proximal portion of the talus and decreases distally in the talar neck and head.

   a. The densest portion of bone of the talar head is the lateral aspect.

C. Imaging

Talar neck fractures:

1. Standard radiographs include anteroposterior (AP), lateral, and oblique views of the foot and ankle. Modified AP radiographs may also be useful in assessing, but typically CT scan has replaced these specialty views:

   a. Varus/valgus displacement—place ankle in maximum dorsiflexion, pronate foot 15 degrees and position the radiograph beam at 75-degree angle cephalad.

   b. Axial deviation of talar neck: Canale view; pronate foot 15 degrees and position the radiograph beam at 45-degree angle caudally.

   c. Talonavicular joint assessment—dorsoplantar view of the foot with the radiograph beam angled 20 degrees caudally.

2. Copious X-rays can be exchanged for a CT scan with coronal, axial, and sagittal reconstruction.

3. MRI scans are not helpful in preoperative planning.

Talus body fractures:

1. Standard radiographs include AP, lateral, and oblique views of the foot and ankle.

2. Lateral process fractures can be viewed with standard radiography, including the mortise view (AP view with 10-degree internal rotation of the foot).

3. CT scans with coronal, axial, and sagittal reconstruction are needed to confirm degree of displacement and fracture planes.

Talar head fractures:

1. The clearest view of the talar head can be seen with the foot positioned in maximum equinus and pronated 15 degrees with the radiograph beam angled 70 degrees cephalad.

2. A CT scan will be able to confirm a suspected talar head fracture.

D. Classification

Talar neck fractures:

1. The most frequently used classification of talar neck fractures was proposed by Hawkins, and later modified by Canale and Kelly. The Hawkins classification has been shown to be prognostic with respect to final outcome, but only includes talar neck fractures.

   a. Type I: nondisplaced.

   b. Type II: dislocation at the subtalar joint (▶ **Fig. 46.3**).

   c. Type III: dislocation at the subtalar joint and tibiotalar joint.

   d. Type IV: dislocation at the subtalar joint, tibiotalar joint, and talonavicular joint.

2. The Orthopaedic Trauma Association (OTA) has additional classifications based on the number of joints involved. The OTA classification system can also be used for all talus fractures.

   a. Type A: extra-articular fractures—includes talar process fractures.

   b. Type B: partial intra-articular fractures—includes small osteochondral fractures.

   c. Type C: complete intra-articular fractures—includes crush fractures.

Talus body fractures:

1. For classification of talar body fractures and the OTA system, see above section on talus neck fractures: classification.

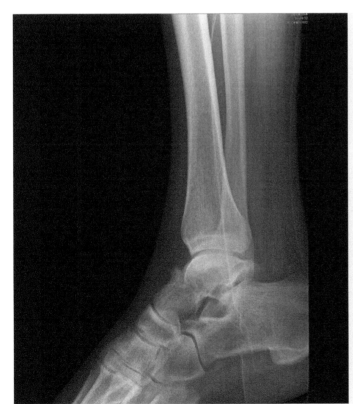

Fig. 46.3 Lateral ankle radiograph demonstrating a Hawkins type II talar neck fracture with subtalar dislocation.

II. Treatment

A. Initial management

Talar neck fractures:

1. Thirteen percent of all talus fractures are open; primary operative treatment is indicated in all open fractures.

2. Closed reduction, typically under conscious sedation, can be attempted in the emergency room for select talus fracture dislocations.

    a. Often successful for Hawkins' type II.

        i.   Medial subtalar dislocation—foot may appear supinated. Reduction can be blocked by lateral structures: peroneal tendons, extensor digitorum brevis.
        ii. Lateral subtalar dislocation—foot may appear pronated. Reduction can be blocked by medial structures: posterior tibial tendon, flexor hallucis longus, and flexor digitorum longus.

    b. Reduction difficult with Hawkins' types III and IV:

        i.   Consider attempting reduction when skin is compromised and/or there may be a delay in taking the patient to the operating room such as physiologic instability.

B. Definitive management

1. Nonoperative treatment

    Talar neck fractures:

    a. Hawkins' type I talar neck fractures do not typically require surgery. CT scan evaluation is indicated to confirm no displacement:

        i.   Foot and ankle can be cast in neutral position and kept non–weight bearing for 6 to 12 weeks.
        ii.   Progression to full weight bearing is allowed after complete radiographic union or other evidence of healing (~8–10 weeks).
        iii. Some consider surgery a relative indication to allow early ROM and accelerated weight bearing.

    b. Hawkins' type II:

        i.   As noted above, closed reduction may be attempted if the patient is relaxed: plantar flexion with traction to realign head and body of talus and varus/valgus force to realign neck in the transverse plane. CT scan evaluation is indicated to confirm no displacement.
        ii. If reduction is anatomic, may be treated like Hawkins I with cast.

    Talus body fractures:

        i.   As with nondisplaced talar neck fractures, nondisplaced talar body fractures may be treated nonoperatively by casting the foot and ankle in the neutral position for 6 to 8 weeks.
        ii. Lateral process fractures with minimal displacement or comminution.

    Talar head fractures:

        i.   Similar to other talus fractures, nondisplaced fractures may be treated nonoperatively in a short leg cast, non–weight bearing, for 6 to 12 weeks. Weight bearing is allowed after complete radiographic union or other evidence of healing.

2. Operative management and fixation

    Talar neck fractures:

        i.   Hawkins' type I fracture—nondisplaced fractures can be fixed via percutaneous screw fixation and allow for early ROM.
        ii.   Hawkins' type II fracture—open reduction should be considered in all displaced fractures.
        iii. Hawkins' type III and IV fractures—surgical emergency if there is a an extruded talus or significant subluxation putting soft tissues (skin, nerve, or artery) at risk.
        iv.   Surgery is indicated in all open fractures.

Talus body fractures:

    i.   Most displaced talar body fractures.

    ii. Lateral process fractures that are displaced greater than 2 to 5 mm (controversial) and sufficiently large enough to hold mini-fragment fixation (>8–10 mm fragment).

Talar head fractures:

1. Treatment options:

    a.   Fractures with less than 50% of head involvement heal well with excision. Injuries with greater than 50% head involvement require ORIF with mini-fragment screw fixation.

    b.   External fixation is an alternative option as definitive treatment for comminuted fractures with soft-tissue compromise. The external fixator is typically left in place for 6 to 8 weeks.

C. Surgical approaches and fixation techniques

Talar neck fractures:

1. For the vast majority of Hawkins' type II to IV fractures, a medial and lateral approach will be necessary to avoid malrotation and achieve anatomical reduction.

    a.   Anteromedial approach (▶ **Fig. 46.4**):

        i.   Incision should begin at the anterior aspect of the medial malleolus and be brought down in a curved line to the dorsal aspect of the navicular tuberosity—halfway between the tendons of the tibialis posterior and anterior.

        ii. To expose the talar dome, extend the incision proximally and perform a medial malleolar osteotomy. Care must be taken to avoid dissecting the deltoid artery.

        iii. Dissection of the talonavicular and tibionavicular ligaments will expose the fracture to the talar neck.

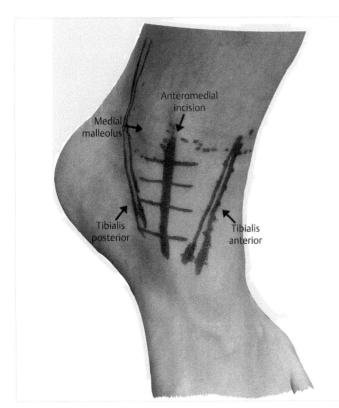

Fig. 46.4 Anteromedial surgical approach to the talus between the tibialis anterior tendon and tibialis posterior tendon.

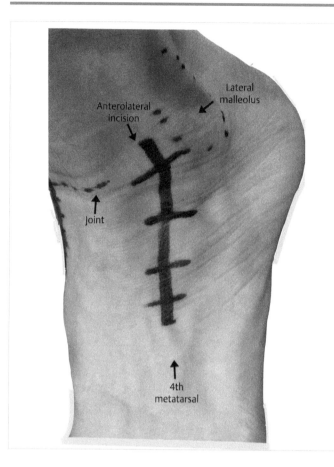

Fig. 46.5 Anterolateral surgical approach to the talus in line with the fourth metatarsal.

b. Lateral approaches:
  i. Anterolateral approach (▶ **Fig. 46.5**)—incision begins at the lateral malleolus and is brought down in a curved line.
  ii. Lateral sinus tarsi approach (▶ **Fig. 46.6**)—incision runs obliquely in front of the lateral malleolus over the sinus tarsi; begin just distal to the tip of the fibular extending over the anterior process of the calcaneus.
  iii. To expose the lateral aspect of the talus, the inferior extensor retinaculum is dissected and the extensor digitorum brevis muscle is reflected superiorly.
  iv. During the lateral approach, take care not to sever the peroneal tendons and the superficial peroneal nerve.

2. Following anatomical reduction of the talus, fixation of the neck of the talus can be achieved.
  a. Controversial, 3.5-mm cortical screws, 4.0-mm cancellous screws, 4.5-mm screws, headless screws, and mini-fragment plates are all routinely used.
    i. Stability is increased if screws are inserted in a convergent manner.
    ii. Avoid placing screws too close to the sinus tarsi so avoid interrupting the sinus tarsi artery, which supplies the talar body.
    iii. Distal talar neck fractures may require the screws to be countersunk into the head of the talus.
  b. The use of titanium screws may allow for postoperative MR imaging.
  c. Alternatively, 2.0-mm mini-fragmentary plates may be applied along the medial or lateral neck surfaces.
    i. Plate fixation is helpful when lateral comminution is present.

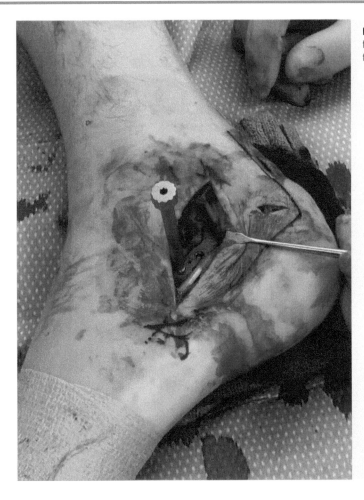

Fig. 46.6 Lateral sinus tarsi approach for open reduction and internal fixation of a calcaneus fracture.

Talus body fractures:

1. The vast majority require a medial and lateral approach, with medial malleolar osteotomy (▶ **Fig. 46.7a–c**).

2. Displaced posterior talar body fractures can be addressed by a posteromedial approach with the patient in the prone position.

3. Displaced lateral talar process fractures are addressed through a lateral approach.

D. Complications

Talar neck fractures:

1. Infection—occurs primarily after an open fracture.

2. Avascular necrosis (AVN): 50% of all talar neck fractures result in AVN.

   a. Hawkins' type I fractures: 0 to 13%; type II fractures: 20 to 50%; type III fractures: 70 to 100%; and type IV: nearly 100%.

   b. Open fractures have an increased risk for AVN.

   c. Hawkins' sign (▶ **Fig. 46.8**): AP ankle radiograph shows presence of subchondral lucency of the talar dome.

      i. A positive Hawkins' sign at 6 weeks postoperation is predictive of vascularity and therefore unlikely to develop AVN later.

      ii. A negative Hawkins' sign at 6 weeks postoperation does not confirm or predict AVN but suggests possible vascular insufficiency.

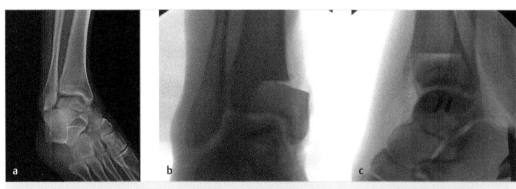

Fig. 46.7 Talar body fracture and fixation. **(a)** Oblique ankle radiograph of a talar body fracture. **(b)** Intraoperative anteroposterior image of talar body fracture fixation through a medial malleolar approach (osteotomy). **(c)** Intraoperative lateral image of talar body fracture fixation through a medial malleolar approach.

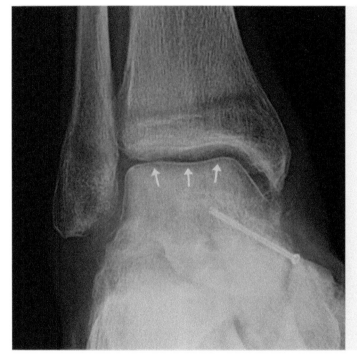

Fig. 46.8 Anteroposterior ankle radiograph demonstrating a positive Hawkins sign. *Arrows* pointing to the subchondral lucency representing vascular resorption indicating adequate blood supply. (This image is provided courtesy of George R. Matcuk Jr., M.D.)

3. Malunion of the talus and malalignment of the joint are seen in up to one-third of talus fracture cases, predominantly following closed treatment:
    a. Malunions of the talar neck and body lead to foot deformities and joint instability.
    b. The most common deformity is varus malunion of the talar neck, which decreases subtalar and mid-tarsal motion.

Talus body fractures:

1. Prognosis is typically worse for fractures of the talar body than those of the neck.
2. AVN:
    a. Body fracture without dislocation: 10 to 25%.
    b. Body fracture with dislocation: 25 to 50%.

3. Nonunion risk with nonoperatively treated displaced lateral process talus fractures.

    a. May go on to become symptomatic with or without post-traumatic arthritis.

Talar head fractures:

1. Avascular necrosis occurs in up to 10% of talar head fractures, likely because the blood supply to the talar head is ample.

E. Outcomes

Talar neck fractures:

1. Talar neck fractures that are not complicated by AVN or post-traumatic arthritis have minimal impact on ROM and ability to return to work, though a fraction of patients have reported aching pain.

2. Talar neck fractures complicated with AVN routinely result in pain. ROM can be decreased significantly with both plantar flexion and dorsiflexion.

3. Post-traumatic arthrosis is common and predominantly affects the subtalar joint

Summary

Talar fractures are relatively uncommon, making up only 0.32% of all fractures and 3.4% of all foot fractures. These injuries typically occur in the third decade of life, approximately three times more often in men than in women. Over 90% of talar fractures result from high-energy motor vehicle accidents or falls from a height. For nondisplaced talar fractures, the timing of internal fixation does not affect the functional outcome of the surgery. Dislocations require surgical fixation and should be treated as a medical emergency. With early fixation and early rehabilitation, good outcomes are expected in the majority of cases.

Suggested Readings

Canale ST, Kelly FB Jr. Fractures of the neck of the talus. Long-term evaluation of seventy-one cases. J Bone Joint Surg Am 1978;60(2):143–156

Hawkins LG. Fractures of the neck of the talus. J Bone Joint Surg Am 1970;52(5):991–1002

Higgins TF, Baumgaertner MR. Diagnosis and treatment of fractures of the talus: a comprehensive review of the literature. Foot Ankle Int 1999;20(9):595–605

JA III, Leucht P. Fractures of the talus: current concepts and new developments. Foot Ankle Surg 2018;24(4):282–290

Jordan RK, Bafna KR, Liu J, Ebraheim NA. Complications of talar neck fractures by Hawkins classification: a systematic review. J Foot Ankle Surg 2017;56(4):817–821

Rammelt S, Zwipp H. Talar neck and body fractures. Injury 2009;40(2):120–135

47 Midfoot Fractures and Dislocation (Lisfranc's Injuries)

John Ketz and Meghan Kelly

Introduction

Midfoot fracture dislocations (Lisfranc's injuries) represent a spectrum of injuries resulting in the disruption of the midfoot architecture. These injuries can range from subtle low-energy mechanisms and sprains to high-energy mechanisms such as motor vehicle collisions. Lisfranc's injuries are often missed on initial evaluation and can result in midfoot destabilization and significant long-term disability. A well-performed physical examination, appropriate imaging, and a high index of suspicion are important for evaluation of these injuries. Subsequent treatment ranges from nonoperative management of subtle sprains to open reduction and internal fixation (ORIF) or primary arthrodesis for more significant injuries (▶Video 47.1).

Keywords: LisFranc, tarsometatarsal, foot, crush, fusion

I. Preoperative

A. History and physical examination

    1. Mechanisms of injury:

        a. **Direct**—force applied directly to the tarsometatarsal (TMT) joint.

            i. Usually associated with significant soft-tissue injuries—MVCs, crush injury—more prone to compartment syndrome.

            ii. Displacement related to direction of force (can be plantar or dorsal).

        b. **Indirect**—twisting or axial loading on a plantar flexed foot—fall from height, athletic injuries. Dorsal displacement due to weaker dorsal ligaments versus plantar ligaments.

        c. Can also occur due to atraumatic or repeated microtrauma in neuropathic patient, such as those with evidence of Charcot's neuropathy.

        d. Associated fractures.

            i. Lisfranc's equivalent: fractures of contiguous metatarsal bases.

            ii. Tarsal fractures (cuboid/navicular fractures).

            iii. Cuboid fractures: often associated with twisting mechanism. Nutcracker injury: cuboid fracture associated with Lisfranc's injury when cuboid is fractured between the fourth and fifth metatarsals and calcaneus (▶Fig. 47.1).

    2. Examination findings:

        a. Significant swelling.

        b. Inability to weight bear.

        c. Tender along TMT joints.

        d. Plantar arch ecchymosis.

        e. Testing.

            i. Pain with passive pronation and abduction.

            ii. Piano key test: dorsal force applied to forefoot while grasping metatarsal heads.

B. Anatomy

    1. Lisfranc's joint complex (▶Fig. 47.2a):

        a. **Plantar** TMT **ligaments**—transverse instability with injury to ligament between medial cuneiform and the second/third metatarsal.

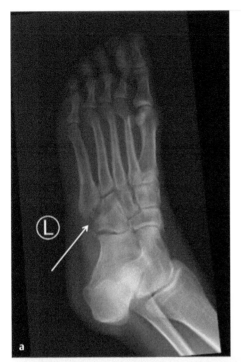
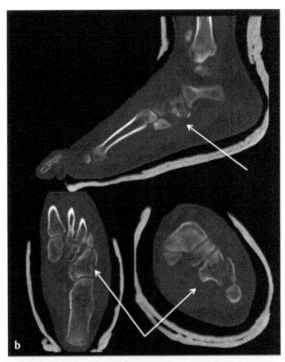

Fig. 47.1 Multiple (second to fourth) metatarsal neck fractures with an associated cuboid fracture (*white arrows*) viewed on **(a)** X-ray and **(b)** CT.

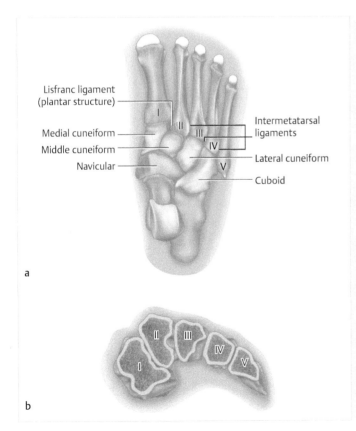

Fig. 47.2 **(a)** Anatomy of lisfranc's ligamentous complex and surrounding structures. **(b)** View of metatarsal bases demonstrating Roman arch structure.

Lisfranc ligament (plantar structure)

Medial cuneiform

Middle cuneiform

Navicular

Intermetatarsal ligaments

Lateral cuneiform

Cuboid

  b. **Dorsal** TMT **ligaments**—weaker than plantar, displacement more often dorsal.

  c. **Intermetatarsal ligaments**—no direction connection between the first and second metatarsals.

  d. Lisfranc's **ligament**—lateral aspect of the medial cuneiform to medial base of the second metatarsal; tightens with pronation and forefoot abduction.

 2. Role of the second metatarsal base (▶ **Fig. 47.2b**):

  a. Recessed proximally; forms mortise in medial and middle cuneiform.

  b. Acts as keystone in Roman arch formation of metatarsal bases.

 3. Associated structures:

  a. **Dorsal pedis artery**—runs between the first and second metatarsals; can be damaged during injury or repair.

  b. **Deep peroneal nerve**—can become interposed during reduction maneuver.

  c. **Anterior tibial tendon**—inserts into the first metatarsal base and medial cuneiform; can obstruct reductions of lateral dislocations.

  d. **Peroneus longus tendon**—inserts into the plantar aspect of the first metatarsal base.

  e. **Interossei/plantar fascia**—provides additional plantar support.

C. Imaging

 1. Anteroposterior (AP), lateral, and oblique X-rays: **20% go unrecognized:**

  a. AP—best for the first and second TMT joints.

  b. Oblique—best for the third, fourth, and fifth TMT joints.

  c. Best if weight bearing.

   i. If clinical suspicion remains, obtain comparison films of the contralateral foot.

   ii. Many times, a patient cannot bear weight the day of injury due to pain. Repeat weight bearing films the following week may be helpful in these circumstances.

 2. X-ray assessment for midfoot stability:

  a. AP view (▶ **Fig. 47.3a**):

   i. Up to 3 mm between the first and second metatarsal bases.

   ii. Lateral base of the first metatarsal in line with the lateral aspect of the medial cuneiform.

   iii. Medial base of the second metatarsal in line with the medial aspect of the middle cuneiform.

  b. Oblique view (▶ **Fig. 47.3b**):

   i. Medial base of the third metatarsal is in line with the medial aspect of the lateral cuneiform.

   ii. Medial base of the fourth metatarsal is in line with the medial aspect of the cuboid.

  c. Lateral view (▶ **Fig. 47.3c**): The metatarsal is in line with the tarsal bone (no dorsal subluxation).

 3. Other radiographic signs:

  a. Second metatarsal base fractures.

  b. Widening of the first intermetatarsal space (check contralateral limb for asymmetry): best if films are **weight bearing** (▶ **Fig. 47.4**).

  c. **"Fleck sign"**—avulsion of Lisfranc's ligament (▶ **Fig. 47.5a**).

 4. Additional imaging:

  a. CT—high-energy or for preoperative planning.

  b. MRI—rarely useful, but can be utilized if other imaging is negative and clinical suspicion remains.

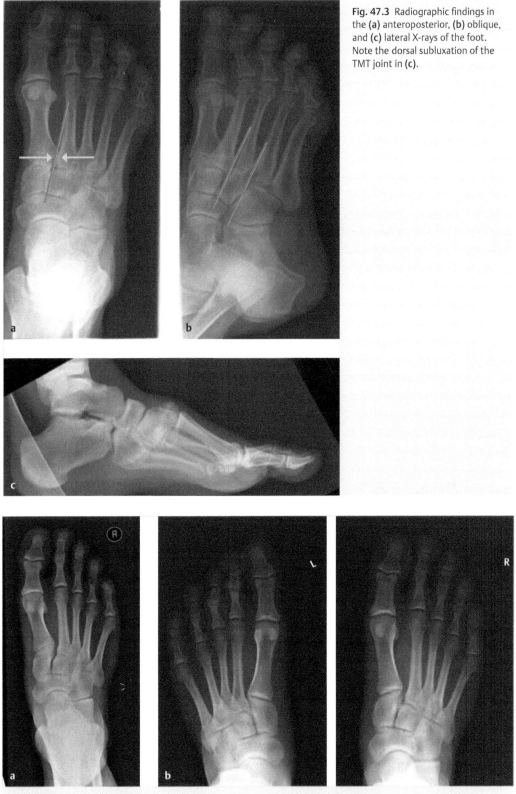

Fig. 47.3 Radiographic findings in the **(a)** anteroposterior, **(b)** oblique, and **(c)** lateral X-rays of the foot. Note the dorsal subluxation of the TMT joint in **(c)**.

Fig. 47.4 (a) Subtle widening of the first and second metatarsals, with **(b)** widening more apparent in weight-bearing bilateral foot X-rays.

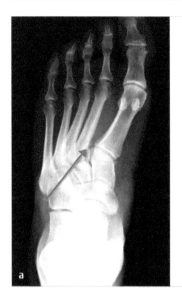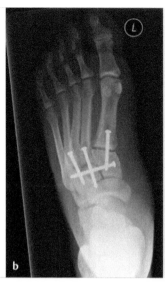

Fig. 47.5 **(a)** Lisfranc's injury with a *red arrow* indicating a "fleck" sign and **(b)** postoperative films following open reduction and internal fixation.

D. Classifications: have not been determined to have prognostic value

  1. Quenu and Kuss (modified by Hardcastle):

    a. Homolateral—all five metatarsals displaced in one direction (typically laterally).

    b. Isolated—one or two metatarsals displaced.

    c. Divergent—the first metatarsal displaced medially and the second to fifth metatarsals displaced laterally. There is displacement in both the sagittal and coronal planes.

II. Treatment

A. Initial management

  1. Immobilization—strict non–weight bearing.

  2. Attempt closed reduction if skin compromise is imminent:

    a. Improves joint alignment and soft tissue.

    b. If closed reduction is unsuccessful and there is impending skin compromise, the patient should be taken to surgery for closed reduction under anesthesia with temporary percutaneous pinning or open reduction to improve soft-tissue integrity.

  3. May require placement of external fixator with significant soft-tissue injury for temporization (i.e., open wounds, ballistic injuries, etc.):

    a. A 4.0-mm Schanz pin in the calcaneus (or talus or navicular).

    b. A 2.5- to 3.0-mm Schanz pin in the first and fifth metatarsals.

    c. Typically need a "small" external fixation tray rather than the more common large tray.

    d. Can also utilize spanning plates as temporary fixation typically placed with a minimally invasive technique.

    e. Definitive fixation once tissues are amenable.

B. Definitive management

  1. Nonoperative:

    a. Poor surgical candidates (insensate foot, peripheral vascular disease, and nonambulatory).

    b. Stable on physical examination.

    c. No clinical or radiographic evidence of instability (< 2 mm widening with weight-bearing films).

d. Cast immobilization for 8 weeks. Progress to weight bearing in boot or other rigid sole to limit midfoot motion; also, consider rocker bottom shoe modification.

2. Operative management:

   a. Indications—unstable injury (> 2 mm shift), open fracture, vascular compromise, compartment syndrome.

   b. Treatment can be delayed until swelling subsides (presence of skin wrinkles).

3. ORIF versus primary arthrodesis (PA):

   a. Controversial.

   b. Must take into account all joints involved. For example, cuneiform stability—requires fixation to navicular.

   c. Considerations for ORIF (▶ **Fig. 47.5a, b**):

      i. Best for bony fracture dislocations, minimal articular comminution: "subtle Lisfranc's injury."

      ii. Implants are frequently symptomatic and many patients benefit from hardware removal:

      • Lateral column K-wires typically removed at 4 to 6 weeks.
      • Medial column stabilization: screws typically not removed before 3 months.

      iii. Advantages:

      • Preserves all joints.
      • May spare some motion compared to arthrodesis.
      • Improved healing potential (in setting of multiple fractures).

      iv. Disadvantages:

      • Requires anatomic reduction for success.
      • Often requires additional procedures (hardware removal).
      • Progression of arthrosis.

   d. Considerations for primary arthrodesis (▶ **Fig. 47.6a,b**):

      i. Relative indications:

      • Delayed presentation.
      • Purely ligamentous injury.
      • Chronic deformity.
      • Articular comminution (unsalvageable joint).

      ii. Fuse the first, second, and third TMT joints, **never** fuse the fourth and fifth TMT joints.

      iii. Advantages:

      • Possible lower rate of hardware removal.
      • Anatomic reduction is not critical.
      • Minimal motion in midfoot joints at baseline.

      iv. Disadvantages:

      • Loss of motion at medial midfoot.

   e. What to do with the fourth and fifth rays:

      i. Lateral column is the mobile segment of the midfoot. Reduction often occurs with medial column reduction.

      ii. If unstable, can pin with K-wires.

   f. Closed reduction percutaneous fixation:

      i. Limited role—poor surgical candidates; significant skin or soft-tissue compromise.

      • Comminuted metatarsal fractures.
      • Can be used as temporizing with external fixation until definitive management can occur.

      ii. Reduction under fluoroscopy—small incisions and indirect reduction techniques used to preserve soft tissues.

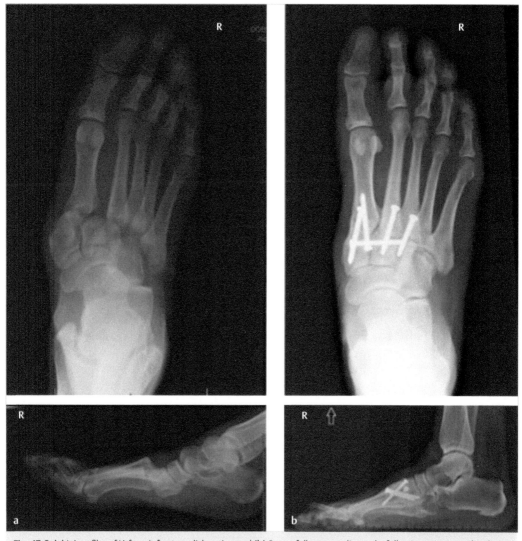

Fig. 47.6 (a) Injury film of Lisfranc's fracture dislocation and (b) 8-year follow-up radiographs following primary arthrodesis.

4. Implants:

   a. Screws:

      i. Small fragment 3.5- to 4.0-mm cortical or cannulated screws.

      ii. Allows for direct reduction and/or compression.

      iii. Countersink to avoid fracture of dorsal cortex.

   b. Plates:

      i. Small fragment (3.5 mm) or mini-fragment fixation (2.0–2.7 mm).

      ii. Used in setting of comminution.

      iii. Considered "joint sparing."

      iv. Can break over time.

   c. Additional fixation:

      i. Medial column spanning plate:

         • Added stability for medial column injuries, Chopart's injuries, navicular fractures and comminution of the first metatarsal.

         • Maintains medial column length.

      ii. Suture button—limited use due to inability to control midfoot joints.

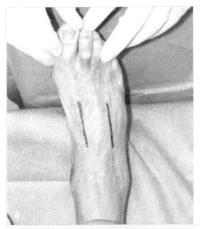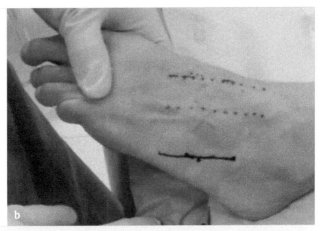

Fig. 47.7 (a) Primary and secondary incisions for the surgical approach for Lisfranc's fixation. (b) Primary and secondary incisions for surgical approach for Lisfranc's injury (*dotted lines*) as well as an additional lateral approach (*solid line*) for the displaced fourth and fifth metatarsal fractures.

C. Surgical approaches
1. Primary incision—centered over the first TMT joint, lateral to extensor hallucis longus, and medial to extensor hallucis brevis (▶ **Fig. 47.7a**):
    a. Medial dorsal cutaneous nerve is proximal.
    b. Dorsalis pedis artery and deep peroneal nerve are lateral.
    c. Full-thickness skin flaps needed.
2. Secondary incision—centered over the fourth ray (▶ **Fig. 47.7a**)—allows for access to the third TMT joint and lateral rays.
3. Lateral incision can be used in addition to the primary and secondary incisions for the displaced fourth and fifth metatarsals (▶ see **Fig. 47.7b**).

D. Operative reduction and fixation techniques
1. ORIF:
    a. Reduce intercuneiform joints: may need to be reduced to navicular if still unstable.
    b. Reduce and fix second metatarsal base to cuneiforms.
    c. Reduce the remaining TMT joints (medial then lateral).
    d. Lateral TMT joints often reduce once the medial column is reduced. K-wire fixation of the fourth and fifth TMT joints if still unstable.
2. Arthrodesis:
    a. Similar order as ORIF.
    b. Each joint is then sequentially taken down in a medial-to-lateral fashion and denude cartilage prior and allow for compression and stabilization across joint.

E. Complications
1. Post-traumatic arthritis–**most common:**
    a. Often related to poor reduction, loss of reduction, or articular comminution.
    b. Radiographic evidence reported to be as high as 100% (range reported 16–100%); however, it is not always symptomatic. One study noted a significant decrease in post-traumatic arthritis in patients with an anatomic reduction.
    c. Conservative management (nonsteroidal anti-inflammatory diseases, bracing).
    d. Surgical treatment:
        i. Fuse the first to third TMT joints ; more difficult as a salvage procedure than primary fusion.
        ii. Resection arthroplasty for fourth and fifth TMT joints.

2. Symptomatic hardware.

3. Nonunion—requires revision if symptomatic. Difficult operation and may require bone grafting.

4. Infection—need for long-term antibiotics, hardware removal, and can result in amputation.

5. Compartment syndrome:

    a. Seen more often in high-energy injuries, especially in the unconscious patient.

    b. If untreated, it may result in clawed toes, forefoot contractures, and a painful foot.

6. Skin complications:

    a. More likely to occur in crush injuries.

    b. Local wound care, vacuum-assisted dressings, or myocutaneous flaps.

7. Neuritis/complex regional pain syndrome (CRPS):

    a. Pain management, physical therapy.

    b. Regional anesthesia/sympathetic nerve block.

    c. No formal recommendations for vitamin C supplementation to prevent CRPS; however, it may be of benefit.

    d. More often observed in delayed diagnosis or lack of reduction.

F. Rehabilitation

1. ORIF:

    a. Splint for 2 weeks.

    b. Transition to walking boot for 2 to 10 weeks.

        i. Begin range of motion exercises at 2 weeks.
        ii. Remove K-wires 4 to 6 weeks.

    c. Advance weight bearing at 6 to 10 weeks.

    d. Return to sports once hardware is removed. Timing based on symptoms.

2. Fusions:

    a. Splint/cast for 6 weeks: Non–weight bearing. Transition to walking boot at 6 weeks and begin range of motion exercises.

    b. Progress to weight bearing at 6 to 10 weeks.

    c. Return to normal shoe wear by 10 to 12 weeks post-op.

G. Outcomes

1. Mechanisms of injury—direct high-energy injuries have poorer outcomes than low-energy injuries. Faster recovery with low-energy injuries.

2. ORIF versus primary fusion—equal functional outcomes:

    a. Decreased rate of hardware removal and revision surgery in fusions.

    b. One study noted that, in purely ligamentous injuries, fusion results in higher return to prior activities at 2 years (but not at prior time points); however, other studies have been unable to detect a significant difference in outcomes.

3. Medial column TMT fusion superior to medial and lateral TMT fusion.

    a. Lateral TMT fusions do poorly.

    b. Resection arthroplasty may be a better salvage procedure for lateral TMT arthritis.

4. ORIF and primary arthrodesis outcomes improved with anatomic reduction.

Summary

Midfoot fractures are typically recognized with plain films but subtle midfoot dislocations can be missed especially if bilateral weight bearing films are not obtained. In the Emergency Department setting immediately following injury, the safest course is to splint and keep the patient non-weightbearing if midfoot injury is suspected and have the patient return to see an Orthopaedic surgeon within a week to obtain bilateral (for comparison) foot weight bearing films when the patient is able to complete this dynamic study. Treatment remains controversial (ORIF vs. fusion) for 1st through 3rd TMT joint dislocations but ORIF is always indicated for acute 4th and 5th TMT dislocations.

Suggested Readings

Hawkinson MP, Tennent DJ, Belisle J, Osborn P. Outcomes of Lisfranc injuries in an active duty military population. Foot Ankle Int 2017;38(10):1115–1119

Henning JA, Jones CB, Sietsema DL, Bohay DR, Anderson JG. Open reduction internal fixation versus primary arthrodesis for lisfranc injuries: a prospective randomized study. Foot Ankle Int 2009;30(10):913–922

Kuo RS, Tejwani NC, Digiovanni CW, et al. Outcome after open reduction and internal fixation of Lisfranc joint injuries. J Bone Joint Surg Am 2000;82(11):1609–1618

Lewis JS Jr, Anderson RB. Lisfranc injuries in the athlete. Foot Ankle Int 2016;37(12):1374–1380

Ly TV, Coetzee JC. Treatment of primarily ligamentous Lisfranc joint injuries: primary arthrodesis compared with open reduction and internal fixation. A prospective, randomized study. J Bone Joint Surg Am 2006;88(3):514–520

48 Forefoot Fractures

Matthew I. Rudloff

Introduction

Forefoot fractures are frequently encountered in the clinical setting. The forefoot contributes to the intricate biomechanical performance of the foot during gait, and injuries to this anatomic area can result in significant disability. While many injuries to the forefoot can be successfully managed by nonoperative means, surgical intervention may be preferred in some circumstances.

Keywords: phalanx, phalanges, metatarsal, Jones, pseudo-Jones

I. History and Physical Examination

A. A careful history should not only include the mechanism of injury but also any remote injury, previous surgery, ambulatory status, and medical or social comorbidities that may influence decision-making, such as diabetes, neuropathy, or peripheral vascular disease.

B. Injury mechanisms typically are direct trauma or torsional for the metatarsals and phalanges, whereas a hyperextension moment is responsible for most metatarsophalangeal (MTP) dislocations.

C. Physical examination should include systematically inspecting and palpating the foot. Comparison to the contralateral foot can aid in identifying focal abnormalities.

D. A thorough neurovascular examination should be performed. Consider monofilament testing when concerns for underlying neuropathy exist.

E. Soft-tissue condition should be noted, particularly any impending compromise from fracture displacement, or open injuries.

F. Excessive or worsening pain should alert one to the potential for foot compartment syndrome and subsequent treatment.

II. Anatomy

A. First metatarsal

1. Shorter and wider.

2. Responsible for bearing one-third of the body's weight, in conjunction with its respective sesamoids.

3. Anterior tibialis and peroneus longus insert upon the first metatarsal, creating deforming forces when fractured.

4. No distal intermetatarsal ligament to provide stability.

B. Second through fourth metatarsals

1. Inherent stability afforded by the distal intermetatarsal ligaments.

C. Fifth metatarsal

1. Peroneus brevis and lateral band of plantar fascia insertion result in avulsion fractures with inversion injuries (pseudo-Jones' fracture; ▶Fig. 48.1).

2. Metatarsal metaphysis is supplied by retrograde nutrient vessel flow, creating a relatively avascular watershed area that can predispose to healing difficulties (Jones' fracture; ▶Fig. 48.1).

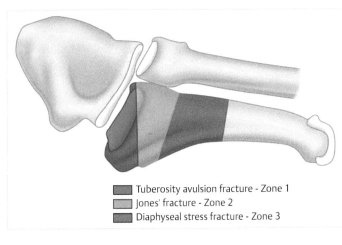

Fig. 48.1 Lawrence and Botte classification of the proximal fifth metatarsal fractures.

Tuberosity avulsion fracture - Zone 1
Jones' fracture - Zone 2
Diaphyseal stress fracture - Zone 3

D. Metatarsophalangeal joints
1. Stabilized primarily by the dorsal capsule, and plantar plate complex.
2. First MTP further stabilized by the extensor hallucis longus, flexor hallucis longus, and brevis tendons.

III. Imaging

A. Three-view radiographic evaluation
1. Anteroposterior, oblique, and lateral.
2. Weight-bearing radiographs.
3. Contralateral comparison films.
B. Computed tomography
1. CT may be used to further evaluate fracture comminution for surgical planning, particularly for the first metatarsal.
C. Magnetic resonance imaging
1. MRI is useful in evaluation of suspected stress fractures.

IV. Classification

A. First through fourth metatarsals
1. Location (neck, shaft, and base).
2. Displacement.
3. Comminution.
4. Angulation.
5. Articular involvement/dislocation.
B. Fifth metatarsal
1. Dancer fracture: distal spiral fracture of the fifth metatarsal (▶ **Fig. 48.2**).
2. Proximal (Lawrence and Botte; ▶ **Fig. 48.1**).
   a. Pseudo-Jones' fracture.
   b. Jones' fracture.
C. First metatarsophalangeal joint dislocation (▶ **Table 48.1**)
D. Lesser metatarsophalangeal joint dislocations and phalangeal fractures: descriptive classification.

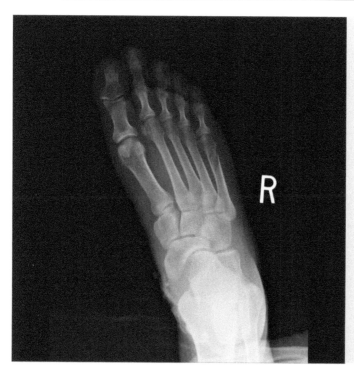

Fig. 48.2 Distal diaphyseal fracture of the fifth metatarsal.

Table 48.1 Jahss' classification for dislocations of the first metatarsophalangeal joint

Type I	Proximal phalanx is dislocated dorsally, and intersesamoid ligament is intact
Type IIA	Proximal phalanx is dislocated dorsally, and intersesamoid ligament is disrupted
Type IIB	Dislocation with associated sesamoid fracture

V. Treatment

A. Goal is to maintain or restore anatomy to permit normal load distribution across the foot.

B. First metatarsal fractures

1. Displacement disrupts the first metatarsal's critical role in forefoot weight bearing, and therefore little coronal or sagittal malalignment is tolerated.

2. Initial management: open or impending soft-tissue injury may warrant reduction or temporizing provisional Kirschner's wire fixation, or external fixation in select circumstances (▶ Fig. 48.3).

3. Definitive management:

   a. Nonoperative treatment is appropriate for minimally displaced or nondisplaced fractures.

   b. Malunion can result in transfer metatarsalgia, in which the normal physiologic load is shifted laterally to the lesser toes resulting in painful weight bearing. Therefore, operative intervention is indicated in displaced injuries.

4. Surgical approach:

   a. Dorsal approach—skin incision in line with the first ray. Deep interval is between the extensor hallucis longus and hallucis brevis. Protect the dorsomedial cutaneous nerve to the hallux medially, and the digital branch of the deep peroneal nerve to the second toe.

   b. Medial approach—skin incision in line with the first ray. The internervous interval is between the dorsomedial cutaneous nerve and the medial plantar hallucal nerve. The abductor hallucis muscle is retracted plantarly.

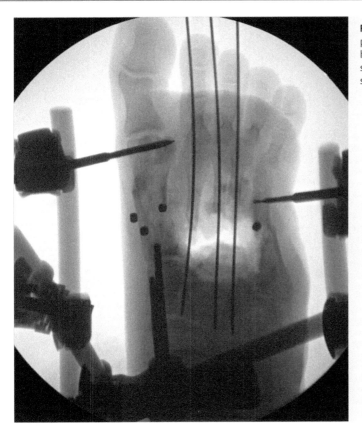

Fig. 48.3 External fixation can provide provisional stability for higher energy fractures with significant soft-tissue disruption, such as this ballistic injury.

5. Fixation technique:
   a. If anatomic closed reduction can be achieved, or significant soft-tissue injury precludes a formal surgical approach, then closed reduction and stabilization with Kirschner's wires can be performed.
   b. Otherwise, internal fixation with interfragmentary lag screws, neutralization plating, or bridge plating may be performed with low-profile small fragment (3.5-mm), mini-fragment (2.7-mm), or anatomic plates.
   c. Fractures with proximal articular involvement can be addressed with fixation extending across the tarsometatarsal joint (▶ **Fig. 48.4**).
6. Complications—hardware prominence.
7. Rehabilitation:
   a. Nonoperatively managed fractures can be initially immobilized with a cast or boot, immediate weight bearing as tolerated versus non-weight bearing for 4 to 6 weeks.
   b. Following operative stabilization, a splint can be applied until the surgical wound is appropriate, and then subsequent conversion to a cast or boot. Non–weight bearing for 4 to 6 weeks, followed by gradual progression.
C. Second through fourth metatarsals
   1. Definitive management:
      a. Central metatarsal fractures can frequently be managed nonoperatively with a hard-sole orthosis and weight bearing as tolerated when isolated and minimally displaced.
      b. Operative treatment should be considered for greater than 4 mm of displacement, greater than 10 degrees of sagittal plane deformity, and multiple metatarsal fractures.

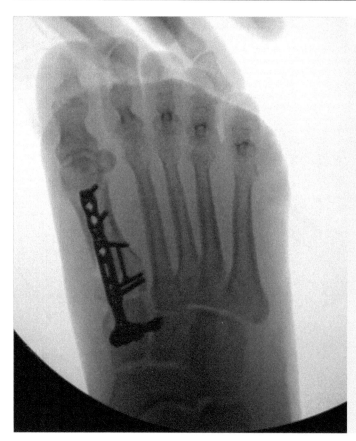

Fig. 48.4 Comminuted first metatarsal shaft with proximal articular extension.

    c. Coronal malalignment is better tolerated than displacement in the sagittal plane. The typical dorsal angulation results in the plantar flexion of the distal metatarsal, thus resulting in abnormal loading and transfer metatarsalgia.

    d. Metatarsal shaft fractures, unless multiple, or with significant sagittal plane displacement, can be managed nonoperatively.

    e. Metatarsal base fractures often are inherently more stable and can be treated nonoperatively, provided a more significant injury to the Lisfranc articulations can be ruled out.

2. Surgical approach:

    a. Percutaneous incisions, localized under fluoroscopy, can facilitate closed reduction maneuvers for fixation.

    b. Dorsal intermetatarsal approach:

        i. Exposure to the second and third metatarsals—make a longitudinal incision in this web space. The deep interval is then between the long and short toe extensor tendons.

       ii. Exposure to the fourth metatarsal—the incision is located along the dorsolateral aspect.

      iii. Fourth metatarsal base fractures—the deep interval lateral to the long extensor of the fifth toe, whereas for more distal fractures, deep dissection occurs between the long extensor of the fourth and fifth toes.

3. Fixation technique:

    a. Metatarsal fractures can be stabilized with mini-fragment plates (▶ **Fig. 48.5**), screws, or Kirschner's wires (▶ **Fig. 48.6**). Joint spanning plates can be utilized in the setting of extensive comminution of the base.

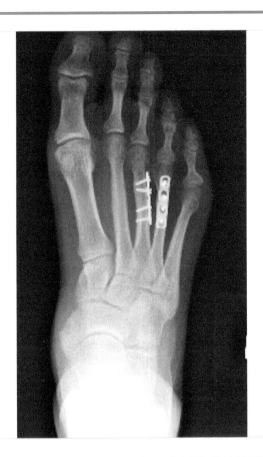

Fig. 48.5 Mini-fragment fixation for open multiple metatarsal fractures.

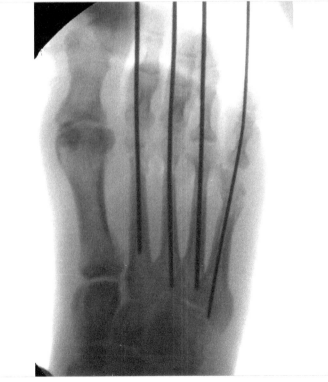

Fig. 48.6 Intramedullary Kirschner's wire fixation for multiple displaced metatarsal fractures.

    b. Most lesser metatarsal neck and shaft fractures can be stabilized with intramedullary Kirschner's wires, and less commonly mini-fragment devices.

    c. Adjuvant Kirschner's wires or a percutaneously placed dental pick can aid in reduction prior to fixation.

    d. Intramedullary Kirschner's wires can be placed retrograde, or through limited exposures in an antegrade/retrograde fashion.

    e. When using the retrograde technique, dorsiflexion of the toe can facilitate a central starting point on the metatarsal head, but can result in extension of the toe. Alternatively, the wire can be inserted into the base of the proximal phalanx, in line with the medullary canal of the metatarsal.

  4. Complications: Toe stiffness can occur with wire fixation. Malunion can lead to transfer metatarsalgia.

  5. Rehabilitation:

    a. Isolated, nondisplaced, or minimally displaced fractures can be treated with a hard-sole orthosis and permitted to weight bear as tolerated.

    b. Fractures treated with intramedullary Kirschner's wires typically are protected in a splint, and converted to a cast. Heel weight bearing is allowed. Pins are typically removed between 4 and 6 weeks once radiographic progression of healing is noted.

D. Fifth metatarsal

  1. Definitive management:

    a. Distal fractures can be managed similar to the central metatarsals. Significant angulation resulting in malunion can impact shoe wear.

    b. Proximal fractures require greater attention given the propensity for nonunion complications.

    c. Zone 1 (avulsion: pseudo-Jones') fractures can typically be managed nonoperatively, unless the fragment has extensive involvement and is displaced greater than 2 mm and greater than 30% of the metatarsal cuboid articulation.

    d. Zone 2 (metadiaphyseal: Jones') fractures managed nonoperatively require cast immobilization and non–weight bearing for minimum of 6 weeks, followed by gradual progression. Displaced fractures or those in younger, high-demand individuals benefit from operative fixation. Fractures that are subacute, stress fractures, or refractures are best treated surgically.

  2. Surgical approaches:

    a. Percutaneous approach—the appropriate starting portal is at the center of the base of the metatarsal.

    b. Lateral approach to the fifth metatarsal—skin incision begins just proximal to the styloid, proceeding distally. Incise the abductor digiti quinti fascia, retracting the musculature plantarly, exposing the metatarsal.

  3. Fixation techniques:

    a. This is typically performed by percutaneous placement of an intramedullary screw in acute fractures. Screw size should permit engagement of the threads into the diaphyseal cortical bone, without disrupting it.

    b. Alternative modalities include mini-fragment plates and tension band constructs but necessitate larger surgical exposures.

  4. Complications:

    a. Nonunion up to 20% of nonoperatively treated fractures.

    b. Implant-related complications include hardware prominence, hardware penetration, and secondary screw removal. Nonunion and refracture can also occur.

  5. Rehabilitation:

    a. Immobilization in a non–weight bearing cast or boot for a minimum of 6 weeks, potentially longer depending upon radiographic progression.

b. Time to union of nonoperatively managed metadiaphyseal fractures has been reported to be 16 weeks, whereas those treated acutely in a surgical manner heal in 7 to 8 weeks. Operative intervention in this subset of fractures permits earlier return to function.

E. First metatarsophalangeal joint dislocation

1. Definitive management: Urgent closed reduction should be attempted under local digital block anesthesia. If unsuccessful, operative open reduction should be undertaken. Typically, these are Jahss' type I injuries, where the first metatarsal head has become incarcerated with the plantar plate complex (▶ Table 48.1).

2. Surgical approach: Dorsal approach to the MTP joint—skin incision medial to the extensor hallucis longus tendon. The plantar plate, which may require release, can then be reduced from the metatarsal head. Residual instability may rarely require Kirschner's wire fixation.

3. Complications—stiffness, nonconcentric reduction, and osteoarthritis from chondral injury.

4. Rehabilitation—Immobilization with a hard-sole orthosis, with dorsiflexion limitation for 4 weeks. If Kirschner's wire fixation is necessary, wires can be removed at 4 weeks.

F. Lesser toe metatarsophalangeal dislocations (▶ Fig. 48.7)

1. Definitive management: similar to dislocations of the first MTP.

G. Phalangeal fractures

1. Definitive management:

a. Almost all phalangeal fractures can be managed by nonsurgical means. Nondisplaced or minimally displaced fractures can be effectively treated with buddy taping and a hard-sole orthosis.

b. Displaced fractures with visible deformity of the toe can be closed under digital anesthesia with longitudinal traction and correction of angulation.

c. Operative intervention considered for displaced intra-articular fractures of hallux.

2. Complications: Malunion can occur; however, it is rarely symptomatic.

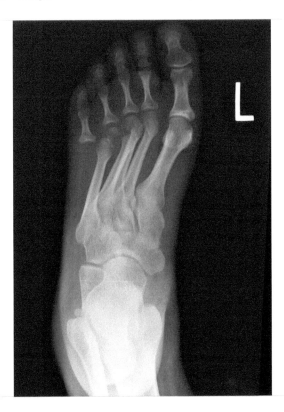

Fig. 48.7 Irreducible fifth metatarsophalangeal dislocation with associated the fourth metatarsal neck fracture, requiring open reduction.

Summary

Many forefoot fractures can be treated nonoperatively. In general, the more displaced the fracture or when multiple fractures are present, the more likely surgery might be beneficial. In the Emergency department setting, the safest course for anything other than a simple phalanx fracture is to splint and make non weight-bearing until the patient is evaluated by an Orthopaedic surgeon. Isolated closed phalangeal fractures can typically be made immediate WBAT and buddy tape for comfort.

Suggested Readings

Dean BJ, Kothari A, Uppal H, Kankate R. The jones fracture classification, management, outcome, and complications: a systematic review. Foot Ankle Spec 2012;5(4):256–259

Jahss MH. Traumatic dislocations of the first metatarsophalangeal joint. Foot Ankle 1980;1(1):15–21

Lawrence SJ, Botte MJ. Jones' fractures and related fractures of the proximal fifth metatarsal. Foot Ankle 1993;14(6):358–365

Mologne TS, Lundeen JM, Clapper MF, O'Brien TJ. Early screw fixation versus casting in the treatment of acute Jones fractures. Am J Sports Med 2005;33(7):970–975

Wiener BD, Linder JF, Giattini JFG. Treatment of fractures of the fifth metatarsal: a prospective study. Foot Ankle Int 1997;18(5):267–269

Zwitser EW, Breederveld RS. Fractures of the fifth metatarsal; diagnosis and treatment. Injury 2010;41(6):555–562

49 Cervical Spine Trauma

Carlo Bellabarba, Haitao Zhou, and Richard J. Bransford

Introduction

Injuries of the cervical spine, particularly when associated with spinal cord injury (SCI), rank among the costliest to society. The treatment of spine fractures should be tailored to each patient based on fracture pattern, comorbidities, and other patient factors. This chapter aims to provide an overview of the evaluation and preferred treatment of the more common injuries of the upper and subaxial cervical spine (▶Video 49.1).

Keywords: cervical, C-spine, neck, Hangman's, spinal cord injury

I. Preoperative

A. History and physical examination
   1. Preliminary evaluation:
      a. The highest priority in patients with cervical spine injury is to establish and maintain the airway, restore ventilation, and maintain blood pressure.
      b. Hypotension in trauma patients is typically due to insufficient blood volume, and responds to fluid resuscitation and transfusion. Patients with SCI may also have neurogenic shock from loss of sympathetic function, manifested as hypotension with bradycardia, which may be treated with vasopressors and atropine.
      c. Maintaining adequate spinal cord perfusion by keeping the mean arterial pressure at 80 mm Hg or higher may be a factor in minimizing the extent of SCI, and in promoting greater functional recovery.
   2. Clinical evaluation:
      a. After completing the primary survey, sensorimotor function of the extremities and the integrity of the spinal column are assessed in detail as part of the secondary survey.
      b. The neurological examination involves documentation of the American Spinal Injury Association (ASIA) Impairment Scale (AIS), the level of neurological injury, and the ASIA motor score, based on manual muscle testing of five key muscle groups in each of the four extremities (▶Fig. 49.1).
      c. Sensation to pinprick and light touch in all dermatomes and vibration or position sense are evaluated. Deep tendon reflexes in both arms and legs should be performed and pathologic responses recorded.
      d. Perineal function is assessed by evaluation of perianal pinprick sensation, voluntary anal sphincter contraction, and the bulbocavernosus reflex. Intact perianal function may be the only indication of an incomplete lesion and, in addition to having significant prognostic value, may influence the timing of surgical intervention.
      e. The use of high-dose methylprednisolone in adult patients within 8 hours of SCI due to nonpenetrating trauma is controversial. Particularly in patients with comorbidities, it may do more harm than good.

B. Imaging and cervical spine clearance
   1. Asymptomatic patients:
      a. The clinical evaluation is often key to assessing for potential spine injury.
      b. Important elements of the clinical examination include the presence of a neurological deficit, neck or back pain, or a palpable abnormality in spinal alignment.
      c. In alert, nonelderly patients with low-energy mechanisms and no distracting injuries, the absence of neck tenderness or pain through a physiologic range of motion is typically considered sufficient to clear the cervical spine without imaging.

ASIA impairment scale (AIS)

A = Complete: No sensory or motor function is preserved in the sacral segments S4–5.

B = Sensory incomplete: Sensory but not motor function is preserved below the neurological level and includes the sacral segments S4–5 (light touch or pin prick at S4–5 or deep anal pressure) and no motor function is preserved more than three levels below the motor level on either side of the body.

C = Motor incomplete: Motor function is preserved at the most caudal sacral segments for voluntary anal contraction (VAC) or the patient meets the criteria for sensory incomplete status (sensory function preserved at the most caudal sacral segments (S4–S5) by LT, PP or DAP), and has some sparing of motor function more than three levels below the ipsilateral motor level on either side of the body. (This includes key or non-key muscle functions to determine motor incomplete status.) For AIS C–less than half of key muscle functions below the single NLI have a muscle grade ≥ 3.

D = Motor incomplete: Motor incomplete status as defined above, with at least half (half or more) of key muscle functions below the single NLI having a muscle grade ≥ 3.

E = Normal: If sensation and motor function as tested with the ISNCSCI are graded as normal in all segments, and the patient had prior deficits, then the AIS grade is E. someone without an initial SCI does not receive an AIS grade.

Using ND: To document the sensory, motor and NLI levels, the ASIA Impairment Scale grade, and/or the zone of partial preservation (ZPP) when they are unable to be determined based on the examination results.

Fig. 49.1 American Spinal Injury Association International Standards for Neurological Classification of Spinal Cord Injury.

2. Symptomatic and obtunded patients:

   a. Patients who do not match the above description require radiographic screening, which consists of any variety of institutionally standardized methods designed to exclude fracture and confirm anatomic cervical alignment (▶ **Fig. 49.2**).

   b. The question of how cervical spine clearance should be undertaken in the comatose patient remains a matter of controversy.

   c. Radiographic evaluation:

      i. In trauma patients, the cross-table lateral plain radiograph has been widely supplanted by advanced imaging due to limited visualization of the cervicothoracic junction by plain films and improved speed of screening CT:

         • Radiographs are widely available and have a relatively high specificity (94%) and sensitivity (96%) in most circumstances.
         • These radiographs must be evaluated for soft-tissue swelling, fractures, and abnormalities in alignment.

      ii. CT scan:

         • High sensitivity (95–99%) and specificity (93%) for detecting cervical spine fractures.
         • Has become the primary screening method in level-one trauma centers.

      iii. MRI:

         • Useful in assessing vertebral column and spinal cord anatomy in patients with neurological deficits, and otherwise undetectable soft-tissue injuries that may influence treatment, such as nondisplaced diskoligamentous injury, disk herniation, and epidural hematoma.
         • Especially helpful in patients with progressive neurological deficits or deficits that do not correspond to CT findings.

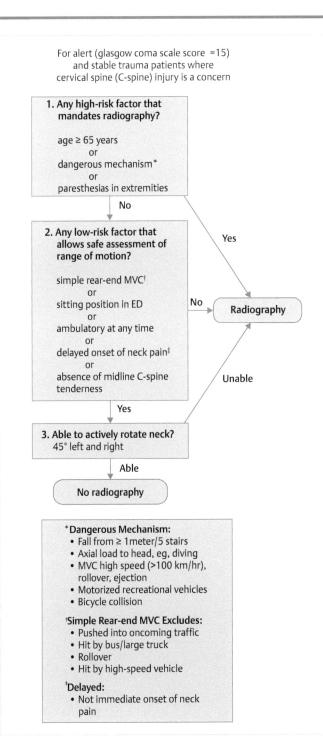

For alert (glasgow coma scale score =15)
and stable trauma patients where
cervical spine (C-spine) injury is a concern

Fig. 49.2 Canadian C-spine rule for cervical spine clearance.

1. Any high-risk factor that mandates radiography?

age ≥ 65 years
or
dangerous mechanism*
or
paresthesias in extremities

No

Yes

2. Any low-risk factor that allows safe assessment of range of motion?

simple rear-end MVC†
or
sitting position in ED
or
ambulatory at any time
or
delayed onset of neck pain‡
or
absence of midline C-spine tenderness

No → Radiography

Unable

Yes

3. Able to actively rotate neck?
45° left and right

Able

No radiography

*Dangerous Mechanism:
- Fall from ≥ 1meter/5 stairs
- Axial load to head, eg, diving
- MVC high speed (>100 km/hr), rollover, ejection
- Motorized recreational vehicles
- Bicycle collision

†Simple Rear-end MVC Excludes:
- Pushed into oncoming traffic
- Hit by bus/large truck
- Rollover
- Hit by high-speed vehicle

‡Delayed:
- Not immediate onset of neck pain

- Spinal cord signal change on MRI may also shed light on the nature of a neurological injury in the absence of osseous injury.
- MRI also allows for prognostic assessment of SCI.
- Although MRI has excellent sensitivity, its poor specificity makes it suboptimal in screening for cervical spine injuries.

iv. CT myelography may be useful if neuroimaging is desirable, but MRI is unavailable or contraindicated.

    v. Patients with high-energy mechanisms should also receive routine imaging of the thoracic and lumbar spine, whether by plain radiographs, helical CT, or reformatted thoracic and abdominopelvic CT.

II. Specific Injury Types by Anatomic Region: Classification, Treatment, Indications for Surgery, Outcomes, and Complications

A. Upper cervical spine (Occiput to C2)

The occipitocervical (O-C) junction is a functional unit that consists of osseoligamentous and neurovascular structures that extend from the skull base to C2. It includes the O-C and atlantoaxial articulations. Stability of the O-C junction is established primarily by its unusual ligamentous anatomy rather than by intrinsic bony stability. Patient outcome often depends more on associated intracranial injury than on the injury to the spine.

1. Occipital condyle fractures:

    a. Classification—occipital condyle fractures may be unstable when they represent bony avulsion of major O-C stabilizers. Anderson described a classification system (▶Fig. 49.3) consisting of three categories:

        • Type I: stable, comminuted axial loading injuries.
        • Type II: potentially unstable injuries caused by a shear mechanism that results in an oblique fracture extending from the condyle into the skull base.
        • Type III: alar ligament avulsion fractures that may be part of an unstable O-C dissociation.

    b. Indications for surgery—operative intervention, in the form of O-C fusion, is generally reserved for type III injuries with O-C instability. Nonoperative management with a cervical collar is recommended for the majority of (stable) type I and II injuries.

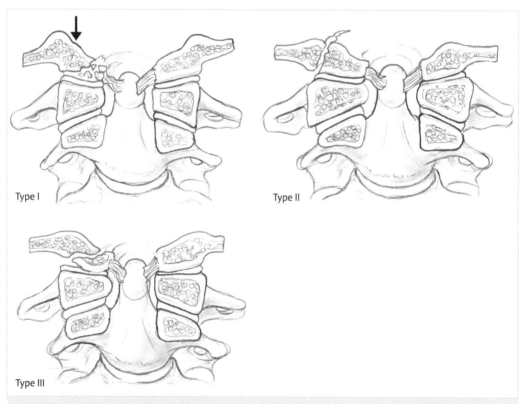

Fig. 49.3 Anderson and Montesano classification of occipital condyle fractures.

   c. Outcomes and complications—symptomatic post-traumatic arthritis resulting in neck pain, occipital headaches, restricted O-C motion, and torticollis.

   d. Palsy of closely associated cranial nerves (IX, X, XI, XII) has been described.

   e. If part of an O-C dissociation, prognosis is worse (see later).

2. OC dissociation:

   a. Classification—the Harborview classification system, based on the extent of instability, may require traction testing of minimally displaced injuries (≤2 mm) to appropriately guide treatment and prognosis.

   b. Indications for surgery: If the basion dens interval (BDI) or basion axis interval (BAI) is greater than 12 mm, O-C dissociation is likely, and should be investigated with MRI.

   c. Displacement of more than 2 mm at the atlantooccipital joint on static imaging or with provocative traction testing (▶Fig. 49.4), or the presence of neurological injury, is an indication for O-C stabilization.

   d. Outcomes and complications—most O-C dissociations are fatal.

   e. The outcome of survivors is dependent on the following:

      i. Type and severity of associated injuries, particularly closed head injuries.

      ii. Severity of neurological injury at the O-C junction.

      iii. Timing of diagnosis and stabilization of O-C dissociation is important. Delayed diagnosis is associated with secondary neurological deterioration and possibly death in up to 75% of patients.

   f. Vertebral artery injury should be considered in any distractive upper cervical injury.

3. Fractures of the atlas:

   a. Classification—classified as either stable or unstable based on the integrity of the transverse alar ligament (TAL).

   b. TAL insufficiency can be diagnosed directly by identifying bony avulsion on CT scan or ligament rupture on MRI, or indirectly by identifying widening of the C1 lateral masses with ≥7 mm lateral overhang relative to the lateral masses of C2 on either open mouth odontoid or coronal CT images (▶Fig. 49.5).

   c. C1 fractures are also classified as (i) axial loading type C1 ring fractures, (ii) lateral mass fractures, and (iii) posterior arch fractures.

   d. Indications for surgery—most C1 fractures are treated nonoperatively.

   e. If upright radiographs with external immobilization show unacceptable lateral mass displacement (≥7 mm) or an anterior atlantodens interval (ADI) of greater than 3 mm, patients are typically treated with posterior C1–C2 or occiput C2 fixation.

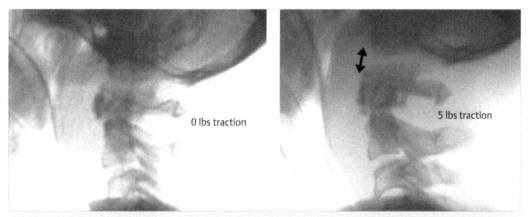

0 lbs traction

5 lbs traction

Fig. 49.4 Positive provocative traction test, manifested as greater than 2 mm of atlantooccipital joint distraction, can be used to confirm the diagnosis of occipitocervical dissociation in a patient with instability that was out of proportion to the amount of initial occipitocervical displacement.

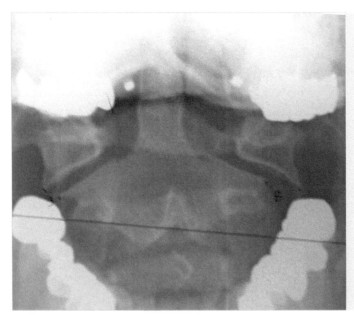

Fig. 49.5 Upright open-mouth anter-oposterior (odontoid view) view demonstrates a cumulative 11-mm overhang bilaterally of the C1 lateral masses beyond the C2 lateral mass, suggesting rupture of the transverse atlantal ligament. Although the C1–C2 overhang can also be measured on coronal CT images, upright open mouth views provide a better measure of stability due to loading of the spine in the upright position.

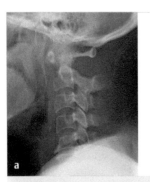
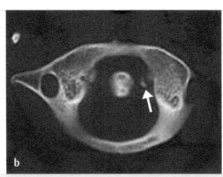
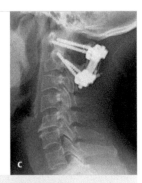

Fig. 49.6 (a) Lateral radiograph demonstrates anterior translation of C1 on C2 with increased atlanto dens interval associated with traumatic transverse atlantal ligament (TAL) disruption. (b) Axial CT shows avulsion fracture of the TAL insertion site (*arrow*), which makes this injury potentially amenable to nonoperative treatment. (c) Due to the high amount of displacement and instability and the patient's multiple injuries, a C1–C2 posterior instrumented arthrodesis was performed as demonstrated on lateral x-ray done 6 months postoperatively.

    f. Surgical stabilization typically consists of posterior C1–C2 instrumented fusion.

    g. Outcomes and complications:

       i. Severe complications are rare.

      ii. Eighty percent incidence of residual neck pain, possibly due to post-traumatic arthritis.

      iii. Seventeen percent nonunion rate.

      iv. Severe malunion of unstable atlas fractures may result in painful torticollis, requiring realignment and O-C fusion.

  4. Atlantoaxial instability:

    a. Classification—three atlantoaxial instability patterns can occur and may coexist.

      i. Type A injuries are rotationally displaced in the transverse plane. These deformities are usually nontraumatic in nature.

      ii. Type B injuries are translationally unstable in the sagittal plane due to TAL insufficiency. Distinguishing a ligamentous TAL tear (type I) from a bony avulsion fracture (type II) may impact treatment (▶Fig. 49.6).

      iii. Type C injuries are distractive injuries that represent a variant of O-C dissociation.

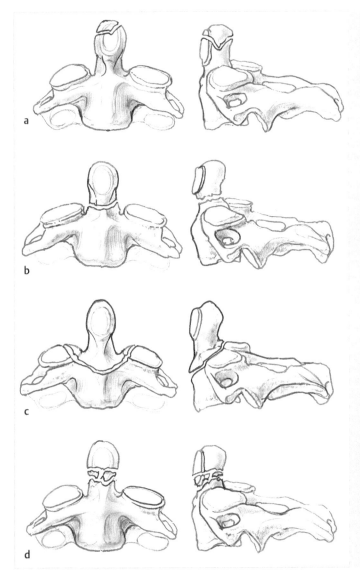

Fig. 49.7 Anderson and D'Alonzo classification of odontoid fractures. (a) Type I. (b) Type II. (c) Type III. (d) Type IIa (segmentally comminuted).

    b. Diagnosis:
        i. Type B: suspect if plain radiographs or CT shows ADI greater than 3 mm.
        ii. Type C: suspect if distraction is noted on imaging studies or if Harris' lines are greater than 12 mm.
    c. Indications for surgery:
        i. Type B: translational instability—posterior atlantoaxial arthrodesis.
        ii. Type C: distraction injuries—posterior atlantoaxial versus O–C stabilization.
    d. Outcomes and complications:
        i. Acute TAL insufficiency is usually fatal.
        ii. In survivors, profound neurological deficits or head injury may be present.
        iii. Syncope and vertigo may result from injury to vertebrobasilar arterial system.
        iv. Atlantoaxial distraction has a similar prognosis to O–C dissociation.
  5. Odontoid fractures:
    a. Classification—three-part classification of Anderson and D'Alonzo (▶ **Fig. 49.7**).
        i. Type I injuries are bony avulsions of the alar ligament, which may result in O–C dissociation.

  ii. Type II injuries at the odontoid waist, which have the highest propensity for pseudar-
    throsis, due to vascular watershed phenomenon and small cancellous bone surface
    area. The IIa subtype consists of a highly unstable, segmentally comminuted fracture.

  iii. Type III fractures extend into the cancellous vertebral body and have wider, well-
    vascularized cancellous fracture surfaces.

 b. Indications for surgery:

  i. Type I:

- The treatment of type I odontoid fractures relates to their impact on O-C stability.
  The indications for surgical management of these injuries are therefore the same as
  those discussed for the treatment of O-C instability.

  ii. Type II:

- Surgical indications remain controversial, but the weight of recent evidence suggests
  decreased mortality and complications with surgery. We advocate surgical stabilization for displaced fractures in patients with functional needs, distractive patterns of
  displacement, or fractures with associated SCI (▶ Fig. 49.8).
- Relative indications include multiply injured patients, associated closed head injury, initial displacement of greater than 4 mm, angulation greater than 10 degrees,
  delayed presentation (>2 weeks), multiple risk factors for nonunion, the inability
  to externally immobilize, associated intracranial or thoracoabdominal injury, other
  medical comorbidities, and the presence of associated upper cervical fractures.
- Displaced, noncomminuted fractures with favorable bone quality and fracture obliquity and appropriate body habitus are ideal for anterior odontoid screw fixation.
- In patients with extensive fracture comminution, compromised bone quality, or with
  technical constraints to anterior odontoid screw trajectory, we favor posterior atlantoaxial fusion using either transarticular screw fixation or segmental C1–C2 fixation.

  iii. Type III:

- Operative stabilization is not commonly required, but is warranted in patients with
  significant/progressive deformity, SCI, or distractive instability patterns.
- Delayed unions or pseudoarthroses occur in up to half of nonoperatively treated
  patients, and are also amenable to posterior C1–C2 or C1–C3 fixation.

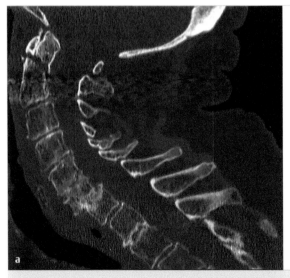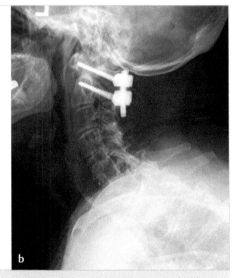

Fig. 49.8 **(a)** Sagittal CT image demonstrates displaced type II geriatric odontoid fracture, which was treated with
posterior reduction and C1–C2 instrumented arthrodesis. **(b)** Postoperative upright lateral X-ray shows restoration of
alignment and stability.

- Posterior C1–C2 versus C3 posterior spinal instrumentation and fusion (PSIF) is the surgical treatment method of choice, since anterior odontoid screw fixation has a high failure rate with type III odontoid fractures.

c. Outcomes and complications:

  i. Associated with significant morbidity and mortality.
  ii. Neurological injury occurs in up to 25% of type II odontoid fractures, and ranges in severity from isolated cranial nerve injury to complete quadriplegia.
  iii. One-year mortality rates for elderly patients with type II odontoid fracture have been reported to be as high as 40%.
  iv. Fracture nonunion and missed injuries are the most common complications.
  v. Risk factors for nonunion include initial nonoperative treatment, displacement of greater than 4 mm, fracture angulation greater than 10 degrees, male gender, older age, and delay in treatment.
  vi. Perioperative complication rate of approximately 30% and a nonunion rate of approximately 10% have been described with odontoid screw fixation.
  vii. C1–C2 fusions have reported nonunion rates of 4% or less using rigid fixation.
  viii. Though considered more benign injuries, nonoperative treatment of type III odontoid fractures is associated with pseudoarthrosis rates of 9 to 13%.

6. Traumatic spondylolisthesis of the axis (hangman's fractures):

a. Classification—three primary injury types and two "atypical" subtypes (▶Fig. 49.9).

  i. Type I: minimally displaced, stable fracture of the pars interarticularis.
  ii. Type IA: atypical unstable, obliquely displaced fracture typically extending through one pars and more anteriorly into the body on the contralateral side.
  iii. Type II: displaced injuries of pars interarticularis with greater than 3 mm C2–C3 translation.
  iv. Type IIA: unstable flexion–distraction injury with associated C2–C3 disk and interspinous ligament disruption. Kyphosis is the prevailing deformity rather than translation (▶Fig. 49.10).
  v. Type III: Unstable injuries in which C2–C3 facet dislocation accompanies pars interarticularis fracture.

b. Indications for surgery:

  i. Operative stabilization is rarely indicated for traumatic spondylolisthesis of the axis, the most common of which are type II injuries.
  ii. Most type I and II injuries are treated with 12 weeks of external immobilization using a rigid collar or halo vest.
  iii. Type IA injuries behave unpredictably and often fail nonoperative treatment.
  iv. Type IIA injuries typically require surgical stabilization:

    - Traction is contraindicated, as it accentuates their kyphotic deformity.
    - A C2–C3 anterior diskectomy and fusion (ACDF) with plating allows for fusion across the least number of levels (▶Fig. 49.10).
    - Posterior stabilization is more stable, but unless adequate purchase is achieved across the fractured C2 pars interarticularis, loss of atlantoaxial motion results from the need to extend fixation to C1.

c. Type III injuries are generally irreducible by traction and require open posterior reduction and stabilization. Stabilization options include the following:

  i. Posterior C1–C3 fusion.
  ii. Posterior C2–C3 fusion using lag screws across the fracture at C2.
  iii. Anterior C2–C3 ACDF if reduction has occurred spontaneously or in the unusual event that reduction occurs by closed methods.

d. Outcomes and complications:

  i. Associated injuries such as upper cervical (15%), subaxial (23%), or head injuries usually have a greater influence on prognosis than the C2 fracture itself.
  ii. Neurological injury has been identified in only up to 10% of patients, but occurs in 60% of type III and 33% of type IA fractures (▶Fig. 49.11).

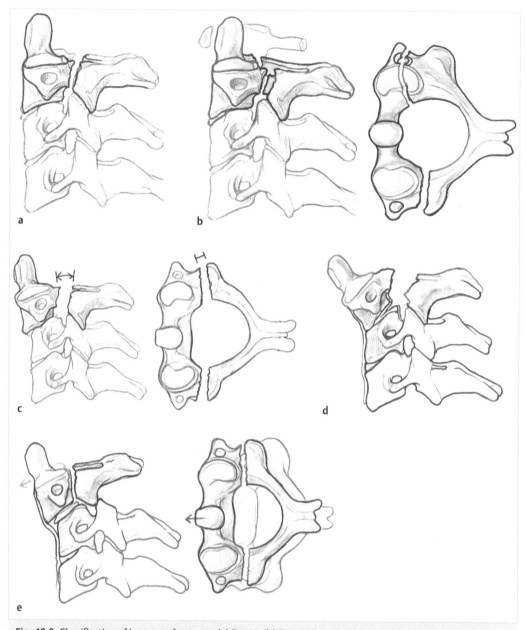

Fig. 49.9 Classification of hangman fractures. **(a)** Type I. **(b)** Type IA (atypical hangman fracture). **(c)** Type II. **(d)** Type IIA. **(e)** Type III.

    iii. Type IA injuries also have a greater potential for vertebral artery injury because of common foramen transversarium involvement.

    iv. Traumatic spondylolistheses of the axis have a 5% pseudoar-throsis rate.

    v. Type IA, IIA and III fractures are more challenging to treat due to either atypical fracture orientation or associated ligamentous injury.

B. Subaxial cervical spine (below C2)

    1. Classification of subaxial cervical spine injuries:

        a. There is no universally accepted classification system for fractures and dislocations of the subaxial cervical spine.

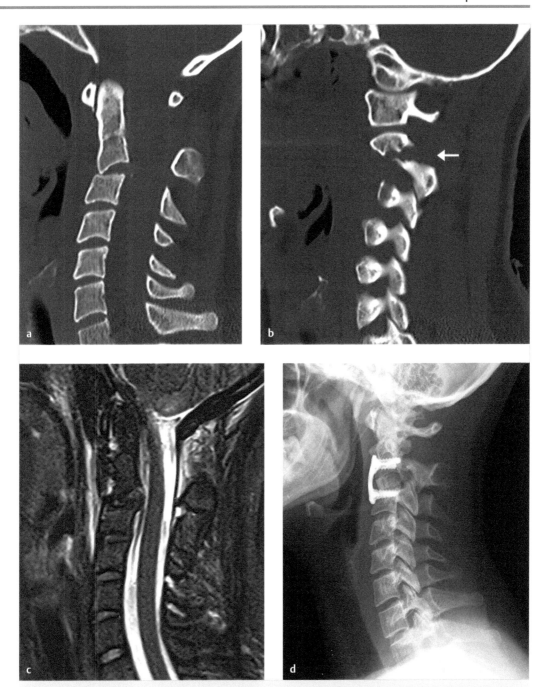

Fig. 49.10 Sagittal CT images at midline **(a)** and through the pars interarticularis **(b)** show kyphosis disproportionate to the degree of anterior translation and a horizontal tension type failure of the pars interarticularis (*arrow*), both of which are hallmarks of the type IIA hangman fracture. This injury typically results from a flexion–distraction mechanism, causing posterior-to-anterior disruption of the C2–C3 disk space, which is illustrated on sagittal T2-weighted MRI **(c)**. **(d)** Lateral X-ray 3 months after anterior diskectomy and fusion shows acceptable alignment.

    b. A recently developed (2016) AO subaxial C-spine injury classification combines morphological features of the injury, type of facet injury, severity of neurological injury, and patient specific modifiers (▶**Fig. 49.12**).

    c. Brief summary of AO classification:

        i. Morphology.

       ii. Type A: compression injuries with intact tension band (AO through A4).

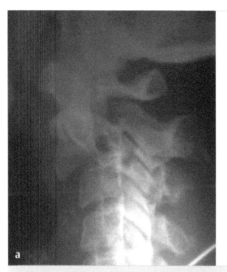
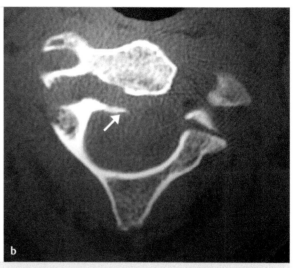

Fig. 49.11 Atypical (type IA) hangman fracture, as seen on **(a)** lateral X-ray and **(b)** axial CT image. Along with type III injuries, type IA injuries have a higher propensity for causing spinal cord injury than other hangman fractures because the fracture pattern may form a spike that impinges on the spinal cord with fracture displacement (*arrow*).

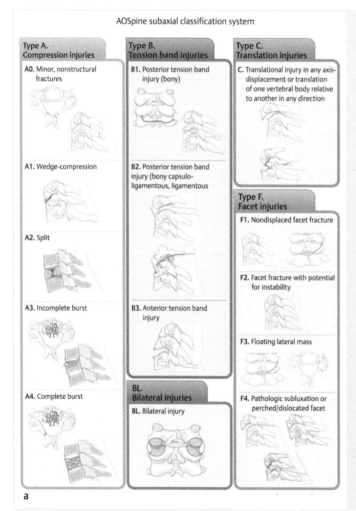

AOSpine subaxial classification system

Type A.
Compression injuries

A0. Minor, nonstructural fractures

A1. Wedge-compression

A2. Split

A3. Incomplete burst

A4. Complete burst

Type B.
Tension band injuries

B1. Posterior tension band injury (bony)

B2. Posterior tension band injury (bony capsulo-ligamentous, ligamentous)

B3. Anterior tension band injury

BL.
Bilateral injuries

BL. Bilateral injury

Type C.
Translation injuries

C. Translational injury in any axis-displacement or translation of one vertebral body relative to another in any direction

Type F.
Facet injuries

F1. Nondisplaced facet fracture

F2. Facet fracture with potential for instability

F3. Floating lateral mass

F4. Pathologic subluxation or perched/dislocated facet

a

Fig. 49.12 (a) AO morphological classification of subaxial cervical spine fractures.

(Continued)

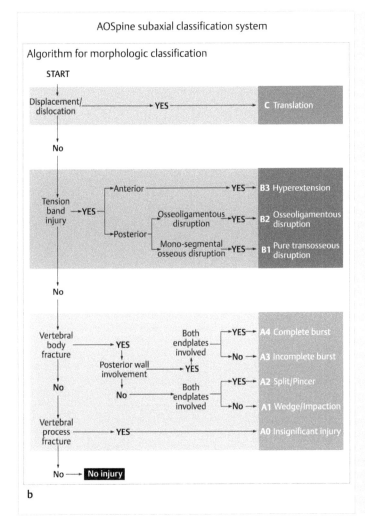

Fig. 49.12 (*Continued*) (b) Algorithm for determining AO subaxial cervical spine injury type. (Acknowledgment of copyright - AOSpine International© AOSpine International, Switzerland Acknowledgment of the AOSpine Knowledge Forum work "AOSpine is a clinical division of the AO Foundation—an independent medically guided nonprofit organization. The AOSpine Knowledge Forums are pathology-focused working groups acting on behalf of AOSpine in their domain of scientific expertise. Each forum consists of a steering committee of up to 10 international spine experts who meet on a regular basis to discuss research, assess the best evidence for current practices, and formulate clinical trials to advance spine care worldwide. Study support is provided directly through AOSpine's Research department and AO's Clinical Investigation and Documentation unit. This figure can be found at www.aospine.org/classification.)

b

   iii. Type B: tension band injuries without spinal discontinuity or translation (B1 vs. B2).

   iv. Type C: displacement or translation of one vertebral body relative to another in any direction; anterior, posterior, lateral translation, or vertical distraction (no subtypes):

- Injuries are classified by level and either C, B, or A in this order.
- Type A (vertebral body) injuries associated with type B or C injuries are then listed, as they may affect treatment or prognosis.

   v. Facet injury descriptors (F1 through F4):

- Describe the specific features of the facet injury.
- F1: nondisplaced facet fracture.
- F2: facet fracture with potential for instability.
- F3: floating lateral mass.
- F4: pathologic subluxation or perched/dislocated facet.

   vi. Neurological examination (Nx and N0 through N4):

- Describes the severity of neurological injury.
- Complimentary to the AIS and ASIA motor scores.

   vii. Case-specific modifiers—patient or injury features that may affect treatment or prognosis:

- M1: evidence of posterior capsuloligamentous complex injury without complete disruption.
- M2: critical disk herniation.

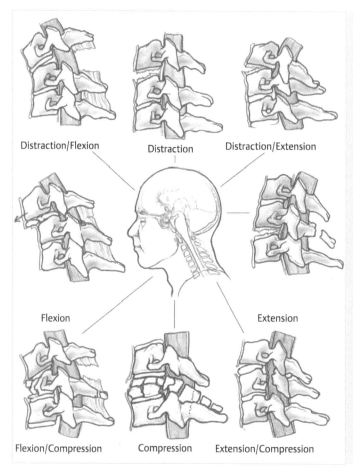

Fig. 49.13 The Allen–Ferguson cervical spine fracture classification is based on the presumed forces applied to the neck at the time of injury, and results in a continuum of fracture patterns based on varying and often combined influence of four primary force vectors: distraction, extension, compression, and flexion. A lateral compression injury pattern was also included, but is not illustrated.

- • M3: ankylosing spine condition.
- • M4: vertebral artery injury.

d. Mechanistic classification systems based on that proposed by Allen et al in 1982 can be valuable in comprehending instability patterns. It is useful to consider the injury mechanism as occurring along a continuum involving four "cardinal" force vectors to which the spine may be subjected: distraction, compression, extension, and flexion (▶ Fig. 49.13).

2. Injury categories:

a. AO type A injuries: vertical compression injuries—burst fractures:

i. General considerations:

- • Vertical compression injuries result from an axial load applied to the top of the head with the cervical spine in a nonflexed position. The fracture pattern, commonly known as a cervical burst fracture if the posterior cortex is involved, is characterized by relatively symmetric loss of anterior and posterior vertebral body height.
- • Uncommon injury with C7 most commonly affected.
- • Distinguished from flexion–compression (flexion teardrop) injuries by relative absence of kyphosis and translational malalignment.
- • Injury to the posterior ligament complex is uncommon.

ii. Treatment:

- • Treatment is largely determined by the presence or absence of SCI, the degree of canal compromise, spinal alignment, and the integrity of posterior soft tissues (▶ Fig. 49.14).

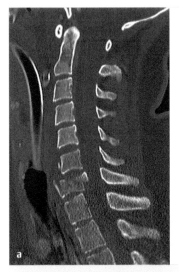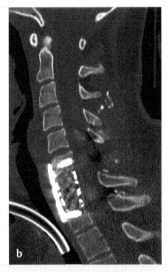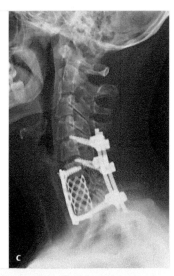

Fig. 49.14 (a) Sagittal CT image demonstrates a C7 burst fracture. These typically occur in the lower cervical spine. Because of the extent of comminution, and the presence of neurological deficits, the patient underwent an anteroposterior reconstruction consisting of C7 corpectomy, C6–C7 laminectomy and C5–T1 posterior arthrodesis, as demonstrated on (b) postoperative sagittal CT image and (c) lateral X-ray 6 months postoperatively.

- If overall architecture of the vertebral body is reasonably well maintained, with minimal retropulsion and no neurological injury, treatment consists of 12 weeks of immobilization with a rigid cervical orthosis, SOMI-type brace or halo vest.
- With more severe loss of vertebral body height, wider centrifugal fracture displacement resulting in greater bony retropulsion into the spinal canal, kyphotic malalignment, and neurological deficit occurs more frequently. Anterior decompression and stabilization with corpectomy, interbody reconstruction, and plating are warranted. Addition of PSIF is appropriate if there is concern about stability of stand-alone anterior reconstruction, particularly in the presence of posterior ligamentous injury (type B injury).

b. AO type B injuries—extension or flexion "bending" injuries without translational displacement.

   i. Caused primarily by a flexion or extension moment, with potential application of compressive or distractive forces that give characteristic morphological features (▶Fig. 49.15, ▶Fig. 49.16).

   ii. More severe stages of these injuries may involve sagittal plane translation, which typically affects treatment and prognosis, thus categorizing them as type C injuries (▶Fig. 49.17).

   iii. Facet injuries are quantified separately (▶Fig. 49.12) based on the severity of the facet injury.

c. AO type C injuries—unilateral facet dislocations and fracture-dislocations with translational displacement.

   i. The defining characteristic is a rotational deformity in the axial plane.

   ii. The rotational deformity in unilateral facet injuries is manifested on sagittal plane images as 25% or less anterolisthesis of the affected vertebral body (▶Fig. 49.18).

   iii. The mechanism of injury involves a flexion injury with resulting distraction of the posterior elements, coupled with a rotational force.

d. AO type C injuries—bilateral facet dislocations and fracture-dislocations with translational displacement.

   i. Typically results in at least 50% anterior vertebral body translation. Facet fractures occur frequently with unilateral and bilateral facet dislocations.

   ii. Reversal of the position of the superior relative to the inferior facets provides the typical appearance of facet dislocation on axial and sagittal CT images.

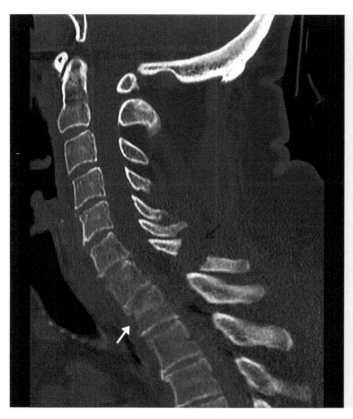

Fig. 49.15 Sagittal CT image demonstrates a C7–T1 flexion–distraction injury, consisting of tension failure of the C7 spinous process (*black arrow*) and compression fracture of the superior end plate of T1 (*white arrow*).

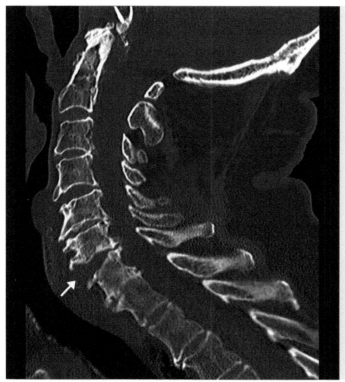

Fig. 49.16 C6–C7 extension fracture in a patient with diffuse idiopathic spinal hyperostosis (DISH). Injuries that have angulation without translation are designated as type B injuries.

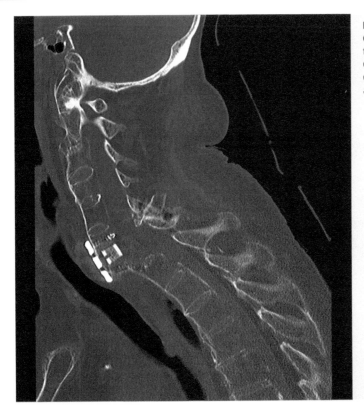

Fig. 49.17 Sagittal CT image of C6–C7 extension fracture with translational malalignment (AO type C) that occurred below a previous C6–C7 fusion in a patient with ankylosing spondylitis.

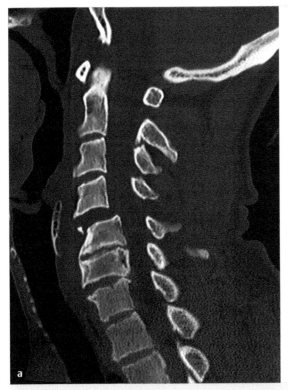
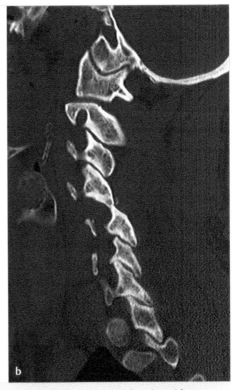

Fig. 49.18 Sagittal CT images along the midline **(a)** and the left facet joints **(b)** show a C4–C5 left unilateral facet dislocation with perched facets. Anterior vertebral body translation of less than 25% at the injury level indicates the presence of unilateral facet dislocation.

    iii. MRI illustrates the soft-tissue injury and degree of spinal cord compression, and is likely to show disruption of the interspinous ligament and facet capsules, with at least partial intervertebral disk disruption in over 60% of cases.

    iv. Disruption of the annulus may result in disk extrusion into the spinal canal, which may have important treatment implications, as discussed in detail later.

    v. MRI also plays a prognostic role in predicting the potential for functional recovery from SCI based on the appearance of the injured spinal cord.

3. The role of prereduction MRI:

    a. Whether an MRI scan to identify disk herniation is required prior to closed reduction of facet dislocations remains a matter of considerable controversy.

    b. Spinal realignment in the presence of posteriorly extruded disk material has been postulated to result in SCI from cord compression, if reduction causes displacement of the disk material into the canal.

    c. However, regardless of the presence of intervertebral disk extrusion, if a patient can participate for neurological examination, closed reduction with clinical monitoring of neurological status has been shown to be safe, with the understanding that the procedure be aborted at the first sign of neurological abnormality.

    d. Conversely, in a patient who is obtunded, anesthetized, or in whom a reliable neurological examination cannot be obtained during the course of reduction, circumstances may dictate that an MRI scan be obtained prior to any attempt at reduction. If the MRI were to demonstrate a concerning disk extrusion, anterior diskectomy could be undertaken prior to spinal realignment and fixation.

    e. Available evidence does not strongly support any treatment standard for facet dislocations.

    f. The risk of neurological worsening during spinal realignment must be weighed against the detrimental effect of delay in spinal realignment on neurological outcome.

4. Treatment:

    a. Closed reduction technique:

       i. Patients who present with a unilateral or bilateral facet dislocation, particularly when associated with neurological injury, should undergo an attempt at closed reduction at the earliest possibility, according to the above guidelines.

      ii. The reduction is ideally performed in a fluoroscopy suite, under mild sedation.

     iii. Traction pulleys are positioned to allow for flexion of the neck during the initial phase of reduction to facilitate disengagement of the dislocated facet.

     iv. After application of the initial 5 to 10 lb of traction, the O-C junction should be scrutinized for undetected unstable ligamentous injuries.

     v. With the addition of subsequent weight, the injured level and all other intervertebral levels should be evaluated for unacceptable distraction.

     vi. A thorough sensorimotor evaluation must be performed after each increase in weight, and the patient should be questioned regarding the presence of new or worsening neurological symptoms. Any such complaints should cause the reduction procedure to be aborted in lieu of an open reduction (see later).

     vii. Weight is added in 5- to 10-lb increments until the dislocated facet appears to have "cleared" its more caudal counterpart. Increasing the extension vector of the traction by lowering the height of the traction pulley or placing an interscapular bump beneath the patient may then facilitate the final phase of reduction.

    viii. Once reduction has been achieved, traction weight is incrementally reduced under fluoroscopic evaluation to between 15 and 25 lb, depending on which level is involved. Higher weights may be required if recurrence of subluxation occurs.

     ix. An MRI of the cervical spine is obtained at the earliest possibility, regardless of whether one was obtained prior to reduction, to evaluate the spinal cord and the presence of any compressive lesions.

     x. If an objective neurological deficit occurs, the inciting event should be reversed. Although controversial, methylprednisolone might be administered according to institutional protocol. Imaging studies should be obtained to assess for potential causes.

   b. Definitive surgical treatment:

      i. Cervical facet dislocations and fracture-dislocations require operative stabilization.

     ii. In the absence of anterior compressive lesions on postreduction MRI, posterior stabilization is appropriate, and may be superior biomechanically to anterior fixation.

   iii. Even in the absence of disk herniation, ACDF is acceptable and sometimes preferable, particularly in patients whose care could be compromised by prone positioning, or in whom ACDF might spare a fusion level.

   iv. Although biomechanically inferior to PSIF, treatment with ACDF has been largely equivalent for (fracture-)dislocations, with fusion rates exceeding 90%.

    v. In the presence of significant disk herniation on postreduction MRI, particularly with associated neurological deficits, ACDF is the most appropriate treatment.

   vi. Although not always necessary after ACDF, adding PSIF may be appropriate for highly unstable injuries or in patients otherwise prone to failure of fixation due to osteoporosis or other medical comorbidities.

  vii. The inability to successfully reduce a facet dislocation with closed techniques may complicate the choice of anterior versus posterior approach.

 viii. Traditionally, in the absence of disk herniation, unreduced flexion–distraction injuries have been realigned and stabilized through a posterior approach.

   ix. Conventional treatment for unreduced injuries with MRI evidence of disk herniation has been anterior diskectomy followed by prone positioning and posterior reduction and stabilization, possibly followed by anterior interbody fusion.

    x. If an anterior approach is warranted for unreduced dislocations, the authors prefer to complete the reduction and stabilization entirely from the anterior approach, when possible. Once the diskectomy has been performed, reduction can safely be performed by various means, such as Gardner–Wells tong traction, or direct manipulation of the vertebral bodies with a Cobb elevator, lamina spreader, or Caspar pins.

   xi. Surgical procedures requiring reduction are performed with spinal cord monitoring.

C. Flexion–Compression (flexion teardrop) injuries

  1. General considerations:

    a. Axial loading injuries with an associated flexion force vector, typically caused by diving injuries, football spearing injuries, and motor vehicle collisions.

    b. Consistent injury pattern with varying degrees of severity:

      i. In more severe stages, the primary fracture line separates the anteroinferior corner of the vertebral body (the so-called teardrop), which remains aligned with the caudal intervertebral disk and vertebra, from the remaining, posteriorly displaced vertebral body.

     ii. The severity of retrolisthesis and canal compromise, the presence of which qualifies the injury as AO type C, correlates with risk of SCI. Injuries with greater than 3 mm of retrolisthesis have greater than 90% likelihood of SCI, over half of which are complete.

   iii. The axial compression results in an associated sagittal split through the vertebral body in up to two-thirds of cases, as well as bilaminar fracture. The combination of sagittal vertebral body split with neural arch fracture is usually associated with a severe SCI.

    c. The flexion component threatens the integrity of the posterior ligamentous structures.

  2. Classification:

    a. The severity of flexion–compression injuries is contingent on the degree of vertebral comminution, kyphosis, and retrolisthesis.

    b. Radiographs and CT scan should be scrutinized for evidence of interspinous or facet widening, and MRI should be obtained to assess the status of the interspinous ligament, facet capsules, and ligamentum flavum.

    c. Lower-grade injuries without gross angular or translational malalignment or compromise of the posterior ligamentous complex (PLC) are best classified as AO type A injuries.

    d. Moderate-grade injuries with disruption of the PLC and kyphosis, without retrolisthesis, are best classified as AO type B injuries (**Fig. 49.19**).

    e. The highest grade injuries, in which PLC injury and kyphosis are associated with retrolisthesis, are best classified as AO type C injuries (**Fig. 49.20**).

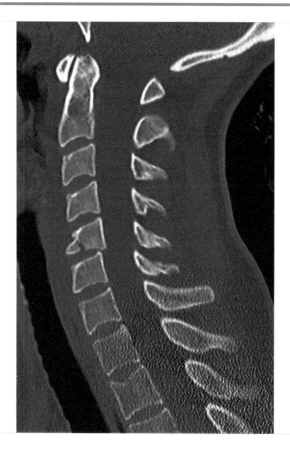

Fig. 49.19 Sagittal CT image of C5 flexion teardrop fracture in a neurologically normal patient. Because there is minimal retrolisthesis and kyphosis, and no evidence of severe posterior element injury, an anterior-only reconstruction was performed.

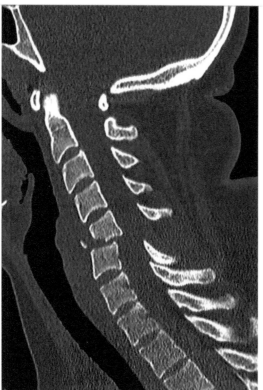

Fig. 49.20 Sagittal CT image of a C5 flexion teardrop fracture with severe retrolisthesis and posterior ligamentous complex disruption with kyphosis in patient with quadriplegia.

3. Treatment:

   a. Patients with SCI or injuries qualifying as AO type B or C require surgery.

   b. Low-grade (type A) injuries—in the absence of neurological deficits, nonoperative treatment with 12 weeks of rigid external immobilization:

      i. The potential for progressive kyphosis and instability after nonoperative treatment is high, and requires careful radiographic follow-up.

      ii. Flexion–extension radiographs should be obtained after 12 weeks, when external immobilization is discontinued.

      iii. Anterior corpectomy and instrumentation are required in the presence of SCI.

   c. Moderate- to high-grade (types B and C) injuries: operative intervention is required in the presence of SCI or PLC injury:

      i. Corpectomy with anterior instrumentation is the surgical treatment of choice, for flexion teardrop injuries, and is superior to rigid immobilization in maintaining sagittal alignment and minimizing treatment failures.

      ii. Supplemental posterior fixation may be required in more severe injuries, in the presence of metabolic bone disease, if stability remains a concern due to extensive posterior injury, or if a posterior approach is required for the purpose of spinal cord decompression.

4. Outcomes—high-fusion and functional neurological recovery rates in patients with incomplete SCI have been reported with anterior treatment of flexion–compression injuries, with few approach-related complications.

D. Extension injuries

1. General consideration:

   a. Extension injuries usually result from a blow to the face or forehead.

   b. The degree to which extension is combined with a distraction or compression force vectors influences both the injury morphology and subsequent treatment.

   c. In extension–distraction injuries, the sequence of injury to the spinal column progresses from the anterior through the middle column to the posterior column. Simultaneous compressive forces across the posterior elements may result in fractures involving the neural arch, lateral masses, or pedicles.

   d. Extension injuries typically result from high-energy mechanisms in younger patients with nonspondylotic cervical spines, or from seemingly trivial injuries in older patients with spondylotic or ankylosed spines. Treatment for these two groups can differ significantly.

   e. Injuries are broadly divided into those that result in obvious compromise of the osseoligamentous elements of the cervical spine, and those with SCI but no obvious radiographic evidence of musculoskeletal injury or spinal instability.

   f. Injuries with radiographic signs of a vertebral column lesion are classified and treated according to the severity of hyperextension deformity and sagittal plane translation, which also correlate with the likelihood of SCI.

   g. Extension injuries are classified as AO type B3 in the absence of translation (usually retrolisthesis) and as AO type C injuries if associated with translation/retrolisthesis. SCI occurs with higher frequency in patients with retrolisthesis due to compression between the posteroinferior end plate of the posteriorly displaced vertebral body and the anterosuperior lamina of the more caudal vertebra.

   h. Cervical SCI not accompanied by radiographic signs of osseoligamentous injury are typical of central cord syndrome and SCWIORA (SCI without radiographic abnormality).

2. Examples of extension injuries:

   a. Extension teardrop fractures:

      i. Malrotated avulsion fracture of anteroinferior end plate, most often of C2.

      ii. Should be differentiated from the more severe flexion teardrop fracture.

      iii. External immobilization for 6 to 12 weeks is successful in most patients.

    b. Disruptions of the anterior longitudinal ligament (ALL) and intervertebral disk:

        i. Purely diskoligamentous injuries involving the ALL, intervertebral disk, and possibly the posterior ligaments.

        ii. Lack of a visible fracture may present a diagnostic dilemma, particularly in injuries that reduce spontaneously on supine imaging.

        iii. Retrolisthesis indicates a more unstable injury with compromise of the posterior longitudinal ligament.

        iv. Anterior cervical diskectomy and fusion with plating is effective as either a primary form of treatment or in patients with dynamic instability after nonoperative treatment.

    c. Special circumstances—extension injuries in ankylosed spines:

        i. Patients with ankylosed spines secondary to DISH (diffuse idiopathic skeletal hyperostosis) or seronegative inflammatory spondyloarthropathies (e.g., ankylosing spondylitis) have poor tolerance for even nominal extension forces and typically sustain either AO type B3 (hyperextension *without* translation [▶Fig. 49.16] or AO type C [with translation]; ▶Fig. 49.17) injuries.

        ii. These fractures usually occur in the lower cervical spine and can be highly unstable despite being minimally displaced and difficult to identify. The resulting delay in diagnosis can result in potentially catastrophic neurologic consequences.

        iii. Patients with ankylosis of the cervical spine who present with neck pain and no obvious acute injury on initial radiographic assessment should be evaluated with a thorough imaging workup including CT and possibly MRI.

        iv. If a spine fracture is identified in this patient population, noncontiguous injuries should be sought with multiplanar CT and possibly MRI of the entire spine.

3. Treatment of hyperextension injuries in patients with ankylosing spine conditions:

    a. Patients with ankylosing conditions who sustain extension injuries should be treated with urgent decompression of the spinal canal, if warranted, which can usually be achieved through closed spinal realignment techniques.

    b. Standard longitudinal tong traction should be avoided because of the potential to further extend and potentially distract these three column injuries.

    c. Provisional immobilization in a halo vest after realignment of the spine to its native, usually kyphotic position or support on a stack of towels can be useful.

    d. Due to their elevated risk of developing epidural hematoma, patients with ankylosing spondylitis or DISH and neurological deficits should have an MRI of the cervical spine at the earliest opportunity.

    e. Mortality rates of greater than 30%, neurological morbidity rates of greater than 50%, and a high likelihood of pulmonary complications have been reported in patients with ankylosing spondylitis who sustain cervical spine fractures, all of which increase in elderly patients.

    f. Because of the high complication rates in nonoperatively treated patients, however, an aggressive surgical approach is recommended.

    g. Canal decompression and stabilization is best achieved by posterior multisegmental instrumentation using plate or rod–screw systems.

    h. Anterior fixation alone is generally not recommended due to the difficulty with achieving adequate screw fixation in the usually osteoporotic vertebral bodies.

4. Extension injuries without radiographic abnormality—central cord syndrome:

    a. Forced neck hyperextension may cause SCI from compression of the spinal cord between the infolded ligamentum flavum posteriorly and diskosteophytes anteriorly.

    b. SCI can be complete or incomplete.

    c. Although central cord syndrome is the most common SCI under these circumstances, other types of incomplete SCI may result.

d. The diagnosis of central cord syndrome is contingent on substantially worse upper than lower extremity function.

e. The prognosis for recovery after central cord syndrome is thought to be good, although patients frequently have significant residual hand dysfunction and spasticity.

f. Treatment is contingent on the severity of SCI and canal compression.

g. Initial nonoperative treatment is appropriate in patients with minor, improving neurological deficits, although eventual surgical intervention is typically required to address the causative underlying stenosis.

h. Early surgical intervention is appropriate in patients with ongoing compression who have severe, progressive, or nonimproving neurological deficits.

   i. The surgical approach depends on the location of compression (e.g., anterior vs. posterior), the number of levels involved, cervical alignment, associated instability patterns, and preexisting conditions (e.g., metabolic bone disease, comorbidities).

E. Additional subaxial spine injuries: Distraction injuries

1. Distraction injuries of the subaxial cervical spine are extremely unstable high-energy injuries that result in tension failure of all three columns (▶Fig. 49.21).

2. Diskoligamentous injury with or without avulsion fracture is most common.

3. Their severity and associated translational displacement classifies them as AO type C injuries.

4. In addition to resuscitation measures, early treatment should focus on the evaluation and treatment of spinal cord and vertebral artery injury.

5. Surgical stabilization is invariably required, with posterior reduction and stabilization being the preferred method.

6. Secondary anterior cervical diskectomy and interbody fusion may be considered, but are not routinely necessary.

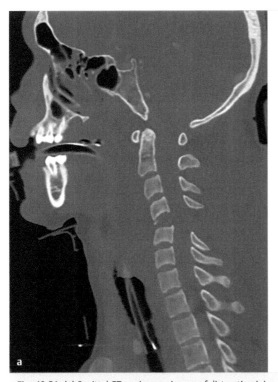 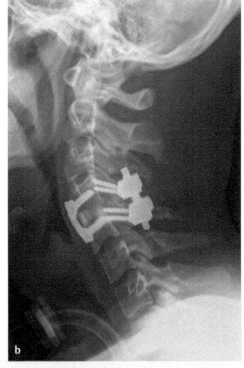

Fig. 49.21 (a) Sagittal CT angiogram image of distraction injury at C4–C5 with associated quadriplegia. (b) Radiographs 1 year postoperatively demonstrate a healed fusion with acceptable cervical alignment.

F. Additional subaxial spine injuries: Lateral compression injuries

1. Lateral compression injuries are unusual and occur mainly as a result of motor vehicle collisions and sports-related mechanisms.

2. They typically involve unilateral arch fracture with ipsilateral vertebral body compression, with possible contralateral posterior facet widening..

3. SCI is unusual, though the causative mechanism of lateral flexion of the neck results in frequent traction injuries of the contralateral nerve roots and brachial plexus.

4. Higher-grade injuries with more severe coronal plane deformity and associated facet subluxation may require operative intervention.

Summary

1. Cervical spine fractures remain a significant public health issue.

2. With appropriate diagnostic and treatment protocols, outcomes can be optimized.

3. Recent developments in C-spine injury classification have been geared toward increasing relevance toward treatment, prognosis, and communication/research.

4. A better understanding of any specific cervical spine injury allows for an improved appreciation of the optimal treatment approach, and helps prevent complications.

5. Approximately 15,000 patients per year sustain SCI in the United States and Canada.

6. The prognosis for survival and recovery is improving, with decreasing mortality rates for severe spinal cord injuries. However, except in rare cases, a complete cervical cord injury is associated with little chance of functional recovery.

7. Prevention of SCI therefore plays a key role, through improved industrial, vehicular, and sports-related safety measures and education.

8. However, further efforts are needed, and should focus on fall prevention in the elderly, the use of protective equipment in higher-risk activities, rule enforcement in contact sports such as football, and improvements in road safety.

9. Technological advances are being made to bring forth treatments for SCI. Several clinical trials involve the use of stem cell therapy, and medications designed to mitigate or reverse the extent of secondary injury to the spinal cord.

Suggested Readings

Allen BL Jr, Ferguson RL, Lehmann TR, O'Brien RP. A mechanistic classification of closed, indirect fractures and dislocations of the lower cervical spine. Spine 1982;7(1):1–27

Bohlman HH. Acute fractures and dislocations of the cervical spine. An analysis of three hundred hospitalized patients and review of the literature. J Bone Joint Surg Am 1979;61(8):1119–1142

Clark CR, White AA III. Fractures of the dens. A multicenter study. J Bone Joint Surg Am 1985;67(9):1340–1348

Fehlings MG, Vaccaro A, Wilson JR, et al. Early versus delayed decompression for traumatic cervical spinal cord injury: results of the Surgical Timing in Acute Spinal Cord Injury Study (STASCIS). PLoS One 2012;7(2):e32037

Fehlings MG, Arun R, Vaccaro AR, Arnold PM, Chapman JR, Kopjar B. Predictors of treatment outcomes in geriatric patients with odontoid fractures: AOSpine North America multi-centre prospective GOF study. Spine 2013;38(11):881–886

Vaccaro AR, Koerner JD, Radcliff KE, et al. AOSpine subaxial cervical spine injury classification system. Eur Spine J 2016;25(7):2173–2184

50 Thoracolumbar Spine Trauma

Joseph P. Gjolaj and Alexander Ghasem

Introduction

Trauma to the thoracic and lumbar spine mechanistically falls on a continuum. Current treatment algorithms for thoracolumbar spinal trauma are in part guided by evaluation of injury to a multitude of anatomical structures comprising the posterior ligamentous complex, fracture pattern, and neurological compromise. Objectives following treatment of thoracolumbar injury include the maintenance or restoration of spinal alignment and stability, preservation of neurologic status, early patient mobilization, and assistance with comanagement of other injuries in the setting of polytrauma. While there is not always consensus regarding selection of operative versus nonoperative intervention, we review in this chapter the basic concepts of management of thoracolumbar spinal injuries (▶Video 50.1).

Keywords: thoracolumbar, burst fracture, Chance fracture, posterior ligamentous complex, spinal instability, corpectomy, posterior instrumentation

I. History and Physical Examination

A. Mechanism of injury

1. Usually high-energy mechanism with greater than 50% of thoracolumbar spine injuries occurring as a result of motor vehicle accidents.

2. Five to 20% have concomitant noncontiguous spinal injuries.

3. Identifying mechanism of injury provides information in regard to classification of injury pattern: *Primary directional forces*—axial compression, lateral compression, flexion, extension, distraction, shear, and rotation.

4. Association with pelvic and extremity fractures, head trauma, chest, and intra-abdominal injuries.

B. Relevant past history

1. Inquire about patient's history of congenital and acquired conditions:

    a. Coagulopathy.

    b. Prior spine surgery.

    c. Spondyloarthropathy.

    d. Ankylosing spondylitis/diffuse idiopathic skeletal hyperostosis.

C. Physical examination

1. Maintain spinal precautions during inspection for lacerations, ecchymosis, tenderness to palpation, swelling, and step-off between spinous processes.

2. Secondary and tertiary survey for associated injuries.

3. **Neurologic examination findings:**

    a. Motor examination graded 0 to 5 based on resistance, monitoring for new-onset weakness (▶Table 50.1).

    b. Sensory function examined by dermatomal distribution for decreased sensation.

    c. Altered reflexes (i.e., abdominal, cremasteric, patellar, Achilles tendon).

    d. Sustained clonus and positive Babinski's sign: lateral aspect of the plantar surface of foot is stroked with an upgoing great toe.

    e. Pain and temperature changes may be tested with sterile needle and alcohol swab.

4. Consideration given to patient experiencing spinal shock in the setting of complete spinal injury and should be reexamined when bulbocavernosus reflex is present.

Table 50.1 Motor strength testing

Numerical motor grade	Corresponding motor function
0	No muscle contraction
1	Muscle movement visible but insufficient to cause joint motion
2	Movement of the joint but muscle strength cannot overcome gravity
3	Muscle strength can overcome gravity but not against resistance
4	Movement against resistance, but muscle strength is not fully normal
5	Normal muscle strength against full resistance

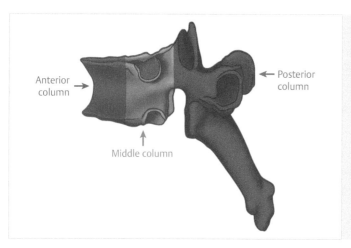

Fig. 50.1 Three-column theory depicted in the thoracic spine as derived from the Denis classification.

II. Anatomy

A. **Three-column theory** requires two-column destabilization prior to instability (▶**Fig. 50.1**).

 1. Anterior column: anterior longitudinal ligament (ALL), anterior two-thirds annulus, and anterior two-thirds vertebral body.

 2. Middle column: posterior one-third annulus, posterior one-third vertebral body, and posterior longitudinal ligament (PLL).

 3. Posterior column: neural arch, ligamentum flavum, facet joint, lamina, spinous process, and posterior ligamentous complex (PLC).

B. Thoracic spine

 1. Increased intrinsic stability as a result of rib cage, which produces long rigid lever arm during traumatic insult.

 2. Smallest pedicle width at T4, T5, and T6.

 3. Center of gravity located anterior to spine placing posterior elements under tension, while anterior/middle columns undergo axial compression.

 4. Kyphosis in thoracic spine ranges from 20 to 45 degrees with transitional thoracolumbar junction having 0 to 3 degrees of lordosis.

C. Lumbar spine

 1. Most lordosis (20–80 degrees) in the lumbar spine originates from L4/L5 and L5/S1. Important to restore sagittal alignment upon surgical stabilization.

 2. Very mobile in flexion/extension as a result of facets oriented in the sagittal plane, which become more coronal when moving caudally.

3.   L3 or L4 pedicles are generally oriented perpendicular to the floor when patient is prone.

4.   L1 pedicle has 5 degrees of medial convergence with general rule of additional 5 degrees per level when moving caudally.

III. Imaging

A.   Radiographs

1.   **Anteroposterior (AP) radiographs:** Visualize coronal alignment, interpedicular distance, and for operative purposes, endplate overlap as well as position of spinous processes for instrumentation.

2.   **Lateral radiographs and flexion/extension views:** Useful for vertebral body height, sagittal alignment, evaluation of posterior column, and dynamic instability.

B.   Computed tomography scan

1.   Advantage of improved bony detail and fracture characterization (25% of burst fractures are missed on X-ray; ▶Fig. 50.2).

2.   Review fracture morphology and pedicle dimensions prior to operative intervention.

3.   Facet widening, splayed spinous processes, and body translation could be indicators of instability.

C.   Magnetic resonance imaging

1.   Damage to soft tissues and PLC seen on T2 sequence.

2.   Correlation of neurologic deficits with sources of compression (i.e., hematoma).

3.   May have role in prognostic implications in the setting of spinal cord injury.

IV. Classification

A.   Common fracture morphology described in the Denis classification (▶Table 50.2).

B.   Mechanical and neurologic stability incorporated into the Thoracolumbar Injury Classification Severity (TLICS) score. Cumulative score greater than 4 warrants surgical intervention (▶Table 50.3).

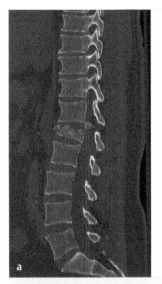
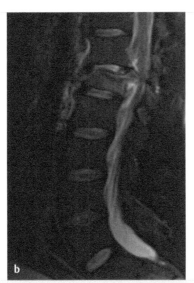
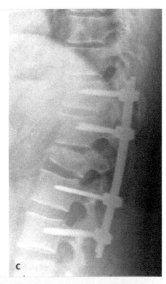

Fig. 50.2 L1 burst fracture with a retropulsed fragment resulting in conus syndrome visualized on sagittal CT (**a**) and MRI (**b**). The patient underwent a transpedicular decompression with posterior stabilization seen on postoperative radiographs (**c**).

Table 50.2 Common thoracolumbar fracture patterns: based on Denis' classification

Fracture pattern	Mechanism of injury	Columns involved
Compression	Axial loading, anterior burst (stable and unstable), flexion/axial loading	Anterior and middle
Seat-belt injury (Chance)	Flexion-distraction	Anterior, middle, posterior
Fracture-dislocation	Rotation/shear/translation	Anterior, middle, posterior

Table 50.3 Thoracolumbar injury classification severity (TLICS) score

Fracture morphology	PLC	Neurologic injury
Compression (1) (Burst [+1])	Intact (0)	No deficits (0)
Translational/rotational (3)	Possible injury (2)	Nerve root injury (2)
Distraction (4)	Injured (3)	Cord/conus complete (2)
		Cord/conus incomplete (3)
		Cauda equina (3)

Source: Data from Vaccaro AR, Lehman RA Jr, Hurlbert RJ, et al. A new classification of thoracolumbar injuries: the importance of injury morphology, the integrity of the posterior ligamentous complex, and neurologic status. Spine (Phila Pa 1976) 2005;30(20):2325–2333.

V. Initial Management

A. Maintain strict spinal precautions during advanced trauma life support (ATLS) trauma evaluation.

B. Avoid hypotension with fluid resuscitation and vasopressors in setting of hemorrhagic or neurogenic shock.

C. Adjuvant therapy for spinal cord injury

   1. Steroids are controversial.

   2. GM1 (monosialotetrahexosylganglioside) ganglioside.

   3. Systemic hypothermia.

VI. Definitive Management

A. Nonoperative treatment

   1. Particular fracture patterns (i.e., compression, burst, and isolated posterior element fractures) without evidence of instability can be treated with bracing.

   2. Bracing:

     a. Acts to immobilize above and below the level of injury.

     b. Bracing levels:

       i. Above T6—cervicothoracic orthosis.

       ii. T6 to L3—thoracolumbar orthosis (Jewett's or custom molded).

       iii. Below L3—TLSO (thoracolumbosacral orthosis) with thigh inclusion.

B. Operative treatment

   1. Laminectomy alone without stabilization usually inadequate in treating thoracolumbar trauma and will result in late kyphosis and instability.

   2. Patients at high risk of failure with bracing may be treated with percutaneous versus open approach internal fixation. Various methods are discussed in the fixation section.

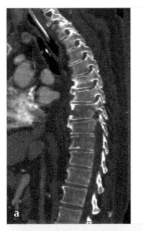 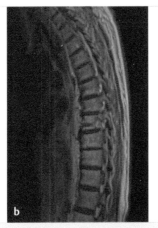 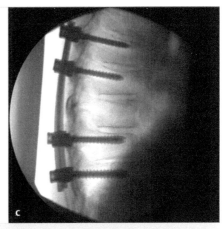

Fig. 50.3 Osseous Chance fracture of the thoracic spine viewed on sagittal CT **(a)** and MRI **(b)** and subsequent stabilization with a long segment construct. Postinstrumented imaging and final fracture alignment is seen on fluoroscopy **(c)**.

3. Surgical indications:
   a. Absolute indications:
      i. Progressively worsening neurologic deficit is a surgical emergency.
      ii. Incomplete stable neurologic deficits are surgical indications but should be addressed as soon as the patient is medically optimized.
      iii. High-energy penetrating injuries to the spine require formal debridement.
   b. Relative indications:
      i. Patient has contraindication to bracing such as concomitant chest/intra-abdominal injuries or excessively large body habitus.
      ii. Compression and burst fractures with 30-degree focal kyphosis or greater than 50% loss of height, although controversial in absence of mechanical and neurologic instability.
      iii. Greater than 15 degrees of kyphosis in Chance fractures (▶ **Fig. 50.3**). Chance fracture—flexion/distraction injury characterized by an anterior wedge fracture of the vertebral body and a transverse fracture of the posterior elements or widening of the facet joints and interspinous processes.
      iv. Increased proportion of ligamentous damage generating instability as opposed to osseous injury (i.e., Chance variant).

VII. Surgical Approaches

A. Posterior approach
   1. Most commonly used approach for thoracic and lumbar fractures (▶ **Fig. 50.4**).
   2. Extensile approach that is very familiar to spine surgeons and gives the ability to apply biomechanically rigid instrumentation via pedicle screws.
   3. Superior approach for fracture dislocations as well as significant PLC injury.
   4. Performed using midline incision and dissection down to the level of fascia guided by palpation of spinous processes.
   5. Subsequent full-thickness division of the fascia and subperiosteal elevation of the paraspinal musculature to the level of the transverse processes are conducted.

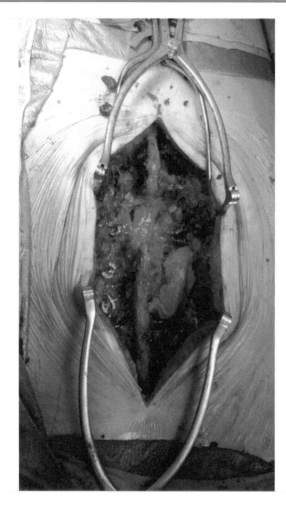

Fig. 50.4 Posterior approach to the thoracolumbar spine. Note: laminectomies have already been performed at multiple levels with placement of posterior instrumentation.

6. Contraindication include posterior traumatic wounds and neurologic compromise secondary to anterior/middle column retropulsion.

7. Posterior percutaneous approach may be useful in complete spinal injury for reduced operative time or in tandem with anterior stabilization.

B. Anterior approach

1. May require the assistance of an approach surgeon and is often difficult to visualize multiple levels.

2. Primarily indicated in the setting of burst fracture retropulsion with neurologic deficit for purposes of decompression.

3. Assists in augmentation of anterior column in the setting of significant comminution.

4. Classic contraindications include fracture-dislocations and multilevel fracture involvement.

VIII. Fixation Techniques

A. Decompression

1. Posterior sources of compression should be decompressed through laminectomy.

2. Pathology ventral to thecal sac may be addressed anteriorly with corpectomy or posteriorly through costotransversectomy as well as transpedicular decompression.

B. Instrumentation

1. Pedicle screws remains the mainstay of treatment and allows for three-column fixation at multiple levels with the potential for direct deformity manipulation.

2. Posterior instrumentation in the absence of PLC stability, provides tension band effect.

3. Anterior grafts or interbody cages can be used synergistically with posterior instrumentation or as a stand-alone means of fixation.

4. Spinal stabilization without fusion is an alternative means of fixation that preserves motion but requires a secondary surgery for hardware removal.

C. Construct length

1. Long segment constructs with two to three levels above and below the level of injury may be required for unstable fracture patterns (i.e., burst fractures that are unstable to axial loading; ▶Fig. 50.2c, ▶Fig. 50.3c).

2. Short segment constructs that extend one level above and below fracture are used for axially stable patterns such as Chance fractures to preserve mobility.

3. Load Sharing Score (LSS) is helpful for identifying poor candidates for short segment construct.

IX. Complications

A. Local complications

1. Screw malpositioning, traumatic durotomies, spinal cord and nerve root injury, iatrogenic flat back, hardware failure, wound infection, and hematoma.

B. General complications

1. Ileus, thromboembolic disease, decubitus ulcers, and pneumonia.

X. Rehabilitation

A. Patients mobilized immediately: rotation and bending limited by surgeon preference.

B. Upright bracing may be performed for 3 to 6 months or more based on extent of injury.

XI. Outcomes

A. Burst fractures with no neurologic compromise have comparable clinical results when treated with or without surgery.

B. Incomplete cord injuries from burst fractures have greater than 95% probability of at least one grade of neurologic improvement following decompression.

XII. Special Considerations for Geriatric Patients

A. Percutaneous balloon-assisted reduction with cement augmentation (also known as kyphoplasty) combined with minimally invasive pedicle screw instrumentation has proven to be a viable option in the geriatric population.

B. This combined procedure may be suitable for severe compression fractures with significant kyphosis in the setting of diminished bone density such as osteoporosis or osteopenia. This technique may not be suitable for burst fractures, as the cement could leak through the fracture gap involving the posterior vertebral body and could adversely affect the neural elements by compressing the spinal canal or through the exothermic reaction associated with cement hardening.

1. Vertebral augmentation with percutaneous instrumentation provides anterior column support while concomitantly reducing the surgical physiological burden of an open approach.

2. Long-term clinical and radiographic results show acceptable outcomes.

C.   Traditional vertebral augmentation procedures (vertebroplasty or kyphoplasty) without instrumentation placement may be adequate for select patients.

D.   This technique may provide pain relief for severely symptomatic osteoporotic compression fractures not associated with severe kyphosis in elderly patients or for those geriatric patients who may not tolerate instrumentation placement (placed in a minimally invasive or open fashion) due to medical comorbidities.

E.   The treatment of uncomplicated osteoporotic compression fractures with vertebroplasty or kyphoplasty is a still matter of debate.

1.   Most of these types of fractures in the geriatric population do not require surgical intervention but instead may heal adequately over time with activity restrictions, optimization of bone metabolic factors, and treatment of underlying osteoporosis.

2.   Bracing may provide symptomatic relief but may not be required as senile compression fractures are not considered frankly unstable.

Summary

Thoracolumbar spine trauma encompasses a wide spectrum of injuries. Accurate diagnosis involves consideration of mechanism of injury, relevant past history, neurological status and imaging studies. Classification systems such as TLICSS incorporate these factors and provide a framework to guide management. Treatments are based on neurological status, fracture pattern and other associated injuries, since these details can help determine whether the injury should be treated non-operatively versus operatively, and if operative, which surgical approach is most appropriate. The goals of treatment should include the maintenance or restoration of spinal alignment and stability, preservation or restoration of neurologic status, early patient mobilization to avoid postoperative complications, and a multidisciplinary approach in the setting of polytrauma.

Suggested Readings

Bohlman HH. Treatment of fractures and dislocations of the thoracic and lumbar spine. J Bone Joint Surg Am 1985;67(1):165–169

Cantor JB, Lebwohl NH, Garvey T, Eismont FJ. Nonoperative management of stable thoracolumbar burst fractures with early ambulation and bracing. Spine 1993;18(8):971–976

Chu JK, Rindler RS, Pradilla G, Rodts GE Jr, Ahmad FU. Percutaneous instrumentation without arthrodesis for thoracolumbar flexion-distraction injuries: a review of the literature. Neurosurgery 2017;80(2):171–179

Schroeder GD, Harrop JS, Vaccaro AR. Thoracolumbar trauma classification. Neurosurg Clin N Am 2017;28(1):23–29

Index

Note: Page numbers set in **bold** or *italic* indicate headings or figures, respectively.